ORTHOPAEDIC ISSUES in OSTEOPOROSIS

ORTHOPAEDIC ISSUES *in* OSTEOPOROSIS

Edited by

Yuehuei H. An, M.D.

Associate Professor and Director
Orthopaedic Research Laboratory
Department of Orthopaedic Surgery
Medical University of South Carolina
Charleston, South Carolina

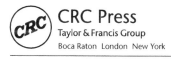

CRC Press
Taylor & Francis Group
Boca Raton London New York

CRC Press is an imprint of the
Taylor & Francis Group, an **informa** business

Cover Art (left to right): Lateral radiograph showing two cannula (partially overlapping) in place for vertebroplasty (see Chapter 21); a femoral intertrochanteric fracture (see Chapter 17); a proximal four-part humerus fracture that was reduced through an open procedure and stabilized using a plate and screws (see Chapter 15); and Colles' fracture of the distal radius in a woman with osteoporosis (see Chapter 6).

CRC Press
Taylor & Francis Group
6000 Broken Sound Parkway NW, Suite 300
Boca Raton, FL 33487-2742

© 2017 by Taylor & Francis Group, LLC
CRC Press is an imprint of Taylor & Francis Group, an Informa business

No claim to original U.S. Government works

ISBN-13: 978-0-849-31033-1 (hbk)
ISBN-13: 978-0-367-39575-9 (pbk)

This book contains information obtained from authentic and highly regarded sources. While all reasonable efforts have been made to publish reliable data and information, neither the author[s] nor the publisher can accept any legal responsibility or liability for any errors or omissions that may be made. The publishers wish to make clear that any views or opinions expressed in this book by individual editors, authors or contributors are personal to them and do not necessarily reflect the views/opinions of the publishers. The information or guidance contained in this book is intended for use by medical, scientific or health-care professionals and is provided strictly as a supplement to the medical or other professional's own judgement, their knowledge of the patient's medical history, relevant manufacturer's instructions and the appropriate best practice guidelines. Because of the rapid advances in medical science, any information or advice on dosages, procedures or diagnoses should be independently verified. The reader is strongly urged to consult the relevant national drug formulary and the drug companies' and device or material manufacturers' printed instructions, and their websites, before administering or utilizing any of the drugs, devices or materials mentioned in this book. This book does not indicate whether a particular treatment is appropriate or suitable for a particular individual. Ultimately it is the sole responsibility of the medical professional to make his or her own professional judgements, so as to advise and treat patients appropriately. The authors and publishers have also attempted to trace the copyright holders of all material reproduced in this publication and apologize to copyright holders if permission to publish in this form has not been obtained. If any copyright material has not been acknowledged please write and let us know so we may rectify in any future reprint.

Except as permitted under U.S. Copyright Law, no part of this book may be reprinted, reproduced, transmitted, or utilized in any form by any electronic, mechanical, or other means, now known or hereafter invented, including photocopying, microfilming, and recording, or in any information storage or retrieval system, without written permission from the publishers.

For permission to photocopy or use material electronically from this work, please access www.copyright.com (http://www.copyright.com/) or contact the Copyright Clearance Center, Inc. (CCC), 222 Rosewood Drive, Danvers, MA 01923, 978-750-8400. CCC is a not-for-profit organization that provides licenses and registration for a variety of users. For organizations that have been granted a photocopy license by the CCC, a separate system of payment has been arranged.

Trademark Notice: Product or corporate names may be trademarks or registered trademarks, and are used only for identification and explanation without intent to infringe.

Visit the Taylor & Francis Web site at
http://www.taylorandfrancis.com

and the CRC Press Web site at
http://www.crcpress.com

Preface

Metabolic bone diseases, such as osteoporosis, osteomalacia, hyperparathyroidism, and Paget's disease, are usually associated with osteoporotic or soft skeleton, especially in the elderly patient. Orthopaedic procedures in elderly patients are costly and with the increasing age of the population these costs will continue to escalate. Great challenges are often encountered when internal fixation is needed for fractures or osteotomies to osteoporotic bone. This book conveys basic and clinical essentials of osteoporosis and related orthopaedic issues on applied research and surgical treatment. Potential readers include orthopaedic surgeons, orthopaedic residents, orthopaedic researchers, fellows, and graduate students, as well as implant designers who work in orthopaedic departments or companies. The book will also be of interest to anyone working in the fields of clinical orthopaedics, orthopaedic research, or implant manufacture, and to internal medicine physicians who see patients with osteoporosis. This is the first inclusive and organized reference book on orthopaedic relevance to osteoporotic conditions, a topic that has not been covered adequately by any existing books.

Yuehuei H. An, M.D.
Charleston, South Carolina

About the Editor

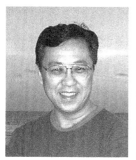

Yuehuei H. (Huey) An, M.D., graduated from the Harbin Medical University, Harbin, Northeast China in 1983 and trained in orthopaedic surgery at the Beijing Ji Shui Tan Hospital (Residency), and in hand surgery at Sydney Hospital (Clinical Fellow), Australia. In 1991, Dr. An joined with Dr. Richard J. Friedman in the Department of Orthopaedic Surgery at the Medical University of South Carolina to establish the MUSC Orthopaedic Research Laboratory, which is now a multifunctional orthopaedic research center.

Dr. An has published more than 100 scientific papers and book chapters and more than 100 abstracts. He has edited five books: *Animal Models in Orthopaedic Research* (1999) and *Mechanical Testing of Bone and the Bone–Implant Interface* (2000), both published by CRC Press, *Handbook of Bacterial Adhesion* (2000), *Handbook of Histology Methods for Bone and Cartilage* (2002), and *Internal Fixation in Osteoporotic Bone* (2002).

Dr. An has a wide range of research interests. He is an active member of eight academic societies in the fields of orthopaedics, biomaterials, biomechanics, and tissue engineering. He enjoys art and has created many of the line drawings and images used in his books and articles.

Contributors

Yuehuei H. An, M.D.
Associate Professor and Director
Orthopaedic Research Laboratory
Department of Orthopaedic Surgery
Medical University of South Carolina
Charleston, South Carolina
and
Adjunct Assistant Professor
Department of Bioengineering
Clemson University
Clemson, South Carolina

Richard M. Aspden, Ph.D.
Senior MRC Research Fellow
Department of Orthopaedic Surgery
University of Aberdeen
Foresterhill
Aberdeen, Scotland

Stephen M. Belkoff, Ph.D.
Assistant Professor and Director
Orthopaedic Instrumentation Laboratory
Department of Orthopaedic Surgery
The Johns Hopkins University/
Johns Hopkins Bayview Medical Center
Baltimore, Maryland

Christopher V. Bensen, M.D.
Department of Orthopaedic Surgery
Medical University of South Carolina
Charleston, South Carolina

Earl R. Bogoch, M.D., FRCSC
Professor
Department of Surgery
University of Toronto
Mobility Program
St. Michael's Hospital
Toronto, Ontario, Canada

Ermanno Bonucci, Ph.D.
Professor
Department of Experimental Medicine
  and Pathology
University "La Sapienza"
Rome, Italy

Ricardo F. Capozza, Ph.D.
Centro de Estudios de Metabolismo
  Fosfocalcico (CEMFoC)
Hospital del Centenario
Universidad Nacional de Rosario
Rosario, Argentina

Gustavo R. Cointry, Ph.D.
Centro de Estudios de Metabolismo
  Fosfocalcico (CEMFoC)
Hospital del Centenario
Universidad Nacional de Rosario
Rosario, Argentina

Hervé Deramond, M.D.
Professor
Service de Radiologie A
Centre Hospitaliere Universitaire
Amiens, France

Harry A. Demos, M.D.
Assistant Professor
Department of Orthopaedic Surgery
Medical University of South Carolina
Charleston, South Carolina

Daniele Diacinti, M.D.
Department of Clinical Sciences
University "La Sapienza"
Rome, Italy

Bryon Dickerson, M.D.
Department of Radiology
Wake Forest University School of Medicine
Winston-Salem, North Carolina

Donald G. Eckhoff, M.D., M.S.
Professor
Department of Orthopaedics
University of Colorado Health Sciences
Denver, Colorado

Ryland B. Edwards III, D.V.M, M.S.
Comparative Orthopaedic Research Laboratory
Department of Medical Sciences
School of Veterinary Medicine
University of Wisconsin–Madison
Madison, Wisconsin

Lisa A. Ferrara, M.Sc.
Director
Spine Research Laboratory
Department of Neurosurgery
Cleveland Clinic Foundation
Cleveland, Ohio

José Luis Ferretti, Ph.D.
Director
Centro de Estudios de Metabolismo
 Fosfocalcico (CEMFoC)
Hospital del Centenario
Universidad Nacional de Rosario
Rosario, Argentina

Angela N. Fontana, M.S.N., R.N., ANP
Assistant Professor
Department of Orthopaedic Surgery
University of South Carolina School
 of Medicine
Columbia, South Carolina

Abbas Fotovati, D.V.M., Ph.D.
Research Fellow in Orthopaedic Research
Laboratory of Haradoi Hospital
Department of Orthopaedic Surgery
Faculty of Medicine, Fukuoka University
Medical Institute of Bioregulation
Faculty of Medicine, Kyushu University
Fukuoka, Japan

Harold M. Frost, M.D., D.Sc.
Department of Orthopaedic Surgery
Southern Colorado Clinic
Pueblo, Colorado

Emanuel Gautier, M.D.
Department of Orthopaedic Surgery
Hôpital Cantonal
Fribourg, Switzerland

Leon J. Grobler, M.D., FACS
Research Institute International, Inc.
Phoenix, Arizona

Dagmar K. Gross, M.Sc.
President
MedSci Communications & Consulting
 Company
Toronto, Ontario, Canada

Giuseppe Guglielmi, M.D.
Department of Radiology
Scientific Institute Hospital "Casa Sollievo della
 Sofferenza"
San Giovanni Rotondo, Italy

Kazuo Hayashi, M.D.
Department of Orthopaedic Surgery
Faculty of Medicine
Fukuoka University
Haradoi Hospital
Fukuoka, Japan

Kathleen A. Hogan, M.D.
Department of Orthopaedic Surgery
Medical University of South Carolina
Charleston, South Carolina

Roland P. Jakob, M.D.
Department of Orthopaedic Surgery
Hôpital Cantonal
Fribourg, Switzerland

Qian K. Kang, M.D.
Orthopaedic Research Laboratory
Department of Orthopaedic Surgery
Medical University of South Carolina
Charleston, South Carolina

Pekka Kannus, M.D., Ph.D.
The UKK Institute for Health Promotion
 Research
Tampere, Finland

Samir S. Kulkarni, M.D.
Research Institute International, Inc.
Phoenix, Arizona

**Raymond Lau, M.D., MRCP (U.K.),
FAMS (Singapore)**
Institute of Bone and Joint Research
University of Sydney
Royal North Shore Hospital
Sydney, New South Wales, Australia

Jes Bruun Lauritzen, M.D.
Professor
Department of Orthopaedic Surgery
University of Copenhagen, Bispebjerg Hospital
Copenhagen, Denmark

Leon Lenchik, M.D.
Department of Radiology
Wake Forest University School of Medicine
Winston-Salem, North Carolina

Mandi J. Lopez, D.V.M., Ph.D.
Comparative Orthopaedic Research Laboratory
Department of Medical Sciences
School of Veterinary Medicine
University of Wisconsin–Madison
Madison, Wisconsin

Gary L. Lowery, M.D., Ph.D.
Research Institute International, Inc.
Phoenix, Arizona

Mark D. Markel, D.V.M., Ph.D.
Professor
Comparative Orthopaedic Research Laboratory
School of Veterinary Medicine
University of Wisconsin–Madison
Madison, Wisconsin

John M. Mathis, M.D., M.Sc.
Chairman
Department of Radiology
Lewis-Gale Medical Center
Salem, Virginia

William E. McCormick, M.D.
Department of Neurosurgery
Cleveland Clinic Foundation
Cleveland, Ohio

Onno G. Meijer, M.D., Ph.D.
Faculty of Human Movement Sciences
Vrije Universiteit
Amsterdam, the Netherlands

Tsuyoshi Ohishi, M.D.
Department of Orthopaedic Surgery
Hamamatsu University School of Medicine
Hamamatsu, Japan

Thomas F. Oppelt, Pharm.D.
Clinical Assistant Professor
Department of Pharmacy Practice
College of Pharmacy
University of South Carolina
Columbia, South Carolina

Dariusz Palczewski, M.D., Ph.D.
Department of Orthopaedics and Traumatology
Regional Hospital Siedlce
Siedlce, Poland

Meinrad Peterlik, M.D., Ph.D.
Department of Pathophysiology
University of Vienna Medical School
Vienna, Austria

Peter Pietschmann, M.D.
Department of Pathophysiology
University of Vienna Medical School
  and Ludwig Boltzmann Institute
  of Aging Research
Vienna, Austria

Heinrich Resch, M.D.
Ludwig Boltzmann Institute of Aging Research
  and Department of Medicine II
St. Vincent Hospital
Vienna, Austria

Subrata Saha, Ph.D.
Professor
Biomedical Materials Engineering Science
  Program
New York State College of Ceramics
  at Alfred University
Alfred, New York

Philip N. Sambrook, M.D., B.S., FRACP
Professor
Institute of Bone and Joint Research
University of Sydney
Royal North Shore Hospital
Sydney, New South Wales, Australia

Christine M. Schnitzler, M.D., FRCS (Edin.)
MRC Mineral Metabolism Research Unit
  and Department of Orthopaedic Surgery
Baragwanath Hospital
University of the Witwatersrand
Johannesburg, South Africa

H. Del Schutte, Jr., M.D.
Associate Professor
Department of Orthopaedic Surgery
Medical University of South Carolina
Charleston, South Carolina

Walter H. Short, M.D.
Professor
Department of Orthopaedic Surgery
Musculoskeletal Research Laboratory
Upstate Medical University
Syracuse, New York

Joseph A. Spadaro, Ph.D.
Professor
Department of Orthopaedic Surgery
Musculoskeletal Research Laboratory
Upstate Medical University
Syracuse, New York

Khalid Syed, M.D.
Resident
Division of Orthopaedic Surgery
University of Toronto
Toronto, Ontario, Canada

Masaaki Takahashi, M.D.
Department of Orthopaedic Surgery
Hamamatsu University School of Medicine
Hamamatsu, Japan

Ilkka Vuori, M.D.
Professor
The UKK Institute for Health Promotion
  Research
Tampere, Finland

Stephan W. Wachtl, M.D.
Department of Orthopaedic Surgery
Hôpital Cantonal
Fribourg, Switzerland

Jeffrey M. Walker, M.Sc.
Department of Bioengineering
Clemson University
Clemson, South Carolina

Michael S. Wildstein, M.D.
Department of Orthopaedic Surgery
Medical University of South Carolina
Charleston, South Carolina

Paul I. Wuisman, M.D.
Professor
Department of Orthopaedic Surgery
Vrije Universiteit Medical Center
Amsterdam, the Netherlands

Dedication

To Q. Kay Kang, M.D.
Without her love, inspiration, and support,
this book would not have been possible.

Yuehuei H. An, M.D.

Contents

Part VII
Prevention and Management of Osteoporotic Conditions

Part I

Basic Science and Clinical Essentials

1 Etiology and Pathogenesis of Osteoporosis

Peter Pietschmann, Heinrich Resch, and Meinrad Peterlik

CONTENTS

I. INTRODUCTION

Bone is a dynamic tissue that serves two highly specialized functions: it has a fundamental biomechanical role in locomotion, and it is essential for the maintenance of mineral homeostasis. Thus, chronic disturbances of local or systemic regulation of bone turnover inevitably result in clinically overt metabolic bone diseases including primary and secondary osteoporosis, Paget's disease, osteomalacia, hyperparathyroidism, and renal osteodystrophy. Osteoporosis is defined as a "systemic skeletal disease characterized by low bone mass and microarchitectural deterioration of bone tissue with a consequent increase in bone fragility and susceptibility to fracture."[1] Primary, i.e., involutional, osteoporosis is clearly the most frequent and also, clinically, the most important bone disease. This chapter provides a condensed review on our present knowledge of regulatory processes involved in normal bone turnover, which should be useful for a better understanding of the numerous pathophysiologic aspects of osteoporosis.

0-8493-1033-4/02/$0.00+$1.50

II. BONE PHYSIOLOGY

A. STRUCTURE AND COMPOSITION OF BONE

Regardless whether bones are typically long bones, e.g., femur, tibia, etc., or are of rather flat appearance such as iliac or skull bones, their external part is built as a compact structure (cortical bone), whereas their interior comprises a three-dimensional network of rather fine trabeculae (spongy or cancellous bone).[2] Approximately 80% of the adult human skeleton consists of cortical bone and 20% trabecular bone. Trabecular bone is considered metabolically far more active than cortical bone and thus more responsive to disturbances of mineral homeostasis. Histologically, woven and lamellar bone can be distinguished; woven bone is typically formed during fetal and postnatal skeletal development. In the adult organism only lamellar bone is formed, except under some conditions of enhanced bone formation such as fracture healing or in Paget's disease, where predominantly woven bone is built.[3]

Bone is composed of mineral, organic matrix, cells, and water. Bone mineral, which accounts for approximately two thirds of its dry weight, consists mainly of calcium phosphate in the form of crystalline hydroxyapatite, but also contains other mineral ions such as magnesium, strontium, carbonate, citrate, and fluoride.[3] The main components of the organic matrix are proteoglycans and proteins, of which 90% consist of collagen (predominantly collagen type I). Deposition of normal collagen in sufficient amounts is necessary for achieving an adequate bone mass and mineral density during skeletal development, and is thus critical for optimal biomechanical properties of bone. Otherwise, mutational defects in the procollagen-α(I) genes have been identified as cause for the various forms of osteogenesis imperfecta.

Bone tissue contains also a small amount of noncollagenous proteins such as osteocalcin, bone sialoprotein, osteopontin, and osteonectin. Although the function of these proteins is not yet fully understood, they seem to be involved in the process of matrix mineralization.

Bone is constantly renewed not only during skeletal development (bone modeling) but also in later life (bone remodeling). The four major types of bone cells involved in bone turnover are osteoblasts, bone lining cells, osteocytes, and osteoclasts.

1. Osteoblasts and Bone Lining Cells

Osteoblasts are fully differentiated cells of mesenchymal origin that are able to produce not only the various components of the organic matrix but also a number of factors that are required to initiate and promote the mineralization process of the osteoid, i.e., nonmineralized tissue. Osteoblasts are cuboidal cells with a round nucleus at the base of the cell, a strongly basophilic cytoplasm, and a prominent Golgi complex, which form a continuous single-cell layer on bone surfaces.[2]

The following stages of development of osteoblasts have been identified: mesenchymal stem cell, stromal mesenchymal cell (inducible osteoprogenitor), osteoprogenitor (determined), committed pre-osteoblast, osteoblast, and osteocyte.[4] The progression of maturation of bone-forming cells requires the sequential activation and/or suppression of specific genes that encode phenotypic and regulatory proteins — c-fos, procollagen-α(I), alkaline phosphatase, osteopontin, osteocalcin. Factors that promote differentiation of precursor cell populations include various bone morphogenic proteins (BMPs, e.g., BMP-2), transforming growth factor-β (TGF-β), fibroblast growth factor, parathyroid hormone (PTH), PTH-related peptide, 1,25-dihydroxyvitamin D_3 (1,25-$(OH)_2D_3$) and insulin-like growth factor-1 (IGF-1).[4] Cbfa1, Msx-2, c-fos, and fra-2 are examples of transcription factors that have been identified as key regulators of bone formation.[4] Cbfa1 (Osf2) is the first osteoblast-specific transcription factor that has been described; the central role for Cbfa1 in bone formation is highlighted by the fact that null mutation mice completely lack mineralization of cartilage tissue.[5,6]

Osteoblasts on bone surfaces that are not actively involved in the process of bone formation are termed lining cells. These "resting osteoblasts" can be recruited, if necessary, for a new round of bone formation through appropriate stimuli from bone-active hormones, e.g., PTH.[7]

2. Osteocytes

Osteocytes are nonproliferative cells at the terminal stage of differentiation of osteoblasts, which in course of formation of new bone have become entrapped in the mineralized matrix.[2] Nevertheless, osteocytes are in contact with osteoblasts and lining cells on the bone surface as part of a syncytium-like functional network: long cytoplasmic processes protruding from osteocytes run through a system of canaliculi that permeates the entire bone matrix, and establish cell–cell contacts through gap junctions with osteoblasts or lining cells, respectively.

The functional role of osteocytes is only incompletely understood. Osteocytes, through their ability to exchange Ca^{2+} with the surrounding extracellular fluid, may play a role in the regulation of plasma calcium homeostasis; moreover, because osteocytes respond to fluid sheer stress by the release of bone-active prostaglandins, they could possibly transduce mechanical loads into appropriate stimuli of bone remodeling.[3]

3. Osteoclasts

The osteoclast is the cell type responsible for the resorption of bone. Osteoclasts are giant multinucleated cells containing as many as 20 nuclei. They are attracted to the surface of cortical or trabecular bone and activated by stimuli from calcemic hormones, growth factors, cytokines, or prostaglandins. Active osteoclasts are often found within a lacuna (Howship's lacuna) resulting from their own resorptive activity. Usually only one or two osteoclasts are found at the same resorptive site. A very characteristic ultrastructural feature of active osteoclasts is the "ruffled border" made up of deep infoldings of the plasma membrane in the area facing the bone matrix.[2] The ruffled border is surrounded by the so-called clear zone, a peripheral ring of tight adherence between the cell and the bone surface, which seals off the resorptive site from the surrounding extracellular fluid compartment. Through secretion of H^+ ions and lysosomal enzymes, including collagenase, cathepsin, tartrate-resistant acid phosphatase, osteoclasts are able to resorb both bone mineral and organic matrix.

It is now well established that the osteoclast derives from a multipotent hemopoietic precursor of the mononuclear/phagocytic lineage. Differentiation into either monocytes/macrophages or osteoclasts may occur at the early promonocyte stage; nevertheless, osteoclasts have also been generated from peripheral blood monocytes or resident macrophages. In contrast to monocytes/macrophages, osteoclasts do not express Fc receptors but express receptors for calcitonin and vitronectin ($\alpha_v\beta_3$ integrin). The extent of osteoclastic bone resorption is determined by two distinct processes: (1) formation of new osteoclasts (osteoclastogenesis), and (2) recruitment and activation of already existing mature, so-called resting osteoclasts. Both processes are controlled by a multitude of cytokines, growth factors, and hormones, which will be described in more detail below.

B. BONE REMODELING

In the adult skeleton, bone is constantly remodeled throughout life. This process is fundamental for the adaptation of bone to changes in mechanical conditions and to the requirements of calcium and inorganic phosphate homeostasis. Bone resorption and bone formation do not occur at random; in the normal adult skeleton, new bone is formed only after old bone has been resorbed. The sequence of events at a so-called bone remodeling unit in cancellous bone is as follows: the remodeling cycle is initiated by osteoclastic bone resorption. The duration of the resorptive phase has been estimated at 43 days.[8] This is followed by the reversal phase, in which pre-osteoblasts enter the excavation site (7 days), and finally by the phase of bone formation (145 days). In this period, pre-osteoblasts differentiate into mature osteoblasts, which through deposition and mineralization of bone matrix fill the resorption cavity with new bone. Finally, as the result of the remodeling cycle a "bone structural unit" is rebuilt, which then enters into a resting phase. The remodeling of cortical bone follows the same principles as described above for trabecular bone.

Cortical bone is removed primarily by endosteal resorption and resorption within the Haversian canals,[9] whereby osteoclasts create an advancing tunnel, which is subsequently refilled with new bone formed by osteoblasts.

The duration of one complete remodeling cyle at each remodeling site has been estimated at approximately 3 months in cortical bone, and 6 months in cancellous bone.[2]

1. Local Regulation of Bone Remodeling by Cytokines and Growth Factors

Because of the cyclic course of the bone remodeling process, bone formation is tightly coupled to bone resorption (the "coupling phenomenon"). Bone remodeling is subject to control by systemic hormones as well as by a number of local factors such as growth factors, cytokines, and prostaglandins, which are produced within the bone remodeling unit by (pre)osteoblasts, and which act on the various types of bone cells in an autocrine/paracrine fashion. It is important to note that with the exception of calcitonin, specific plasma membrane or nuclear receptors for these bone-active hormones and factors are predominantly found in osteoblasts. This explains why effective generation of osteoclasts eventually requires the presence of cells of the osteoblastic lineage and, consequently, how under physiologic conditions an equilibrium between formation and resorption of bone can be maintained.

Very recently significant progress in our understanding of bone remodeling has been made by the identification of two final effectors of osteoclast formation: the osteoclast differentiation factor (ODF), which is expressed on cells of the osteoblast lineage, and osteoprotegerin (OPG), which is also produced by osteoblasts and functions as its soluble decoy receptor.

ODF, also termed osteoprotegerin ligand (OPGL), was identified independently by Yasuda et al.[10] and Lacey et al.[11] This factor has been demonstrated to be identical to tumor necrosis factor-related activation-induced cytokine (TRANCE) and receptor activator of nuclear factor-κB ligand (RANKL).[12,13] RANKL (ODF/OPGL/TRANCE) is a member of the tumor necrosis factor (TNF) ligand family and is a polypeptide of 317 amino acids. Steady-state mRNA levels of RANKL are highest in skeletal and lymphoid tissue; lower levels have been detected in heart, skeletal muscle, lung, stomach, placenta, and thyroid gland.[14] The RANKL gene promotor contains vitamin D and glucocorticoid response elements, and a binding site for the osteoblast-specific transcription factor Cbfa1.[15,16] RANKL has been demonstrated to stimulate the differentiation, survival, and fusion of osteoclast precursor cells, to activate mature osteoclasts, and to inhibit osteoclast apoptosis.[17] The central role of RANKL in the skeletal and the immune system has been demonstrated in RANKL knockout mice: these animals completely lack osteoclasts, have severe osteopetrosis, and exhibit defects in early differentiation of T and B lymphocytes.[18]

In the presence of macrophage colony–stimulating factor (M-CSF), expression of no factor other than RANKL is required for osteoclast differentiation and activation.[11] The op/op variant of murine osteopetrosis is a recessive mutation characterized by defective bone resorption due to the lack of osteoclast formation as a consequence of an impaired production of M-CSF; the administration of M-CSF corrects *in vivo* the impaired bone resorption of this animal.[19]

While the effects of M-CSF are mediated by c-fms, the receptor for RANKL is a receptor activator of nuclear factor-κB (RANK).[17] RANK, which has also been termed osteoclast differentiation and activation receptor (ODAR), is expressed by osteoclasts, dendritic cells, T cells, B cells, and fibroblasts.[17] RANK knockout mice suffer from osteopetrosis and immune defects.[20,21]

In 1997, OPG was independently discovered by two groups.[10,22,23] OPG has also been named osteoclastogenesis inhibitory factor (OCIF), TNF receptor–related molecule-1 (TR-1), and follicular dendritic cell receptor-1 (FDCR-1). OPG is a propeptide of 401 amino acids and a member of the TNF receptor superfamily. High levels of OPG mRNA have been detected in a variety of tissues including bone, lung, heart, kidney, intestine, and thyroid.[14] In bone tissue OPG is predominantly produced by cells of the osteoblastic lineage.[24,25] OPG is a decoy receptor for RANKL and thus inhibits the differentiation, survival, and fusion of osteoclast precursor cells, inhibits the activation of mature osteoclasts, and induces osteoclast apoptosis.[14] The overexpression of OPG in transgenic animals results in severe osteopetrosis, which — in contrast to RANK or RANKL knockout mice — is not associated with immune abnormalities.[22] OPG knockout mice suffer from severe osteoporosis.[26,27] In animal experiments, recombinant OPG has been demonstrated to have potent antiresorptive effects and currently is under investigation for human bone diseases.[17]

Recently, Hofbauer and co-workers[14] introduced a "convergence hypothesis" for the regulation of osteoclast functions by hormones and cytokines. This hypothesis proposes that a variety of "upstream" hormones and cytokines alters the pool size of active osteoclasts by converging at the level of RANKL and OPG expression. The balance of these two "downstream" factors regulates bone resorption by modulating osteoclastogenesis, osteoclast activation, and osteoclast apoptosis.

Interleukin-1 (IL-1), produced by activated monocytes, osteoblasts, and tumor cells, is among the most powerful stimulators of bone resorption and an inhibitor of bone formation.[28] There are two independent species of IL-1 (IL-1α and IL-1β), which exert the same biologic effects and act through the same receptor. IL-1 appears to be relevant for the pathophysiology of postmenopausal osteoporosis as an increased monocytic production of this cytokine after natural and surgical menopause, which is decreased by hormone replacement therapy, has been demonstrated.[29]

TNF-α is another proinflammatory cytokine with potent bone resorptive activities. TNF-α has been demonstrated to be involved in tumor- and nontumor-induced osteopenia and is secreted in higher amounts by mononuclear cells from postmenopausal than from premenopausal women.[28]

Interleukin-6 (IL-6) is the third "classical" bone resorptive cytokine. There is indirect evidence that production of IL-6 by mononuclear cells is under estrogen control in humans[30] and also experimental animals. IL-6 has been thus implicated in the increased rate of osteoclastogenesis observed in ovarectomized mice.[31] Although it is obvious that IL-6 acts on hemopoietic precursors rather than on mature osteoclasts,[32] the exact mechanism by which IL-6 induces osteoclast formation is only partially understood. IL-6 exerts its effects via a heterodimeric cell surface receptor that consists of a ligand binding chain (IL-6R) and a signal transducing unit known as gp130. There is evidence that activation of the IL-6/IL-6R system provides co-stimulatory signals for the osteoclast inducive action of bone-resorbing agents such as 1,25-$(OH)_2D_3$, PTH, or PGE_2.[33]

TGF-β is produced not only by cells of the immune system but also by osteoblasts, and hence is abundant in the extracellular bone matrix. In most systems, TGF-β interferes with osteoclastogenesis by blocking both proliferation and differentiation of osteoclast precursors. Moreover, TGF-β inhibits the activity and enhances apoptosis of mature osteoclasts.[9] In addition, TGF-β has potent stimulatory effects on osteoblasts and thus appears to be a pivotal factor in the regulation of bone remodeling. It should be noted that expression of TGF-β in osteoblastic cells is under positive control from anabolic sex steroids.[34]

IGF-1 seems to be of particular importance for local regulation of bone remodeling because IGF-1 enhances proliferation of pre-osteoblasts and augments bone matrix synthesis in more mature osteoblasts. Upregulation of IGF-1 by triiodothyronine[35] may at least in part explain the well-known stimulatory action of thyroid hormones on bone formation.

Prostaglandins (PGs) play an important role in skeletal metabolism in health and disease (for a detailed review, see Reference 36). Early work on the effects of prostaglandins on bone resorption demonstrated that particularly prostaglandins of the E series are potent activators of bone degradation.[37] Prostaglandins thus appear to be important mediators of bone loss in various diseases such as in rheumatoid arthritis or periodontal disease, for example. With respect to osteoporosis, estrogen withdrawal in rats is associated with an increased prostaglandin production in bone, which can be reversed by estrogen replacement.[38] It should be noted that prostaglandins, like many other bone-active factors, appear to have a dual effect on bone remodeling. They promote replication and differentiation of osteoblast precursors and thus faciltate bone formation, although they also inhibit collagen synthesis in mature osteoblasts.[36]

2. Regulation of Bone Turnover by Systemic Hormones

$1,25\text{-}(OH)_2D_3$ increases the intestinal absorption of calcium and phosphate as well as the renal tubular absorption of calcium. Moreover, the steroid hormone promotes osteoblast proliferation, differentiation, and function. The expression of several bone matrix proteins such as type I collagen, osteocalcin, and osteopontin in osteoblasts is upregulated by $1,25\text{-}(OH)_2D_3$. In addition to its action on osteoblasts, the hormone also promotes the generation of osteoclasts from undifferentiated hematopoetic precursor cells.

PTH is responsible for the short-term regulation of serum calcium levels. It increases the renal tubular absorption of calcium and enhances bone resorption by promoting differentiation, recruitment, and activation of osteoclasts. PTH apparently also has a role in bone formation inasmuch as the hormone is able to induce the proliferation of (pre)osteoblasts.

Calcitonin is an inhibitor of the activity of mature osteoclasts; nevertheless, the physiologic role of this hormone in the regulation of bone turnover in humans is unclear.

The importance of estrogens in the regulation of bone turnover has been demonstrated by the clinical observation that estrogen deficiency leads to enhanced bone resorption. Estrogens suppress osteoclast formation through negative effects on signaling from the IL-6/IL-6R system[31,33] as well as through upregulation of OPG expression in osteoblasts.[39] Estrogens also inhibit the activity of osteoclasts[40] and promote TGF-β-mediated apoptosis of osteoclasts.[41]

The importance of androgens for the maintenance of bone mass is underscored by the fact that castration leads to very rapid bone loss.[42] Like estrogens, androgens are apparently able to stimulate osteoblast proliferation and, more importantly, also to inhibit induction of osteoclast formation by calcemic hormones.

Thyroid hormones promote bone formation through acceleration of osteoblastic differentiation, in particular through upregulation of IGF-1 expression.[35] In organ cultures triiodothyronine stimulates bone resorption;[43] data from our laboratory demonstrate that triiodothyronine augments $1,25\text{-}(OH)_2D_3$-induced osteoclastogenesis.[44] Clinically, the excessive production of thyroid hormones is associated with bone demineralization.

Glucocorticoids have complex actions on both bone formation and resorption, among which inhibition of collagen type I synthesis in bone-forming cells seems to be predominant. Stimulation of osteoclast formation, induction of hypercalciuria, as well as inhibition of vitamin D–independent intestinal calcium absorption apparently contribute also to the gross negative effect of the steroids on bone mass and mineral density.

C. EXTRASKELETAL REGULATION OF CALCIUM HOMEOSTASIS

Calcium homeostasis in the body is achieved by the action and interaction of calcemic hormones such as $1,25\text{-}(OH)_2D_3$ and PTH on their three classical target organs: bone, (small) intestine, and kidney. Consequently, hormonal regulation of calcium absorption from the intestinal lumen as well as of renal handling of calcium is a major determinant of bone mineral density in health and disease.

In humans and in many other species, the small intestine is the most important site of calcium absorption, whereas the large bowel is only of minor significance. Calcium is absorbed from the intestinal lumen via a paracellular as well as a transcellular route. The paracellular pathway, which involves migration through intercellular tight junctions, displays characteristics of passive transfer inasmuch as it is not regulated, and the extent to which calcium is transferred depends solely on its intraluminal concentration. Calcium transfer across the enterocyte is a sequential multistep process that shows saturation kinetics, and encompasses calcium entry via specific calcium channels in the brush border membrane (ECaC-1[45] and CaT-1[46]), intracellular diffusion after binding to the calcium-binding protein (calbindin-9kD[47]), and extrusion across the basolateral aspect of the cell predominantly via an ATP-driven calcium pump (Ca^{2+}-ATPase[48]). It is important to note that transcellular calcium transport is highly vitamin D-dependent due to the stimulatory action of

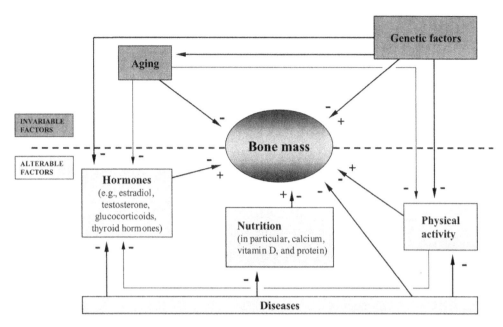

FIGURE 1.1 Factors that influence the accrual and involution of bone mass. (Adapted from Ziegler, R. et al., *J. Nutr.,* 125, 20335, 1995.)

$1,25\text{-}(OH)_2D_3$ on each individual transfer step. Consequently, in vitamin D deficiency, when transcellular calcium transport is downregulated, the paracellular pathway could become the more important route of intestinal calcium absorption.

Evidence is also accumulating that estrogens play a role in regulation of calcium absorption from the small intestinal lumen, although the exact mechanism by which sex hormones could enhance transepithelial Ca^{2+} transport has not yet been elucidated.[49]

The major role of the kidney in calcium homeostasis is to conserve body calcium; only approximately 0.5% of the calcium cleared by glomerular filtration is excreted in the urine. More than 60% of calcium is reabsorbed in the proximal convoluted tubule under the influence of PTH; other sites of PTH-mediated calcium reabsorption are the thick ascending limb and the collecting duct, while in the distal convoluted tubule $1,25\text{-}(OH)_2D_3$ stimulates calcium reabsorption in a fashion identical to that in the small intestine.[50]

III. OSTEOPOROSIS

Osteoporosis is a pathologic condition of the entire skeleton and is characterized by a low bone mass in combination with microarchitectural changes, particularly of the cancellous bone; both add to the fragility of bone at distinct sites of the axial as well as the perpendicular skeleton. As detailed before, bone remodeling both in cortical and trabecular bone proceeds in an orderly fashion with bone resorption tightly coupled to bone formation. Osteoporosis must therefore be viewed as the consequence of a specific imbalance of bone remodeling, which leads to net bone loss because formation of new bone by osteoblasts for several reasons does not match the extent of bone resorbed by osteoclast activity.

There are two major determinants of bone mass and mineral density in later life: (1) the extent of peak bone mass in early adulthood, and (2) the rate of involutional bone loss thereafter. Both determinants are governed by complex interactions of genetic, environmental, nutritional, hormonal, age-related, and lifestyle factors (Figure 1.1).

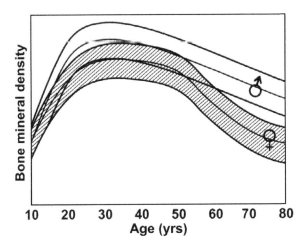

FIGURE 1.2 Schematic representation of changes in bone mineral density (means ± SD) with age in women (shaded area) and men (open area). (Adapted from Pietschmann, P. and Peterlik, M., *Wien. Med. Wschr.,* 149, 454, 1999.)

A. DETERMINANTS OF PEAK BONE MASS

The increase in bone mass that occurs during childhood and puberty results from a combination of enchondral bone formation (bone growth at the end plates) and of bone modeling (appositional bone growth). The early rapid increase in bone mass at puberty is associated with an increase in sex hormone levels and the closure of the growth plates. The resulting peak bone mass is achieved by the age of 20.[51] There exists an important sexual dimorphism in this respect inasmuch as males accrue a significantly higher peak bone mass than females (Figure 1.2).

Genetic factors are the main determinants of the peak bone mass.[52] This has been shown by studies on twins[53] and on mother–daughter pairs.[54] The genetic disposition appears to account for about 50 to 80% of the variance in bone mass, depending on the skeletal site. It is likely that several genes regulate bone mass, each with a moderate effect; likely candidates include the genes for type 1 collagen and for the vitamin D receptor.[52] The nongenetic factors that determine peak bone mass include, as well as sex hormones, calcium intake, body weight at maturity, sedentary lifestyle, and age at puberty.[55]

B. AGE-RELATED BONE LOSS IN MEN AND WOMEN

Within the third decade of life the skeletal mass begins to diminish at a rate of about 0.5% per year in both sexes. Involution of bone mass and mineral density is a truly age-related process because it proceeds invariably at a constant rate even in the absence of any disease or nutritional or hormonal deficiency. In males, bone loss proceeds continously into senescence at the same low rate, and generally reaches the "fracture threshold" at a more advanced age than in women. The reason that the fracture threshold in women is reached much earlier than in men is twofold: first, peak bone mass in females, as mentioned before, is generally lower than in males, and, second, when entering the menopause, due to cessation of ovarian function bone loss is acclerated to about 3% per year (particularly in cancellous bone, e.g., in the spine; Figure 1.2). After this phase of rapid bone loss that lasts for approximately 5 to 10 years, the skeletal mass is diminished at cancellous and cortical sites at a much slower rate, which is similar to that observed also in men.[56]

Riggs et al.[56] have proposed a "unitary model" for involutional osteoporosis in postmenopausal women and in aging men (Figure 1.3): the rapid phase of cancellous bone loss at the beginning of the menopause reflects the loss of the effective restraint that high circulating levels of estrogens are thought to have on bone cell functions. The ensuing slow phase of proportionate bone loss at cortical and cancellous sites may be caused by the effects of loss of estrogen on extraskeletal sites,

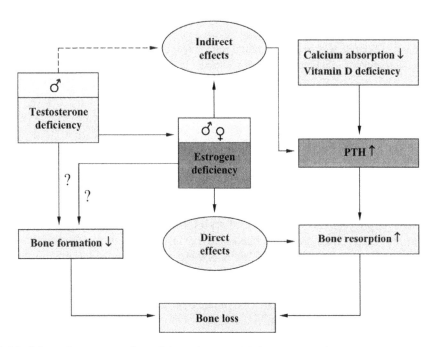

FIGURE 1.3 Schematic representation of the unitary model for bone loss in postmenopausal women and aging men as proposed by Riggs, Khosla, and Melton. (Adapted from Riggs, B.I., *Bone Miner. Res.,* 13, 763, 1998.)

e.g., intestinal calcium absorption, and is certainly aggravated (in both sexes) by progressive secondary hyperparathyroidism. Notably, low levels of bioavailable estrogen may be responsible for deterioration of bone mass also in aging men.

C. Estrogen Deficiency/Postmenopausal Osteoporosis

Clinically the most frequent consequences of the accelerated bone loss present during the first years after menopause are vertebral deformities, compression fractures of the spine, and distal forearm fractures ("type I osteoporosis," according to Riggs and Melton[57]).

At the time of the menopause, blood levels of circulating estradiol decrease by 90%. Estrogen deficiency is the most important mechanism of the rapid phase of bone loss as can be inferred from the fact that postmenopausal bone loss can be prevented by hormone replacement therapy.[58] As described above, estrogens inhibit both the generation and activation of osteoclasts; estrogen deficiency thus results in an imbalance between the processes of bone resorption and bone formation.[59] This remodeling imbalance is magnified by an increase in the rate of initiation of new bone-remodeling cycles, also called activation frequency. Estrogens act partly through the osteoblast[60] by the synthesis of osteoprotegerin or IGF and partly through monocytes in the bone marrow environment by decreasing the synthesis of IL-1 and TNF α.[32] Thus, an enhanced production of cytokines such as IL-1 in response to estrogen deficiency may account for a more rapid bone loss.

Estrogen deficiency increases the sensitivity of the skeletal system to parathyroid hormone and, perhaps, to other resorption-inducing agents,[61] and thereby further augments the remodeling imbalance. As a consequence of the skeletal outflow of calcium into extracellular fluids, urinary calcium excretion increases and intestinal calcium absorption declines.[62] Thus, although there is a trend toward slightly decreased levels, serum PTH in early postmenopausal women remains within the normal range.[63] In this context it should be mentioned that hormone replacement therapy results in increased serum PTH levels, suggesting that there is a slight decrease in PTH secretion in the steady state.[56,64]

D. SENILE OSTEOPOROSIS

The slow phase of bone loss (previously called type II osteoporosis[37]) involves comparable deficits of both trabecular and cortical bone and can be attributed to age-related factors including an increase in PTH levels and osteoblast senescence.[56] The major fractures associated with this process are those of the proximal femur and vertebral fractures.[65]

In both males and females PTH levels increase with aging.[66,67] PTH concentrations correlate with biochemical markers of bone remodeling; bone resorption parameters may be returned to those found in young people by intravenous infusions of calcium.[68] The increase in PTH levels seen with aging results from decreased renal calcium reabsorption and impaired intestinal calcium absorption.[69] The latter may be a consequence of vitamin D deficiency especially in housebound elderly subjects,[70] decreased 1α-hydroxylase activity in the kidney resulting in decreased synthesis of $1,25\text{-}(OH)_2D_3$, or resistance to vitamin D. Whatever the cause, in elderly subjects a diet high in calcium returns both PTH and bone turnover markers to levels found in healthy young adults.

It has been suggested that the age-related increase in PTH levels could be a consequence of indirect effects of estrogen deficiency.[56] This hypothesis is based on the following evidence: in older women estrogen treatment results in (1) a decrease in bone turnover markers and PTH levels; (2) an increase in intestinal calcium absorption, possibly mediated by an increase in $1,25\text{-}(OH)_2D_3$; (3) an increase in the PTH-independent calcium reabsorption in the kidney; and, finally, (4) a decrease in the parathyroid secretory reserve.[56]

The late postmenopausal phase of bone loss is primarily due to excessive bone resorption; nevertheless, as demonstrated by histomorphometry,[71] decreased bone formation also is a contributing factor. Impaired bone formation with aging has been linked to a decreased production of several locally acting growth factors,[72] and low serum levels of growth hormone and insulin-like growth factor.[73]

A number of risk factors have been associated with low bone mass and osteoporotic fractures in population studies and could perhaps aid in risk assessment.[74] For example, later age at menopause, estrogen or thiazide use, non-insulin-dependent diabetes, and greater height, weight, and strength are all positively associated with peripheral bone density in the Study of Osteoporotic Fractures,[75] whereas greater age, smoking, high caffeine intake, prior gastric surgery, and a maternal history of fracture were negatively associated. Slosman[76] was able to show that in women entering menopause, multiple factors, including age, height, weight, alcohol intake, tobacco use, frame size, and markers of bone turnover, could be used to identify only two thirds of women with low bone mass.

E. OSTEOPOROSIS IN MEN

Although osteoporotic fractures are less common in men than in postmenopausal women, osteoporosis in men is a severe condition more frequent than generally thought. In later life in men the incidence of fractures due to low-energy trauma increases rapidly with aging.[77] The Dubbo Osteoporosis Epidemiology Project[78] suggested that the lifetime risk of a low-trauma fracture is as high as 25% in men with an average age of 60 years. Vertebral fracture risk in the second half of life is 5% for males and 16% for females of the same age.[79] The incidence of hip fracture rises exponentially in men with aging, but the age at which the increase begins is slightly higher in men than in women.[80] Perhaps as a result of a higher prevalence of concomitant disease, the mortality associated with a hip fracture in elderly men is considerably higher than in women;[81] thus, one of the strongest predictors of mortality after a hip fracture is gender.[82]

As mentioned before, the average bone loss at the spine in the second half of life is lower for males than for females. Also in men there is a negative correlation between the risk of fracture and bone mass;[78] thus, the age-related decline in bone mass that occurs in men is likely to contribute to the increase in fracture rates in elderly people. Moreover, the fracture threshold is higher for males than for females.[83] In this context, Mosekilde[84] found that, while bone density is not particularly different in older men and women, the microarchitectural pattern of trabecular bone is distinct. It is also known that men have bigger bones than women, because they have 2 years longer prepubertal growth.

Approximately 30% of men seen for evaluation of fractures have idiopathic osteoporosis.[85] In a group of men with vertebral fractures due to idiopathic osteoporosis we found an elevated urinary excretion of hydroxyproline indicating excessive bone resorption.[86] Recently, a link between idiopathic osteoporosis and low levels of IGF-1, or IGF-1-binding protein 3 (IGFBP-3) levels, was postulated.[87]

Systemic diseases, certain medications, and lifestyle factors may increase the risk of osteoporosis. The majority of men with osteoporotic fractures are found to have one or more of these secondary causes of metabolic bone disease.[88,89]

Hypogonadism is a well-established cause of osteoporosis in males and of failure to achieve peak bone mass.[42] One of the prominent clinical symptoms of testosterone deficiency in men is a significant decrease in bone mineral density.[89] Ringe et al.[85] found secondary osteoporosis due to androgen deficiency in 20% of their study group of male patients with osteoporosis. These data are in accordance with our unpublished data on 120 males suffering from osteoporosis, where bone mineral density was assessed by quantitative computed tomography at the lumbar spine. Our observations indicated that lower serum testosterone levels correlate with decreased spinal bone mass.

Serum testosterone concentrations decline with increasing age in some but not in all men; androgen deficiency may be accelerated by illness, medication, and stress. In a longitudinal study on male aging, annual decreases of 0.4% in total testosterone and 1.2% in free testosterone were found.[90] These declines may contribute to decreases in muscle mass, muscle strength, and bone mass that often occur in elderly men. Little is known about the amount of androgen required to maintain bone mass in men; moreover, it is not known whether the beneficial effect of androgen is due to the androgen itself or to the consecutively produced estrogen. As the testes produce both sex hormones and testosterone can be converted in peripheral tissues to estrogen, a deficiency of either could mediate postorchiectomy bone loss. Furthermore, human osteoblasts contain both estrogen[60] and androgen receptors.[91]

In human males, skeletal dependency on estrogen is supported by several studies. Khosla et al.[68] demonstrated in a large population-based sample by multivariate analysis that both in men and postmenopausal women serum bioavailable estrogen levels were consistent, independent predictors of bone mineral density. In one of our studies, male patients with idiopathic osteoporosis and vertebral fractures had significantly decreased estradiol levels.[92] It appears that both estrogens and androgens are required for the growth and maintenance of the adult male bone. If there are low levels of either class of sex hormones, skeletal maturation is impaired and peak bone mass during growth is not optimal, and skeletal involution in later life may lead to an increased fracture risk.

F. SECONDARY OSTEOPOROSIS

The term *secondary osteoporosis* has been used in the presence of specific conditions, diseases, lifestyle factors, and the use of medications that are responsible for bone loss (Table 1.1). We have found[86] one or more of these factors present in about 20% of females and 50% of males presenting with vertebral or peripheral fractures. Young patients with an osteoporotic fracture are more likely to have underlying illness, and patients with secondary osteoporosis are likely to have fractures at a somewhat younger age. Especially common secondary causes of osteoporosis are hypogonadism (see above), subtotal gastrectomy,[93,94] hyperthyroidism,[95] immobilization,[96] chronic obstructive lung disease,[97] and the use of glucocorticoids[98] or anticonvulsant drugs.[99]

One of the most important causes for secondary osteoporosis is glucocorticoid-induced bone loss. The true incidence of osteoporosis-related fractures in these patients is unknown, but available

---

TABLE 1.1
Some Important Causes of Secondary Osteoporosis

Glucocorticoid-induced osteoporosis
Hypogonadism
Immobilization
Thyroid disease
Gastrointestinal disorders
Hyperparathyroid bone disease
Defects of bone development (osteogenesis imperfecta)
Other connective tissue diseases
Hematologic disorders
Alcoholism
Chronic heparin administration
Rheumatoid arthritis
Post-transplantation osteoporosis
Osteoporosis associated with pregnancy

---

data suggest that the incidence is between 30 and 50%.[100] Prolonged exposure to glucocorticoid medication decreases cell replication, differentiation of osteoblasts, and proliferation of periostal precursor cells resulting in inhibition of bone formation.[98] Glucocorticoids have a biphasic effect on osteoclasts. Physiologic concentrations are required for the late stages of differentiation and function, whereas the generation of new osteoclasts is inhibited and apoptosis of future osteoclasts is increased by high doses and prolonged exposure.[101] The urinary excretion of markers of bone resorption is increased in glucocorticoid-treated patients. Glucocorticoid-induced enhanced resorption may be due to secondary hyperparathyroidism, which increases the amount of bone remodeling units and probably also augments the amount of bone resorbed at each site.[102,103] Glucocorticoids inhibit pituitary secretion of gonadotropins, ovarian and testicular secretion of estrogen and testosterone, and adrenal secretion of androstendione dehydroepiandrosterone.[104] Because these hormones decrease bone resorption, their absence accelerates glucocorticoid-induced bone loss. Furthermore, glucocorticoids inhibit gastrointestinal absorption[103] and increase renal excretion of calcium.

Negative calcium balance and, perhaps, failure to transport calcium into the parathyroid cell cause an increase in secretion of PTH,[105] increasing the number of sites undergoing bone remodeling. In conclusion, the combination of an increased number of sites undergoing remodeling and a decrease in bone formation at each site may cause rapid bone loss as a result of glucocorticoid treatment.

REFERENCES

1. Anonymous, "Consensus Development Conference: Prophylaxis and treatment of osteoporosis," *Am. J. Med.,* 94, 646, 1993.
2. Baron, R., "Anatomy and ultrastructure of bone," in *Primer on the Metabolic Bone Diseases and Disorders of Mineral Metabolism*, 4th ed., Favus, M.J., Ed., Lippincott-Williams & Wilkins, Philadelphia, 1999, 3.
3. Fleisch, H., *Bisphosphonates in Bone Disease. From the Laboratory to the Patient,* 3rd ed., Parthenon, New York, 1997.
4. Lian, J.B., Stein, G.S., Canalis, E., et al., "Bone formation: osteoblast lineage cells, growth factors, matrix proteins, and the mineralization process," in *Primer on the Metabolic Bone Diseases and Disorders of Mineral Metabolism*, 4th ed., Favus, M.J., Ed., Lippincott-Williams & Wilkins, Philadelphia, 1999, 14.

5. Ducy, P., Zhang, R., Geoffroy, V., et al., "Osf2/Cbfa1: a transcriptional activator of osteoblast differentiation," *Cell*, 89, 747, 1997.

6. Otto, F., Thornell, A.P., Crompton, T., et al., "Cbfa1, a candidate gene for cleidocranial dysplasia syndrome, is essential for osteoblast differentiation and bone development," *Cell*, 89, 765, 1997.

7. Dobnig, H. and Turner, R.T., "Evidence that intermittent treatment with parathyroid hormone increases bone formation in adult rats by activation of bone lining cells," *Endocrinology*, 136, 3632, 1995.

8. Eriksen, E.F., Axelrod, D.W., and Melsen F., *Bone Histomorphometry*, Raven Press, New York, 1994.

9. Mundy, G.R., "Bone remodeling," in *Primer on the Metabolic Bone Diseases and Disorders of Mineral Metabolism*, 4th ed., Favus, M.J., Ed., Lippincott-Williams & Wilkins, Philadelphia, 1999, 30.

10. Yasuda, H., Shima, N., Nakagawa, N., et al., "Osteoclast differentiation factor is a ligand for osteoprotegerin/osteoclastogenesis-inhibitory factor and is identical to TRANCE/RANKL," *Proc. Natl. Acad. Sci. U.S.A.*, 95, 3597, 1998.

11. Lacey, D.L., Timms, E., Tan, H.L., et al., "Osteoprotegerin (OPG) ligand is a cytokine that regulates osteoclast differentiation and activation," *Cell*, 93, 165, 1998.

12. Anderson, M.A., Maraskovsky, E., Billingsley, W.L., et al., "A homologue of the TNF receptor and its ligand enhance T-cell growth and dendritic cell function," *Nature (London)*, 390, 175, 1994.

13. Wong, B.R., Rho, J., Arron, J., et al., "TRANCE is a novel ligand for the tumor necrosis factor receptor family that activates c-Jun N-terminal kinase in T cells," *J. Biol. Chem.*, 272, 25190, 1997.

14. Hofbauer, L.C., Khosla, S., Dunstan, C.R., et al., "The roles of osteoprotegerin and osteoprotegerin ligand in the paracrine regulation of bone resorption," *J. Bone Miner. Res.*, 15, 2, 2000.

15. Gao, Y.H., Shinki, T., Yuase, T., et al., "Potential role of cbfa1, an essential transcription factor for osteoblast differentiation, in osteoclastogenesis: regulation of mRNA expression for osteoclast differentiation factor (ODF)," *Biochem. Biophys. Res. Commun.*, 252, 697, 1998.

16. Kitazawa, R., Kitazawa, S., and Maeda, S., "Promotor structure of mouse RANKL/TRANCE/OPGL/ODF gene," *Biochim. Biophys. Acta*, 1445, 134, 1999.

17. Hofbauer, L.C. and Heufelder, A.E., "The role of receptor activator of nuclear factor-κB ligand and osteoprotegerin in the pathogensis and treatment of metabolic bone disease," *J. Clin. Endocrinol. Metab.*, 85, 2355, 2000.

18. Kong, Y.Y., Yoshida, H., Sarosi, I., et al., "OPGL is a key regulator of osteoclastogenesis, lymphocyte development and lymph-node organogenesis," *Nature (London)*, 397, 315, 1999.

19. Felix, R., Cecchini, M.G., and Fleisch, H., "Macrophage colony stimulating factor restores *in vivo* bone resorption in the op/op osteopetrotic mouse," *Endocrinology*, 127, 2592, 1990.

20. Dougall, B., Glaccum, M., Charrier, K., et al., "RANK is essential for osteoclast and lymph node development," *Genes Dev.*, 13, 2412, 1999.

21. Li, J., Sarosi, I., Yan, X.Q., et al., "RANK is the intrinsic hematopoietic cell surface receptor that controls osteoclastogenesis and regulation of bone mass and calcium metabolism," *Proc. Natl. Acad. Sci. U.S.A.*, 97, 1566, 2000.

22. Simonet, W.S., Lacey, D.L., Dunstan, C.R., et al., "Osteoprotegerin: a novel secreted protein involved in the regulation of bone density," *Cell*, 89, 309, 1997.

23. Tsuda, E., Goto, M., Mochizuki, S.I., et al., "Isolation of a novel cytokine from human fibroblasts that specifically inhibits osteoclastogenesis," *Biochem. Biophys. Res. Commun.*, 234, 137, 1997.

24. Hofbauer, L.C., Dunstan, C.R., Spelsberg, T.C., et al., "Osteoprotegerin production by human osteoblast lineage cells is stimulated by vitamin D, bone morphogeneic protein-2, and cytokines," *Biochem. Biophys. Res. Commun.*, 250, 776, 1998.

25. Hofbauer, L.C., Gori, F., Riggs, B.L., et al., "Stimulation of osteoprotegerin ligand and inhibition of osteoprotegerin production by glucocorticoids in human osteoblastic lineage cells: potential paracrine mechanisms of glucocortiocid induced osteoporosis," *Endocrinology*, 140, 4382, 1999.

26. Bucay, N., Sarosi, I., Dunstan, C.R., et al., "Osteoprotegerin-deficient mice develop early onset osteoporosis and arterial calcification," *Genes Dev.*, 12, 1260, 1998.

27. Mizuno, A., Amizuka, N., Irie, K., et al., "Severe osteoporosis in mice lacking osteoclastogenesis inhibitory factor/osteoprotegerin," *Biochem. Biophys. Res. Commun.*, 247, 610, 1998.

28. Pacifici, R., "Aging and cytokine production," *Calcif. Tissue Int.*, 65, 345, 1999.

29. Pacifici, R., Rifas, L., McCracken, R., et al., "Ovarian steroid treatment blocks a postmenopausal increase in blood monocyte interleukin-1 release," *Proc. Natl. Acad. Sci. U.S.A.*, 86, 2398, 1989.

30. Ralston, S.H., Russell, R.G., and Gowen, M., "Estrogen inhibits release of tumor necrosis factor from peripheral blood mononuclear cells in postmenopausal women," *J. Bone Miner. Res.*, 5, 983, 1990.

31. Jilka, R.L., Hangoc, C., Girasole, G., et al., "Increased osteoclast development after estrogen loss: mediation by interleukin-6," *Science*, 257, 88, 1992.

32. Pacifici, R., "Postmenopausal osteoporosis: how the hormonal changes of menopause cause bone loss," in *Osteoporosis*, Marcus, R., Feldman, D., and Kelsey, J., Eds., Academic Press, London, 1996, 727.

33. Schiller, C., Gruber, R., Redlich, K., et al., "17β-Estradiol antagonizes effects of 1α,25-dihydroxy-vitamin D_3 on interleukin-6 production and osteoclast-like cell formation in mouse bone marrow cell cultures," *Endocrinology*, 138, 4567, 1997.

34. Komm, B.S., Terpening, C.M., Benz, D.J., et al., "Estrogen binding, receptor mRNA, and biologic response in osteoblast-like osteosarcoma cells," *Science*, 241, 81, 1988.

35. Klaushofer, K., Varga, F., Glantschnig, H., et al., "The regulatory role of thyroid hormones in bone cell growth and differentiation," *J. Nutr.*, 125, 1996S, 1995.

36. Pilbeam, C., Harrison, J.R., and Raisz, L.G., "Prostaglandins and bone metabolism," in *Principles of Bone Biology*, Bilezikian, J.P., Raisz, L.G., and Rodan, G.A., Eds., Academic Press, San Diego, 1996, 715.

37. Raisz, L.G. and Martin, T.J., "Prostaglandins in bone and mineral metabolism," in *Bone and Mineral Research*, Annual 2, Excerpta Medica, Amsterdam, 1983, 286.

38. Feyen, J.H.M. and Raisz, L.G., "Prostaglandin production from sham operated and oophorectomized rats: effect of 17β-estradiol *in vivo*," *Endocrinology*, 121, 819, 1987.

39. Hofbauer, L.C., Khosla, S., Dunstan, C.R., et al., "Estrogen stimulates gene expression and protein production in human osteoblastic cells," *Endocrinology*, 140, 4367,1999.

40. Oursler, M.J., Osdoby, P., Pyfferoen, J., et al., "Avian osteoclasts as estrogen target cells," *Proc. Natl. Sci. Acad. U.S.A.*, 88, 6613, 1991.

41. Hughes, D.E., Dai, A., Tiffee, J.C., et al., "Estrogen promotes apoptosis of murine osteoclasts mediated by TGF-β," *Nat. Med.*, 2, 1132, 1996.

42. Stepan, J.J., Lachman, M., Zverina, J., and Pacovsky, V., "Castrated men exhibit bone loss: effect of calcitonin treatment on biochemical parameters of bone remodeling," *J. Clin. Endocrinol. Metab.*, 69, 523, 1989.

43. Klaushofer, K., Hoffmann, O., Gleispach, H., et al., "Bone resorbing activity of thyroid hormones is related to prostaglandin production in neonatal mouse calvaria," *J. Bone Miner. Res.*, 4, 305, 1989.

44. Schiller, C., Gruber, R., Ho, G.M., et al., "Interaction of triiodothyronine with 1α,25-dihydroxyvitamin D_3 on interleukin-6-dependent osteoclast-like cell formation in mouse bone marrow cell cultures," *Bone*, 22, 341, 1998.

45. Hoenderop, J.G.J., van der Kemp, A.W.C.M., Hartog, A., et al., "Molecular identification of the apical Ca^{2+} channel in 1,25-dihydroxyvitamin D_3-responsive epithelia," *J. Biol. Chem.*, 274, 8375, 1999.

46. Peng, J.B., Chen, X.Z., Berger, U.V., et al., "Molecular cloning and characterization of a channel-like transporter mediating intestinal calcium absorption," *J. Biol. Chem.*, 274, 22739, 1999.

47. Wasserman, R.H., Corradino, R.A., and Taylor, A.N., "Vitamin D-dependent calcium binding protein: purification and some properties," *J. Biol. Chem.*, 243, 3978, 1968.

48. Bronner, F., "Intestinal calcium transport: the cellular pathway," *Miner. Electrolyte Metab.*, 16, 94, 1990.

49. Arjmandi, B.H., Hollis, B.W., and Kalu, D.N., "*In vivo* effect of 17β-estradiol on intestinal calcium absorption in rats," *Bone Miner.*, 26, 181, 1994.

50. Bronner, F., "Renal calcium transport: mechanisms and regulation — an overview," *Am. J. Physiol.*, 257, F707, 1989.

51. Gilsanz, V., Gibbens, D.T., Roe, T.F., et al., "Vertebral bone density in children: effect of puberty," *Radiology*, 166, 847, 1988.

52. Ralston, S.H., "Osteoporosis," *Br. Med. J.*, 315, 469, 1997.

53. Kelly, P.J., Nguyen, T., Pocock, N., et al., "Genetic determination of changes in bone density with age: a twin study," *J. Bone Miner. Res.*, 8, 11, 1993.

54. Soroko, S., Barrett Condor, E., Edelstein, S.L., et al., "Family history of osteoporosis and bone mineral density at the axial skeleton: the Rancho Bernardo Study," *J. Bone Miner. Res.*, 9, 761, 1994.

55. Johnston, C.C., Miller, J.Z., Slemenda, C.W., et al., "Calcium supplementation and increases in bone mineral density in children," *N. Engl. J. Med.*, 327, 82, 1992.

56. Riggs, B.L., Khosla, S., and Melton, L.J., III, "A unitary model for involutional osteoporosis: estrogen deficiency causes both type I and type II osteoporosis in postmenopausal women and contributes to bone loss in aging men," *Bone Miner. Res.*, 13, 763, 1998.

57. Riggs, B.I. and Melton, L.J., III, "Evidence for two distinct syndromes of involutional osteoporosis," *Am. J. Med.*, 75, 899, 1983.

58. Lindsay, R., Aitkin, J.M., Anderson, J.B., et al., "Long-term prevention of postmenopausal osteoporosis by estrogen," *Lancet*, 1, 1038, 1976.

59. Parfitt, A.M., Mundy, G.R., and Roodman, G.D., "A new model for the regulation of bone resorption, with particular reference to the effects of bisphosphonates," *J. Bone Miner. Res.*, 11, 150, 1996.

60. Eriksen, E.F., Colvard, D.S., Berg, N.J., et al., "Evidence of estrogen receptors in normal human osteoblast-like cells," *Science*, 241, 84, 1988.

61. Cosman, F., Shen, V., and Xie, F., "Estrogen protection against bone resorbing effects of parathyroid hormone infusion," *Ann. Intern. Med.*, 118, 337, 1993.

62. Heaney, R.P., Recker, R.R., and Saville, P.D., "Menopausal changes in calcium balance performance," *J. Lab. Clin. Med.*, 92, 953, 1978.

63. Scharla, S.H., Minne, H.W., Waibel-Treber, S., et al., "Bone mass reduction after estrogen deprivation by long-acting gonadotropin-releasing hormone agonists and its relation to pretreatment serum concentrations of 1,25-dihydroxyvitamin D3," *J. Clin. Endocrinol. Metab.*, 70, 1055, 1990.

64. Khosla, S., Atkinson, E.J., Melton, L.J., III, et al., "Effects of age and estrogen status on serum parathyroid hormone levels and biochemical markers of bone turnover in women: a population-based study," *J. Clin. Endocrinol. Metab.*, 82, 1522, 1997.

65. Riggs, B.L. and Melton, L.J., III, "Medical progress series: involutional osteoporosis," *N. Engl. J. Med.*, 314, 1676, 1986.

66. Eastell, R., Yergey, A.L., Vicira, N., et al., "Interrelationship among vitamin D metabolism, true calcium absorption, parathyroid function and age in women: evidence of an age-related intestinal resistance to 1,25-(OH)$_2$D action," *J. Bone Miner. Res.*, 6, 125, 1991.

67. Resch, H., Pietschmann, P., Kudlacek, S., et al., "Influence of sex and age on biochemical bone metabolism parameters," *Miner. Electrolyte Metab.*, 20, 117, 1994.

68. Khosla, S., Melton, L.J., III, Atkinson, E.J., et al., "Relationship of serum sex steroid levels with bone mineral density in aging women and men: a key role for bioavailable estrogen," *J. Clin. Endocrinol. Metab.*, 86, 821, 1998.

69. Avioli, L.V., McDonald, J.E., and Lee, S.W., "The influence of age on the intestinal absorption of ^{47}Ca in women and its relation to ^{47}Ca absorption in postmenopausal osteoporosis," *J. Clin. Invest.*, 44, 1960, 1965.

70. Krexner, E., Resch, H., Pietschmann, P., et al., "Vitamin D status in residents of a long-term-care geriatric hospital in Vienna," *Osteologie*, 5, 13, 1996.

71. Lips, P., Courpron, P., and Meunier, P.J., "Mean wall thickness of trabecular bone packets in the human iliac crest: changes with age," *Calcif. Tissue Res.*, 26, 13, 1978.

72. Marie, P.J., Hou, M., Launay, J.M., et al., "*In vitro* production of cytokines by bone surface-derived osteoblastic cells in normal and osteoporotic postmenopausal women: relationship with cell proliferation," *J. Clin. Endocrinol. Metab.*, 77, 824, 1993.

73. Vermeulen, A., "Nyctohemeral growth hormone profiles in young and aged men: correlation with somatomedin-C levels," *J. Clin. Endocrinol. Metab.*, 64, 884, 1987.

74. Cummings, S.R., Kelsey, J.L., Nevitt, M.C., et al., "Epidemiology of osteoporosis and osteoporotic fractures," *Epidemiol. Rev.*, 7, 178, 1985.

75. Bauer, D.C., Browner, W.S., Cauley, J.A., et al., "For the Study of Osteoporotic Fractures Research Group. Factors associated with appendicular bone mass in older women," *Ann. Intern. Med.*, 118, 657, 1993

76. Slosman, D.O., Rizzoli, R., and Donath, A., "Vertebral bone mineral density measured laterally by dual energy X-ray absorptiometry," *Osteoporos. Int.*, 1, 23, 1990.

77. Donaldson, L.J., Cook, A., and Thomson, R.G., "Incidence of fractures in a geographicly defined population," *J. Epidemiol. Commun. Health*, 44, 241, 1990.

78. Nguyen, T.V., Eisman, J.A., and Kelly, P.J., "Risk factors for osteoporotic fractures in elderly men," *Am. J. Epidemiol.*, 144, 258, 1996.

79. Melton, L.J., III, "Epidemiology of spinal osteoporosis," *Spine*, 22, 2, 1997.

80. Farmer, M.E., White, L.R., Brody, J.A., et al., "Race and sex differences in hip fracture incidence," *Am. J. Public Health*, 74, 1374, 1984.

81. Poor, G., Atkinson, E.J., and O'Fallon, W.M., "Determinants of reduced survival following hip fractures in men," *Clin. Orthop.*, 319, 260, 1995.

82. Schurch, M.A., Rizzoli, R., and Mermillod, B., "A prospective study on socio-economic aspects of fracture of the proximal femur," *J. Bone Miner. Res.,* 11, 1935, 1996.

83. Kudlacek, S., Schneider, B., Resch, H., et al., "Differences in bone mineral density and fractures between women and men," *Maturitas*, 36/3, 173, 2000.

84. Mosekilde, L., "Sex differences in age related bone loss of vertebral trabecular bone mass and structure — biochemical consequences," *Bone*, 10, 325, 1989.

85. Ringe, J.D., Dorst, A.J., and Faber, H., "Osteoporosis in men — clinical assessment of 400 patients and 205 controls by risk factor analysis, densitometry and X-ray findings," *Osteologie,* 6, 81, 1997.

86. Resch, H., Pietschmann, P., Woloszczuk W., et al., "Bone mass and biochemical parameters of bone metabolism in men with spinal osteoporosis," *Eur. J. Clin. Invest.*, 22, 542, 1992.

87. Rosen, J.C., "Insulin-like growth factors and bone: implications for the pathogenesis and treatment of osteoporosis," in *Osteoporosis in Men*, Orwoll, E.S., Ed., Academic Press, London, 1999, 157.

88. Kelepouris, N., Harper, K.D., and Gannon, F., "Severe osteoporosis in men," *Ann. Intern. Med.*, 123, 452, 1995.

89. Hermann, F., Behre, M., and Kliesch, S., "Long-term effect of testosterone therapy on bone mineral density in hypogonadal men," *J. Clin. Endocrinol. Metab.*, 82, 2386, 1997.

90. Gray, A., Feldman, H.A., and McKinley, J.B., "Age, disease and changing sex hormone levels in middle-aged men. Results of the Massachusetts Male Aging study," *J. Clin. Endocrinol. Metab.*, 72, 1016, 1991.

91. Colvard, D.S., Eriksen, E.F., and Keeting, P.E., "Identification of androgen receptors in normal human osteoblast-like cells," *Proc. Natl. Acad. Sci. U.S.A.*, 86, 854, 1989.

92. Bernecker, P., Willvonseder, R., and Resch, H., "Decreased estrogen levels in patients with primary osteoporosis," *J. Bone Miner. Res.*, 10, T364, 1995.

93. Resch, H., Pietschmann, P., and Bernecker, P., "The influence of partial gastrectomy on biochemical parameters of bone metabolism and bone density," *Clin. Invest.,* 70, 426, 1992.

94. Aukee, S., Alhava, E.M., and Karjalainen, P., "Bone mineral after partial gastrectomy II," *Scand. J. Gastroenterol.,* 10, 165, 1975.

95. Eriksen, E.F., Mosekilde, L., and Melsen, F., "Trabecular bone remodeling and bone balance in hyperthyroidism," *Bone*, 6, 421, 1985.

96. Alffram, P.-A., "An epidemiologic study of cervical and trochanteric fractures of the femur in an urban population: analysis of 1,664 cases with special reference to etiologic factors," *Acta Orthop. Scand. Suppl.,* 65, 1, 1964.

97. Praet, J.-P., Peretz, A., Rozenberg, S., et al., "Risk of osteoporosis in men with chronic bronchitis," *Osteoporos. Int.*, 2, 257, 1992.

98. Canalis, E.M., "Effect of cortisol on periosteal and nonperiosteal collagen and DNA synthesis in cultured rat calvariae," *Calcif. Tissue Int.,* 36,158, 1984.

99. Barden, H.S., Mazess, R.B., Chesney, R.W., et al., "Bone status of children receiving anticonvulsant therapy," *Metab. Bone Dis. Relat. Res.*, 4, 43, 1982.

100. Adinoff, A.D. and Hollister, J.R., "Steroid-induced fractures and bone loss in patients with asthma," *N. Engl. J. Med.*, 309, 265, 1983.

101. Gronowicz, G., McCarthy, M.B., and Raisz, L.G., "Glucocorticoids stimulate resorption in fetal rat parietal bones *in vitro*," *J. Bone Miner. Res.*, 5, 1223, 1990.

102. Bikle, D.D., Halloran, B., Fong, L., et al., "Elevated 1,25-dihydroxyvitamin D levels in patients with chronic obstructive pulmonary disease treated with prednisone," *J. Clin. Endocrinol. Metab.*, 76, 456, 1993.

103. Fucik, R.F., Kukreja, S.C., Hargis, G.K., et al., "Effect of glucocorticoids on function of the parathyroid glands in man," *J. Clin. Endocrinol. Metab.*, 40, 152, 1975.

104. Crilly, R.G., Cawood, M., Marshall, D.H., et al., "Hormonal status in normal, osteoporotic and corticosteroid-treated postmenopausal women," *J. R. Soc. Med.*, 71, 733, 1978.

105. Caniggia, A., Nuti, R., Lorè, F., et al., "Pathophysiology of the adverse effects of glucoactive corticosteroids on calcium metabolism in man," *J. Steroid Biochem.*, 15, 153, 1981.

106. Ziegler, R., Scheidt-Nave, C., and Scharla, S., "Pathophysiology of osteoporosis: unresolved problems and new insights," *J. Nutr.*, 125, 2033S, 1995.

107. Pietschmann, P. and Peterlik, M., "Pathophysiologie der Osteoporose," *Wien. Med. Wschr.*, 149, 454, 1999.

2 Histomorphology of Osteoporosis

Christine M. Schnitzler

CONTENTS

I. INTRODUCTION

The skeleton serves two major functions: (1) to provide structural support for the body and (2) to act as mineral reservoir. Histomorphology is predominantly concerned with bone structure. The skeleton changes its structure through modeling and remodeling. Whereas modeling alters the external shape of bones during growth, remodeling maintains skeletal competence throughout life by replacing old bone with new, adjusting the internal microarchitecture of bone, and controlling

0-8493-1033-4/02/$0.00+$1.50

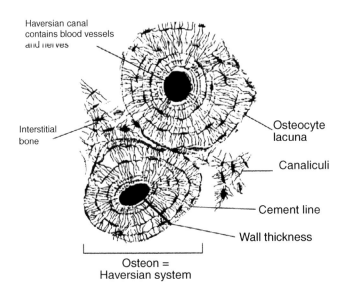

FIGURE 2.1 Diagram of the histologic features of a transverse section through cortical bone showing cortical osteons (Haversian systems). The wall thickness of osteons is the mean distance between the cement line and the surface of the Haversian canal.

bone gain and loss. Histomorphology is concerned with bone remodeling and its structural consequences.

The human skeleton is made up of 85% cortical bone and 15% trabecular (cancellous) bone. Bone mass peaks around age 30 years, which is followed by a slow linear decline of 1% a year, with an acceleration of bone loss in women during the 10 years around the menopause. Women can expect to lose about 35% of cortical and 50% of trabecular bone; men lose about two thirds of these amounts.[1] These are physiologic changes, and the bone loss of osteoporosis secondary to other causes is superimposed on this loss. The clinical manifestations of osteoporosis due to aging and those that are secondary to other causes are the same: low bone mass and fragility fractures. However, the derangements of bone remodeling that lead to the osteoporosis differ depending on the etiology. Bone marrow also changes with age: by age 25 years the marrow of the peripheral skeleton has lost its high cellularity and consists predominantly of fat.[2] Moreover, its vascularity declines.[3] These marrow changes are thought to interact with bone remodeling,[4] because marrow cellularity correlates positively with bone turnover.[5]

II. NORMAL BONE HISTOMORPHOLOGY

A. CORTICAL BONE

Cortical bone is made up of longitudinally arranged, branching, and anastomosing osteons,[6] also referred to as Haversian systems (Figure 2.1). Osteons are the basic building blocks of bone. An osteon is a packet of bone formed by a team of osteoblasts during a remodeling cycle. The interstitial bone between the Haversian systems is the unremodeled part of old Haversian systems. A Haversian system consists of a thick-walled tube of bone around a narrow central canal (Haversian canal). The Haversian canal contains blood vessels, lymph vessels, and nerves. The wall of the Haversian system is made up of concentrically arranged layers of lamellar bone with osteocytes embedded in it. The thickness of the wall of the Haversian system is referred to as wall thickness. This is the distance between the Haversian canal and the cement line (junction of the Haversian system and surrounding bone). Wall thickness is an important indicator of bone loss and gain. It reflects the efficiency of the team of osteoblasts that formed the osteon during its remodeling cycle.[7]

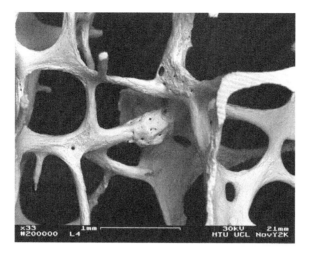

FIGURE 2.2 Scanning electron microscopic image of trabecular bone showing changes of bone loss. A few remnants of trabecular plates are present; the remainder has been converted to rods by perforations. Most trabecular rods are thin, and several have been perforated, leaving only disconnected stumps. The notched trabecula (bottom center) is in danger of being perforated. The roughened, scalloped surfaces are unrepaired resorption sites. The fusiform bulge on one trabecula (center) is the microcallus of a healing trabecular microfracture. (Courtesy of Alan Boyde.)

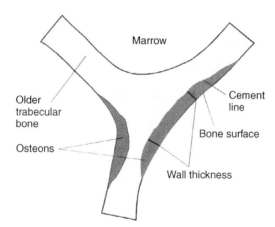

FIGURE 2.3 Diagram of trabecular bone showing two osteons. The wall thickness of the osteons is measured as the distance between the cement line and the bone surface, as in cortical bone.

B. TRABECULAR BONE

Trabecular bone consists of an interconnected network of plates and rods (Figure 2.2). Trabecular architecture is determined at the growth plate during childhood; in the first 15 years of life trabecular thickness increases but trabecular number remains unchanged.[8] As bone loss sets in after peak bone mass has been attained around age 30 years, trabecular plates are perforated by resorption and gradually become converted to rods. Trabecular osteons correspond to cortical Haversian systems cut in half longitudinally. Trabecular osteons are thus concavo-convex packets of bone (Figure 2.3). Like Haversian systems, they consist of parallel layers of lamellar bone with embedded osteocytes. As in the cortex, wall thickness of the trabecular osteons is the distance between the bone surface and the cement line. Wall thickness determines trabecular thickness. The spaces between the

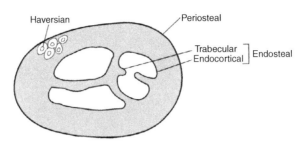

FIGURE 2.4 Diagram of the remodeling envelopes.

trabecular plates and rods are filled with bone marrow, blood vessels, lymph vessels, and nerves. The bone marrow is a rich source of cells, growth factors, and cytokines that assist in bone remodeling and repair.

C. The Lacunar–Canalicular System

The cell body of each osteocyte lies in a lacuna from which canaliculi lead to other canaliculi and lacunae. The long, slender cell processes of the osteocyte reach into the canaliculi where they connect, by means of gap junctions, with the processes of neighboring osteocytes, and also with the lining cells of the Haversian canals and of endosteal surfaces.[9] This facilitates signal traffic between cells. Within this interconnected lacunar–canalicular system the osteocytes and their processes are bathed in interstitial fluid, which carries nutrients, waste, minerals, and other chemicals, and which transmits the pulsatile fluid flow generated by loading. Osteocytes are the mechanotransducers in bone that contribute to the control of initiation of the remodeling cycles[9] (see below).

III. BONE REMODELING IN NORMAL BONE

A. The Remodeling Process

Bone loss and gain as well as microarchitectural alterations are achieved by bone remodeling. Bone remodeling takes place on bone surfaces, also referred to as envelopes. These are the periosteal, intracortical (Haversian), endocortical, and trabecular surfaces (Figure 2.4). The endocortical and trabecular surfaces combined are also referred to as the endosteal surface. On the endosteal surface bone remodeling is greater than on the intracortical surface because of the greater bone surface area available for remodeling activities. The periosteal surface shows little remodeling.

Bone remodeling, or turnover, is a lifelong physiologic process that constantly replaces minute quantities of old bone with new to adapt the skeleton to changes in mechanical stresses, and to ensure that fatigue-damaged bone does not accumulate, and weaken bone.[10,11] In healthy human adults approximately 1 million remodeling sites are operating at any one time.[12] On trabecular and endocortical surfaces, bone remodeling takes place in a trench (up to 60 µm in depth[13] and 2 to 3 mm in greatest dimension[14]) (Figure 2.5), and in the cortex in tunnels (about 100 to 200 µm in diameter and up to 10 mm in length[13]) (Figure 2.6). Bone remodeling proceeds in an orderly sequence of bone resorption, followed by bone formation. The histologic unit that carries out remodeling is referred to as the basic multicellular unit (BMU).[15] It comprises osteoclasts, mononuclear cells, pre-osteoblasts, and osteoblasts, in that temporal order.[14] Osteoclasts first excavate a resorption cavity that advances by 10 to 20 µm a day along the bone surface of trabecular bone, and in a tunnel in cortical bone. Then mononuclear cells smooth the cavity. The floor of the cavity to which the new osteon will be cemented is referred to as the cement line (Figures 2.5 and 2.6).

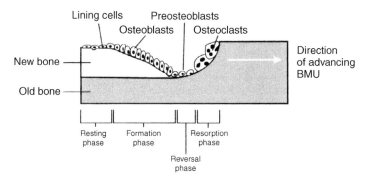

FIGURE 2.5 Diagram of a BMU in trabecular bone. Osteoclasts dig a trench in the trabecular bone surface, and osteoblasts refill it with new bone. The trabecular BMU corresponds to a cortical BMU, cut in half longitudinally.

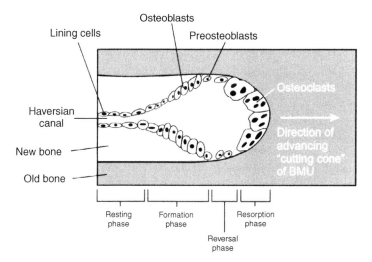

FIGURE 2.6 Diagram of a BMU in cortical bone. Osteoclasts cut a tunnel, and osteoblasts refill it with new bone. The reconstructed bone packet is a Haversian system.

At any one point of the advancing BMU, resorption takes approximately 10 days. Next, pre-osteoblasts (small cells) line the cavity for about 1 week (reversal phase), and then differentiate to osteoblasts (large cells) that lay down osteoid, consisting of collagen, non-collagenous proteins, glycoproteins, and proteoglycans.[16] After 10 to 20 days osteoblasts initiate mineralization (an active process) by releasing exocytosed, membrane-bound bodies into the osteoid. Further crystal growth around these bodies is a passive process under the control of non-collagenous proteins.[17]

Mineralization is accomplished in two phases: approximately 70% of the bone mineral is deposited within days of the start of mineralization (primary phase), and the remainder is added slowly over years (secondary phase).[18] Recently deposited bone is therefore less dense than older bone.[19] For this reason high turnover bone, i.e., bone with an increased number of recently completed osteons, as in children, has lower bone mineral density (BMD) than lower turnover bone in adults. As unremodeled bone becomes increasingly mineralized, it becomes more brittle. Bone formation at any one point of the BMU takes 3 to 4 months to complete in adults. On completion of the remodeling cycle in young adults the same amount of bone is present as before resorption started, i.e., the remodeling process is balanced. However, in elderly individuals and in bone-losing conditions, less bone is formed than was resorbed, so that the remodeling process is in imbalance, or negative balance. If formation does not take place at all, uncoupling of formation from resorption exists. Imbalance and uncoupling lead to increasing cortical porosity and to thinning of trabecular plates and rods.

B. SIGNALS CONTROLLING THE BONE REMODELING CYCLE

Osteocytes are thought to be the mechanosensors and tranducers in bone[9,20] that contribute to the control of the initiation of the remodeling cycle. Osteocyte cell bodies in the lacunae, and their cellular processes in the canaliculi, are bathed in interstitial fluid, which undergoes pulsatile fluid flow generated by loading.[9,20] Fluid flow over the cell surface subjects the cell to two kinds of stimuli, namely, fluid shear stress and streaming electrical potentials. The osteocyte is able to sense these perturbations and to transduce them into signal molecules (mechanotransduction) that are communicated via the lacunar–canalicular system to lining cells on the bone surfaces.[9] Following the appropriate signal, the lining cells retract, and remodeling can begin. The signal molecules involved in this communication remain to be identified but production by osteocytes of prostaglandin, nitric oxide (NO), and insulin-like growth factor-1 (IGF-1) is thought to play a role.[9,20] Furthermore, osteocyte apoptosis (programmed cell death*)[21] in the vicinity of fatigue-damaged bone appears to also stimulate osteoclast differentiation; this serves to remove fatigue-damaged bone by remodeling.[22]

Upon receipt of the activation signal, hemopoietic pluripotent mononuclear precursors proliferate, and under the influence of monocyte–macrophage colony–stimulating factor (M-CSF) they differentiate to osteoclast precursors. These cells fuse under the stimulus provided by the cytokine interleukin-1 (IL-1) and the hormones PTH and 1,25-dihydroxy vitamin D to form mature multinucleate osteoclasts, which commence resorbing bone. The spatial and temporal extent of resorption is limited by osteoclast apoptosis, which is induced by transforming growth factor beta (TGF-β) and by estrogens. TGF-β is set free locally during the resorption process from the resorbed and degraded bone matrix. On the other hand, estrogen deficiency and the associated increase in IL-1, IL-6, and PTH delay osteoclast apoptosis so that resorption cavities can become excessively deep, and trabecular perforations result.[23-25] Mechanical forces appear to influence the direction of the resorption cavity.[13] In normal bone remodeling, formation is coupled to resorption, which means that bone formation is induced by the foregoing bone resorption. Resorption either sets coupling factors free from resorbed bone, or induces other cells to produce coupling factors that initiate bone formation. These coupling factors are TGF-β, BMPs, IGF-I and -II, platelet-derived growth factor (PDGF), fibroblast growth factors (FGFs),[1] and the mounting mechanical strain generated by the increasing depth of the resorption cavity.[13]

The bone formation process is a cascade of complex interactions between growth factors and the cells of the osteoblast lineage.[1] The coupling factors attract mesenchymal stem cells to the remodeling site by chemotaxis, and these cells then proliferate and become osteoblast precursors under the influence of TGF-β, IGF-I and -II, PDGF, and FGFs. Differentiation of these preosteoblasts to mature osteoblasts occurs under the influence of BMP-2 and IGF-I. Bone formation is terminated by a combination of (1) osteoblasts encasing themselves in bone as osteocytes (approximately 15% of osteoblasts),[26] (2) osteoblasts becoming lining cells on bone surfaces, and (3) osteoblast apoptosis (initiated by, e.g., IL-6).[27]

---

* Apoptosis causes single cells to "shrivel up," whereas necrotic cells rupture.

C. The Regional Acceleratory Phenomenon

Any perturbation of bone (e.g., injury, surgery, infection, tumor) leads to an increase in bone remodeling in the region of the perturbation. This means that additional remodeling cycles of resorption followed by formation are activated. This phenomenon has been referred to by Frost[28] as the regional acceleratory phenomenon (RAP). It is thought to be due to the paracrine effects of local cytokines and growth factors. A RAP can be identified by increased uptake in the affected bone region of the radionuclide tracer technetium-99 methylenediphosphonate (^{99}Tc-MDP), which seeks growing bone crystals at new bone formation sites. Clinical examples are the increased radionuclide uptake around a recent total hip arthroplasty, a loose or infected arthroplasty prosthesis, a stress fracture (even before radiographic evidence), a healing fracture, metastases, and any site of a bony surgical procedure. A RAP may take months to subside, i.e., at least one formation period of the remodeling cycle (3 to 4 months) after the last perturbation.

IV. DISORDERED BONE REMODELING AND HISTOMORPHOLOGY IN OSTEOPOROSIS

"Osteoporosis is a disease characterized by low bone mass and microarchitectural deterioration of bone tissue, leading to enhanced bone fragility and a consequent increase in fracture risk."[29] This current definition of osteoporosis encompasses the two main structural faults of the disorder, namely, low bone mass and microarchitectural deterioration. Both result from disordered bone remodeling, and they always go together. There is, however, evidence that bone matrix also deteriorates: with increasing age the stability of trabecular collagen has been found to decline,[30] and proteoglycan components of bone have been shown to exhibit altered molecular orientation.[31]

A. Trabecular Bone

Although the skeleton contains more cortical than trabecular bone, the manifestations of bone loss are first evident in trabecular bone because of its larger surface area on which disordered bone remodeling can wreak havoc.

Hence, sites consisting of a high proportion of trabecular bone, e.g., vertebral bodies, proximal femur, and distal radius, show the highest fragility fracture rates. The derangements of remodeling pose a "triple threat" to trabecular bone: trabeculae become fewer, thinner, and longer.[32] Only one, or at most two, phases of the remodeling cycle have to be deranged to bring about the devastating changes of osteoporosis: increased bone resorption, or decreased bone formation, or both. Bone resorption may be increased by a greater number of resorption sites and/or an increase in resorption depth, e.g., as a result of estrogen deprivation.[23] An increase in resorption depth may cause perforation and disconnection of trabecular plates and rods. Decreased bone formation results from impaired osteoblast recruitment and/or premature osteoblast apoptosis.[7] Impaired osteoblast recruitment may be due to stem cell depletion, preferential differentiation of marrow stromal stem cells to adipocytes rather than to osteoblasts, deficient microcirculation, and other derangements.[7] The decline in bone formation with age is reflected in decline in wall thickness of osteons with age,[33] which results in a reduction of trabecular thickness.[34] The structural consequence of these remodeling derangements is bone loss. Two thirds of this loss has been attributed to removal of trabecular structures, i.e., perforations of trabeculae, and one quarter to trabecular thinning.[34,35] The space vacated by bone is taken up by fatty bone marrow. The rate of bone loss increases with bone turnover because each cycle ends with a deficit; therefore, the more cycles, the faster the loss. However, high bone turnover is a bad thing only if it is associated with a negative remodeling balance. On the contrary, in children high bone turnover leads to an increase in bone mass because of a positive remodeling balance.[8]

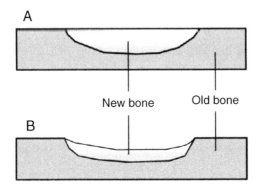

FIGURE 2.7 Diagrams showing balance (A) and imbalance (B) during bone remodeling. In young adults the amount of bone formed during bone remodeling equals the amount of bone resorbed: no bone is lost (B). In elderly people and in osteoporosis less bone is formed than was resorbed: some bone is lost in every remodeling cycle, and as a result trabeculae become thinner (B).

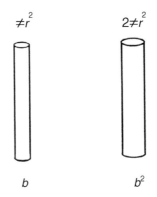

FIGURE 2.8 Diagram of two trabecular rods showing the relationship between trabecular cross-sectional area (πr^2) and resistance to buckling (b). A mere 41% increase in thickness doubles the cross-sectional area of the thin rod on the left; this increases its resistance to buckling not by a factor of 2, but by a factor of $2^2 = 4$, i.e., exponentially. Thus a small increase in trabecular thickness confers a disproportionately greater benefit.

The microarchitectural changes resulting from imbalance or uncoupling at the BMU in trabecular bone are (1) thinning of trabeculae, (2) perforation of trabeculae leading to disconnection of the trabecular network, (3) fatigue damage, and (4) lattice irregularity (see Figure 2.2).

1. Thinning of Trabecular Plates and Rods

Imbalance at the remodeling cycle and uncoupling of formation from resorption lead to a reduction in wall thickness, and thereby to progressive thinning of trabecular plates and rods (Figure 2.7). The higher the bone remodeling rate, the faster this bone loss progresses. Thinning of a trabecula leads to disproportionate loss of bone strength: reduction of the cross-sectional area of a trabecular rod by half is associated with a decrease in the buckling load, not to one half but to one quarter.[36] In other words, there is an exponential relationship between decreasing trabecular cross-sectional area and loss of bone strength (Figure 2.8). When the bone remodeling rate is high, many trabeculae bear the notches of resorption sites. At these sites the trabeculae have reduced thickness. Because a rod is only as strong as its thinnest part, trabecular bone is weaker in a high than in a low turnover state, given similar bone mass.

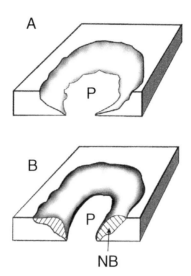

FIGURE 2.9 Bone loss by trabecular plate perforation. Resorption on an already thin trabecular plate (A) has penetrated the plate and created a plate perforation (P). As new bone can only be laid down on existing bone, the remodeling site is repaired by new bone formation (NB) only on the edges of the perforation (B). The remainder of the perforation fills in with bone marrow.

2.   Perforation and Disconnection of Trabeculae

As a result of increased resorption depth or reduction in trabecular thickness, subsequent resorption will eventually perforate the plate or rod[37] (Figure 2.9). This event constitutes a critical phase in bone loss because perforations are not repaired: when resorption switches to formation, new bone will be deposited only on the edge of the perforation, whereas the center of the gap fills with bone marrow. This bone loss is irreversible[38] because in our current state of knowledge no remedy exists that will repair trabecular perforations, or rebuild trabeculae in marrow. Moreover, at the perforation site, bone surface area is lost as potential scaffolding for new bone deposition during anabolic therapy. Hence, the importance of early prevention, i.e., before the trabecular network is disconnected.

In vertebrae, perforations affect horizontal trabeculae before vertical ones, especially in women.[39] Perforation of horizontal struts results in longer free-standing segments of vertical trabeculae. This elongation is associated with an exponential loss of bone strength because an increase in length of an unsupported rod, e.g., by a factor of 3, reduces the buckling load not threefold, but by a factor of 9. In other words, a small loss of bone at a horizontal perforation produces a disproportionately greater loss of bone strength in the vertical trabeculae[36] (Figure 2.10). Because the small amount of bone removed at trabecular perforations is unlikely to initially cause a significant drop in BMD, the associated loss in bone strength will not be reflected in BMD measurements. Indeed, between ages 20 and 80 years vertebral ash density declines by 50%, whereas bone strength declines by more than 80%.[40] Eventually, the disconnected remnants of perforated rods will be resorbed as well because they are not loaded.[37] Then, BMD would be expected to drop.

Perforations of the few remaining vertical trabeculae in an already osteoporotic vertebra deprive the top plate of its support so that it may cave in, and lead to a vertebral fracture (Figure 2.11). Here, too, a small loss of bone leads to a critical loss of structural integrity. Trabecular microarchitecture has indeed been found to be a major and independent determinant of vertebral fractures.[41,42] This is further borne out by the finding that on antiresorptive therapy fracture rates declined

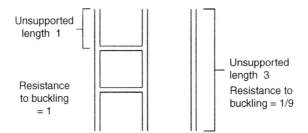

FIGURE 2.10 Diagram showing the relationship between free-standing length of trabeculae and their resistance to buckling. Removal of the two horizontal ties (representing horizontal trabeculae) elongates the free-standing length of the vertical structure by a factor of 3. The buckling load of the now elongated structure is not 3 but $3^2 = 9$, i.e., exponentially, weaker than the supported structure.

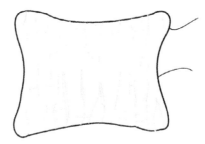

FIGURE 2.11 Diagram showing perforations in the few remaining vertical trabeculae of an already osteoporotic vertebra. A load placed on the unsupported top plate will not be transmitted to the bottom plate. The top plate may cave in, leading to a vertebral fracture.

together with resorption markers, unrelated to the magnitude of change in BMD. This effect is attributed to inhibition of trabecular plate perforation and concomitant loss of connectivity.[43] Moreover, trabeculae are no longer weakened by an excessive number of resorption sites.

3. Fatigue Damage

Repeated loading of bone, even if the load remains below the ultimate failure load (where complete fracture would occur), can lead to fatigue failure in the form of microfractures, microcracks, and stress fractures (see below).

4. Lattice Irregularity

Perforations and microfractures lead to increasing lattice irregularity of the trabecular network. This is associated with marked progressive loss of bone strength, although bone mass may be little changed initially. The loss of bone strength is due to a change from simple compression forces to a mixture of compression and bending forces.[44]

B. CORTICAL BONE

Although cortical bone is also lost in osteoporosis, cortical bone (e.g., the shafts of long bones) is not a common site for osteoporotic fractures because loss proceeds more slowly than in trabecular bone, and microarchitectural disorganization plays a lesser role. Bone loss in cortical bone occurs on both the endocortical and the intracortical (Haversian) surfaces. Cortical bone loss is due to the same derangements of the remodeling cycle as in trabecular bone. In each cycle less bone is formed than was resorbed, and the rate of bone loss rises with increasing bone remodeling rates.

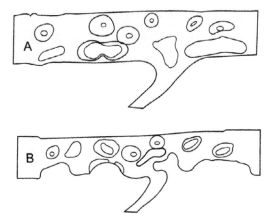

FIGURE 2.12 Diagrams showing cortical bone loss. (A) Cancellization of the subendocortical cortex: large cavities within this portion of the cortex give it a semblance of cancellous bone. (B) Thinning of the cortex: the large subendocortical cavities have been incorporated into the medullary cavity by resorption of the remaining thin plates that separated them from the marrow cavity. Moreover, cortical porosity has increased through incomplete or failed bone formation in Haversian systems.

1. Endocortical Bone Loss

Remodeling on the endocortical envelope takes place in trenches on the flat surface, as it does in trabecular bone (see Figure 2.5). On completion of each cycle, the cortex is a little thinner, and the marrow cavity a little wider because less bone was formed than was resorbed.

2. Intracortical (Haversian) Bone Loss

Bone resorption is initiated from an existing Haversian canal, which contains a blood vessel that brings in the necessary cell precursors. The sequence of events, the time frame, and the derangements of the remodeling cycle are similar to those in trabecular bone, except that the process takes place in a tunnel within solid bone rather than on a flat surface (Figure 2.6). On completion of new bone formation, the new Haversian canal is wider because formation was incomplete. This results in increasing cortical porosity. These intracortical cavities do not fill again with bone. The larger cavities contain fatty bone marrow. This results from a switch in the differentiation pathway of marrow stromal stem cells from osteoblastogenesis to adipogenesis.[4,45] In due course, intracortical cavities will coalesce to form very large marrow spaces within the cortex. This process is most pronounced in the subendocortical region of the cortex, i.e., adjacent to the marrow cavity, perhaps because of the proximity of the bone marrow with its abundant supply of blood vessels, cytokines, and growth factors that support bone remodeling. Since the subendocortical portion of the cortex now resembles trabecular bone, this process is referred to as cancellization of the cortex (Figure 2.12). This change may be evident on plain radiographs as a loss of distinction at the cortico-cancellous and cortico-medullary junction. It is a sign of cortical bone loss. Finally, a plate perforation of the thin plate of bone separating the subendocortical cavity from the marrow cavity will join the two cavities, thus further thinning the cortex and widening the marrow cavity.

The periosteal envelope shows little remodeling activity, but a small amount of bone is added to this envelope throughout life.[46,47] This leads to a minimal but measurable increase in bone size with age that may compensate, in part, for loss of bone strength consequent upon bone loss on the other envelopes. Despite the small amount of bone deposited, maximal strength is derived because this bone is biomechanically advantageously placed, namely, farthest away from the center of the bone.

C. MICROFRACTURES, MICROCRACKS, STRESS FRACTURES, AND MICROPETROSIS

The term *microfracture* is conventionally reserved for such lesions in *trabecular* bone, presumably because a trabecular microfracture shows the characteristic features of a healing long bone fracture, namely, a complete fracture of the trabecula, and healing by callus formation (see Figure 2.2). It is not clear whether these lesions in trabecular bone are the result of fatigue damage or of instantaneous overload.[32,48] The hallmark of the trabecular microfracture is the spindle-shaped or globular mass of callus,[37] approximately 500 μm in diameter,[49] surrounding the microfracture site (see Figure 2.2). Trabecular microfractures have been observed in the proximal femur[50,51] and in vertebral bodies.[52] Cortical fatigue damage, on the other hand, is referred to as microcracks. These lesions lack the resemblance to a microfracture seen in trabecular bone. Instead, short cracks develop within the cortical bone substance. Microcracks are found predominantly in interstitial bone, which happens to be the oldest (unremodeled), most highly mineralized, and therefore most brittle bone.[11] Healing of microcracks by callus formation within compact cortical bone is obviously not possible because of a lack of space around the crack. Instead, the microcrack stimulates local bone remodeling so that the bone containing the crack is resorbed and replaced with new bone.[10] The number of both microfractures in trabecular bone and microcracks in cortical bone increases exponentially with age[11] because of increases in bone strain as a result of bone mass depletion, focal changes in material properties, decreased ability of bone to perceive microdamage, and an inability of bone remodeling to keep pace with the appearance of new lesions, or the propagation of existing ones. This adds to progressive weakening of bone with age.

At what point microcracks and microfractures become stress fractures is probably a matter of degree. Whereas small numbers of microcracks and microfractures are mostly asymptomatic, stress fractures (i.e., propagated cortical microcracks; many trabecular microfractures) are symptomatic.

The development of a stress fracture is determined by a number of interdependent factors:

1. *The load.* The likelihood of failure rises with increasing load. Stress fractures are seen almost exclusively in the lower limbs because of the load of weight bearing.
2. *Number of loading cycles per unit time.* Non-ambulant patients rendered ambulant following a total hip or knee arthroplasty may develop a stress fracture in the same limb, or in the pelvis because recently normalized gait has allowed an increase in loading cycles.
3. *Bone mass.* With declining bone mass, the stress fracture risk rises.[53]
4. *Remodeling.* Incipient microdamage is removed by normal bone remodeling. Low remodeling rates may not be able to remove fatigue-damaged bone as fast as lesions develop.
5. *Microarchitectural deterioration of trabecular bone.* The more deranged the microarchitecture, particularly by erosion, the greater is the trabecular stress fracture risk.[54]

The healing of trabecular stress fractures differs from that in cortical bone, as does the healing of the microscopic lesions that precede them. Trabecular stress fractures heal by callus formation around each of its component microfractures, and occasionally also by periosteal new bone formation at the level of the fracture site. Attempts at remodeling, as in cortical microcracks, usually end in plate perforation as osteoclasts remove the bone bearing the trabecular microfracture.[55] On the other hand, cortical stress fractures heal by a combination of remodeling and periosteal (and endocortical) new bone formation.

Trabecular stress fractures occur most commonly in the metaphyses of tibia and femur, and in the posterior portion of the calcaneum of osteoporotic individuals.[56,57] Because they occur in abnormal bone under normal load, namely, gait, trabecular stress fractures are referred to as "insufficiency fractures," with the insufficiency the osteoporosis. In contrast, cortical stress fractures occur most commonly in the shafts of long bones of the lower limbs, and in the inferomedial cortex of the femoral neck of athletes and military recruits engaging in strenuous, unaccustomed, repetitive activity. Stress fractures of the pars interarticularis of lumbar vertebrae may afflict young ballet dancers. Cortical stress fractures are referred to as "fatigue fractures" because they occur in normal bone under fatiguing abnormal load, i.e., under the reverse bone/load relationship of that in trabecular stress fractures.[57] Cortical stress fractures develop as a result of the inability of normal cortical bone to respond sufficiently rapidly to increased repetitive loading with additional new bone formation, and with increased bone remodeling to replace damaged bone. The reason lies in the low surface area available for such corrective activity in cortical bone.

Demonstration of trabecular and cortical stress fractures by plain radiography depends on callus formation. Callus becomes radiologically visible about 3 weeks from the onset of symptoms. In trabecular bone it typically presents as an about 2-cm-wide, radiodense band across the metaphysis, at right angles to the compressive trabeculae.[56,57] In cortical bone a spindle-shaped mass of callus surrounds the bone at the level of the stress fracture. The stress fracture itself is rarely obvious. Computerized tomography (CT), however, may reveal the crack during this early phase. A presumptive early diagnosis can be made more readily from a radionuclide bone scan using the bone tracer ^{99}Tc-MDP. This will show increased uptake in the region of the stress fracture. The area of uptake extends beyond the extent of the stress fracture, or its callus, as a result of the RAP induced by the fracture. Magnetic resonance imaging (MRI) also shows early changes: it demonstrates the bone marrow edema accompanying the stress fracture. MRI may also show the stress fracture itself.[57]

Micropetrosis refers to the calcification of lacunae and canaliculi following osteocyte apoptosis. Osteocytes, the mechanotransducers of bone, have a life span of about 20 to 25 years[28] if the bone in which they are encased is not remodeled earlier. Their life is terminated by apoptosis. Premature osteocyte apoptosis occurs around microfractures, in the vicinity of resorption sites, and as a result of glucocorticoid therapy.[12] The lacunae and canaliculi of apoptotic osteocytes fill with highly calcified material, a condition referred to as micropetrosis by Frost.[58] Micropetrosis thus adds to the hypermineralization and brittleness of bone. Bone quality is further compromised through the loss of mechanotransduction, and initiation of remodeling, that would have been the task of the apoptotic osteocytes. This is borne out by the negative correlation between osteocyte viability and the number of microfractures.[59]

D. REMODELING DISORDERS

The osteoporotic state, presenting clinically with low bone mass and fragility fractures, is reached through a variety of different derangements of bone remodeling, depending on the underlying disorder. The nature of this derangement has been elucidated in a number of conditions.

1. Menopause- and Age-Related Bone Loss

The derangements of bone remodeling in hypogonadal (menopause-related) bone loss differ from those in age-related bone loss.[7] Menopause-related bone loss is due to a combination of an increase in bone turnover and a negative remodeling balance between bone resorption and formation. Osteoclast birth rate and life span (delayed apoptosis) are increased.[23] This results in deeper erosion pits, perforations, and therefore loss of connectivity of the trabecular network. This bone loss is rapid. In age-related bone loss, on the other hand, bone turnover is not increased, but osteoblast recruitment is defective so that at each remodeling site less bone is formed than was resorbed. This manifests as reduced wall thickness of osteons,[7] which in turn leads to reduced trabecular thickness. This bone loss is not as rapid as hypogonadal bone loss. Thus, hypogonadal bone loss is due mainly to an osteoclast problem, and age-related bone loss to an osteoblast problem. In combination, these two derangements are destructive.

2. Steroid Osteoporosis

Steroid osteoporosis results from a combination of severely impaired bone formation and increased resorption. Osteoblast proliferation and function are decreased and apoptosis is increased. Resorption is increased as a result of a prolonged life span of osteoclasts.[12] Later, resorption is also depressed and bone turnover becomes very low. Furthermore, glucocorticoid excess causes widespread osteocyte apoptosis, and with it a loss of mechanotransduction: fatigue-damaged bone accumulates because it is not remodeled. These abnormalities result in skeletal disintegration: fracture rates rise,[60] and the subchondral bone of convex joint surfaces may fragment. The terms *osteonecrosis* or *avascular necrosis* for this condition are now considered misnomers because the condition is caused by osteocyte apoptosis and not by necrosis or avascularity.[12]

3. Hyperparathyroid Bone Disease

The radiographic manifestations of primary hyperparathyroidism, namely, osteoporosis, fractures, and brown tumors, are features of advanced disease that are infrequently seen nowadays because in most cases the diagnosis of primary hyperparathyroidism is made early by routine serum calcium estimation. For this reason, too, the histologic picture of osteitis fibrosa cystica is now rarely encountered.[61] Nevertheless, even asymptomatic patients without radiographic skeletal changes have reduced cortical thickness.[62] Cortical bone is lost predominantly from the endocortical surface,[63] and to a lesser extent from the periosteal surface.[64] Histological abnormalities are seen long before fractures occur. Hyperparathyroid bone disease is characterized by high bone turnover and a negative remodeling balance leading to reduced wall thickness and to trabecular thinning.[65] The remodeling imbalance is due to an increase in resorption depth, especially on the endocortical envelope, where it leads to cortical thinning.[63] Cancellous bone is generally better preserved than cortical bone.[62,66,67]

4. Hyperthyroidism

Hyperthyroidism, both endogenous and iatrogenic, leads to progressive bone loss at trabecular and cortical sites.[68,69] Bone loss is due to a combination of high bone turnover and a negative remodeling balance.[70] The clinical and histologic pictures of osteoporosis due to hyperthyroidism closely resemble those of postmenopausal ostoeporosis but long bone shaft fractures may also occur. If superimposed on postmenopausal bone loss, the osteoporosis may become severe.[69]

5. Chronic Alcohol Abuse

Osteoporosis is common in chronic alcohol abuse,[71] and develops before severe liver damage occurs.[72] Bone turnover is generally low. The mechanism of bone loss is decreased bone formation[72-75] in the presence of normal[74-76] or increased bone resorption.[72] The decrease in bone formation is not only due to a decreased number of remodeling sites[75] but also to impaired efficiency of teams of osteoblasts.[7,72,74-76] Direct toxicity to osteoblasts by alcohol,[77] and by its metabolite acetaldehyde,[78] has been demonstrated *in vitro*. Moreover, the low serum values of the bone formation marker osteocalcin in drinkers[72,79] corroborate these findings. A decline in serum osteocalcin was apparent within 2 hours of alcohol ingestion, and was dose dependent. Raised hydroxyproline excretion rates in alcohol abuse reflect increased bone resorption.[74,80] Numerous other biochemical abnormalities reflecting disordered bone metabolism have been reported in alcohol abuse.[71]

6. Immobilization

The bone loss of immobilization for orthopaedic conditions, paralysis, or during prolonged bed rest affects whatever part is immobilized. Bone loss commences as soon as immobilization is instituted, progresses rapidly before reaching a plateau after some months, and rarely recovers completely after remobilization.[81] A 50% loss of bone mineral in the head of the humerus and no reversal after recovery were found in patients suffering from a frozen shoulder.[82] Immobilization for 12 to 18 weeks for fracture of the tibia led to a decrease in ipsilateral bone density of 9 and 6% in the trochanter and femoral neck, respectively. By 12 months, the trochanteric loss had increased to 15% despite remobilization.[83] During this period of unloading a small loss of bone had occurred also in the contralateral hip and in the spine. Another study found that 9 years after fracture of the shaft of the tibia, patients had a significantly lower BMD than normal controls, not only in the entire affected limb but also in the opposite leg, and in the lumbar spine.[84] A 10 to 18% reduction in tibial bone mineral content within 12 weeks of ligamentous knee injuries and no subsequent recovery[85] have been recorded. Femoral neck BMD was found to have declined by 28% following above-knee amputations.[86] Lumbar spinal bone loss progressed at 2% a week following scoliosis surgery,[87] and at 0.9% a week in patients treated with bed rest for lumbar disc disease.[88] The latter study reported only partial recovery.

Biochemical markers of bone resorption were elevated,[89-92] and bone formation markers either unchanged or also raised,[91] the latter presumably as a result of coupling. Bone histomorphometric data on the effects of immobilization in humans are scant.[90,92-94] These studies were based on iliac crest bone biopsies either in patients para/quadriplegic from spinal cord injuries[92] or in healthy volunteers on bed rest.[90,93,94] In the study of 28 patients with para/quadriplegia, bone volume decreased by approximately 33% in the first 25 weeks, after which no further bone loss took place.[92] The rate of bone loss had thus initially increased approximately 70-fold over the normal age-related bone loss of 1% per year. Cortical thickness declined by about 50%. Bone loss was due to an increase in bone resorption and a decrease in bone formation. Osteoclastic surfaces were high in the first 16 weeks but had returned to normal values by 40 weeks. Osteoblast function remained severely depressed throughout as judged by a very low calcification rate.[92] The histomorphometric studies on volunteers undergoing bed rest from 7 days to 4 months[90,93,94] showed less bone loss, but in one study there was a reduction in the number of trabeculae. Bone resorption was elevated in one study,[90] and unchanged in the other two, but bone formation was decreased in all. Thus, the bone loss of immobilization comes about through bone formation not being able to keep up with bone resorption.

Experimental work in dogs suggests that following remobilization the reversibility of disuse osteoporosis diminishes with the duration of immobilization and with age.[95] The concern is that with increasing duration of disuse, trabecular perforations will occur that lead to irreversible bone loss. If, however, remobilization commences before perforations have disconnected the trabecular network, bone loss is expected to recover as erosion cavities fill in with new bone — provided, of course, bone formation resumes.

There is both experimental and clinical evidence that antiresorptive therapy with bisphosphonates during immobilization prevents bone loss.[96,97] This is expected to prevent trabecular perforations that lead to irreversible loss of whole structural elements of bone.

7. Idiopathic Juvenile Osteoporosis

Idiopathic juvenile osteoporosis[98] is diagnosed when other conditions that may cause osteoporosis in childhood have been excluded. This rare systemic disorder affects prepubertal boys and girls for a period of several years and may leave lifelong impairment. It is characterized by low bone volume, few and thin trabeculae, and low bone turnover. The bone loss is due to insufficient performance by teams of osteoblasts at remodeling sites, in the presence of a lesser reduction of bone resorption. Thus, too little bone is formed at each remodeling cycle with the result that wall thickness declines, and as trabeculae become thinner they may be perforated.

REFERENCES

1. Mundy, G.R., "Bone remodeling," in *Bone Remodeling and Its Disorders*, Martin Dunitz, London, 1995, chap. 1.
2. Wickramasinghe, S.N., *Human Bone Marrow*, Blackwell Scientific Publications, Oxford, 1975, 36.
3. Burkhardt, R., Kettner, G., Bohm, W., et al., "Changes in trabecular bone, hematopoiesis and bone marrow vessels in aplastic anemia, primary osteoporosis, and old age: a comparative histomorphometric study," *Bone*, 8, 157, 1987.
4. Nuttall, M.E. and Gimble, J.M., "Is there a therapeutic opportunity to either prevent or treat osteopenic disorders by inhibiting marrow adipogenesis?" *Bone*, 27, 177, 2000.
5. Martin, R.B. and Lucas, P.A., "Bone marrow fat content in relation to bone remodeling and serum chemistry in intact and ovariectomized dogs," *Calcif. Tissue Int.*, 46, 189, 1990.
6. Davies, D.V. and Coupland, R.E., Eds., *Gray's Anatomy*, 34th ed., Longmans, Green, London, 1972, 39.
7. Parfitt, A.M., Villanueva, A.R., Foldes, J., and Rao, D.S., "Relations between histologic indices of bone formation: implications for the pathogenesis of spinal osteoporosis," *J. Bone Miner. Res.*, 10, 466, 1995.
8. Parfitt, A.M., Travers, R., Rauch, F., and Glorieux, F.H., "Structural and cellular changes during bone growth in healthy children," *Bone*, 27, 487, 2000.
9. Burger, E.H. and Klein-Nulend, J., "Mechanotransduction in bone — role of the lacuno-canalicular network," *FASEB J.*, 13, S101, 1999.
10. Mori, S. and Burr, D.B., "Increased intracortical remodeling following fatigue damage," *Bone*, 14, 103, 1993.
11. Schaffler, M.B., Choi, K., and Milgrom, C., "Aging and matrix microdamage accumulation in human compact bone," *Bone*, 17, 521, 1995.
12. Manolagas, S.C. and Weinstein, R.S., "New developments in the pathogenesis and treatment of steroid-induced osteoporosis," *J. Bone Miner. Res.*, 14, 1061, 1999.
13. Smit, T.H. and Burger, E.H., "Is BMU-coupling a strain-regulated phenomenon? A finite element analysis," *J. Bone Miner. Res.*, 15, 301, 2000.
14. Parfitt, A.M., "Osteonal and hemi-osteonal remodeling: the spatial and temporal framework for signal traffic in adult human bone," *J. Cell. Biochem.*, 55, 273, 1994.
15. Frost, H.M., *Bone Remodeling and Its Relationship to Metabolic Bone Diseases*, Charles C Thomas, Springfield, IL, 1973, 28.
16. Baron, R.E., "Anatomy and ultrastructure of bone," in *Primer on the Metabolic Bone Diseases and Disorders of Mineral Metabolism*, 4th ed., Favus, M.J., Ed., Lippincott-Raven, Philadelphia, 1996, chap. 1.
17. Termine, J. and Robey, P.G., "Bone matrix proteins and the mineralization process," in *Primer on the Metabolic Bone Diseases and Disorders of Mineral Metabolism*, 3rd ed., Favus, M.J., Ed., Lippincott-Raven, Philadelphia, 1996, chap. 4.
18. Parfitt, A.M., "The physiologic and clinical significance of bone histomorphometric data," in *Bone Histomorphometry: Techniques and Interpretation*, Recker, R.R., Ed., CRC Press, Boca Raton, FL, 1983, chap. 9.
19. Jowsey, J., "Age changes in human bone," *Clin. Orthop.*, 17, 210, 1960.
20. Nijweide, P.J., Burger, E.H., Klein-Nulend, J., and van der Plas, A., "The osteocyte," in *Principles of Bone Biology*, Bilezikian, J.P., Raisz, L.G., and Rodan, G.A., Eds., Academic Press, San Diego, 1996, chap. 9.
21. Boyce, B.F., "Role of apoptosis in local regulation," in *Principles of Bone Biology*, Bilezikian, J.P., Raisz, L.G., and Rodan, G.A., Eds., Academic Press, San Diego, 1996, chap. 53.
22. Verborgt, O., Gibson, G.J., and Schaffler, M.B., "Loss of osteocyte integrity in association with microdamage and bone remodeling after fatigue *in vivo*," *J. Bone Miner. Res.*, 15, 60, 2000.
23. Jilka, R.L., "Cytokines, bone remodeling, and estrogen deficiency: a 1998 update," *Bone*, 23, 75, 1998.
24. Mundy, G.R., "Bone resorbing cells," in *Primer on the Metabolic Bone Diseases and Disorders of Mineral Metabolism*, 3rd ed., Favus, M.J., Ed., Lippincott-Raven, Philadelphia, 1996, chap. 3.
25. Parfitt, A.M., Mundy, G.R., Roodman, G.D., et al., "A new model for the regulation of bone resorption, with particular reference to the effects of bisphosphonates," *J. Bone Miner. Res.*, 11, 150, 1996.
26. Puzas, J.E., "Osteoblast cell biology — lineage and function," in *Primer on the Metabolic Bone Diseases and Disorders of Mineral Metabolism*, 3rd ed., Favus, M.J., Ed., Lippincott-Raven, Philadelphia, 1996, chap. 2.

27. Jilka, R.L., Weinstein, R.S., Bellido, T., et al., "Osteoblast programmed cell death (apoptosis): modulation by growth factors and cytokines," *J. Bone Miner. Res.*, 13, 793, 1998.

28. Frost, H.M., *Bone Remodeling Dynamics,* Charles C Thomas, Springfield, IL, 1963.

29. Consensus Development Conference: Prophylaxis and treatment of osteoporosis, *Am. J. Med.*, 90, 107, 1991.

30. Oxlund, H., Mosekilde, Li., and Ørtoft, G., "Alterations in the stability of collagen from human trabecular bone with respect to age," in *Osteoporosis 1987*, Christiansen, C., Johansen, J.S. and Riis, B.J., Eds., Osteopress ApS, Copenhagen, 1987, 313.

31. Ferris, B.D., Klenerman, L., Dodds, R.A., et al., "Altered organization of non-collagenous bone matrix in osteoporosis," *Bone*, 8, 285, 1987.

32. Snyder, B.D., Piazza, S., Edwards, W.T., and Hayes, W.C., "Role of trabecular morphology in the etiology of age-related vertebral fractures," *Calcif. Tissue Int.*, 53(Suppl. 1), S14, 1993.

33. Lips, P. and Meunier, P.J., "Mean wall thickness of trabecular bone packets in the human iliac crest: changes with age," *Calcif. Tissue Res.*, 26, 13, 1978.

34. Weinstein, R.S. and Hutson, M.S., "Decreased trabecular width and increased trabecular spacing contribute to bone loss with aging," *Bone*, 8, 137, 1987.

35. Parfitt, A.M., Mathews, C.H., Villanueva, A.R., et al., "Relationships between surface, volume, and thickness of iliac trabecular bone in aging and in osteoporosis," *J. Clin. Invest.*, 72, 1396, 1983.

36. Bell, G.H., Dunbar, O., Beck, J.S., and Gibb, A., "Variations in strength of vertebrae with age and their relation to osteoporosis," *Calcif. Tissue Res.*, 1, 75, 1967.

37. Mosekilde, Lis, "Consequences of the remodeling process for vertebral trabecular bone structure: a scanning electron microscopy study (uncoupling of unloaded structures)," *Bone Miner.*, 10, 13, 1990.

38. Parfitt, A.M., "Trabecular bone architecture in the pathogenesis and prevention of fracture," *Am. J. Med.*, 82(Suppl. 1B), 68, 1987.

39. Mosekilde, Lis, "Sex differences in age-related loss of vertebral trabecular bone mass and structure — biomechanical consequences," *Bone*, 10, 425, 1989.

40. Mosekilde, Li., Mosekilde, Le., and Danielsen, C.C., "Biomechanical competence of vertebral trabecular bone in relation to ash density and age in normal individuals," *Bone*, 8, 79, 1987.

41. Legrand, E., Chappard, D., Pascaretti, C., et al., "Trabecular bone microarchitecture, bone mineral density, and vertebral fractures in male osteoporosis," *J. Bone Miner. Res.*, 15, 13, 2000.

42. Oleksik, A., Ott, S.M., Vedi, S., et al., "Bone structure in patients with low bone mineral density with or without vertebral fractures," *J. Bone Miner. Res.*, 15, 1368, 2000.

43. Delmas, P.D., "How does antiresorptive therapy decrease the risk of fracture in women with osteoporosis?" *Bone*, 27, 1, 2000.

44. Jensen, K.S., Mosekilde, Lis, and Mosekilde, L., "A model of vertebral trabecular bone architecture and its mechanical properties," *Bone*, 11, 417, 1990.

45. Maurin, A.C., Chavassieux, P.M., Frappart, L., et al., "Influence of mature adipocytes on osteoblast proliferation in human primary cocultures," *Bone*, 26, 485, 2000.

46. Mosekilde, Lis and Mosekilde, L., "Sex differences in age-related changes in vertebral body size, density and biomechanical competence in normal individuals," *Bone*, 11, 67, 1990.

47. Beck, T.J., Looker, A.C., Ruff, C.B., et al., "Structural trends in the aging femoral neck and proximal shaft: analysis of the third National Health and Nutrition Examination Survey dual-energy X-ray absorptiometry data," *J. Bone Miner. Res.*, 15, 2297, 2000.

48. Fyrhie, D.P. and Schaffler, M.B., "Failure mechanisms in human vertebral cancellous bone," *Bone*, 15, 105, 1994.

49. Fazzalari, N.L., "Trabecular microfracture," *Calcif. Tissue Int.*, 53(Suppl. 1), S143, 1993.

50. Koszyca, B., Fazzalari, N.L., and Vernon-Roberts, B., "Trabecular microfractures. Nature and distribution in the proximal femur," *Clin. Orthop.*, 244, 208, 1989.

51. Todd, R.C., Freeman, M.A.R., and Pirie, C.J., "Isolated trabecular fatigue fractures in the femoral head," *J. Bone Joint Surg.*, 54B, 723, 1972.

52. Vogel, M., Hahn, M., and Delling, G., "Relation between two- and three-dimensional architecture of trabecular bone in the human spine," *Bone*, 14, 199, 1993.

53. Schnitzler, C.M., Wing, J.R., Mesquita, J.M., et al., "Risk factors for the development of stress fractures during fluoride therapy for osteoporosis," *J. Bone Miner. Res.*, 5(Suppl. 1), S195, 1990.

54. Schnitzler, C.M., Mesquita, J.M., Gear, K.A., et al., "Iliac bone biopsies at the time of periarticular stress fractures during fluoride therapy: comparison with pretreatment biopsies," *J. Bone Miner. Res.*, 5, 141, 1990.

55. Schnitzler, C.M. and Solomon, L., "Histomorphometric analysis of a calcaneal stress fracture: a possible complication of fluoride therapy for osteoporosis," *Bone*, 7, 193, 1986.

56. Schnitzler, C.M., Wing, J.R., Gear, K.A., and Robson, H.J., "Bone fragility in the peripheral skeleton during fluoride therapy for osteoporosis," *Clin. Orthop.*, 261, 268, 1990.

57. Resnick, D., Goergen, T.G., and Niwayama, G., "Physical injury: concepts and terminology," in *Diagnosis of Bone and Joint Disorders,* Resnick, D., Ed., 3rd ed., W. B. Saunders, Philadelphia, 1995, chap. 67.

58. Frost, H. M, "Micropetrosis," *J. Bone Joint Surg.*, 42A, 144, 1960

59. Wong, S.Y., Kariks, J., Evans, R.A., et al., "The effect of age on bone composition and viability in the femoral head," *J. Bone Joint Surg.,* 67A, 274, 1985.

60. Manolagas, S., "Corticosteroids and fractures: a close encounter of the third cell kind," *J. Bone Miner. Res.*, 15, 1001, 2000.

61. Marcove, R.C. and Arlen, M., "Metabolic diseases," in *Atlas of Bone Pathology*, Marcove, R.C. and Arlen, M., Eds., J.B. Lippincott, Philadelphia, 1992, chap. 3.

62. Silverberg, S.J., Shane, E., de la Cruz, L., et al., "Skeletal disease in primary hyperparathyroidism," *J. Bone Miner. Res.*, 4, 283, 1989.

63. Parfitt, A.M., Kleerekoper, M., Rao, D., Stanci, J., and Villanueva, A.R., "Cellular mechanisms of cortical thinning in primary hyperparathyroidism," *J. Bone Miner. Res.*, 2(Suppl. 1), abstr. 384, 1987.

64. Resnick, D. and Niwayama, G., "Parathyroid disorders and renal osteodystrophy," in *Diagnosis of Bone and Joint Disorders,* 3rd ed., Resnick, D., Ed., W.B. Saunders, Philadelphia, 1995, chap. 57.

65. Eriksen, E.F., Mosekilde, L., and Melsen, F., "Trabecular bone remodeling and balance in primary hyperparathyroidism," *Bone,* 7, 213, 1986.

66. Christiansen, P., Steiniche, T., Mosekilde, L., et al., "Primary hyperparathyroidism: changes in trabecular bone remodeling following surgical treatment — evaluated by histomorphometric methods," *Bone*, 11, 75, 1990.

67. Parisien, M., Cosman, F., Mellish, R.W., et al., "Bone structure on postmenopausal hyperparathyroid, osteoporotic, and normal women," *J. Bone Miner. Res.*, 10, 1393, 1995.

68. Meunier, P.J., S.-Bianchi, G.G., Edouard, C.M., et al., "Bony manifestations of thyrotoxicosis," *Orthop. Clin. North Am.*, 3, 745, 1972.

69. Resnick, D., "Thyroid disorders," in *Diagnosis of Bone and Joint Disorders*, 3rd ed., Resnick, D., Ed., W. B. Saunders, Philadelphia, 1995, chap. 56.

70. Eriksen, E.F., Mosekilde, L., and Melsen, F., "Trabecular bone remodeling and bone balance in hyperthyroidism," *Bone,* 6, 421, 1985.

71 Seeman, F., "The effects of tobacco and alcohol use on bone," in *Osteoporosis*, Marcus, R., Feldman, D., and Kelsey, J., Eds., Academic Press, San Diego, 1996, chap. 26.

72. Diez, A., Puig, J., Serrano, S., et al., "Alcohol-induced bone disease in the absence of severe chronic liver damage," *J. Bone Miner. Res.*, 9, 825, 1994.

73. Bikle, D.D., "Bone disease in alcohol abuse," *Ann. Intern. Med.*, 103, 42, 1985.

74. Diamond, T., Stiel, D., Lunzer, M., et al., "Ethanol reduces bone formation and may cause osteoporosis," *Am. J. Med.*, 86, 282, 1989.

75. Lindholm, J., Steiniche, T., Rasmussen, E., et al., "Bone disorder in men with chronic alcoholism: a reversible disease?" *J. Clin. Endocrinol. Metab.*, 73, 118, 1991.

76. de Vernejoul, M.C., Bielakoff, J., Herve, M., et al., "Evidence for defective osteoblast function," *Clin. Orthop.*, 179, 107, 1983.

77. Friday, K. and Howard, G.A., "Ethanol inhibits bone cell proliferation and function *in vivo*," *Metabolism*, 40, 562, 1991.

78. Hurley, M.M., Martin, D.L., Kream, B.E., and Raisz, L.G., "Effects of ethanol and acetaldehyde on collagen synthesis, prostaglandin release and resorption of fetal rat bone in organ culture," *Bone*, 11, 47, 1990.

79. Nielsen, H.K., Lundby, L., Rasmussen, K., et al., "Alcohol decreases serum osteocalcin in a dose-dependent way in normal subjects," *Calcif. Tissue Int.*, 46, 173, 1990.

80. Pepersack, T., Fuss, M., Otero, J., et al., "Longitudinal study of bone metabolism after ethanol withdrawal in alcoholic patients," *J. Bone Miner. Res.*, 7, 383, 1992.

81. Kiratli, B.J., "Immobilization osteopenia," in *Osteoporosis*, Marcus, R., Feldman, D., and Kelsey, J., Eds., Academic Press, San Diego, 1996, chap. 42.

82. Lundberg, B. and Nilsson, B., "Osteopenia in the frozen shoulder," *Clin. Orthop.*, 60, 187, 1968.

83. Van der Wiel, H.E., Lips, P., Nauta, J., et al., "Loss of bone in the proximal part of the femur following unstable fractures of the leg," *J. Bone Joint Surg.*, 76A, 230, 1994.

84. Kannus, P., Jarvinen, M., Sievanen, H., et al., "Osteoporosis in men with a history of tibial fracture," *J. Bone Miner. Res.*, 9, 423, 1994.

85. Andersson, S. and Nilsson, B., "Changes in bone mineral content following ligamentous knee injuries," *Med. Sci. Sports*, 11, 351, 1979.

86. Rush, P.J., Wong, J.S., Kirsh, J., and Devlin, M., "Osteopenia in patients with above knee amputation," *Arch. Phys. Med. Rehabil.*, 75, 112, 1994.

87. Hansson, T., Roos, B., and Nachemson, A., "Development of osteopenia in the fourth lumbar vertebra during prolonged bedrest after operations for scoliosis," *Acta Orthop. Scand.*, 46, 621, 1975.

88. Krølner, B. and Toft, B., "Vertebral bone loss: an unheeded side effect of therapeutic bed rest," *Clin. Sci.*, 64, 537, 1983.

89. LeBlanc, A., Schneider, V., Spector, E., et al., "Calcium absorption, endogenous excretion, and endocrine changes during and after long-term bed rest," *Bone*, 16, 301S, 1995.

90. Zerwekh, J.E., Ruml, L.A., Gottschalk, F., and Pak, C.Y., "The effects of twelve weeks of bed rest on bone histology, biochemical markers of bone turnover, and calcium homeostasis in 11 normal subjects," *J. Bone Miner. Res.*, 13, 1594, 1998.

91. Lueken, S.A., Arnaud, S.B., Taylor, A.K., and Baylink, D.J., "Changes in markers of bone formation and resorption in a bedrest model of weightlessness," *J. Bone Miner. Res.*, 8, 1433, 1993.

92. Minaire, P., Meunier, P., Edouard, C., et al., "Quantitative histologic data on disuse osteoporosis," *Calcif. Tissue Int.*, 17, 57, 1974.

93. Palle, S., Vico, L., Bourrin, S., and Alexandre, C., "Bone tissue response to four-month antiorthostatic bedrest: a bone histomorphometric study," *Calcif. Tissue Int.*, 51, 189, 1992.

94. Arnaud, S.B., Sherrard, D.J., Maloney, N., et al., "Effects of 1-week head-down tilt bed rest on bone formation and the calcium endocrine system," *Aviat. Space Environ. Med.*, 63, 14, 1992.

95. Jaworski, Z.F.G. and Uhthoff, H.K., "Reversibility of nontraumatic disuse osteoporosis during its active phase," *Bone*, 7, 431, 1986.

96. Mosekilde, Lis, Thomsen, J.S., Mackey, M.S., and Phipps, R.J., "Treatment with risedronate or alendronate prevents hind-limb immobilization-induced loss of bone density and strength in adult female rats," *Bone*, 27, 639, 2000.

97. Minaire, P., Depassio, J., Berard, E., et al., "Effects of clodronate on immobilization bone loss," *Bone*, 8(Suppl. 1), S63, 1993.

98. Rauch, F., Travers, R., Norman, M.E., et al., "Deficient bone formation in idiopathic juvenile osteoporosis: a histomorphometric study of cancellous iliac bone," *J. Bone Miner. Res.*, 15, 957, 2000.

3 Biomechanics of Osteoporotic Bone

Richard M. Aspden

CONTENTS

I. INTRODUCTION

The health problem most commonly associated with osteoporosis is bone fracture, and the feature that distinguishes osteoporosis-related fractures from others is that they generally occur with minimal or no trauma. The sites where most fractures occur are the spine, the hip, and the wrist. In the spine, crushing of the vertebrae, experienced while performing everyday activities, results in an increased kyphosis and loss of height, seen externally in the classical "Dowager's hump." Wrist (Colles' fracture) and hip fractures commonly follow a fall from standing. The mechanics of these fractures, which are determined by the magnitude and location of the force applied to the bone, are discussed elsewhere. Clearly, the strength of the bone is an important factor in whether it will sustain a fracture under a given set of forces. This strength is determined by geometric factors, the size, shape, and internal structure of the bone itself, as well as material factors, such as its composition. In cancellous bone the distinction between material and structure is not always easy to define and treating it as a cellular material has met with a considerable degree of success.[1,2]

0-8493-1033-4/02/$0.00+$1.50

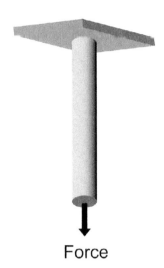

Force

FIGURE 3.1 A force applied to the end of a rod will stretch it, in proportion to its stiffness. At the same time its radius will decrease. For a given force the stiffness of the object (its resistance to deformation) will depend not only on the stiffness of the material from which it is made (its material elastic modulus) but also on the dimensions of the object.

This chapter addresses the basic mechanical and geometric concepts needed to understand the factors that contribute to bone strength. Each factor is described briefly to assist those who have little biomechanics background. Changes that have been measured in these properties of bone as a consequence of osteoporosis will then be reviewed to identify which are believed to be important for the loss of bone strength. Mechanics is a deceptive discipline for the unwary: at its simplest level it can be understood with no more than high-school mathematics and many of the ideas are intuitive. Unfortunately, a full treatment requires concepts, such as tensors, that are not generally met until well through a physics or engineering degree course, and this enormous leap can pose significant problems for those requiring a deeper understanding. An added complexity for biological tissues is that the properties of the materials often depend not just on the forces or deformations that are applied but also on how they are applied. Tissues often offer more resistance to rapidly applied forces, i.e., appear stiffer, than to those applied slowly or over long periods. Fortunately, for bone, these effects are small and little mention will be made of them, although impact loading on bone has been little studied. This chapter concentrates on osteoporotic bone, or the effects of aging where these cannot be distinguished, and other sources (such as *Bone Mechanics Handbook*[3] or the chapters in *Skeletal Tissue Mechanics*[4]) are suggested for those wanting more detail on bone mechanical properties in general.

II. FACTORS AFFECTING THE PROPERTIES OF A BONE

A. MATERIAL PROPERTIES

1. Stiffness

When forces act on a fixed object they alter its shape and size. For example, a force applied to the end of the rod in Figure 3.1 will alter its length and its radius. The resistance offered by the object to this deforming force is determined by its stiffness. However, it is often useful to be able to separate the stiffness of the material of which the object is made from the stiffness of the object itself, which will also depend upon its dimensions. For example, a hip may fracture because either

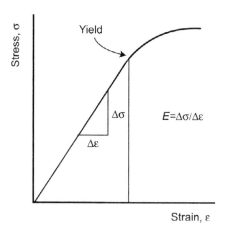

FIGURE 3.2 If tested carefully, the stress and the strain in a piece of bone appear to be linearly related, shown schematically here. The slope of that relationship is the Young's or elastic modulus. The point where the slope starts to decrease is the elastic limit or yield point. Fracture does not occur until the stress and strain increase still further.

the bone material is too weak or the shape and size of the femoral neck have changed, or both. In a similar way, the deformation of an object will depend on its dimensions and on the magnitude of the force in comparison with those dimensions. So, to remove this dependency on the dimensions it is essential to define the stiffness of a material in terms of stress and strain, rather than force and deformation. When this is done, the stiffness of the material is conventionally called the elastic, or Young's, modulus.

Stress may be considered as the intensity of the force and, in simple terms, is defined as the force divided by the area over which it acts. A force of 1 newton (N) acting over an area of 1 square meter (m^2) corresponds to a stress of 1 pascal (Pa). Given that an apple weighs about 1 N it can be seen that this is a very small stress. More common units are megapascals (1 MPa = 1 million Pa) and gigapascals (1 GPa = 1 billion Pa). The symbol for stress is the Greek letter sigma, σ.

Strain is defined as the change in dimension, however this is caused, divided by the original dimension. If a rod with a length of 1 m is stretched by 1 mm this is a strain of 0.001. This is sometimes expressed as a percentage (0.1% in this case) and is clearly dimensionless. The symbol for strain is either the letter e or the Greek letter epsilon, ε. In bone mechanics, where strains are typically of this magnitude, it is common to use the concept of microstrain: 1 microstrain ($\mu\varepsilon$) is a fractional change in length of 10^{-6}, or 0.0001%. So then a strain of 0.1% is equivalent to 1000 microstrain. This is often written 1000 $\mu\varepsilon$, which can be confusing because it looks as though strain now has a dimension. The force applied to the rod in Figure 3.1 will not only increase its length but will also result in a reduction in radius. The ratio of the lateral strain to the axial strain is called Poisson's ratio and is denoted by the Greek letter nu, ν.

If the strain produced in a material is linearly proportional to the applied stress, then the slope of this line is the elastic modulus and is denoted by the letter E (Figure 3.2). This is a property of the material and is independent of the dimensions of the object. Elastic means that when the stress is removed the specimen returns to its original dimensions. Often in biological materials, the relationship between stress and strain is not linear and the material does not have a unique Young's modulus; it becomes a function of the strain (or stress). If a small cylinder or cube of bone is tested in compression in a materials testing machine and the stress and the strain recorded, the result is generally nonlinear. The curve is often J shaped with a region near the origin in which the elastic modulus increases. Recent studies in which the samples are carefully mounted have indicated that this region is an artifact of the method.[5] The studies showed that bone is linearly elastic and has the same elastic modulus in tension as in compression.

So far only a simple stress has been considered, such as that shown in Figure 3.1. For completeness, there are other types of stress and strain: shear stresses and strains, which in their pure form cause a change in shape but not in volume, and bulk stresses and strains, which cause a change in volume but not in shape. These all have similar definitions to those given above but need not be considered further here, except to say that shear is often an important factor in the failure of materials and hence in fracture.

2.   Static Strength

This is the stress at which a material will fail if it is loaded relatively slowly. If a piece of cancellous bone is subjected to a slowly increasing stress in a materials testing machine, then the relationship between stress and strain will generally look similar to that shown schematically in Figure 3.2. The stress and strain will increase linearly, as described above, until a point is reached at which the stress will start to increase more slowly than the strain and the line will start to bend over. The point at which the slope of the line starts to decrease is called the yield point and marks the onset of failure in the material. After this point the deformation is called plastic because if the stress is removed now, the specimen will exhibit a residual deformation, and it will not return completely to its original dimensions. As the strain increases further, the stress rises only a little more before reaching a maximum. The stress at this point is often used to describe the strength of the material. Cancellous bone then displays a plateau region, during which the trabeculae are breaking and the whole cellular material is crushing, sometimes referred to as densification. Once crushing is complete, the stress starts to rise again as the crushed bone matrix itself starts to resist the applied stress. Cortical bone does not display this plateau region but fails completely once its strength is exceeded. The way in which it fails will depend on how it is loaded (e.g., bending, tension, or compression). The static strength of cortical bone is about 250 MPa in compression and 150 MPa in tension.[6] The strength of bone is different when loaded in different directions, i.e., it is anisotropic. The yield strength of cancellous bone is between about 1 and 10 MPa in compression and tension.

3.   Dynamic Strength and Toughness

Bone fractures are rarely caused by slow applications of load. Trauma is the main cause, although in patients with osteoporosis this trauma may be minimal, even resulting from a fall from a standing position. This results in an impulse force applied over a short time period. In this case it is not only the strength of the material but also the energy imparted to it that is of interest. As a material is deformed, it stores the energy put into it as strain energy, a form of potential energy. The amount of energy stored per unit volume at the yield point for a linear material, such as bone, may be found from the stress–strain graph and is half the yield stress multiplied by the strain at that point, i.e., the area under the line. If a crack starts to form, this energy can be released as the material at either side of the crack then becomes unloaded. To form the crack, two new surfaces have to be created where there was none before and this takes up the energy. If the amount of energy released is less than that required to form a crack, then the crack will stop, as there is not enough energy available to feed it, irrespective of how high the stresses are. Otherwise it will spread, often catastrophically. This is true however rapidly a load is applied. The main reason that an impact can be more damaging than a slowly applied load is that a high stress is often generated over a localized area. This stress is transmitted very rapidly through the material (at approximately the speed of sound) and may be reflected back by any surfaces and interfaces. In this way stresses can be focused and magnified into specific regions.

The ability of the material to resist fracture is its toughness. This is often expressed as the work of fracture and is a measure of the amount of energy that is required to cause a fracture surface, although it is not easy to quantify. The opposite of tough is brittle, and osteoporosis is often accused of causing bones to become brittle. The evidence for this is scanty and has arisen largely by confusing the concepts of strength and toughness (brittleness). Some examples may help to clarify this. Glass is strong but brittle; once a crack starts it propagates rapidly across the whole piece and the crack surface is smooth. Pottery, cookies, and even jello (jelly in the United Kingdom) are brittle (demonstrated by how easy it is to create cracks in them) but clearly have different strengths. The energy stored in the deformed material is greater than that required to create the new surfaces and as it is released more cracks may form explosively as stress waves bounce around inside and the object may be seen to shatter. In contrast, glass-reinforced plastic (fiberglass) is strong and tough; cracks do not spread and crack surfaces are very irregular, right down to the level of the individual glass fibers, which can often be seen protruding from the crack surface. An enormous amount of energy has been dissipated creating a surface around the fibers and is not therefore available for propagating the crack. Bone and wood are similarly tough; cracks are forced to keep deviating around structures within the material. Glass and aluminum have approximately the same tensile strength, but if dropped it is clear why one is used for tableware while the other can be taken on camping expeditions! Paradoxically, weaker materials may be tougher than strong materials because weak interfaces within the material result in larger fracture surfaces and hence better crack resistance.

4. Fatigue

Repetitive loading at a stress that may be considerably below the strength of a material may also cause fracture if sustained over a long period. For example, not many people can tear an aluminum drink can in half. But if it is squashed in the middle and repeatedly bent backward and forward, then there are not many who could fail to end up with two pieces. Repeated loading damages the material in some way, possibly by forming microcracks, until eventually a fatal crack develops and the material fails.

B. GEOMETRIC PROPERTIES

The properties described above have all been normalized for specimen size and shape and are related only to the material. This was done so that the material properties of bone can be considered separately from the properties of a whole bone. In the clinic, however, it is not just the material that is important, but whether the whole bone is likely to break. In this case it is not simply the stress in some part of the bone that is important but the load that the bone as a whole is capable of supporting. Two bones will be able to support the same load even though the bone material of one is half as strong as that of the other, providing the weaker bone has twice the cross-sectional area to support the load. In this case the bone with the stronger material may even be more likely to fracture because there is less thickness of bone to absorb a crack and the stronger material may be less tough. The following sections will consider the effects of geometric factors on load bearing and fracture. Once this is done we shall be in a good position to consider what is happening in real osteoporotic bones.

1. Bone Shape

If loads are applied to an object along an axis of symmetry, such as in Figure 3.1, then stresses may be calculated very simply. Clearly, bones have much more complicated shapes, and forces are rarely applied along such simple axes. Off-axis loads can result in bending moments and shear stresses. The hip is a clear example of forces being applied away from the axis of the femur and

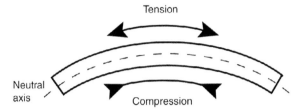

FIGURE 3.3 An initially straight rod, bent as shown, will be in tension along its upper surface, as this is stretched, and in compression along the lower surface. Along the center, the bending axis, there is no strain. For this reason hollow cylinders, such as long bones, are almost as effective as solid rods for resisting bending but with considerable saving of weight.

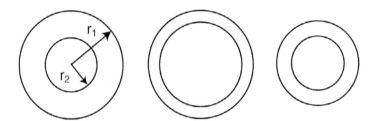

FIGURE 3.4 The shaded regions represent cross sections through hollow cylinders and the two on the right both have half the cross-sectional area of that on the left. However, the middle one has the same outer radius but has lost material from the center, whereas the rightmost has the same inner radius and has lost material from the outside. Table 3.1 shows how the relative bending stiffness is more drastically reduced by loss of material from the outside.

the angle and length of the neck of the femur might be expected to be factors in determining fracture risk.

2. Bending and Buckling

A slightly modified concept of stiffness is important when considering the bending or buckling of a rod. Failure in this case does not depend so much on the strength of the material as on its stiffness and how the material is arranged around the bending axis. Considering bending first, a straight rod, bent as shown in Figure 3.3, will be in tension along its upper surface, as this is stretched, and in compression along the lower surface. Along the center, strictly the bending axis, there is no strain. It is immediately obvious that material in the center is really not doing anything constructive to resist the bending. This is the reason hollow tubes can be used in place of solid rods where bending is the main factor, with consequent weight saving. The bending stiffness of such a rod is dependent on both the stiffness of the material, E, and on a measure of the geometry called the second moment of area, I, and is defined as the product of these two factors. The effects of changing the inner and outer radii of such a hollow cylinder, without changing the cross-sectional area, are shown in Figure 3.4 and Table 3.1, and the more serious effects of losing material from the outer surface can be seen.

Buckling is a particular form of bending that occurs when compression is applied to the end of a rod that is either too slender or not stiff enough. This can be seen, for example, when pushing down on the end of a slender stick, such as a cane, which will cause the center to deflect sideways in a bow once a certain force is exceeded. If the force is increased still further the bowing will increase until the stick breaks. Although, in the end, failure is determined by the strength of the material, it is the buckling that makes this inevitable and, therefore, the stiffness that is the main factor in the initial failure. The same definition of bending stiffness governs this type of behavior.

TABLE 3.1
The Effects of Changing the Inner and Outer Radii of a Hollow Cylinder

Outer Radius, r_1	Inner Radius, r_2	Relative Area	Relative Bending Stiffness
2	1	1	1
2	1.58	0.5	0.65
1.58	1	0.5	0.35

Note: The bending stiffness of a rod is given by the product of the elastic modulus of the material from which it is made and the second moment of area, *I*, which itself is proportional to the fourth power of the radius. Starting with the hollow cylinder on the left in Figure 3.4, the cross-sectional area of the material is halved by first increasing the inner radius while the outer radius is unchanged, then reducing the outer radius leaving the inner radius unchanged. The initial area and bending stiffness are assigned values of unity for ease of comparison and the radii are given as a ratio. This shows clearly that losing material on the outside has far more severe consequences than losing it from the inside.

3. Internal Structure

Wolff's famous law relating structure to function of cancellous bone[7] describes how internal structure, in terms of the arrangement of the trabeculae, is adapted to the prevailing loads. Loss of this structure is then likely to affect the ability of the bone to support those loads, and may be even more important when loads are applied from an unusual direction, such as experienced in a fall. This structure has directional properties, i.e., bone is anisotropic, which needs to be taken into account when measuring mechanical properties. Modeling of cancellous bone as a cellular material has been very successful in describing the origin of some of its properties, but assume, as a first approximation, an isotropic arrangement of cells. In a cellular material there are two factors that are important for relating the material to the mechanical properties: the density of the material from which it is made (the material density) and the overall density of the cellular material itself (the apparent density). For example, in a cylindrical sample, the apparent density is the mass divided by the total volume occupied by the cylinder, whereas the material density is the same mass (assuming the cells are empty) divided by the volume occupied by the struts or cell walls themselves. According to models of cancellous bone as a cellular material, the stiffness and strength of the bone are proportional to the square of the relative density (apparent density/material density). Assuming no change in material density, halving the amount of bone would result in a reduction in the stiffness and strength by a factor of four.

4. Stress or Strain?

So far in this chapter, and in most papers and in engineering as a whole, stress has been considered to be the main factor determining the failure of a material. Contrary to this popular belief, however, it is probably the strain in bone, and in most biological materials, that is more important than the stress for maintaining tissue homeostasis and determining its mechanical behaviour. Stress in any material can only be inferred by measuring some other property; it can never be measured directly. Even engineers commonly measure stress by using devices sensitive to strain calibrated against known forces. At the most fundamental level, deformation of a material causes stretching of the chemical bonds between atoms and it is the nature of these bonds that will determine the intrinsic stiffness and strength. The strain energy stored in the material, discussed above, is stored in these bonds. Fracture is ultimately caused by separating these atoms by a sufficient distance such that the bond is effectively broken and cannot be reformed.

It has been proposed that in soft connective tissues, strain is the factor that relates the properties of the tissue to joint movement.[8] The stresses involved are far less well defined. The situation in bone is slightly more complicated, but recent studies on cancellous bone have shown that even though there is a considerable anisotropy in stiffness and strength, due to structural anisotropy, the yield strains were isotropic.[9] Trabecular damage, a possible cause of loss of bone stiffness and strength, has also been attributed to strain rather than stress.[10] In addition, the cells that produce and maintain the connective tissues of the body, soft and hard, are known to be responsive to mechanical stimuli. It is difficult to imagine ways in which they could detect stress directly but deformation of the cell *in vivo* and *in vitro* has been shown to elicit a signaling or metabolic response in many different cell types. Taken together, these factors indicate that strains and deformations are more important than stresses and forces when it comes to determining how bone behaves mechanically and how it is regulated by the cells.

III. OSTEOPOROTIC BONE

A. INTRODUCTION

Cancellous bone is most affected by osteoporosis, but most testing of age-related changes has been conducted on cortical bone because it is much easier to machine suitable specimens and the results are not complicated by the associated changes in internal structure. It has proved remarkably elusive to separate changes due to aging from changes that are attributable to osteoporosis. This may be a consequence of the somewhat arbitrary definition of osteoporosis formulated by the World Health Organization (WHO). By measuring the absorption of X-rays by bone in a patient, a measure of bone quantity can be derived called the bone mineral density (BMD). Patients are then said to be osteoporotic if they have a BMD value that is 2.5 standard deviations from the mean of the statistical distribution describing the BMD values of a young adult population. While this definition has been of enormous benefit for the diagnosis of progressive bone loss, it is of little help in trying to identify pathophysiologic changes in the bone itself. Osteoporosis results in a reduction in the quantity of bone, an alteration in its structural organization, and, possibly, changes in the material properties of the bone matrix. In combination these result in a loss of stiffness and strength in the whole tissue. Separating and quantifying them, however, is not trivial. In addition, there may be changes in the overall shape and dimensions of the bone. Here, the material properties of osteoporotic bone are first considered before the changes in internal structure are described. Finally, some of the findings regarding the overall shape, especially of the proximal femur, are summarized.

B. MATERIAL PROPERTIES

Skeletal maturity is believed to be achieved at about 35 years of age. After this the elastic properties and failure strength of bone deteriorate in both men and women.[11-13] The majority of studies of bone concentrate on understanding bone as a material, summarized, for example, by Cowin.[3] There are numerous investigations of age-related changes in mechanical properties[14-18] and geometric factors (see next section) but surprisingly few that expressly investigate bone from patients with osteoporosis. Clearly, there are difficulties in, first, being able to identify suitable patients and, then, to obtain bone from them. Two options are available for the former: either using the WHO definition in terms of BMD or a clinical definition. The WHO definition requires access to some means of measuring BMD and, because this is defined in patients not isolated bones, is difficult to do postmortem. Alternatively, some studies have used a clinical definition, using as evidence a fracture sustained with minimal trauma. While femoral heads can be obtained in this way from patients having a hemiarthroplasty, it is not so easy to obtain bone from other sites.

Cancellous bone was obtained from the femoral head and neck region of patients having a hemiarthroplasty following an osteoporotic fracture of the femoral neck. It was shown to have a

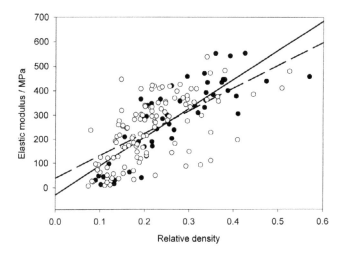

FIGURE 3.5 The elastic modulus of cancellous bone from the femoral heads of patients who had sustained a fractured neck of femur appeared to be linearly related to the relative density (dashed line), although the correlation is not strong ($R^2_{adj} = 0.38$). Bone from an age- and sex-matched control group was not significantly different (continuous line).

lower apparent density and, consequently, a reduced stiffness and strength compared with an age- and sex-matched group with no evidence of disease.[19,20] The median stiffness was reduced from 310 MPa in the control group to 247 MPa in the osteoporosis (OP) group and the yield strengths were reduced from 3.3 to 2.5 MPa. The groups were all skewed, however, with lower values overrepresented compared with a normal distribution. Plotting elastic modulus against relative density showed a linear increase in modulus with density over the range of densities measured but no significant difference in the slope of the relationship between the OP group and the controls (Figure 3.5). The regression equation for the OP group is

$$E = 40 + 930 \; \rho^* \quad R^2_{adj} = 0.38$$

where ρ^* is the relative density. Although theory suggests that stiffness should be proportional to the square of the density and a statistical analysis of pooled data on normal cancellous bone has suggested this is a reasonable model,[21] correlation in this case was weaker ($R^2_{adj} = 0.30$) between stiffness and the square of the relative density.

No differences were found between the material densities of the OP and the control group. However, there was a small but significant correlation between the apparent and material densities in the OP group, which was not found in the control group (Figure 3.6). The regression is described by

$$\rho_{app} = 1.0 - 0.35 \; \rho_{mat} \quad R^2_{adj} = 0.14$$

Similar results were obtained in a preliminary study by Zioupos and Aspden.[22] The regression relationship had a similar slope, but a difference in intercept needs further exploration. Both results, however, suggest that there may be some mechanism linking the properties of the bone material with those of the tissue; that as bone is lost and the apparent density declines there is an increase in mineralization. An increase in density would be expected to result in an increase in stiffness and strength but indentation testing of the same specimens suggested that there was a decline in elastic modulus with increasing bone loss.[22] These relationships are being investigated further. A study of bone from the iliac crest of osteoporotic patients using scanning acoustic microscopy indicated that

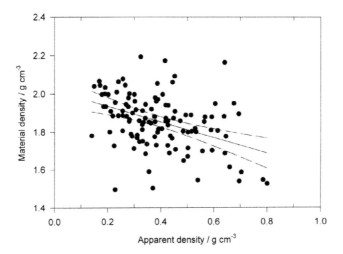

FIGURE 3.6 In the osteoporotic cancellous bone there appeared to be a relationship between the material and the apparent densities, which was not found in the control group. Shown are the regression line and its 95% confidence limits (dashed lines).

the OP bone was 6% less stiff than an age-matched, postmenopausal group with no evidence of OP.[23] This suggests that there may be a more complicated relationship between composition and properties in OP bone than has been inferred from studies of normal bone. In this study, however, the postmenopausal control group had more bone with a higher acoustic stiffness than a premeno-pausal group and this is hard to explain.

In a study of the subchondral bone plate of the femoral head it was found that the stiffness and the density were both lower than in the control group.[24] The subchondral bone plate underlies the articular cartilage and, although immediately adjacent to the cancellous bone, its relatively solid structure makes it more akin to cortical than to cancellous bone. However, its proximity to the cancellous bone may result in its being affected by the same processes affecting the cancellous bone and this may provide insight into the changes described above. The material density was reduced from 1.79 to 1.64 g/cm³, which was a consequence of a reduction in mineral content from 48 to 43% of the wet mass. No changes were found in the amounts of organic material or water and so it would appear that this is a reduction in mineralization. Perhaps surprisingly, the densities and mineral contents of the subchondral bone plate were less than those of the cancellous bone material whose densities were control 1.89 g/cm³; OP 1.86 g/cm³; and mineral contents, 54 and 53%, respectively. The stiffness of the bone plate (measured using 10 MHz ultrasound) reduced from a median value of 19.8 GPa in the control group to 14.9 GPa in the OP group, so in this case the reduction in stiffness is what might be expected from a reduced mineralization.

Studies of the individual components of bone matrix have investigated changes in the collagen and in crystal morphology. Post-translational modifications to the collagen type I have been reported with an increase in hydroxylation and a reduction in intermediate cross-links.[25-28] It was suggested that these were indicative of a faster turnover of the collagen and, hence, of a more rapid turnover of the bone matrix. A similar increase in reducible cross-links was found in vitamin B_6-deficient chicks and the long bones were found to have decreased yield and fracture loads.[29] Because proper cortical bone mineralization appeared to have occurred, it was suggested that it was the alterations to the collagen that resulted in changes to the mechanical performance of the bone. Such results suggest that a similar reduction in fracture properties may be expected in osteoporotic bone. Changes in the mineral component, however, have been less conclusive with reports of increased, decreased, or unaltered crystallite size,[30-35] suggesting that changes in the mineral component itself are not responsible for any alterations in the bone matrix.

C. GEOMETRIC PROPERTIES

1. Structure

The three-dimensional architecture of trabecular bone varies from bone to bone and the particular organization is adapted to the mechanical loading to which that bone is subject; this is Wolff's eponymous law.[7] Trabecular bone is generally described as being composed of interconnected rods or plates with a gross porosity of greater than 30%,[36,37] and there have been recent attempts to quantify the relative amounts of rod- or plate-likeness using a structure model index.[38] Numerous methods have been proposed to characterize the organization of trabeculae and to try to relate this to mechanical properties.[39-43] One of the aims of this has been to test hypotheses for explaining the optimization strategies adopted by bone that result in Wolff's law. But another, more relevant to this chapter, is the attempt to identify which features of trabecular morphology are crucial for the mechanical integrity of bone and, hence, to understand the effects of osteopenic disease. It has been noted that structural changes affect the strength of bone more than the reduction in the amount of bone by itself would suggest.[44]

Trabecular thickness is probably the most obvious structural factor and is one of the main histomorphometric parameters used to characterize trabecular bone. However, obtaining unbiased estimates is not trivial and the published results vary from site to site, and even within sites. Trabeculae from the femur[45] and lumbar vertebrae[46] have been reported to thin with aging, although another study suggested that vertically oriented trabeculae in the vertebrae did not change and that thinning, therefore, was anisotropic.[47] Results for iliac crest are conflicting in that some reported no change with aging[46] whereas others suggested that thinning of trabecular plates was significant in males with OP but not females.[48] This same study suggested that reduced plate density was more significant for the loss of bone volume and that this was caused by total removal of trabeculae rather than their thinning. It was proposed that the process of removal is initiated by increased depth of osteoclastic resorption cavities leading, in turn, to focal perforation of trabecular plates. Progressive enlargement of the perforations converts trabecular plates to rods. The resulting structural changes were thought to be more severe in patients with osteoporosis than in normal subjects, but to have been completed in most patients before they develop symptoms.[48] These changes would result in changes in anisotropy and in one study it was shown that more than 80% of the variance in the stiffness modulus could be explained by bone volume fraction and trabecular orientation; this was not materially improved by including measures of connectivity or trabecular plate number.[49] Studies of cancellous bone from the femoral neck of patients who had sustained an osteoporotic fracture showed no significant differences in the architecture compared with a comparable post-mortem group with no fracture.[50]

In addition to the obvious measurements of dimensions, spacings, and angles in two- or three-dimensional images of bone, more abstract methods have been devised in an attempt to quantify structure, including fractals and Fourier spectral methods. Fractal methods have been used on images from radiographs,[51-53] biopsies,[53,54] and magnetic resonance imaging (MRI),[55] although few studies have tried to compare these measures directly with stiffness or strength. Some have reported that including a fractal measure of architecture along with porosity[56] or BMD[57] can increase the correlation with Young's modulus. However, another study reported that after controlling for BMD, no association could be detected between measures of fractal dimension and elastic modulus in the craniocaudal direction of human vertebral bodies.[58] This could be a problem with the particular methods chosen to determine the fractal dimension, as this has been shown to have an effect on the predictive ability of the linear model.[57] Fourier methods, to identify features that occur with some degree of regularity, are being used to assess cancellous structure.[59,60] Combining these with statistical and neural network classification techniques has been used to predict the load at fracture and the ultimate stress of radii, with correlation coefficients of 0.91 and 0.93, respectively.[61] Similar methods are being assessed as a means of improving the prediction of fracture risk in patients.[59]

Changes in cortical bone with aging, thinning of cortices, and increasing porosity are not generally regarded as significant factors underlying osteoporotic fractures because the most common fractures occur in areas rich in trabecular bone, i.e., the wrist, hip, and spine. Indeed, a study comparing femoral neck cortical width in patients who had fractured a hip with those who had not found no significant difference.[50] However, recent studies on the cortex surrounding the femoral neck have suggested that increased porosity and thinning of the inferoanterior to superoposterior region could weaken the cortex in regions believed to be maximally loaded on impact due to falling.[62] An additional role of the cortex, which is often overlooked, is how it works in combination with the cancellous bone to enhance the apparent properties of the tissue. By restricting some of the dimensional changes that normally occur with loading (the Poisson's ratio effects) the cortical bone could cause the cancellous bone to appear stiffer than results from testing an isolated sample would suggest.[63,64] Some loss of this constraint could have a detrimental effect on the femoral neck as a whole, more than might be expected simply from loss of cortical bone.

2. Shape Factors

The shape of a bone may have important consequences for how it responds to forces, especially if those forces are not along an axis of symmetry. Clearly, the hip is an obvious place where this might be important, whereas for vertebrae and the radius geometric changes may not be so significant and have been little studied.

As for trabecular architecture, most approaches adopted have concentrated on specific, measurable features such as the width of the femoral neck, the so-called hip-axis length, which is the distance from greater trochanter to the inner pelvic brim, and the angle between the femoral neck and the shaft of the femur. In a study of over 8000 women, a longer hip-axis length was associated with an increased risk of both femoral neck — odds ratio (OR) = 1.9; 95% confidence interval (CI) 1.3, 3.0 — and trochanteric fractures (OR 1.6; CI 1.0, 2.4) in the 164 who fractured over the ensuing 1.6 years after recruitment. No significant association was found between the neck width (OR 1.1; CI 0.8, 1.5) or the neck/shaft angle (OR 1.4; CI 0.9, 2.2) and risk of hip fracture.[65] In another study, 111 postmenopausal women with a hip fracture were found to have a longer hip-axis length and a more valgus (more obtuse) neck-shaft angle. However, the hip-axis length correlated significantly with neck-shaft angle, femoral neck width, and age. Standardized logistic regression showed that the hip axis length and the neck-shaft angle predicted fracture independently of BMD after correction for age, weight, and femoral neck BMD.[66]

This study indicates something of the confusion that can be caused by the interrelationship of geometric factors. This is compounded in the literature by *ex vivo* studies, which showed that geometric factors correlated only weakly with femoral strength, with a value for R^2 of just over 0.2 for both neck axis length and neck width,[67] and a study of Polynesian women, which found they have longer femoral necks but a low incidence of hip fracture.[68] Taken together the evidence suggests that the shape of the proximal femur almost certainly plays some role in fracture risk, but exactly what features are important is as yet unclear. A study of trends in hip geometry over the period between approximately 1960 and 1990 found that the ratio of hip-axis length to femoral width (to allow for differences in radiographic technique) increased by 2.3%, although this was not statistically significant. They concluded that there has been a small apparent change in geometric measurements of the hip during the past 36 years and extrapolated this, albeit cautiously, to suggest that such a change may explain up to one-third of the increase in incidence of hip fracture observed during this period.[69] A study of femurs from the northeast of Scotland found an increase of about 9% in femoral neck length in a modern group compared with a group from the turn of the century.[70] This increase was highly significant and considerably more than the percentage increases found in the femoral length (1.6%), neck width (5%), and head diameter (3.5%). A longer femoral neck will increase the lever arm between the femoral head and the shaft, and it has been suggested that an increase in length of one standard deviation will double the risk of fracture.[65] This is about the size of the increase reported in the Scottish study over a period of just under a century.

On the assumption that the shape of the proximal femur may be an important factor we recently used active shape modeling (ASM)[71] to describe the outline of the proximal femur in radiographs from a group of 54 patients, 29 of whom had suffered a hip fracture.[72] ASM is an image processing technique in which the computer is trained to recognize the shape of interest in one set of images and then, when presented with another set, can model that shape and obtain a statistical measure of, for example, how close it is to a chosen "perfect" shape or how one group of shapes differs from another group. Some medical applications are shapes that have common features, but are subject to natural variation, such as vertebrae[73] or proximal femurs with hip replacements.[74] Its advantages are that it is trained by the "expert" and it makes no direct measurements of specific distances or angles; these are all included in the overall description of shape. The patients had all had measurements made of BMD at various sites in the proximal femur and a pelvic radiograph. In the fracture group we used the contralateral hip for measurement. We found that BMD in Ward's triangle area was the best single predictor, predicting 80% of the fracture group. Combining shape with BMD predicted over 90% of the fracture group. This study is limited by the relatively small number of patients, but if confirmed in larger groups will provide a powerful tool to assist in identifying patients at risk of hip fracture.

In summary, there are clearly changes in internal architecture and an overall loss of bone in patients with osteoporosis, which are very well documented. However, surprisingly little appears to be known of the detailed nature of these changes. There appears to be an overall change in the shape of the femur, which will alter the stress distribution arising from impact loading during a fall. There may also be subtle, but very important, changes in the organic and mineral phases of the matrix. These could impair the ability of the bone to absorb energy or decrease the work of fracture, either or both of which could result in increased fragility.

ACKNOWLEDGMENTS

The author thanks the Medical Research Council for the award of a Senior Fellowship and the Arthritis Research Campaign, The Sir Halley Stewart Trust, the PPP Foundation, and the Engineering and Physical Sciences Research Council for additional funding.

REFERENCES

1. Gibson, L.J., "The mechanical behavior of cancellous bone," *J. Biomech.*, 18, 317, 1985.
2. Gibson, L.J. and Ashby, M.F., *Cellular Solids*, Pergamon Press, Oxford, 1988.
3. Cowin, S.C., *Bone Mechanics Handbook*, CRC Press, Boca Raton, FL, 2001.
4. Martin, R.B., Burr, D.B., and Sharkey, N.A., *Skeletal Tissue Mechanics*, Springer-Verlag, New York, 1998.
5. Keaveny, T.M., Guo, X.E., Wachtel, E.F., et al., "Trabecular bone exhibits fully linear elastic behavior and yields at low strains," *J. Biomech.*, 27, 1127, 1994.
6. Cowin, S.C., *Bone Mechanics*, CRC Press, Boca Raton, FL, 1989.
7. Wolff, J., *Das Gesetz der Transformation der Knochen,* Hirschwald, Berlin, 1892.
8. Hukins, D.W.L., Aspden, R.M., and Hickey, D.S., "Strain relates connective tissue properties to joint movement," *Clin. Biomech.*, 4, 3, 1989.
9. Chang, W.C., Christensen, T.M., Pinilla, T.P., and Keaveny, T.M., "Uniaxial yield strains for bovine trabecular bone are isotropic and asymmetric," *J. Orthop. Res.*, 17, 582, 1999.
10. Wachtel, E.F. and Keaveny, T.M., "Dependence of trabecular damage on mechanical strain," *J. Orthop. Res.*, 15, 781, 1997.
11. Burstein, A.H., Reilly, D.T., and Martens, M., "Aging of bone tissue: mechanical properties," *J. Bone Joint Surg.*, 58A, 82, 1976.
12. Lindahl, O. and Lindgren, A.G., "Cortical bone in man. II. Variation in tensile strength with age and sex," *Acta Orthop. Scand.*, 38, 141, 1967.

13. Lindahl, O. and Lindgren, G.H., "Cortical bone in man. 3. Variation of compressive strength with age and sex," *Acta Orthop. Scand.*, 39, 129, 1968.

14. Boyce, T.M. and Bloebaum, R.D., "Cortical aging differences and fracture implications for the human femoral neck," *Bone*, 14, 769, 1993.

15. Currey, J.D., "Changes in the impact energy absorption of bone with age," *J. Biomech.*, 12, 459, 1979.

16. Currey, J.D., Brear, K., and Zioupos, P., "The effects of aging and changes in mineral content in degrading the toughness of human femora," *J. Biomech.*, 29, 257, 1996.

17. McCalden, R.W., McGeough, J.A., Barker, M.B., and Court-Brown, C.M., "Age-related changes in the tensile properties of cortical bone — the relative importance of changes in porosity, mineralization, and microstructure," *J. Bone Joint Surg.*, 75A, 1193, 1993.

18. Simmons, E.D., Pritzker, K.P.H., and Grynpas, M.D., "Age related changes in the human femoral cortex," *J. Orthop. Res.*, 9, 155, 1991.

19. Li, B. and Aspden, R.M., "Material properties of bone from the femoral neck and the calcar femorale of patients with osteoporosis or osteoarthritis," *Osteoporos. Int.*, 7, 450, 1997.

20. Li, B. and Aspden, R.M., "Composition and mechanical properties of cancellous bone from the femoral head of patients with osteoporosis or osteoarthritis," *J. Bone Miner. Res.*, 12, 641, 1997.

21. Rice, J.C., Cowin, S.C., and Bowman, J.A., "On the dependence of the elasticity and strength of cancellous bone on apparent density," *J. Biomech.*, 21, 155, 1988.

22. Zioupos, P. and Aspden, R.M., "Density, material quality and quantity issues in OP cancellous bone," in *Proceedings of the 12th Conference of the European Society of Biomechanics*, Prendergast, D.J., Lee, T.C., and Carr, A.J., Eds., Royal Academy of Medicine in Ireland, Dublin, 2000, 327.

23. Hasegawa, K., Turner, C.H., Recker, R.R., et al., "Elastic properties of osteoporotic bone measured by scanning acoustic microscopy," *Bone*, 16, 85, 1995.

24. Li, B. and Aspden, R.M., "Mechanical and material properties of the subchondral bone plate from the femoral head of patients with osteoarthritis or osteoporosis," *Ann. Rheum. Dis.*, 56, 247, 1997.

25. Bailey, A.J., Wotton, S.F., Sims, T.J., and Thompson, P.W., "Post-translational modifications in the collagen of human osteoporotic femoral head," *Biochem. Biophys. Res. Commun.*, 185, 801, 1992.

26. Bailey, A.J., Wotton, S.F., Sims, T.J., and Thompson, P., "Biochemical changes in the collagen of human osteoporotic bone matrix," *Connect. Tissue Res.*, 29, 119, 1993.

27. Oxlund, H., Mosekilde, L., and Ortoft, G., "Reduced concentration of collagen reducible cross links in human trabecular bone with respect to age and osteoporosis," *Bone*, 19, 479, 1996.

28. Smith, F.G., "Aspects of bone quality in osteoporosis and osteoarthritis: collagen post-translational modification and mechanical factors," Ph.D. thesis, University of Aberdeen, 1999.

29. Masse, P.G., Rimnac, C.M., Yamauchi, M., et al., "Pyridoxine deficiency affects biomechanical properties of chick tibial bone," *Bone*, 18, 567, 1996.

30. Baud, C.A., Very, J.M., and Courvoisier, B., "Biophysical study of bone mineral in biopsies of osteoporotic patients before and after long-term treatment with fluoride," *Bone*, 9, 361, 1988.

31. Baud, C.A., Pouezat, J.A., and Tochon-Danguy, H.J., "Quantitative analysis of amorphous and crystalline bone tissue mineral in women with osteoporosis," *Calcif. Tissue Res.*, 21, S452–S456, 1976.

32. Cohen, L. and Kitzes, R., "Infrared spectroscopy and magnesium content of bone mineral in osteoporotic women," *Isr. J. Med. Sci.*, 17, 1123, 1981.

33. Thompson, D.D., Posner, A.S., Laughlin, W.S., and Blumenthal, N.C., "Comparison of bone apatite in osteoporotic and normal Eskimos," *Calcif. Tissue Int.*, 35, 392, 1983.

34. Paschalis, E.P., Betts, F., DiCarlo, E., et al., "FTIR microspectroscopic analysis of human iliac crest biopsies from untreated osteoporotic bone," *Calcif. Tissue Int.*, 61, 487, 1997.

35. Mkukuma, L.D., Imrie, C.T., Skakle, J.M.S., et al., unpublished observations.

36. Whitehouse, W.J., "The quantitative morphology of anisotropic trabecular bone," *J. Microsc.*, 101, 153, 1974.

37. Singh, I., "The architecture of cancellous bone," *J. Anat.*, 127, 305, 1978.

38. Hildebrand, T. and Rüegsegger, P., "Quantification of bone microarchitecture with the structure model index," *Comput. Methods Biomech. Biomed. Eng.*, 1, 15, 1997.

39. Ulrich, D., van Rietbergen, B., Laib, A., and Rüegsegger, P., "The ability of three-dimensional structural indices to reflect mechanical aspects of trabecular bone," *Bone*, 25, 55, 1999.

40. Goulet, R.W., Goldstein, S.A., Ciarelli, M.J., et al., "The relationship between the structural and orthogonal compressive properties of trabecular bone," *J. Biomech.*, 27, 375, 1994.

41. Hildebrand, T. and Rüegsegger, P., "A new method for the model-independent assessment of thickness in three-dimensional images," *J. Microsc.*, 185, 67, 1997.

42. Ulrich, D., Hildebrand, T., van Rietbergen, B., et al., "The quality of trabecular bone evaluated with micro-computed tomography, FEA and mechanical testing," *Stud. Health Technol. Inf.*, 40, 97, 1997.

43. Pugh, J.W., Rose, R.M., and Radin, E.L., "A structural model for the mechanical behavior of trabecular bone," *J. Biomech.*, 6, 657, 1973.

44. Parfitt, A.M., "Age-related structural changes in trabecular and cortical bone: cellular mechanisms and biochemical consequences," *Calcif. Tissue Int.*, 36, S123-S128, 1984.

45. McCalden, R.W., McGeough, J.A., and Court-Brown, C.M., "Age-related changes in the compressive strength of cancellous bone. The relative importance of changes in density and trabecular architecture," *J. Bone Joint Surg.*, 79A, 421, 1997.

46. Dempster, D.W., Ferguson-Pell, M.W., Mellish, R.W., et al., "Relationships between bone structure in the iliac crest and bone structure and strength in the lumbar spine," *Osteoporos. Int.*, 3, 90, 1993.

47. Bergot, C., Laval-Jeantet, A.M., Preteux, F., and Meunier, A., "Measurement of anisotropic vertebral trabecular bone loss during aging by quantitative image analysis," *Calcif. Tissue Int.*, 43, 143, 1988.

48. Parfitt, A.M., Mathews, C.H., Villanueva, A.R., et al., "Relationships between surface, volume, and thickness of iliac trabecular bone in aging and in osteoporosis. Implications for the microanatomic and cellular mechanisms of bone loss," *J. Clin. Invest.*, 72, 1396, 1983.

49. Goldstein, S.A., Goulet, R., and McCubbrey, D., "Measurement and significance of three-dimensional architecture to the mechanical integrity of trabecular bone," *Calcif. Tissue Int.*, 53, S127, 1993.

50. Hordon, L.D. and Peacock, M., "The architecture of cancellous and cortical bone in femoral neck fracture," *Bone Miner.*, 11, 335, 1990.

51. Buckland-Wright, J.C., Lynch, J.A., et al., "Fractal signature analysis of macroradiographs measures trabecular organization in lumbar vertebrae of postmenopausal women," *Calcif. Tissue Int.*, 54, 106, 1994.

52. Buckland-Wright, J.C., Lynch, J.A., and Bird, C., "Microfocal techniques in quantitative radiography: measurement of cancellous bone organization," *Br. J. Rheumatol.*, 35, 18, 1996.

53. Lespessailles, E., Roux, J.P., Benhamou, C.L., et al., "Fractal analysis of bone texture on os calcis radiographs compared with trabecular microarchitecture analyzed by histomorphometry," *Calcif. Tissue Int.*, 63, 121, 1998.

54. Fazzalari, N.L. and Parkinson, I.H., "Fractal dimension and architecture of trabecular bone," *J. Pathol.*, 178, 100, 1996.

55. Link, T.M., Majumdar, S., Augat, P., et al., "*In vivo* high resolution MRI of the calcaneus: differences in trabecular structure in osteoporosis patients," *J. Bone Miner. Res.*, 13, 1175, 1998.

56. Hodgskinson, R. and Currey, J.D., "Effects of structural variation on Young's modulus of nonhuman cancellous bone," *Proc. Inst. Mech. Engs. [H], J. Eng. Med.*, 204, 43, 1990.

57. Majumdar, S., Lin, J., Link, T., et al., "Fractal analysis of radiographs: assessment of trabecular bone structure and prediction of elastic modulus and strength," *Med. Phys.*, 26, 1330, 1999.

58. Uchiyama, T., Tanizawa, T., Muramatsu, H., et al., "Three-dimensional microstructural analysis of human trabecular bone in relation to its mechanical properties," *Bone*, 25, 487, 1999.

59. Gregory, J.S., Junold, R.M., Undrill, P.E., and Aspden, R.M., "Analysis of trabecular bone structure using Fourier transforms and neural networks," *IEEE Trans. Inf. Technol. Biomed*, 3, 289, 1999.

60. Wigderowitz, C.A., Abel, E.W., and Rowley, D.I., "Evaluation of cancellous structure in the distal radius using spectral analysis," *Clin. Orthop.*, 152, 1997.

61. Wigderowitz, C.A., Paterson, C.R., Dashti, H., et al., Prediction of bone strength from cancellous structure of the distal radius: can we improve on DXA? *Osteoporos. Int.*, 11, 840, 2000.

62. Bell, K.L., Loveridge, N., Jordan, G.R., et al., "A novel mechanism for induction of increased cortical porosity in cases of intracapsular hip fracture," *Bone*, 27, 297, 2000.

63. Aspden, R.M., "Constraining the lateral dimensions of uniaxially loaded materials increases the calculated strength and stiffness: application to muscle and bone," *J. Mater. Sci. Mater. Med.*, 1, 100, 1990.

64. Bryce, R., Aspden, R.M., and Wytch, R., "Stiffening effects of cortical bone on vertebral cancellous bone *in situ*," *Spine*, 20, 999, 1995.

65. Faulkner, K.G., Cummings, S.R., Black, D., et al., "Simple measurement of femoral geometry predicts hip fracture: the study of osteoporotic fractures," *J. Bone Miner. Res.*, 8, 1211, 1993.

66. Gnudi, S., Ripamonti, C., Gualtieri, G., and Malavolta, N., "Geometry of proximal femur in the prediction of hip fracture in osteoporotic women," *Br. J. Radiol.*, 72, 729, 1999.

67. Cheng, X.G., Lowet, G., Boonen, S., et al., "Assessment of the strength of proximal femur *in vitro*: relationship to femoral bone mineral density and femoral geometry," *Bone*, 20, 213, 1997.
68. Chin, K., Evans, M.C., Cornish, J., et al., "Differences in hip axis and femoral neck length in premenopausal women of Polynesian, Asian and European origin," *Osteoporos. Int.*, 7, 344, 1997.
69. O'Neill, T.W., Grazio, S., Spector, T.D., and Silman, A.J., "Geometric measurements of the proximal femur in U.K. women: secular increase between the late 1950s and early 1990s," *Osteoporos. Int.*, 6, 136, 1996.
70. Duthie, R.A., Bruce, M.F., and Hutchison, J.D., "Changing proximal femoral geometry in north east Scotland: an osteometric study," *Br. Med. J.*, 316, 1498, 1998.
71. Hill, A., Cootes, T.F., and Taylor, C.J., "Active shape models and the shape approximation problem," *Image Vision Comput.*, 14, 601, 1996.
72. Gregory, J.S., Testi, D., Undrill, P.E., and Aspden, R.M., "Shape modeling for predicting hip fracture," *Osteoporos. Int.*, 12, S6, 2001.
73. Smyth, P.P., Taylor, C.J., and Adams, J.E., "Vertebral shape: automatic measurement with active shape models," *Radiology*, 211, 571, 1999.
74. Redhead, A.L., Kotcheff, A.C.W., Taylor, C.J., et al., "An automated method for assessing routine radiographs of patients with total hip replacements," *Proc. Inst. Mech. Eng. [H], J. Eng. Med.*, 211, 145, 1997.

4 Healing of Normal and Osteoporotic Bone

Mandi J. Lopez, Ryland B. Edwards III, and Mark D. Markel

CONTENTS

I. INTRODUCTION

Bones are vital components of the body that serve many functions. They make up the frame of the body, provide protection for soft tissues and vital internal organs, and potentiate locomotion by providing anchoring points for the origin and insertion of tendons and ligaments. Bones also serve as a natural reservoir of calcium and phosphorus, which are released on demand. Normal bone represents one tenth of the body weight and has a breaking strength comparable to medium steel, yet is flexible and elastic enough that it returns to its original form after deformation within its limits of elasticity. Bone absorbs energy imparted by deforming forces until the point of fracture, upon which a well-organized cascade of events occurs to restore the original structure. The dynamic changes that bone normally undergoes can be classified into three major categories: modeling, the process of bone formation during skeletal growth; remodeling, the continuous changes that occur during adult life; and coupling, the process by which bone balances resorption by bone formation. All of these processes occur in a continuum during the process of fracture repair.

55

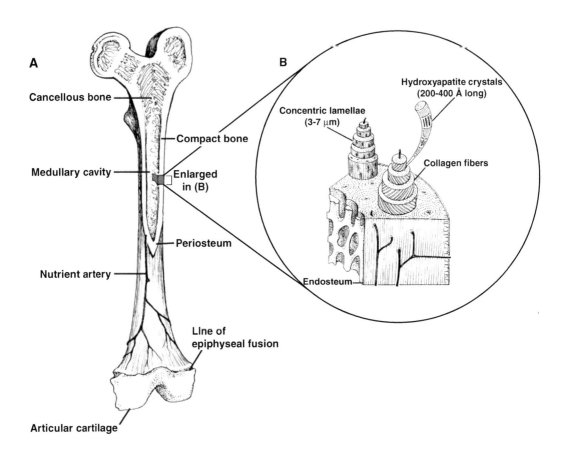

FIGURE 4.1 (A) The structure of mammalian long bones. (B) Enlargement of gray box in Figure 4.1A showing ultrastructure of mammalian long bones. Note the differences in magnification.

II. NORMAL BONE ANATOMY

Bone is one of the few organs capable of spontaneous regeneration rather than simple repair with restoration of structure. The unique structure of bone supports its regenerative and remodeling capacities, both of which are critical for fracture repair. Every structural element of bone from the ultrastructural to the macroscopic level is an integral functional component (Figure 4.1A and B). The typical bone has a composition of approximately 8% water and 92% solid material, which is further divided into approximately 30% organic and 70% inorganic material.[1,2] The organic component includes osteogenic cells and the extracellular matrix while the inorganic component is primarily hydroxyapatite $(Ca_{10}(PO_4)_6(OH)_2)$, a calcium phosphate salt crystal.[1,2]

Extracellular matrix supplies form and supporting structure for the deposition and crystallization of inorganic salts. It is composed of approximately 95% type I collagen with the remainder consisting of ground substance.[1,2] The organization of collagen in individual secondary osteons has been described as parallel to the osteon and bone long axis, circumferential, or alternating.[3] Type I collagen imparts a great deal of mechanical strength to bone, and collagen fibers also serve as the site of mineralization.[3] Hydroxyapatite crystals are aligned parallel to the longitudinal axis of the collagen fiber in a band pattern with the collagen fibril (Figure 4.1B).[1,4] Ground substance, composed of glycosaminoglycans and proteoglycans, composes the remainder of the organic matrix. Glycosaminoglycans are attached as side chains to the central protein core of proteoglycans.

Osteoblasts, osteocytes, and osteoclasts are the osteogenic cells responsible for bone maintenance and repair. Osteoblasts are found in systems of bone formation. They originate from undifferentiated mesenchymal cells located on the inner layer of the periosteum and in bone marrow, and deposit unmineralized bone matrix or osteoid along the bone surface.[5] Osteoblasts also control the transport of substrates from the extracellular space into the osteoid seam, and produce alkaline phosphatase, which initiates matrix mineralization. Osteocytes are osteoblasts that have become encased in bone matrix.[1,2,6] They are primarily responsible for the maintenance of bone matrix. The osteocytes exist individually in lacunae and their cytoplasmic processes radiate outward through canaliculi to communicate with other osteocytic cells (Figure 4.1B).

Osteoclasts are large multinucleated cells found within lacunae (Howship's lacunae) at or near the surface of bone. Their role is to resorb bone in areas of active remodeling. It is believed that osteoclasts originate from pluripotential cells of the bone marrow.[2] They form a ruffled border that is the site of bone resorption. Immediately surrounding the ruffled border and in close apposition to the mineralized bone is the sealing area, which permits the concentration of degradative substances that are responsible for osteoclastic activity.

The basic unit of bone is the osteon or Haversian system (Figure 4.1B). In the center of each osteon is the Haversian canal containing vessels, nerve fibers, and lymphatic channels. Mineralized bone is deposited in concentric layers or osteonal lamellae around the central Haversian canal. Within the lamella are lacunae containing osteocytes. A cement line composed of glycosaminoglycans surrounds and separates each osteon from others. Interstitial lamellae bridge the space between osteons. Osteons can be primary or secondary. Primary osteons form during appositional bone growth while secondary osteons are produced throughout life. Primary osteons are parallel to the longitudinal axis of the bone and surrounded by woven bone, which is eventually replaced by primary lamellar bone. Secondary osteons consist of concentric rings of lamellar bone deposited by osteoblasts on the trailing edge of a cutting cone headed by osteoclasts. Secondary osteons are surrounded by interstitial lamellae and not woven bone.

Grossly, bone has been divided into two categories: long bones and flat bones. Long bones are composed primarily of compact cortical bone and make up the majority of the axial skeleton. Flat bones like the skull serve to protect vital soft tissue structures. Adult long bones are further described with a diaphysis, the shaft of the bone, and metaphysis, the segment of bone bridging the diaphysis and each end of the bone. A central medullary cavity courses through the diaphysis of the long bones and contains a vascular and lymphatic supply, fatty marrow, and some hematopoietic cells (Figure 4.1A). The cancellous metaphyses contain most of the hematopoietic components. The surfaces of the long bones are covered by periosteum, with the exception of each end, where articular cartilage and synovium are present. The periosteum is subdivided into an outer fibrous layer and an inner layer known as the cambium layer. Active cell proliferation occurs from the cambium layer during growth and fracture repair. The outer periosteal layer is structurally supportive and carries the vascular and nerve supply to the surface of cortical bone. The marrow cavity is lined with a fibrous sheet called the endosteum, which is also actively involved in fracture repair.

The classification of the vascular anatomy of long bones is based on function rather than location. An afferent and efferent vascular system exists for all long bones. The three primary components of the afferent vascular system are the principal nutrient artery, the proximal and distal metaphyseal arteries, and the periosteal arterioles.[1,2,7,8] Approximately 70% of the afferent blood flow is directed to the cortex, and 30% is directed to the marrow.[2] The endosteal circulation supplies the medullary area and the inner two thirds to three quarters of the compact cortical bone.[1] The periosteal arterioles supply the outer third or quarter of the compact cortical bone only in localized areas that are related to fascial attachments. On a microscopic level, most Haversian canals and cutting cones contain a single capillary (Figure 4.1B).[9] The efferent vascular system includes the large emissary veins and vena comitans of the nutrient veins, which drain the medullary contents exclusively, the cortical venous channels, and the periosteal capillaries. Drainage of blood via the efferent vascular system occurs primarily in a centripetal direction.[10] In bone, the volume of the venous system is six- to eightfold greater than that of the arterial system.[9]

III. BONE FORMATION

Bone formation always involves the same process. It begins when undifferentiated mesenchymal cells assume the appearance of osteoblasts and begin to secrete osteoid. The osteoid mineralizes, and osteoblasts, surrounded by mineralized matrix, become osteocytes. The appearance of osteo-clasts begins the remodeling process that can convert immature woven bone into mature lamellar bone. The mechanism of bone formation may occur within cartilage (endochondral), within a membrane (membranous), or by deposition of new bone on existing bone (appositional).

Endochondral bone formation requires the formation of a cartilage model. The cartilage is gradually resorbed and replaced by new bone.[11] Membranous ossification does not require a cartilage model.[12] Instead, mesenchymal cells condense, the surrounding tissue becomes vascular-ized, and cells differentiate directly into osteoblasts, which lay down osteoid. This is followed by mineralization to form new bone. For appositional bone formation, osteoblasts align on the surface of existing bone and synthesize osteoid, often in successive layers that form lamellae. During growth, periosteum covers the osseous primordia formed by endochondral or intramembranous ossification. Periosteal osteoblasts then add new bone by secreting osteoid on the outer surface of the bone. During the bone-formation phase of bone remodeling, osteblasts secrete a layer of osteoid at the site of osteoclastic resorption of bone.

IV. HEALING OF NORMAL BONE

A bone fracture disrupts skeletal continuity and mechanical function, injures local blood vessels, and initiates the process of fracture repair. Healing of a fractured bone is a complex biologic event leading to the restoration of the whole bone itself. The repair of a fracture requires synthesis of osseous tissue that necessitates some or all of the mechanisms of bone formation. The healing process can be described by three biological stages: inflammation, repair, and remodeling. The stages follow each other in sequence, with some overlap.

A. INFLAMMATION

The inflammatory stage, the shortest stage in the repair process, begins immediately after fracture and lasts between 2 and 3 weeks after injury. The initiating event is the disruption of the vascular supply to the periosteum, underlying bone, and surrounding connective tissue leading to the formation of a hematoma and cell death at the fracture site (Figure 4.2).[3,11,13] Lysosomal enzymes released by dead osteocytes trigger the destruction of the organic matrix.[2] Necrotic material elicits an intense inflammatory reaction. Acute-phase proteins such as interleukin-1 (IL-1) and interleu-kin-6 (IL-6) spread through the area and activate proteolytic enzyme cascades.[2]

The initial hematoma becomes organized and platelets in the blood attach to the site and release vasoactive mediators and growth factors including platelet-derived growth factor (PDGF), transforming growth factor-β (TGF-β), and epidermal growth factor (EGF).[2,11] Acute inflammatory cells arrive at the site and remove necrotic tissue. Polymorphonuclear leukocytes are the first inflammatory cells to arrive, and are followed by macrophages. Macrophages and lymphocytes release angiogenic and cell growth factors.[2] Osteoclasts are found early in the inflammatory phase and begin the process of resorption and removal of dead bone. The necrotic tissue chemotactically attracts primitive mesenchy-mal elements from the cambium layer of the periosteum, endosteum, bone marrow, and the endothelium that differentiate into mature cellular elements such as chondrocytes and osteoblasts, which begin producing the elements of the soft periosteal callus between fracture ends.[1-3,14]

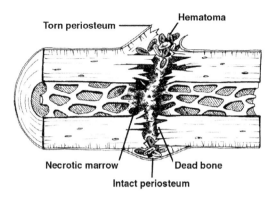

FIGURE 4.2 Inflammatory stage of fracture healing demonstrating trauma to the site and the fracture hematoma.

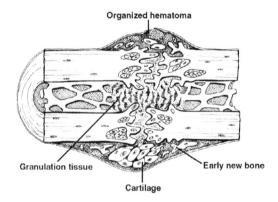

FIGURE 4.3 Reparative stage of fracture healing demonstrating the organized hematoma, granulation tissue, cartilage, and early new bone.

Collagen gene expression analysis has revealed that the granulation tissue matrix of the earliest fracture callus is rich in type III collagen.[13,15] Both chondrogenesis and osteogenesis begin in this matrix rich in type III collagen. The granulation tissue surrounding the fracture site (periosteal callus) forms the foundation for the progressive healing process.[13]

The initial blood supply to the periosteal callus is extraosseous, originating from the surrounding soft tissues.[2] This blood supply is transient and independent of fascial attachments. It is also distinct from normal periosteal arteries. The vessels profuse the periosteal callus and any detached cortical fragments. In spite of the initial vascular proliferation, there is a relative state of hypoxia in the periosteal callus.[1,2] As healing progresses, the contribution of the extraosseous blood supply to further bone healing diminishes.

B. Repair

In all fractures, the reparative phase of healing begins by appositional growth of new woven bone between days 3 and 5, when a majority of the callus still consists of granulation tissue (Figure 4.3).[13] The process of repair consists of the cellular synthesis of new bone, organic matrix, and the ossification of the matrix to form new woven bone.[11] Bone growth in fracture callus proceeds via two routes: intramembranous and endochondral growth. The relative amount of any mechanism of bone formation in the fracture healing process is dependent on the degree of immobilization at the fracture site and physiologic loading.[1,11,13,16] Stable fracture fixation may reduce interfragmentary

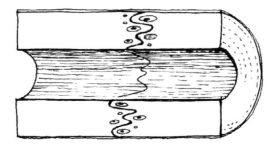

FIGURE 4.4 Schematic representation of primary osteonal healing. Stable fracture fixation may reduce interfragmentary movement to a point where union occurs through primary osteonal healing. This is accomplished by direct growth of secondary osteons from one fragment to another and by bone formation via intramembranous ossification.

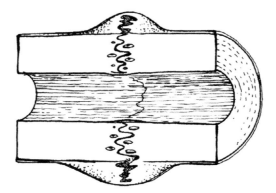

FIGURE 4.5 Schematic representation of endochondral bone formation. If the bone fragments are not well immobilized, endochondral bone formation dominates.

movement to a point where union occurs through osteonal healing of the cortical bone (primary osteonal healing) (Figure 4.4). This is accomplished by direct growth of secondary osteons from one fragment to another and by bone formation via the intramembranous route.[9,13,17] If, on the other hand, the fragments are not well immobilized, endochondral bone formation dominates (Figure 4.5).

Initially, formation of new cancellous bone occurs adjacent to the old bone. A matrix of type III collagen fibers is secreted along the periosteal surface, which serves as a substrate for migration of osteoprogenitor cells and capillary ingrowth, and provides a loose expandable network on which fibroblasts can be further oriented.[18,19] Osteoblasts in the periosteum and in the orifice of the medullary canal form trabeculae without passing through a cartilage stage.[20] An area of crowded irregular cells widens back from the fractured ends, forward to bridge the fracture, and outward from the periosteum.[21] Chondroblasts differentiate and fill most of the free space on the muscle side of the fracture. The chondrocytes become hypertrophic and mineralized matrix is formed. The production of cartilage and fiber bone increases the mechanical stability of the fracture site.[21] This stage of appositional bone growth requires no cartilage intermediate, and is characterized by a marked increase in the level of type I collagen along with the presence of TGF-β, connective tissue growth factor, and osteopontin.[11,21] The next phase of fracture callus development is characterized by a rapid increase in the amount of cartilaginous matrix, type II collagen, and type II collagen mRNA, the amount of which is dependent on the mechanical conditions of the fracture, as mentioned previously.[3,13]

Angiogenesis, mediated by numerous angiogenic factors, occurs throughout the repair process.[2,9] As healing proceeds through both intramembranous and endochondral bone formation, there

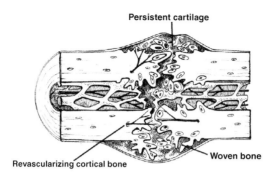

FIGURE 4.6 Remodeling stage of fracture healing demonstrating persistent cartilage, woven bone, and revascularizing cortical bone.

is a proliferation of blood vessels oriented perpendicular to the long axis of the bone on the periosteal side. There is a similar proliferation of vessels oriented parallel on the medullary side of the bone. The capillaries become dilated and full of red blood cells. As stability increases, the medullary blood supply again assumes the primary role of supplying the fibrocartilagenous callus.

The process of bone formation initially requires a biochemical environment with a high concentration of glycosaminoglycans, followed by an increase in collagen and an accumulation of hydroxyapatite crystals.[4] During the latter stages of repair, type I collagen is superimposed on the early collagenous matrix, and types II and III are removed as immature woven bone is remodeled to lamellar bone.[3] Crystals of calcium hydroxyapatite become clustered around the fibrils, eventually forming a rigid callus mass around the fracture.[4] Blood vessels begin to pass through the fibrous callus of one fracture fragment to reunify with those of other fragments. The combination of osteoblasts, cartilaginous matrix, and woven bone is the fracture callus. Formation of a bony bridging callus is the final step in the reparative phase of the fracture healing, and is considered the point of clinical union. The bony callus is the raw material for fracture remodeling.

C. REMODELING

Remodeling is the third and longest biological stage of fracture healing, suggested to last 6 to 9 years after the initial trauma in humans (Figure 4.6).[2,11] During this phase, the mineralized cartilage is transformed into woven bone, which is then modified into lamellar bone.[2] To accomplish this task, osteoclasts on the leading edge of cutting cones remove woven bone, and osteoblasts deposit lamellar bone around a central capillary channel.[22] Bone remodeling is predominantly regulated by the mechanical environment and the resultant piezoelectricity generated in the crystalline environment of the bone.[2,23] Stresses of weight-bearing cause concave surfaces to become electronegative while convex surfaces become electropositive.[24] Osteoblastic activity is enhanced on concave electronegative surfaces, whereas osteoclasts are activated on convex electropositive surfaces.[25] The final result of the remodeling stage is a bone whose organic and mineral phases are better aligned to resist local stresses.[11]

V. BIOMECHANICAL STAGES OF NORMAL FRACTURE HEALING

Biomechanically, four distinct stages in fracture healing characterized by differences in maximum torque and energy to failure have been demonstrated.[26] The types of failure that were observed reflected increasing strength of the healing fracture site as it passed through the three biological stages of healing. In the first biomechanical stage, bones refracture through the original fracture site with low stiffness and large deformation. The mechanical properties of the fracture are similar to those of collagen. In the second stage, the refracture still occurs through the original fracture

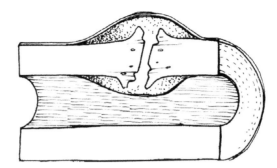

FIGURE 4.7 Schematic representation of defect healing. Initially, a small hematoma develops in the defect, and the surrounding bone becomes necrotic. Granulation tissue gradually replaces the hematoma, and the cambium layer of the periosteum becomes thickened by the proliferation of new osteoblasts, elevating the fibrous layer for some distance from the defect.

site, but with considerably increased stiffness, and less deformation at yield. In biomechanical stage 3 of healing, the refracture occurs partly through the original fracture site, and partly through previously intact bone. The stiffness is similar to stage 2, although the yield strength is greater. In stage 4, the fracture occurs outside the region of injury and with greater strength and energy. A stage 4 refracture pattern indicates that remodeling has restored the original mechanical properties to the injured tissues.

Two effects cause the increase in biomechanical properties during normal fracture healing.[21] The first effect is an increase in the cross-sectional area of bone caused by the periosteal callus. This increases the moment of inertia of the healing region, and therefore its strength and stiffness. The increase in cross-sectional area is of the greatest benefit if the new bone is deposited as far from the central axis as possible. Second, there is a change in the material properties within the healing area. This is due to a decrease in porosity of the bone as it changes from woven to lamellar bone. Another contributing alteration in the material properties is an increase in the mineral content of the healing tissue.

VI. NORMAL HEALING OF OSSEOUS DEFECTS

The process by which small osseous defects heal has been studied primarily in animal models by means of drill holes in bone (Figure 4.7).[1] The healing process is similar to that of normal fracture healing described previously. Initially, a small hematoma develops in the defect, and the surrounding bone becomes necrotic. Polymorphonuclear leukocytes are found in the hematoma almost immediately, followed by plasma cells, lymphocytes, and macrophages. Granulation tissue gradually replaces the hematoma, and the cambium layer of the periosteum becomes thickened by the proliferation of new osteoblasts, elevating the fibrous layer for some distance from the drill site. Transformation of undifferentiated mesenchymal cells seems to occur more rapidly with this type of defect.

Eventually, a bridge resembling the callus of normal fracture healing is formed across the defect on both the periosteal and endosteal surfaces. Intramembranous bone formation occurs within the central portion of the defect with the majority of trabeculae oriented at right angles to the long axis of the bone. Lamellar bone gradually replaces woven bone within the osseous defect, and large intertrabecular spaces are abolished. By 3 weeks after injury, a mixture of fibrous and lamellar bone bridges the gap. There is no evidence of endochondral bone formation in this type of defect healing. Cutting cones gradually replace reactive bone, with new bone oriented along the long axis of the bone. Remodeling of newly formed bone occurs similarly to standard callus remodeling.

TABLE 4.1
Reported Growth Factor Effects on Osteoblasts *in Vitro*

Growth Factor(s)	Cell Proliferation	Alkaline Phosphatase Activity	Collagen Synthesis	Chemotaxis
TGF-β	+++	±	++	+++
BMP-2, -3	0	++	0	+
BMP-7	+	+++	+	?
PDGF isoform BB	++	0	0	+++
PDGF isoform AA	+	0	0	+
IGF-1	++	0	+	+
IGF-2	+	0	0	+
FGF-basic	+	0	0	+
FGF-acidic	0	0	0	0
EGF	+	0	0	0

+ = Activity demonstrated; – = inhibition; 0 = no activity demonstrated; ? = not described.

VII. GROWTH FACTORS INFLUENCING FRACTURE HEALING

Bone growth and remodeling is the result of a balance between bone matrix formation and resorption. These activities are regulated by systemic and local factors. Many polypeptide growth factors have been shown in tissue culture and animal studies to have different effects on cell proliferation, differentiation, and matrix production as related to bone repair.[2,3,16] The effects are mediated by growth factor binding to membrane-bound receptors, leading to a cascade of intracellular events that influence gene expression.[27] On the basis of secretion and actions, growth factors may be divided into three categories: autocrine, factors expressed by a cell that acts on that same cell; paracrine, factors expressed by a cell that act on another cell; and endocrine, factors expressed by a cell at one site that are transmitted by blood to target cells at other sites.[2,16,27] These functional categories are not mutually exclusive, as many factors fit more than one category.

A number of growth factors have important functions during the bone healing process (Table 4.1). Many are integral for the initiation and maintenance of differentiation and proliferation of the osteoprogenitor cells, which contribute to the formation of new bone. Most of the factors have several roles in fracture healing and all of their potential roles have yet to be completely elucidated. Some of the growth factors prominent in fracture healing include TGF-β, bone morphogenetic proteins (BMPs), PDGF, insulin-like growth factors (IGF-I and -II), and fibroblast growth factors (FGF).

The exact sequence of temporally dependent events mediated by growth factors in the process of bone healing has not been precisely defined. A basic outline of the major roles of some of the growth factors involved in fracture repair is as follows.[27] During early healing, TGF-β and PDGF released from platelets in the fracture hematoma initiate differentiation of osteoprogenitor cells toward an osteoblastic lineage. Growth factors are released from the traumatized bone ends, which contribute to continued stimulation of osteoblastic activity. The growth factors released from platelets and bone tissues that initiate fracture healing also stimulate expression and synthesis of growth factors by participating osteoblasts. As fracture healing progresses, BMP is expressed by periosteal osteoblasts. This synthesis contributes to the continuous differentiation of mesenchymal stem cells to osteoblasts. Later, growth factors including TGF-β, FGF, and PDGF are synthesized by osteoblasts to maintain high proliferation and metabolic levels of osteoblasts involved in the healing process. FGFs are probably also important for angiogenesis in newly formed bone. The following are brief summaries of some of the specific roles played by each of these growth factors in fracture healing.

A. TGF-β

TGF-βs belong to a family of related proteins called the TGF-β superfamily, and are divided into five different subtypes.[16,27,28] TGF-βs are probably the most potent multifunctional regulators of bone cell metabolism. They are multifunctional growth factors with a broad range of biological activities including regulation of growth and differentiation of many cell types, and have a general stimulative effect on cells of mesenchymal origin and inhibitory effect on cells of ectodermal origin.[2,16,27-29] The secreted precursor protein, latent TGF-β, is biologically inactive when it is released from degranulating platelets, macrophages, and the extracellar matrix at fracture sites.[16] Its effects begin within 24 hours after injury and last for around 10 days.[16] Activation and cleavage to the mature peptide both occur in the acidic environment of the early fracture wound.[16,27] Bone and platelets contain almost 100 times more TGF-β than any other tissue and osteoblasts bear the highest amount of TGF-β receptors. TGF-β has profound *in vivo* effect on osteoblasts. The effects of TGF-βs on bone cell differentiation are controversial, but in general the *in vivo* data on the ability of TBF-βs to stimulate bone formation are promising.[27-29]

B. BMP

The ability of demineralized bone to induce new cartilage and bone formation in ectopic sites was attributed to a factor named bone morphogenetic protein by Urist in 1965.[30] BMPs, which exert their effects through receptors and are heteromeric complexes of type I and II serine/threonine kinase receptors, now exist in 15 subtypes.[27,31] They are all members of the TGF-β superfamily, with the exception of BMP-1, which is a procollagen C-protease.[31] BMPs are the only growth factors with a known ability to stimulate differentiation of mesenchymal stem cells in a chondro-blastic and osteoblastic direction.[2,3,16,27,31-34] During the healing response, release of BMPs from traumatized bone tissue stimulates differentiation of mesenchymal stem cells that participate in the healing process.[27,32] Other actions attributed to BMPs include cell chemotaxis, mitosis, stimulation of extracellular matrix synthesis, binding to matrix components, maintenance of phenotype, and apoptosis.[35]

Recent studies have demonstrated that BMPs are expressed during the early phases of fracture healing.[27,32,36] *In vivo* studies have focused on the effect of BMPs for stimulating healing of bone defects.[32,37,38] Studies in animal models show the healing of bone defects occurring through a progression of mesenchymal cell proliferation, cartilage differentiation and production, woven bone formation, and lamellar bone formation at 16 weeks.[2] BMP-2, -3, and -7 have been shown to be powerful stimulators of bony healing in nonunions, BMP-2 stimulates bone formation in simian muscle diffusion chambers, and BMP-3 was found to stimulate bony healing of large skull defects in monkeys.[2,27,32] A critical point in the potential use of BMPs to stimulate fracture repair is the development of a suitable carrier or delivery system to immobilize the protein at a particular site for a sufficient amount of time to allow bone induction to occur.[16,27,31,32] The cellular mechanisms for BMP are vaguely understood, but given their *in vivo* bone induction activity, they hold signif-icance as powerful stimulators of fracture healing.[16,17,31]

C. PDGF

PDGFs exist in three isotypes and are potent stimulators of both cellular proliferation and matrix protein synthesis.[2,16,27] They are released from platelet granules and are potent fibroblastic mitogens. PDGF is a competence factor that enables cells to respond to other biological mediators and is associated with increases in type I collagen expression *in vitro*.[2] PDGF also acts as a modulator of local blood flow, and has a significant positive impact on wound healing.[16] PDGF has been shown to promote chemotaxis of inflammatory and mesenchymal cells and to enhance cartilage synthesis.[2] The effects of PDGF may be dose dependent, where some doses have a stimulatory effect on bone healing, but others are inhibitory.[2]

D. IGF

The IGFs promote cell proliferation and matrix synthesis by chondrocytes and osteoblasts.[39] IGF-I and -II are produced by osteoblasts, and have similar biological properties, although IGF-I is four to seven times more potent.[27] Both factors are bound to carrier proteins as inactive forms and are transported via the circulation.[2] An important role of IGF-I is to mediate many of the actions of growth hormone on the skeleton.[39] IGF-II is found at a concentration 10 to 20 times higher than IGF-I in bone matrix. Studies have had limited success using IGFs to stimulate bone healing *in vivo*.[2,27] Additional studies are needed to clarify the role of the IGFs in the fracture healing process.

E. FGF

FGFs are present in bone matrix and are secreted by isolated osteoblasts. They are also released by fibroblasts, chondrocytes, and endothelial cells within the fracture callus.[2] FGF-basic (bFGF) is found in bone matrix at a tenfold higher concentration than FGF-acid (aFGF).[27] In normal bone cells, FGFs are primarily mitogens.[16] bFGF is a chemoattractant and mitogen for chondrocytes and is a key regulator in terminal differentiation of growth plate chondrocytes. It is also expressed by endothelial cells and promotes new vessel formation.[16] The effects of the FGFs are most pronounced on neovascularization and the formation of granulation tissue at the fracture site. Their mitogenic effect is enhanced by heparin and heparin-containing mast cells.[2]

VIII. ENHANCEMENT OF NORMAL FRACTURE HEALING

The process of fracture healing is generally considered to be biologically optimal; however, enhancement of the repair process to ensure rapid restoration of skeletal function would be of great benefit, especially in cases of impaired healing. Biological methods for local stimulation of fracture healing have been evaluated. They include the use of bone grafts, artificial substitutes for bone graft, purified or recombinant molecules with chondrogenic and osteogenic capacities, and local and systemic factors that have been observed to promote bone formation. Mechanical and physical interventions that have been shown to alter fracture healing include static and dynamic methods for post-operative stabilization and the use of noninvasive external stimuli, such as bioelectromagnetic fields and ultrasound.

A. BIOLOGICAL METHODS OF FRACTURE HEALING ENHANCEMENT

Local biological methods for the enhancement of fracture healing include the use of naturally occurring material such as bone grafts.[40-42] Autogenous fresh cancellous and cortical bone is most frequently used, but other common grafts include frozen, freeze-dried, or processed allogeneic cortical, corticocancellous, and cancellous grafts, demineralized bone matrix, and marrow grafts. These grafts have varying capacities to provide cells for active bone formation (osteogenesis), to induce bone formation by cells of the surrounding soft tissue (osteoinduction), and to serve as a substrate for bone formation (osteoconduction). Grafts typically cannot exert their biological activity in isolation, as they are dependent on the surrounding environment for cells to respond to their signals and, sometimes, for blood supply. The mechanical environment of the graft site is also important. Successful graft incorporation requires that an appropriate match be made between the biological activity of a bone graft, the condition of the perigraft environment, and the mechanical environment.

Materials with strictly osteoinductive properties have been investigated to enhance fracture healing.[40] The rationale for the use of these materials is that normal osteoblastic or osteoblast-like cells have the ability to form bone on the appropriate surface. Most investigations on the use of osteoconductive materials have centered on the use of ceramic materials including hydroxyapatite, tricalcium phosphate, calcium-sulfate composite, calcium-aluminate ceramics, and bioactive glasses.[40] Recently, the use of synthetic polymers to promote the healing of osseous defects and combinations of tricalcium phosphate and hydroxyapatite have also been investigated.

As previously described, a number of growth-promoting substances have been identified at fracture sites and are known to participate in the regulation of the associated responses. They can be generally divided into two groups: (1) growth factors, and (2) immunomodulatory cytokines, such as IL-1 and IL-6. With advancements in molecular biology, expression of gene product material in sufficient quantities has enabled investigators to assess effects of these molecules. The relationships among biological regulatory molecules, their temporal profile and concentrations, and the interplay among cells and the local microenvironments make investigation of these molecules difficult. However, despite numerous obstacles, the simulation of fracture healing through the exogenous administration of a number of these substances has been the subject of numerous investigations.[40]

B. Mechanical Methods of Fracture Healing Enhancement

The mechanical environment of a fracture plays an important role in its healing. Hence, fracture healing may be stimulated by strategic manipulation of the environment. Since Wolff hypothesized more than a century ago that bone structure adapts to changes in its stress environment, investigators have studied the response of intact and fractured bone to different forms of mechanical stress. Mechanical modulation of bone fracture repair relies on the fundamental physical concept of modeling according to the type of stress applied to immature or undifferentiated tissue.[43] Variables such as the size of the initial fracture gap, stability of the bone-fixator construct, and the parameters of the applied motion are all important.[44]

Excessive loading and motion of a fracture can delay or prevent healing, and early rigid fixation produces rapid primary bone healing with minimal callus. However, the same fixation rigidity may shield the calcified callus and lead to late resorption and weakening of the bone during the later stages of healing.[21,43] Loading of fracture callus has important effects on the organization and composition of the matrix.[45] There is evidence that controlled loading of a healing fracture stimulates callus formation and remodeling, and accelerates restoration of bone strength.[21,43,45] Work has shown that early or almost immediate loading and movement, including induced micromotion at long bone fracture sites, promotes fracture healing.[21,44,45] Further, delaying the onset of controlled micromotion decreases both bone mineral and fracture gap stiffness. There have been a number of investigations to determine optimum fixation rigidity for bone healing that is rigid enough to prevent excessive initial interfragmentary strain, yet flexible enough to allow load transfer to bone as the callus calcifies. A process to reduce the rigidity of the system by mechanical manipulation as healing progresses, called dynamization, has also been the subject of many studies.[21]

The clinical use of electric and electromagnetic fields for fracture healing applications began in the early 1970s.[46] Since then, several technologies have been developed and shown to promote healing in difficult-to-heal fractures. The development of these devices has been aided in recent years by basic research and several well-controlled clinical trials, although it still is not clear how they work or under what circumstances that they should be used.[46,47] There is a large body of evidence that metabolic activity and mechanical deformation in living bone generate steady, direct current and time-varying electric fields, respectively.[48] Externally supplied direct currents have been used to treat nonunions, appearing to trigger mitosis and recruitment of osteogenic cells. Direct current stimulation of *in vitro* cultured bone cells has been shown to increase intracellular free calcium ion concentration 2.3 times and greatly accelerate the cells' proliferation and calcification.[49] Time-varying electromagnetic fields also have been used to heal nonunions. Their osteogenic capacity does not appear to involve changes in the transmembrane electric potential, but instead seems to require coupling to the cell interior via transmembrane receptor or by mechanical coupling to the membrane itself.[48] Low-intensity pulsed ultrasound, a noninvasive form of mechanical energy transmitted transcutaneously as high-frequency acoustical pressure waves has been suggested to augment fracture healing, especially in cases of delayed healing. Numerous *in vivo* animal studies and prospective double-blind placebo-controlled clinical trials have shown that low-intensity ultrasound is capable of accelerating and augmenting the healing of fresh fractures.[50]

IX. HEALING OF OSTEOPOROTIC BONE

Osteoporosis is a disorder characterized by low bone mass, microarchitectural deterioration of bone, enhanced bone fragility, and increased fracture risk.[51] Although many current therapies are aimed at preventing bone fractures, the hallmark of osteoporosis, it is estimated that one of every two Caucasian women will experience an osteoporotic fracture in her lifetime.[31,32] An understanding of the healing process that occurs following a fracture in osteoporotic bone is important for management of such fractures. A number of studies evaluating fracture healing in osteoporotic bone have been performed using the most widely employed animal model to study osteoporosis, ovariectomized rats.[53]

The events of fracture healing proceed through the normal stages in osteoporotic bone concluding with fracture union. However, the healing process is prolonged. Lindholm[54] demonstrated this with the observation that calcium turnover in fractured tibias in an osteoporotic rat model was initially inhibited and subsequently prolonged. This prolonged healing period is likely not due to lack of bone induction by osteoporotic bone. Bone induction ability in an ovariectomized rat model was normal when decalcified matrix prepared from normal rats was transplanted into model rats; however, there was an absence of osteogenesis with matrix taken from ovariectomized rats and transplanted into normal rats.[55] The investigators also observed that bone matrix taken from ovariectomized donors was incompletely resorbed in both sham-operated and ovariectomized hosts, followed by the reduction of new bone and bone marrow. Instead, chondrogenesis was abundant and delayed. The authors surmised that an altered composition of matrix from ovariectomized rats and a subsequent abnormality in the cell–matrix interaction might be responsible for these effects. Adequate stabilization of fractures in osteoporotic bone is critical during the prolonged healing period, and this is complicated by the fact that osteoporotic bone does not support internal fixation nearly as well as healthy bone.[56-59]

A comparison of the histologic changes that occur during healing of osteoporotic bone fractures contributes to an understanding of the delayed healing process. In a study by Kubo,[60] the histologic changes of healing femoral fractures in normal and osteoporotic rat bones were described. At 6 weeks after fracture, formation of callus and periosteal bone at the fracture areas were found in both the osteoporosis and the control groups, and there were no differences between groups. There also were no histologic differences between groups. However, in the control group 12 weeks after fracture, the endosteal surface of the cortical bone was lined with an appositional layer of lamellar bone and the endosteal surface was lined with flat cells. In the osteoporosis group, clusters of osteoclasts with resorptive lacunae were present on the endosteal surface of the cortical bone, and a newly formed lamellar bone layer was partially present on the endosteal surface. The authors concluded that osteoporotic changes occur in newly generated bones in the period between 6 and 12 weeks after fracture, corresponding to the late reparative phase of fracture healing. In addition, bone mineral density of the new bones decreased at the same time point. The study concluded that osteoporotic changes do not markedly affect the early bone healing process but largely affect the later period. This is critical when considering treatments for osteoporotic fractures.

Several studies have focused on healing fracture strength in osteoporotic bone. Blythe and Buchsbaum[61] determined the tensile strength of healing midfibular fractures in ovariectomized, estrogen-treated, and control rats 5 weeks postfracture, and found no difference in fracture strength between groups. A similar study used the same model to compare the tensile strength of healing tibial bones after 2 weeks, and also found no difference between groups.[62] Using a slightly different osteoporosis model, Nordsletten et al.[63] evaluated tibial fracture healing using three-point cantilever bending 25 days postfracture in rats with and without sciatic neurectomy. To prevent differences in loading between control and nerve-resected animals, the fractured limbs were immobilized with casts. They found that mechanical strength did not differ significantly between legs with sciatic neurectomy and control limbs. Recently, Kubo et al.[60] also determined that the maximum tensile strength of healing femoral fractures after 6 and 12 weeks of healing did not differ significantly between ovariectomized and control rats. All of these studies support the clinical findings that osteoporotic fractures have normal healing potential.[64,65]

Fracture healing in osteoporotic bone progresses through the same stages of healing and ultimately reaches the same end point, fracture union, as normal bone. The time required for bony union, however, is prolonged and this prolongation is not equal in each stage of fracture healing. Appropriate fracture immobilization is required for healing of fractures in osteoporotic bone. This is complicated by the facts that osteoporotic bone does not hold standard stabilization methods well and that a longer period of immobilization is required given the increased fracture healing time. Techniques to enhance fracture healing would clearly be beneficial in the treatment of osteoporotic bone fractures.

REFERENCES

1. Heppenstall, R.B., "Fracture healing," in *Fracture Treatment and Healing,* Heppenstall R., Ed., W. B. Saunders, Philadelphia, 1980, 35.
2. Remedios, A., "Bone and bone healing," *Vet. Clin. North Am. Sm. Anim. Prac.,* 29, 1029, 1999.
3. Liu, S.H., Yang, R.S., al-Shaikh, R., et al., "Collagen in tendon, ligament, and bone healing," *Clin. Orthop.,* 318, 265, 1995.
4. Tencer, A.F., Johnson, K.D., Kyle, R.F., et al., "Biomechanics of fractures and fracture fixation," *Inst. Course Lect.,* 42, 19, 1993.
5. Bruder, S.P., Fink, D.J., and Caplan, A.I., "Mesenchymal stem cells in bone development, bone repair, and skeletal regeneration therapy," *J. Cell. Biochem.,* 56, 283, 1994.
6. Mast, B.A., "Healing in other tissues," *Surg. Clin. North Am.,* 77, 529, 1997.
7. Rhinelander, F.W., "Some aspects of the microcirculation of healing bone," *Clin. Orthop.,* 40, 12, 1965.
8. Rhinelander, F.W., "Normal vascular anatomy," in *Textbook of Small Animal Orthopaedics,* Newton, C.D. and Nunamaker, D.M., Eds., J.B. Lippincott, Philadelphia, 1988, 12.
9. Glowacki, J., "Angiogenesis in fracture repair," *Clin. Orthop.,* 355S, S82, 1998.
10. Trias, A. and Fery, A., "Cortical circulation of long bones," *J. Bone Joint Surg.,* 61A, 1052, 1979.
11. Yaszemski, M.J., Payne, R.G., Hayes, W.C., et al., "Evolution of bone transplantation: molecular, cellular and tissue strategies to engineer human bone," *Biomaterials,* 17, 175, 1996.
12. Ferguson, C.M., Miclau, T., Hu, D., et al., "Common molecular pathways in skeletal morphogenesis and repair," *Ann. N.Y. Acad. Sci.,* 857, 33, 1998.
13. Sandberg, M.M., Aro, H.T., and Vuorio, E.I., "Gene expression during bone repair," *Clin. Orthop.,* 289, 292, 1993.
14. Yoo, J.U. and Johnstone, B., "The role of osteochondral progenitor cells in fracture repair," *Clin. Orthop.,* 355S, S73, 1998.
15. Hiltunen, A., Aro, H.T., and Vuorio, E., "Regulation of extracellular matrix genes during fracture healing in mice," *Clin. Orthop.,* 297, 23, 1993.
16. Hollinger, J.H., "Factors for osseous repair and delivery: Part 1," *J. Craniofac. Surg.,* 4, 102, 1993.
17. Wu, C., "Biomechanical considerations in fracture treatment," *Chang Gung Med. J.,* 20, 251, 1997.
18. Ashhurst, D.E., "Collagens synthesized by healing fractures," *Clin. Orthop.,* 255, 273, 1990.
19. Lane, J.M., Suda, M., von der Mark, K., et al., "Immunofluorescent localization of structural collagen types in endochondral fracture repair," *J. Orthop. Res.,* 4, 318, 1986.
20. Henricson, A., Hulth, A., and Johnell, O., "The cartilaginous fracture callus in rats," *Acta Orthop. Scand.,* 58, 244, 1987.
21. Tencer, A.F. and Johnson, K.D., "The environment for fracture healing," in *Biomechanics in Orthopaedic Trauma,* Tencer, A.F. and Johnson, K.D., Eds., J.B. Lippincott, Philadelphia, 1994, 57.
22. Rahn, B.A., Gallinaro, P., Baltensperger, A., et al., "Primary bone healing. An experimental study in the rabbit," *J. Bone Joint Surg.,* 53A, 783, 1971.

23. Carter, D.R., Beaupre, G.S., Giori, N.J., et al., "Mechanobiology of skeletal regeneration," *Clin. Orthop.*, 355S, S41, 1998.

24. Bassett, C.A.L., "Current concepts of bone formation," *J. Bone Joint Surg.*, 44A, 1217, 1962.

25. Bassett, C.A.L., "Effect of electrical current on bone *in vivo*," *Nature (London)*, 204, 652, 1964.

26. White, A.A., III, Panjabi, M.M., and Southwick, W.O., "The four biomechanical stages of fracture repair," *J. Bone Joint Surg.*, 59A, 188, 1977.

27. Lind, M., "Growth factor stimulation of bone healing," *Acta Orthop. Scand.*, 283S, 6, 1998.

28. Bostrom, M.P.G. and Asnis, P., "Transforming growth factor beta in fracture repair," *Clin. Orthop.*, 355S, S124, 1998.

29. Rosier, R.N., O'Keefe, R.J., and Hicks, D.G., "The potential role of transforming growth factor beta in fracture healing," *Clin. Orthop.*, 355S, S294, 1998.

30. Urist, M.R., "Bone: formation by autoinduction," *Science*, 150, 893, 1965.

31. Croteau, S., Rauch, F., Silvestri, A., et al., "Bone morphogenetic proteins in orthopaedics: from basic science to clinical practice," *Orthopaedics*, 22, 686, 1999.

32. Wang, E.A., "Bone morphogenetic proteins (BMPs): therapeutic potential in healing bony defects," *TIBTECH*, 11, 379, 1993.

33. Bostrom, M.P.G., "Expression of bone morphogenetic proteins in fracture healing," *Clin. Orthop.*, 355S, S116, 1998.

34. Schmitt, J.M., Hwang, K., Winn, S.R., et al., "Bone morphogenetic proteins: an update on basic biology and clinical relevance," *J. Orthop. Res.*, 17, 269, 1999.

35. Reddi, A.H., "Initiation of fracture repair by bone morphogenetic proteins," *Clin. Orthop.*, 355S, 66S,1998.

36. Bostrom, M.P.G. and Camacho, N.P., "Potential role of bone morphogenetic proteins in fracture healing," *Clin. Orthop.*, 355S, S274, 1998.

37. Cook, S.D., "Preclinical and clinical evaluation of osteogenic protein-1 (BMP-7) in bony sites," *Orthopaedics*, 22, 669, 1999.

38. Wolfe, M.W. and Cook, S.D., "Use of osteoinductive implants in the treatment of bone defects," *Med. Prog. Tech.*, 20, 155, 1994.

39. Trippel, S.B., "Potential role of insulinlike growth factors in fracture healing," *Clin. Orthop.*, 355S, S301, 1998.

40. Einhorn, T.A., "Enhancement of fracture healing," *J. Bone Joint Surg.*, 77A, 940, 1995.

41. Stevenson, S., "Enhancement of fracture healing with autogenous and allogeneic bone grafts," *Clin. Orthop.*, 355S, S239, 1998.

42. Connolly, J.F., "Clinical use of marrow osteoprogenitor cells to stimulate osteogenesis," *Clin. Orthop.*, 355S, S257, 1998.

43. Chao, E.Y., Inoue, N., Elias, J.J., et al., "Enhancement of fracture healing by mechanical and surgical intervention," *Clin. Orthop.*, 355S, S163, 1998.

44. Goodman, S. and Aspenberg, P., "Effects of mechanical stimulation on the differentiation of hard tissues," *Biomaterials*, 14, 563, 1993.

45. Buckwalter, J.A. and Grodzinsky, A.J., "Loading of healing bone, fibrous tissue, and muscle: implications for orthopaedic practice," *J. Am. Acad. Orthop. Surg.*, 7, 291, 1999.

46. Ryaby, J.T., "Clinical effects of electromagnetic and electric fields on fracture healing," *Clin. Orthop.*, 355S, S205, 1998.

47. Aaron, R.K. and Ciombor, D.M., "Therapeutic effects of electromagnetic fields in the stimulation of connective tissue repair," *J. Cell. Biochem.*, 52, 42, 1993.

48. Otter, M.W., McLeod, K.J., and Rubin, C.T., "Effects of electromagnetic fields in experimental fracture repair," *Clin. Orthop.*, 355S, S90, 1998.

49. Wang, Q., Zhong, S., Ouyang, J., et al., "Osteogenesis of electrically stimulated bone cells mediated in part by calcium ions," *Clin. Orthop.*, 348, 259, 1998.

50. Hadjiargyrou, M., McLeod, K., Ryaby, J.P., et al., "Enhancement of fracture healing by low intensity ultrasound," *Clin. Orthop.*, 355S, S216, 1998.

51. Lane, J.M., Russell, L., and Khan, S.N. "Osteoporosis," *Clin. Orthop.*, 372, 139, 2000.

52. Lamding, C.L., "Osteoporosis prevention, detection, and treatment," *Postgrad. Med.*, 107, 37, 2000.

53. Kalu, D.N., "Animal models of the aging skeleton," in *The Aging Skeleton,* Rosen, C.J., Glowacki, J., and Bilezikian, J.P., Eds., Academic Press, San Diego, 1999, 37.

54. Lindholm, T.S., "Effects of 1-alpha-hydroxycholecalciferol on osteoporotic changes induced by calcium deficiency in bone fractures in adult rats," *J. Trauma*, 18, 336, 1978.
55. Cesnjaja, M., Stavljenic, A., and Vukicevic, S., "Decreased osteoinductive potential of bone matrix from ovariectomized rats," *Acta Orthop. Scand.*, 62, 471, 1991.
56. Berlemann, U. and Schwarzenbach, O., "Dens fractures in the elderly," *Acta Orthop. Scand.* 68, 319, 1997.
57. Kirk, W.S., Jr., "Risk factors and initial surgical failures of TMJ arthrotomy and arthroplasty; a four to nine year evaluation of 303 surgical procedures," *Oral Surg.*, 16, 154, 1998.
58. Moffet, J.D., "General orthopaedic principles," in *The Aging Skeleton,* Rosen, C.J., Glowacki, J., and Bilezikian, J.P., Eds., Academic Press, San Diego, 1999, 383.
59. Barrios, C., Brostrom, L.A., Stark, A., et al., "Healing complications after internal fixation of trochanteric hip fractures: the prognostic value of osteoporosis," *J. Orthop. Trauma*, 7, 438, 1993.
60. Kubo, T., Shiga, T., Hashimoto, J., et al., "Osteoporosis influences the late period of fracture healing in a rat model prepared by ovariectomy and low calcium diet," *J. Steroid Biochem. Mol. Biol.*, 68, 197, 1999.
61. Blythe, J.G. and Buchsbaum, H.J., "Fracture healing in estrogen-treated and castrated rats," *Obstet. Gynecol.*, 48, 351, 1976.
62. Langeland, N., "Effects of oestradiol-17B benzoate treatment on fracture healing and bone collagen synthesis in female rats," *Acta Endocrinol.*, 80, 603, 1975.
63. Nordsletten, L., Madsen, J.E., Almaas, R., et al., "The neuronal regulation of fracture healing," *Acta Orthop. Scand.*, 65, 299, 1994.
64. Fokter, S.K. and Vengust, V., "Displaced subcapital fracture of the hip in transient osteoporosis of pregnancy," *Int. Orthop.*, 21, 201, 1997.
65. Miyakoshi, N., Sato, K., Murai, H., et al., "Insufficiency fractures of the distal tibiae," *J. Orthop. Sci.*, 5, 71, 2000.

5 Animal Models of Osteoporosis

Kazuo Hayashi and Abbas Fotovati

CONTENTS

I. INTRODUCTION

Using animal models is considered a major method for studying osteoporosis in humans. Limitations in studying on human osteopenic patients, especially regarding new therapeutic methods, leave animal models as the only applicable choice.

There are several animal models with induced osteoporosis, including (1) endocrine deficiency-induced, mostly through ovariectomy (OVX) with the aim of making a model that mimics the postmenopausal woman, and orchiectomy in males; (2) steroid-induced, using exogenous gluco-corticoids; (3) mechanically induced, i.e., immobilization, resulting in disuse osteoporosis; (4) inflammatory-induced, through injection of irritant material into the joints; and recently (5) gene manipulation-induced osteoporosis. Using a calcium/vitamin D-restricted diet or feeding excessive phosphorus and vitamin C also induces osteoporosis. The availability of these methods depends on various factors including animal species. The result achieved using a particular method

TABLE 5.1
Reproductive Parameters of Animal Species Used as Animal Models for Osteoporosis

Species	Age of Puberty	Age of Sexual Maturity	Type of Estrus Cycle	Length of Estrus Cycle
Mouse	4–6(w)	6–8 (w)	Polyestrus	4–6 (d)
Rat	7–10 (w)	8–10 (w)	Polyestrus	4–5 (d)
Guinea pig	7–8 (w)	3–4 (m)	Polyestrus	16.5 (d)
Rabbit	4 (m)	5–9 (m)	Polyestrus	Not regular
Ferret	9–12 (m)	12 (m)	Seasonal (long-day) polyestrus	Not regular
Cat	5–12 (m)	6–12 (m)	Polyestrus	14–21 (d)
Dog	6–12 (m)	6–12 (m)	Unseasonally monoestrus	3 (d)–13 (m)
Sheep	7–10 (m)	10 (m)	Seasonal (short-day) polyestrus	14–19 (d)
Pig	5–8 (m)	10 (m)	Polyestrus	16–56 (w)
Cynomolgus monkey	2–4 (y)	4–5 (y)	Menstrual	28 (d)
Rhesus monkey	2–3.5 (y)	3–5 (y)	Menstrual	28 (d)

Abbreviations: (d) = day; (w) = week; (m) = month; (y) = year

in one species might not be compatible with another species. Each species has its own advantages and disadvantages. Therefore, no single animal species has been recognized as the perfect model that precisely mimics human (especially postmenopausal) osteoporosis.[1]

II. ANIMAL MODELS OF OSTEOPOROSIS
INDUCED BY OVARIECTOMY

Most animals maintain their reproductive capacity throughout their entire lives and never experience natural menopause.[2] Therefore, using them as a model for studying the adverse effects of menopause, including osteoporosis, is not practical for many species. However, as it is observed that women who undergo premenopausal bilateral OVX prematurely experience the symptoms and side effects of menopause soon after surgery, OVX animals can be used as valuable models. Bilateral removal of the ovaries in a middle-aged animal induces a menopausal-like state comparable to human menopause. However, there are some factors that should be considered for development of a reliable model. The model animal should have a cyclic reproduction resembling the human menstrual cycle. In such a model, bone is affected by fluctuations in reproductive hormones during the cycle throughout the year as in humans. Animals with seasonal breeding, which experience reproductive cycles once or twice a year, generally cannot reflect postmenopausal bone changes after OVX.[3] Reproductive characteristics of various animals used as models in osteoporosis are presented in Table 5.1.[4]

A. MOUSE

OVX mice have been used as a model for postmenopausal osteoporosis. They are small, cheap, easy to manage, and have cyclic reproduction. Although OVX mice have been used less frequently than rats, the availability of genetic manipulation in this model is considered an advantage over the rat for future studies (see below). The mechanism and pathogenesis of estrogen deficiency–induced osteoporosis and also therapeutic and diagnostic methods used for treatment and diagnosis of osteoporosis have been studied in OVX mice.

The mechanism of estrogen involvement in bone metabolism has been described in OVX mice. Estrogen is considered the main physiologic regulator of calcium absorption, at least in the C57BL strain of mice, and calcium malabsorption in OVX mice shares many characteristics with intestinal calcium malabsorption and its reversal by estrogen therapy in hypoestrogenic women.[5]

The OVX mouse model showed the central role of estrogen-regulated cytokines, such as tumor necrosis factor (TNF) and interleukins (IL) in the mechanism by which estrogen deficiency causes bone loss.[6] Among these cytokines, TNF is thought to play the most important role.[7] However, infusion of recombinant murine IL-4 (rmIL-4) rapidly inhibits not only bone resorption but also its formation in both sham-operated and OVX growing mice, resulting in a low rate of bone turnover without modulating bone volume.[8]

Although growth hormone (GH) increases bone growth, failure of GH to increase bone mass in OVX mice proved the necessity of intact ovary for GH function.[9]

The effect of various factors on bone metabolism in mice has been investigated in OVX model. For example, cadmium accelerates bone loss in OVX mice, possibly through direct action on bone, which may be the cause of the increased risk of postmenopausal osteoporosis among women who smoke.[10]

The effects of various antiresorptive and bone anabolic agents have also been studied in the OVX model. For example, parathyroid hormone (PTH) restored trabecular network through increased osteoblast activity[11] while estrogen reduced bone loss through decrease in bone resorption in OVX mice.[12]

Integrin ligands such as echistatin showed a rate-limiting role in osteoclastic bone resorption in OVX mice and are suggested as potential therapeutic agents for suppression of bone loss.[13]

Effectiveness of various diagnostic techniques for osteoporosis has also been evaluated in OVX mice. Using dual-energy X-ray absorptiometry (DEXA) and peripheral quantitative computed tomography (pQCT) for evaluation of bone changes in OVX mice before and after treatment with PTH showed that pQCT is more sensitive than DEXA in the detection of bone loss after OVX and increased bone mass after PTH treatment in mice.[14]

In addition to female mice, estrogen withdrawal in male mice also caused osteoporosis. Comparative study on the effects of steroid withdrawal on mandible condyle morphology in both female and male mice through OVX and orchiectomy (ORX), respectively, showed that both methods effectively reduced trabecular bone volume.[15]

Finally, the OVX mouse can aid understanding of some aspects of postmenopausal osteoporosis. Because mice can be genetically manipulated, the mouse is a useful tool for elucidating the role of the factors claimed to be involved in development of osteoporosis in postmenopausal women.

B. Rat

Rats are considered the preferred animal model for studying the bone changes associated with loss of reproductive function.[3] Several hundred studies have used the OVX rat as model for studying various aspects of bone metabolism and osteoporosis. Rats are inexpensive, small in size so easily manageable, and have a short life span enabling studies on the effect of aging on bone metabolism. Additionally, they have reproductive cycles resembling humans. The rat maintained continuously under laboratory conditions will have estrus cycles (so-called polyestrus) of 4 to 5 days duration. Therefore, the rat skeleton will be affected by regular fluctuations in gonadal steroids. This makes rats more sensitive to the loss of ovarian hormones compared to species having only one estrus (monoestrus) cycle per year such as dog.[16] For these reasons, the rat is the most popular animal model used for osteoporosis, especially postmenopausal osteoporosis.

OVX-induced bone loss in the rat and postmenopausal bone loss share many similar characteristics:

1. Increased rate of bone turnover with resorption exceeding formation
2. Initial rapid phase of bone loss following by a much slower phase
3. Greater loss of cancellous than cortical bone
4. Decreased intestinal absorption of calcium
5. Some protection against bone loss by obesity
6. Similar skeletal response to therapy with estrogen, tamoxifen, bisphosphonates, parathyroid hormone, calcitonin, and exercise[17]

After OVX in the rat, there are transient increases in endochondral growth, periosteal apposition, and cancellous bone.[16] Osteopenia is mostly evident in the central metaphyseal cancellous areas of the long bones. Administration of estrogen completely blocks the activation of bone turnover and bone loss. Therefore, increased bone turnover and loss of cancellous bone following OVX is considered a direct result of estrogen deficiency.[18] OVX-induced bone turnover is also age related, more severe in growing young than in aged rats.[18] Changes in the trabecular architecture were different from those that have been observed in the proximal tibia. This difference was a consequence of the much more plate-like structure of the trabecular bone in the vertebrae.[19]

OVX rats also show an increased weight gain. Increased body weight is entirely due to increased body fat and not increased lean body mass.[18] Additionally, OVX rats eat approximately 10% more than sham controls.[20] Increased weight tends to suppress the loss of cancellous bone, possibly because of increased mechanical loads on the skeleton.

Alteration in some biochemical parameters has been observed in OVX rat. Adult OVX rats showed increased urinary calcium excretion similar to postmenopausal woman.[21] Urine hydroxyproline excretion was also positively correlated with calcium.

Therapeutic agents used or proposed to be effective for postmenopausal osteoporosis are mainly divided into two groups: (1) those that reduce bone loss (antiresorptive), which inhibit osteoclasts, e.g., bisphosphonates,[22] calcitonins,[23] estrogens,[24] and (2) selective estrogen receptor modulators (SERMs),[25] which increase new bone growth through osteoblast, e.g., PTH[26,27] and fluoride.[28] Both groups have been tried in OVX osteoporotic rats.

Bisphosphonates have been used in OVX rats and ultrastructural properties of bone mineral have been described.[29] Calcitonin reduced bone loss, especially in the vertebral body, and prevented progress of the OVX-induced osteoporosis.[30] Because the main mechanism of OVX-induced osteoporosis is attributed to estrogen deficiency, estrogen or selective estrogen receptor modulators have been used in rat model.[25]

PTH has been used alone and together with other agents. Concomitant administration of PTH with OPG[31] or GH[32] was more effective in correction of OVX-induced osteoporosis than PTH alone. Several PTH-related peptides have also been tried in this model.[33]

Prostaglandin E2 (PGE2) and its analogues have been reported to produce a bone anabolic response in OVX rat model, and thus may be useful as potential treatments for osteoporosis.[34-36]

Oral prophylactic application of low doses of active vitamin D metabolites can effectively prevent the osteopenia induced by OVX in the axial skeleton of the rat.[37]

There are some other agents claimed to improve osteopenia associated with estrogen deficiency in OVX rats. Systemic administration of activin, a member of the transforming growth factor (TGF) superfamily, increased both bone mass and mechanical strength of vertebral bodies in aged OVX rats. Therefore, it might be considered a possible therapeutic agent for fracture and osteoporosis.[38] Amylin, a peptide co-secreted with insulin by pancreatic beta cells, inhibits bone resorption and stimulates osteoblastic activity in OVX rats.[39]

In addition to chemical therapeutic agents, OVX rats have also been used for evaluation of prosthetic materials including implants, screws, and bone–prosthetic interlocking material, which are commonly used for correction of defects associated with osteoporosis. Because such materials are designed for the patient with osteopenia, their efficacy also should be evaluated in an osteopenic animal model. Authors have evaluated bone reactions to several kinds of prosthetic implants containing hydroxyapatite (HA) or other interlocking materials in OVX rat.[40-42] Results of studies by the authors showed a considerable affinity between osteoporotic bone and HA.

Various diagnostic techniques used for osteoporosis have also been evaluated in OVX rat. DEXA and pQCT were used for detection of bone changes after OVX and treatment with PTH. As observed in OVX mice,[14] pQCT in rat was a more sensitive, reproducible, noninvasive method for monitoring changes in bone mass.[43]

The OVX rat model has been used for studying osteoporosis in oral and maxillofacial bone structures. Areas formed by intramembranous ossification, such as maxillae, sustained fewer effects due to OVX compared to areas formed by endochondral ossification, such as distal femurs.[44] However, increase in masticatory function reported in OVX rats might affect the structure of the mandible.[20] Existing osteoporosis itself may not be capable of causing periodontal destruction.[45] Furthermore, several common therapeutic agents used for general osteoporosis affect osseous tissues in the oral cavity, and this may influence the progression of diseases.[46] For example, systemic intermittent PTH therapy stimulates bone formation in the mandibles in aged OVX rats.[26]

Although using the rat as a model for studying postmenopausal bone changes has many advantages, there are still a few disadvantages preventing its acceptance as a perfect, reliable model. For example, although bone changes after OVX in the short term mimic postmenopausal changes, in the long term (12 months) they are different.[18] Therefore, the results gained in the short term after OVX should be considered carefully.

A sex steroid–deficient model has also been developed in the male rat. Hormone withdrawal symptoms in patients with prostate cancer are accompanied by considerable osteoporosis-related side effects, so an orchiectomized rat model was developed. There was an increased fracture risk in such rats possibly due to reduced bone formation and unchanged bone loss combined with mild metabolic acidosis. Calcium and alkalization seem to be effective prophylaxis for androgen deprivation. [47]

C. Rabbit

Although rabbits are the smallest species known to have Haversian bone remodeling processes, there are only few bone studies in OVX rabbits and the results are confounded by the effects of dietary calcium.[3] However, there are some studies suggesting OVX-induced loss of bone mass at least in some parts of body such as vertebrae.[48] The effects of OVX on the function of the vascular system in bone have been studied. The results showed a relation between altered vascular function after ovarian hormonal withdrawal and the changes in bone turnover associated with osteoporosis.[49]

D. Dog

Although some workers have shown bone loss at least at early phase after OVX,[50-52] generally bone studies conducted on the OVX dog suggest that it is a poor model for menopausal osteoporosis.[53] This might be due to having only one estrus cycle (monestrus) per year in the dog, compared to humans and other animal species that are polyestrus. The obvious reason for considering the OVX dog as a poor model for osteoporosis is that ovariohysterectomy is a very common procedure in pet dogs, but osteoporosis is not a problem in these animals.

In contrast to OVX dog, orchiectomized male dogs showed a loss of bone volume accompanying the fall in sex hormone levels following orchiectomy. Therefore, the orchiectomized dog is suggested as an animal model for studying osteoporosis caused by hypogonadism in men.[54]

The only advantage of dogs in the study of osteoporosis is that they have Haversian systems of cortical bone internal bone remodeling of cortical and trabecular bone similar to that of humans.[55]

E. Swine

Similar reproductive cycle (duration and continuity of reproduction throughout the year) and also similar feeding system, i.e., omnivorous, are advantages of using swine as a model for human osteoporosis. However, there are some disadvantages. Information available on OVX mature pigs used for bone studies is limited: regular pigs have large size and are difficult to manage. Although minipigs are small, they are relatively expensive.[3] Sensitivity of bone density to dietary calcium is another important physiologic limiting factor in this model. OVX in sows did not show any histomorphometric signs of osteopenia/osteoporosis, unless a low calcium diet was used.[56] In minipigs, the structural changes also became more pronounced when OVX was combined with mild calcium restriction.[57]

F. SHEEP

The sheep seems to be a promising large animal model for the bone and cardiovascular systems.[3,55] They are docile, easy to handle and house, relatively inexpensive, available in large numbers, spontaneously ovulate, and have hormone profiles similar to those of women.[55] OVX results in a slight loss of bone from the ovine iliac crest, and biochemical markers such as osteocalcin are well characterized. Physiologic disadvantages are lack of natural menopause, limitation of normal estrus cycles to fall and winter, and having a gastrointestinal system different from humans. Sheep have cortical bone that is plexiform in structure although Haversian remodeling is seen in older animals. When and if biomechanical incompetence of bone follows OVX are still unknown.[55]

The ewe has been suggested as a suitable large animal model for assessment of therapeutic agents for treatment of osteoporosis. Using one or a combination of two or three techniques for producing an osteoporotic model in sheep showed that the induction of severe osteoporosis in sheep is best achieved by combined treatment with OVX, calcium/vitamin D–restricted diet, and steroids. There was a good relationship between density, structural parameters, and mechanical properties of bone.[58] However, using OVX and bone mineral density (BMD) measurement has shown that several complicating factors should be considered during the study including seasonal BMD variation, a correlation between fat/lean ratio and total body BMD together with a reversible reduction in bone mineral content as a result of lactation. Changes in BMD are also affected by age at OVX.[59]

Culture of osteoblasts derived from osteopenic bone of OVX ewe showed that sheep osteoblast cultures can be useful when determining biocompatibility and osteointegration of orthopaedic materials, and also when evaluating for the presence of osteoporosis.[60] Development of oral bone loss in OVX ewe[61] has made sheep an ideal model for workers studying osteoporosis in oral and maxillofacial bones.[62]

According to the experiences of a group studying various complications of menopause in a sheep model, it is too early to promote the sheep as the only model to study estrogen deficiency. The many differences from small animal omnivores and nonhuman primates need to be overcome and a search for more economical models must continue. However, sheep as an animal model may offer the opportunity to study postmenopausal conditions and the safety and efficacy of new therapeutic agents.[61]

G. NONHUMAN PRIMATES

Nonhuman primates include a wide range of diverse species. However, only the suborder of "man-like monkeys" (Anthropoidea) is used as an animal model for studying human diseases. Among them, Old World monkeys such as rhesus, cynomolgus and other macaques, and baboons are most frequently used.[63]

Several factors contributed to the popularity of a nonhuman primate animal model in bone studies:

1. FDA regulations demand "large animal" model data for osteoporosis therapeutics, in addition to the data from rodents.[1]
2. Recently, therapeutic agents have been designed based on the human genome; therefore they are not amenable to test in rodents, whereas nonhuman primates share much genetic and postural similarity with humans.
3. Nonhuman primates have similar ovarian and reproductive endocrinology.[63]

Menstrual cycles and even menopause similar to humans is defined only in Old World monkeys. The latter is a major reason for considering the nonhuman primates an ideal model at least for postmenopausal osteoporosis. Menarche occurs in rhesus monkeys (*Macaca mulatta*), cynomolgus monkeys (*M. fascicularis*), and baboons (*Papio* species) between 2 and 4 years of age (age of puberty); however, sexual maturity (first conception) may delay until 4 to 5 years of age. Both macaques have 28-day cycles, and baboons have 33-day cycles.[63] In these species, profiles of estrogen and progesterone during menstrual cycles and even pregnancy have the same patterns as those of women. Natural menopause starting with declining ovarian function and irregular menstrual cycles has been reported in aged macaques and baboons, after 30 and 15 years of age, respectively. Additionally, in these species, bone resorption and formation are also affected by fluctuations of sex steroids; i.e., bone resorption is significantly decreased when estrogen reaches a maximum, just prior to and during ovulation.[64] For this reason, estrogen deficiency encountered during natural and induced menopause affects bone density. After natural menopause in rhesus[65] and OVX-induced menopause in cynomolgus monkeys, there was a decrease in bone density, an increase in bone turnover and its serum indices such as total alkaline phosphatase, osteocalcin, and acid phosphatase, and reduced bone strength, as happens in postmenopausal women.

This evidence supports using surgical OVX-induced menopause models of these species as a reliable method for evaluation of various osteoporosis preventive agents. Although there are some reports indicating some differences in postmenopausal changes between humans and aged monkeys,[66] and the degree of osteopenia in OVX monkeys is small compared with the profound cancellous osteopenia observed in OVX rats, the monkey data are believed to be more comparable with data from women.[63] Increases in bone loss and indices of bone turnover in these models were prevented by physiologic estrogen replacement therapy.[68]

In addition to surgical methods, chemically induced OVX nonhuman primate models have also been developed in rhesus and cynomolgus monkey using gonadotropin-releasing hormone agonist (GnRHa) and bone turnover was measured using biochemical markers.[69-71] They are suggested as valid models for evaluating antiresorptive therapies.

There are some points that should be considered in making an OVX monkey model. Absolute osteopenia in OVX monkeys develops under certain experimental conditions, including absence of open plates, stable bone mass at the time of OVX (usually after 9 years old), and provision of a lower calcium diet, compared to standard laboratory diet.[67] Additionally, the OVX monkey model does not produce consistent, statistically significant osteopenia and bone fragility, as occurs in human postmenopausal osteopenia.

H. OTHER ANIMALS

1. Avian

Egg production has a special impact on bone metabolism of female birds and osteoporosis is a common problem especially in aged high-producing commercial layer chickens. Therefore, they might be considered as a model for osteoporosis, although they are not yet popular.

2. Guinea Pig

The guinea pig is a very commonly used laboratory animal having a long estrus cycle and spontaneous ovulation like humans. However, since OVX showed no effect on bone volume, it is not considered a useful model for studying postmenopausal osteoporosis of humans.[55] Some workers have used OVX guinea pig, mostly as an animal model for the evaluation of new therapeutics for osteoarthritis rather than osteoporosis. [72]

3. Ferret

As a small animal model, the ferret has been used as a model for bone metabolic unit (BMU)-based remodeling to mimic the bone loss found in postmenopausal women.[73] Estrogen withdrawal in the ferret can be induced by either surgical removal of ovaries or shortening the daylight (since the ferret has a long-day reproductive season).

Ferrets reach skeletal maturity between 4 and 7 months of age as evidenced by closure of the growth plate and maturation of trabeculae from thin rods to thick rods and plates. PTH treatment in the ferret resulted in a marked increase in bone mass accompanied by the PTH-induced tunneling phenomenon known to occur in dogs and humans but not rats. The response to PTH supports the use of the ferret in studies of bone anabolic agents. Bone mass in the proximal tibia was significantly reduced when estrogen depletion was induced by either bilateral OVX or short light/dark cycles (8 hours light, 16 hours dark). Maintenance of intact ferrets under short-light conditions mimicked ovariectomy in terms of serum estrogen levels, uterine weights, and tibia (see above).[73]

4. Cat

Osteoporosis due to using an all-meat diet in growing cats is a common problem of veterinary small animal practice. Therefore, it might be considered as a model for studying osteoporosis. However, using the OVX cat as an osteoporotic model is not seen to be practical, as there is no evidence of increased incidence of osteoporosis in domestic cats, the majority of which are ovario-hysterectomized.[55]

III. ANIMAL MODELS OF STEROID-INDUCED SYSTEMIC OSTEOPOROSIS

Bone loss is the most common and serious side effect of long-term glucocorticosteroid (GC) therapy in humans. GC-mediated reduction in bone density is due to several mechanisms, including (1) direct impairment of osteoblasts and osteocytes; (2) GCs, which antagonize gonadal function and inhibit the osteoanabolic action of sex steroids; and (3) increased renal elimination and reduced intestinal absorption of calcium, leading to a negative calcium balance. This promotes secondary hyperparathyroidism. The effects of PTH might also be more pronounced in the presence of GCs, whereas vitamin D plays a lesser role in the pathogenesis of steroid-induced osteoporosis.[74]

Several small and large animal species have been used as models for steroid-induced osteoporosis.

The mouse is considered a valid and informative model of GC-induced bone disease, not confounded by weight loss or sex steroid deficiency. Many of the effects of chronic GC administration on bone are suggested to be due to decreased development of osteoblast and osteoclast precursors and increased apoptosis of mature osteoblasts and osteocytes.[75]

In rats, GCs decrease endochondral growth and bone formation rates, and at higher doses they reduce osteoclast population.[16] In the growing rat skeleton, GH can counteract most GC-induced side effects, except decreases in the mineralizing surface of cancellous bone of the vertebral body.[76] Administration of cyclosporine to rats also accelerates bone remodeling and causes bone loss.[77]

In rabbits, GCs increase bone resorption and decrease bone formation and mass.[16] Total body bone mineral also decreases. The histomorphometric profile of GC-induced osteoporosis, particularly the lower bone volume and thinner and fewer trabecular plates, has been observed in a rabbit model. Additionally, mechanical tests such as vertebral compression tests show a very significant reduction in bone strength, which is obviously correlated with histomorphometric or densitometric results.[78] Additionally, for testing the hypothesis that systemic GC therapy adversely affects fracture healing, a rabbit ulnar osteotomy model was developed and DEXA confirmed that the bone mineral content was lower in the ulnae of GC-treated rabbits, both within the defect and in adjacent ulnar bone, concluding that chronic GC treatment clearly inhibits bone healing.[79]

Interaction of GC in lipid metabolism and osteoporosis has been studied in rabbit. Induced hypercortisonism in rabbits produces severe hyperlipidemia, fatty liver, systemic fat emboli, terminal vascular obstruction in bone and associated areas of osteocytic death representing avascular necrosis. Osteoporosis develops without fracture.[80] In addition, elevated cholesterol levels are suggested to be involved in this phenomenon through alteration in the osteocyte cell membranes and resulting cell dysfunction. The elevated marrow lipids may also contribute to the development of osteonecrosis by increasing intramedullary pressure and causing venous stasis.[81] Hence, it is suggested that concomitant use of lipid-clearing agents with steroids might have the potential to decrease the severity of steroid-induced osteoporosis.[82]

In addition to skeletal bone, the rabbit with steroid-induced osteoporosis has been used as a model for studying osteoporosis in maxillofacial bone structures. In female rabbit models, mandibular bone mineral density decreases in relation to spinal density and cumulative steroid dose.[83] Osseointegration of titanium implants in the mandible was less affected by steroid-induced osteoporosis, compared with those implanted in skeletal bone.[84] In addition to steroids, heparin has also been studied for induction of osteoporosis in rabbits and the mechanical properties of bones in heparin-treated rabbits indicated osteoporosis.[85]

Larger animals also have been used as models for steroid-induced osteoporosis. In dogs, GCs decreased bone formation and bone mass. However, they did not alter rates of bone formation.[16] Using salmon calcitonin in this model attenuates the early bone loss induced by GCs. However, it failed to prevent GC-induced osteoblast dysfunction.[86]

In sheep, GC therapy reduced biochemical and histomorphometric indices of bone formation.[16] Reduction of bone formation is estimated by some workers to be about 84%.[87] Aged ewes, i.e., more than 9 years old, are considered ideal models.[87]

IV. ANIMAL MODELS OF LOCAL OSTEOPOROSIS

There are some animal models with osteoporosis only induced in a limited area of the body, compared to OVX or steroid-induced osteoporosis, which affect general bone structures. Osteoporosis induced by "disuse" and "joint inflammation" are two common examples of this category of osteoporosis.

A. Disuse Osteoporosis

Low-level mechanical signals are considered key determinants of bone mass and morphology. Therefore, reduction of mechanical stress on bone inhibits osteoblast-mediated bone formation and accelerates osteoclast-mediated bone resorption, leading to so-called disuse osteoporosis. Prolonged therapeutic bed rest, immobilization due to motor paralysis from injury of the central nervous system or peripheral nerves, and application of casts to treat fractures are common etiologies of disuse osteoporosis.[88]

Several species have been used as models for disuse osteoporosis, including mouse, rat, rabbit, turkey, cat, dog, sheep, and monkey. Additionally, various methods have been used for making such models: neurectomy for sciatic nerve,[89] spinal,[90] hind limb tenotomy,[91] casting of limbs,[92] leg bandaging,[93] internal[94] and external[95,96] joint fixation including fixation to the animal's body itself,[97] tail denervation[98] and tail suspension,[99] injection of *Clostridium botulinum* toxin,[100] chair immobilization (semirecumbent) for primates,[101,102] motor activity restriction (hypokinesia),[103] limb lengthening,[104] suspension "hypokinesia/hypodynamia,"[105] and even spaceflight.[106]

In a mouse disuse model, unilateral cast immobilization has a dual negative effect on bone turnover involving both depressed bone formation and enhanced bone resorption.[107] Disuse osteopenia has been studied in mdx mice (X-linked muscular dystrophy) and this model might be useful in understanding the changes in bone mass and muscle–bone attachments in humans with disuse osteoporosis.[108] Induction of disuse by suspension "hypokinesia/hypodynamia" in OVX mouse resulted in extensive trabecular bone loss in association with an increase of osteoclasts.[105]

In rats, limb immobilization was associated with a rapid loss of cancellous bone with transient decreases in bone formation but increases in bone resorption.[16] Histological examination showed rapid and extensive trabecular bone loss, and a substantial part of the decrease in bone mass was due to actual trabecular bone loss and not the reduction of external bone volume.[109] A short period of immobilization significantly distorts the normal allometric scaling relationships between the body weight and femoral bone mineral content (BMC) and BMD in growing male rats. Immobilization during growth may condemn the given bone to a lifetime of relative fragility.[110] Intensified remobilization (more than normal activity) will restore BMC and BMD. However, this hyperactivity probably is needed forever and its termination will halt the recovery process.[111] Very low magnitude mechanical stimuli when used at a high frequency were strongly osteogenic even when applied for very short duration and effectively restore anabolic activity compromised in the disuse-induced rat model.[112] In the sciatic neurectomy model of disuse osteoporosis, applying capacitively coupled electrical signal to the denervated tibia prevented or recovered disuse osteoporosis through increasing the rate of bone formation and not decreasing rate of bone resorption.[113] Kangaroo rats (*Dipodomys ordii*) have been used as a disuse model and they are also suggested as an effective model in the study of disuse osteoporosis.[114]

Short-term limb immobilization in rabbit showed that tibial plateau and femoral condyle of the immobilized limb exhibited prominent subchondral vascular eruptions. Morphological and histochemical evidence collectively suggest that bone loss and remodeling preceded erosive cartilage degradation in immobilized limb of rabbit.[115] In addition, administration of 1,25-dihydroxyvitamin-D_3 exaggerates disuse and prednisolone-induced osteoporosis and impairs fracture healing in rabbits, which is in contrast to what is seen in rat.[116] However, pamidronate, a bisphosphonate, reduced the disuse osteoporosis observed in a limb-lengthening disuse immature rabbit model.[104] An Achilles tendonectomy model is also used and the effects of nandrolone decanoate in preventing, or at least partially correcting, losses of bone mass has been shown.[117]

Disuse osteoporosis developed in a sheep model using hock joint immobilization by an external fixation procedure.[95,96] Although osteoclastic activity was increased in accordance with the usual disuse process, there was an unexpected increase of osteoblastic activity that remains to be defined properly.[96]

In a very interesting study using a sheep model, the mechanism of the adaptability of the skeleton to load bearing was described. Daily mechanical stimulation of adult sheep by very low magnitude, high-frequency vibration significantly increased the density of the spongy (trabecular) bone in the proximal femur. Therefore, using a brief noninvasive stimulus is proposed as a potential way for treating skeletal osteoporosis.[118]

In addition to the above-mentioned animal models, there are a few reports about other animal models. By restraining the monkey in a semirecumbent position, mechanical properties and structural changes in the tibia during the disuse osteoporosis and subsequent recovery have been studied.[101] Progressive changes in compact bone of tibia during osteopenia have also been monitored radiographically.[101]

A turkey disuse model has been developed by functional separation of the ulna, and mechanisms involved in initiation of disuse osteoporosis have been described.[119,120] *In vivo* and *in vitro* results showed that early response of bone to disuse is the upregulation of matrix metalloproteinase-1 activity in osteocytes.[119] Additionally, osteocyte hypoxia and subsequent upregulation of hypoxia-dependent pathways may serve to initiate and mediate disuse-induced bone resorption in this model.[120]

Using cat as a disuse osteoporosis model is limited to two studies,[98,121] one using denervated cat tail as model for disuse osteoporosis.[98]

Finally, although in the all-immobilizing model bone loss occurs, the severity of such response depends on the region and the type of bone examined and also on the duration of immobilization and the age of animal.[97] Thus, the results have to be considered carefully.

B. Joint Inflammation

Chronic inflammatory diseases such as rheumatoid arthritis induce osteoporosis. Several animal models have been used for understanding the pathogenesis of this phenomenon.

An inflammatory model in rat is usually induced by injection of nonspecific irritants. Injection of talc (magnesium silicate) and cotton wool (cellulose) to the rats resulted in loss of bone. Loss of bone was not due to increased PTH secretion, as it also occurred in parathyroidectomized rats, nor due to excessive 1,25-dihydroxyvitamin-D_3 production. In parathyroidectomized rats, this inflammation was associated with significant increase in serum calcium within 4 to 7 days, independent of its cause.[122]

Rats with collagen-induced arthritis (CIA) have been used to clarify the mechanisms of osteoporosis near inflamed joints in patients with early rheumatoid arthritis (RA) and juvenile RA, and the results showed that osteoporosis near inflamed joints is due to an imbalance between bone resorption and formation caused by immune reactions in the CIA rats. Moreover, a decrease in bone formation may, in part, precede the clinical onset of arthritis.[123] Other studies showed that bone loss in adult CIA rats resembles the osteoporosis that develops during the early stage of human rheumatoid arthritis. In addition, adult CIA rats are considered a more appropriate experimental model of secondary osteoporosis due to rheumatoid arthritis than young CIA rats.[124]

Using carrageenan-induced arthritis in rabbit, the effectiveness of pamidronate in the treatment of RA has been investigated. Pamidronate prevented bone loss in this model of experimental inflammatory arthritis by inhibiting the resorptive activity, but not the formation or recruitment of osteoclasts.[125] The skeletal calcium-to-phosphorus (Ca/P) ratio (used as an index of bone quality) in such animals was significantly lower than in controls. In addition, severe alterations were detected at the ultrastructural level in bone and skin collagen fibrils.[126]

Arthritis induced-osteoporosis has also been developed in a dog model. Intra-articular injections of carrageenan induced a generalized osteoporosis of the arthritic limb.[127]

Further studies on models with arthritis, induced by injection of irritant material, will provide valuable information regarding complications of human arthritis including osteoporosis.

V. ANIMAL MODELS OF GENE MANIPULATION–INDUCED OSTEOPOROSIS

Availability of transgenic technology in mice is an important advantage of this model. Mice deficient or overexpressed in factors involved in bone metabolism are increasingly providing valuable information regarding the molecular basis of changes in bone.

Osteopontin (a major noncollagenous bone matrix protein produced by osteoblasts and osteoclasts) knockout mice are resistant to OVX-induced bone resorption.[128] Overexpression of osteoprotegerin (OPG, known also as osteoclastogenesis inhibitory factor) in transgenic mice resulted in severe osteopetrosis,[129] whereas OPG-deficient mice exhibited a generalized osteoporosis due to increased bone resorption associated with increased numbers and activity of osteoclasts and a high incidence of fractures.[130,131] OPG-deficient mice also developed calcified lesions in the aorta and renal arteries,[130] interestingly similar to osteoporosis in humans, which is associated with a higher incidence of arterial calcification. The osteoporosis in these mice is reversible as it is shown that intravenous injection of recombinant OPG protein and transgenic overexpression of OPG in OPG-deficient mice effectively rescue their osteoporotic bone phenotype.[132]

Mice deficient in c-Abl protein, a nonreceptor tyrosine kinase, develop osteoporosis that is not due to accelerated bone turnover but rather to dysfunctional osteoblasts.[133] Biglycan (bgn) is an extracellular matrix component (ECM) proteoglycan that is enriched in bone and other nonskeletal connective tissues and may function in connective tissue metabolism by binding to collagen fibrils and TGF-β. Bgn-deficient mice display a phenotype characterized by a reduced growth rate and decreased bone mass that becomes more obvious with age.[134] Mice deficient in another ECM component, osteonectin, have decreased osteoblast and osteoclast numbers, leading to decreased bone remodeling with a negative bone balance and profound osteopenia. Therefore, these mice may serve as an animal model to study the role of ECM proteins in osteoporosis.[135]

Obesity leads to high bone density and protects individuals from osteoporosis. For understanding the mechanism underlying this phenomenon two mouse models of obesity, leptin-deficient (ob/ob) and leptin receptor-deficient (db/db) mice, have been developed.[136] Both mutant mice have an increased bone formation leading to high bone mass despite hypogonadism and hypercortisolism. Therefore, leptin is identified as a potent inhibitor of bone formation acting through the central nervous system. This indicates the central nature of bone mass control and its disorders. Mice deficient in insulin receptor substrates (IRS) also showed osteopenia. IRS1 (and also IRS2) is essential for intracellular signaling by insulin and IGF-1, anabolic regulators of bone metabolism. Mice lacking the *Irs1* gene have reduced osteoblastic proliferation and differentiation, and osteoclastogenesis is impaired, resulting in severe low-turnover osteopenia.[137] Mice with disrupted klotho locus (KL–/– or *klotho* mouse) exhibit a decrease in bone formation exceeding the decrease in bone resorption, which results in net bone loss.[138] This pathophysiology resembles that of senile osteoporosis in humans.

Although not all of the thus-far-manipulated factors are defined as the important factors involved in human osteoporosis, the future of the mouse as a tool to map the genes that define the osteoporosis syndrome is extremely promising.[139]

In addition to genetically manipulated mice, Senescence-Accelerated Mouse (SAM) strains have been developed by using an inbreeding system.[140] Among SAM strains, SAMP6 mice are considered a murine model for senile osteoporosis. They have low peak bone mass and after 4 or 5 months of age, when bone mass is at peak, they show a slow, constant loss of bone with age. Hence, the elderly mice of this strain are prone to fracture and could be considered valuable models for study of senile osteoporosis seen clinically.[141]

VI. NATURAL ANIMAL MODELS USED FOR STUDYING OSTEOPOROSIS

In addition to the above-mentioned models with induced osteoporosis, there are some natural (non-osteopenic) animal models used for evaluation of therapeutic and diagnostic methods used for human osteoporosis. Sometimes these models are just aged animals showing aging-induced bone changes. Old female sheep, which have a slow bone remodeling activity resembling the bone remodeling of elderly women, are a good model for studying osteoporosis drug therapy in elderly patients.[142] For example, PTH is a stimulator of bone turnover and has an anabolic effect, i.e., increasing trabecular bone mass. However, it has a resorptive side effect, limiting its use in the treatment of osteoporosis. For elimination of the resorptive side effect of PTH, it was coadministered with bisphosphonate, a potent antiresorptive in the old ewe model. Results showed that in old ewes (which have a slow bone remodeling activity that resembles that of elderly women) PTH coadministered with bisphosphonate loses its anabolic effect, in contrast to the results in the growing rat.[142]

Bone changes in aged monkeys have also been studied and they are considered a good model for studying age-related changes in human bone metabolism.[143,144]

Some diagnostic methods have also been evaluated in natural animals. Densitometry techniques have been performed in intact sheep, and it was shown that highly precise, accurate densitometry can be performed on excised small and large sheep bones, supporting studies evaluating the sheep as an animal model of human osteoporosis.[145] Intact pigs have been used for evaluation of ultrasound technique in screening for osteoporosis and the results provide useful indications for interpreting the findings of clinical investigations, most specifically those performed on the phalanx of the hand.[146]

The fixation of fractured bone with screws is important in orthopaedic surgery. However, rigid fixation often cannot be attained in elderly patients with osteoporosis. Hence, an intact rabbit model has been used for evaluation of cements used for augmenting screw fixation. Cancellous screw fixation augmented with CAP, a cement that directly bonds with bone without intervening fibrous tissue, was effective compared with the unaugmented control *in vivo*.[147]

Intact animals have been used for studying side effects of prosthetics such as plates. Plates used for fracture fixation produce vascular injury to the underlying cortical bone. During the recovery of the blood supply, temporary osteoporosis is observed as a result of Haversian remodeling of the necrotic bone. This process temporarily reduces the strength of the bone. Using implants scaled to the size of the bone, a comparable cortical vascular damage was found in the tibia and femur of intact sheep and dog. However, using plates that had a smaller contact area with the underlying bone significantly reduced cortical vascular damage. [148]

Intact dogs have been used as models for studying effectiveness, dosing regimens, or side effects of some therapeutic agents used for osteoporosis. Dosing convenience and safety of long-term administration of alendronate, an aminobisphosphonate, for effective management of osteoporosis have been studied in dog.[149,150] Additionally, toxic side effects of cimadronate, a bisphosphonate with potent inhibitory activity on bone resorption, have also been investigated in the dog.[151] Negative effects of calcitonin, an antiresorptive widely used to prevent and treat osteoporosis, on bone quality have been shown in intact dog models.[152]

Intact mini pigs have also been used for evaluation of the effectiveness of fluoride and bisphosphonates for fracture prevention in osteoporosis.[153]

Normal monkeys have also been used for evaluation of several drugs. A study using S12911, a new agent containing strontium, which has shown positive effects on bone mass in various animal models of osteoporosis, showed the strontium salt did not alter bone mineral in monkey.[154]

VII. SUMMARY

Osteoporosis is considered a major problem of aging especially in postmenopausal woman. Several animals have been used as models for studying etiology, pathogenesis, treatment, and prevention of osteoporosis. There are advantages and disadvantages for each, leaving no single animal species as an ideal model. However, because an animal model is the only reliable method for preclinical trial of therapeutic agents used for humans, using more than one species, e.g., a nonhuman primate in addition to a rodent, might give more reliable data, at least for pre-clinical trial of therapeutic agents. OVX animal models, especially rat, have provided valuable information regarding bone postmenopausal changes in humans. In addition to OVX, other methods including glucocorticoid administration, immobilization, and injection of irritant material into the joints have been used for developing steroid-induced, disuse-induced, and inflammation-induced osteoporosis animal models, respectively. The data gained from these models have elucidated some aspects of related types of osteoporosis in humans. Finally, recent introduction of transgenic technology in mice enlightens mechanisms involved in development of osteoporosis at the molecular level.

REFERENCES

1. Food and Drug Administration (FDA), Guidelines for Pre-clinical and Clinical Evaluation of Agents Used in the Prevention or Treatment of Postmenopausal Osteoporosis, FDA Division of Metabolism and Endocrine Drug Products, Washington, D.C., 1994.
2. Kirkwood, T.B.L., "Comparative and evolutionary aspects of longevity," in *Handbook of the Biology of Aging*, Finch, C.E. and Schneider, E.L., Eds., John Wiley & Sons, New York, 1985, 27.
3. Bellino, F.L., "Nonprimate animal models of menopause: workshop report," *Menopause*, 7, 14, 2000.
4. Morrow, D.A., *Current Therapy in Theriogenology*, 2nd ed., W.B. Saunders, Philadelphia, 1986.
5. Kalu, D.N. and Chen, C., "Ovariectomized murine model of postmenopausal calcium malabsorption," *J. Bone Miner. Res.*, 14, 593, 1999.
6. Kitazawa, R., Kimble, R.B., Vannice, J.L., et al., "Interleukin-1 receptor antagonist and tumor necrosis factor binding protein decrease osteoclast formation and bone resorption in ovariectomized mice," *J. Clin. Invest.*, 94, 2397, 1994.

7. Kimble, R.B., Bain, S., and Pacifici, R., "The functional block of TNF but not of IL-6 prevents bone loss in ovariectomized mice," *J. Bone Miner. Res.*, 12, 935, 1997.

8. Okada, Y., Morimoto, I., Ura, K., et al., "Short-term treatment of recombinant murine interleukin-4 rapidly inhibits bone formation in normal and ovariectomized mice," *Bone*, 22, 361, 1998.

9. Sandstedt, J., Tornell, J., Norjavaara, E., et al., "Elevated levels of growth hormone increase bone mineral content in normal young mice, but not in ovariectomized mice," *Endocrinology*, 137, 3368, 1996.

10. Bhattacharyya, M.H., Whelton, B.D., Stern, P.H., et al., "Cadmium accelerates bone loss in ovariectomized mice and fetal rat limb bones in culture," *Proc. Natl. Acad. Sci. U.S.A.,* 85, 8761, 1988.

11. Alexander, J.M., Bab, I., and Fish, S., "Human parathyroid hormone 1-34 reverses bone loss in ovariectomized mice," *J. Bone Miner. Res.*, 16, 1665, 2001.

12. Bain, S.D., Bailey, M.C., Celino, D.L., et al., "High-dose estrogen inhibits bone resorption and stimulates bone formation in the ovariectomized mouse," *J. Bone Miner. Res.,* 8, 435, 1993.

13. Yamamoto, M., Fisher, J.E., and Gentile, M., "The integrin ligand echistatin prevents bone loss in ovariectomized mice and rats," *Endocrinology*, 139, 1411, 1998.

14. Andersson, N., Lindberg, M.K., and Ohlsson, C., "Repeated *in vivo* determinations of bone mineral density during parathyroid hormone treatment in ovariectomized mice," *J. Endocrinol.*, 170, 529, 2001.

15. Fujita, T., Kawata, T., Tokimasa, C., et al., "Breadth of the mandibular condyle affected by disturbances of the sex hormones in ovariectomized and orchiectomized mice," *Clin. Orthod. Res.*, 4, 172, 2001.

16. Miller, S.C., Bowman, B.M., and Jee, W.S., "Available animal models of osteopenia — small and large," *Bone,* 17, 117S, 1995.

17. Kalu, D.N., "The ovariectomized rat model of postmenopausal bone loss," *Bone Miner.*, 15, 175, 1991.

18. Thompson, D.D., Simmons, H.A., Pirie, C.M., and Ke, H.Z., "FDA guidelines and animal models for osteoporosis," *Bone*, 17, 125S, 1995.

19. Kinney, J.H., Haupt, D.L., Balooch, M., et al., "Three-dimensional morphometry of the L6 vertebra in the ovariectomized rat model of osteoporosis: biomechanical implications," *J. Bone Miner. Res.*, 15, 1981, 2000.

20. Elovic, R.P., Hipp, J.A., and Hayes, W.C., "Ovariectomy decreases the bone area fraction of the rat mandible," *Calcif. Tissue Int.*, 56, 305, 1995.

21. Morris, H.A., O'Loughlin, P.D., Mason, R.A., and Schulz, S.R., "The effects of oophorectomy on calcium homeostasis," *Bone*, 17, 169S, 1995.

22. Francis, R.M., "Oral bisphosphonates in the treatment of osteoporosis: a review," *Curr. Ther. Res. Clin. Exp.*, 56, 831, 1995.

23. Civitelli, R., Gonnelli, S., Zacchei, F., et al., "Bone turnover in postmenopausal osteoporosis — effect of calcitonin treatment, " *J. Clin. Invest.*, 82, 1268, 1988.

24. Turner, R.T., Riggs, B.L., and Spelsberg, T.C., "Skeletal effects of estrogen," *Endocr. Rev.,* 15, 275, 1994.

25. Mitlak, B.H. and Cohen, F.J., "In search of optimal long-term female hormone replacement: the potential of selective estrogen receptor modulators," *Horm. Res.*, 48, 155, 1997.

26. Miller, S.C., Hunziker, J., Mecham, M., and Wronski, T.J., "Intermittent parathyroid hormone administration stimulates bone formation in the mandibles of aged ovariectomized rats," *J. Dent. Res.*, 76, 1471, 1997.

27. Lindsay, R., Nieves, J., Henneman, E., et al., "Subcutaneous administration of the amino-terminal fragment of human parathyroid hormone (1-34): kinetics and biochemical response in estrogenized osteoporotic patients," *J. Clin. Endocrinol. Metab.*, 77, 1535, 1993.

28. Ericksen, E.F., Mosekilde, L., and Melsen, F., "Effects of sodium fluoride, calcium phosphonate, and vitamin D2 on bone balance and remodeling in osteoporosis," *Bone*, 6, 381, 1985.

29. Rohanizadeh, R., LeGeros, R.Z., Bohic, S., et al., "Ultrastructural properties of bone mineral of control and tiludronate-treated osteoporotic rat," *Calcif. Tissue Int.*, 67, 330, 2000.

30. Mochizuki, K. and Inoue, T., "Effect of salmon calcitonin on experimental osteoporosis induced by ovariectomy and low-calcium diet in the rat," *J. Bone Miner. Metab.*, 18, 194, 2000.

31. Kostenuik, P.J., Capparelli, C., Morony, S., et al., "OPG and PTH-(1-34) have additive effects on bone density and mechanical strength in osteopenic ovariectomized rats," *Endocrinology,* 142, 4295, 2001.

32. Mosekilde, L., Tornvig, L., Thomsen, J.S., et al., "Parathyroid hormone and growth hormone have additive or synergetic effect when used as intervention treatment in ovariectomized rats with established osteopenia," *Bone*, 26, 643, 2000.

33. Stewart, A.F., Cain, R.L., Burr, D.B., et al., "Six-month daily administration of parathyroid hormone and parathyroid hormone-related protein peptides to adult ovariectomized rats markedly enhances bone mass and biomechanical properties: a comparison of human parathyroid hormone 1-34, parathyroid hormone-related protein 1-36, and SDZ-parathyroid hormone 893," *J. Bone Miner. Res.*, 15, 1517, 2000.

34. Ma, Y.F., Li, X.J., Jee, W.S.S., and McOsker, J., "Effects of prostaglandin E2 and F2 on the skeleton of osteopenic ovariectomized rats," *Bone*, 17, 549, 1995.

35. Ke, H.Z., Shen, V.W., and Qi, H., "Prostaglandin E2 increases bone strength in intact rats and ovariectomized rats with established osteoporosis," *Bone*, 23, 249, 1998.

36. Soper, D.L., Milbank, J.B., Mieling, G.E., et al., "Synthesis and biological evaluation of prostaglandin-F alkylphosphinic acid derivatives as bone anabolic agents for the treatment of osteoporosis," *J. Med. Chem.*, 44, 4157, 2001.

37. Erben, R.G., Weiser, H., Sinowatz, F., et al., "Vitamin D metabolites prevent vertebral osteopenia in ovariectomized rats," *Calcif. Tissue Int.*, 50, 228, 1992.

38. Sakai, R. and Eto, Y., "Involvement of activin in the regulation of bone metabolism," *Mol. Cell Endocrinol.*, 180, 183, 2001.

39. Horcajada-Molteni, M.N., Davicco, M.J., Lebecque, P., et al., "Amylin inhibits ovariectomy-induced bone loss in rats," *J. Endocrinol.*, 165, 663, 2000.

40. Hayashi, K., Uenoyama, K., Matsuguchi, N., et al., "The affinity of bone to hydroxyapatite and alumina in experimentally induced osteoporosis," *J. Arthroplasty*, 4, 257, 1989.

41. Hayashi, K., Uenoyama, K., Mashima, T., and Sugioka, Y., "Remodeling of bone around hydroxyapatite and titanium in experimental osteoporosis," *Biomaterials*, 15, 11, 1994.

42. Hara, T., Hayashi, K., Nakashima, Y., et al., "The effect of hydroxyapatite coating on the bonding of bone to titanium implants in the femora of ovariectomised rats," *J. Bone Joint Surg. Br.*, 81, 705, 1999.

43. Gasser, J.A., "Assessing bone quantity by pQCT," *Bone*, 17, 145S, 1995.

44. Ishihara, A., Sasaki, T., and Debari, K., "Effects of ovariectomy on bone morphology in maxillae of mature rats," *J. Electron. Microsc. (Tokyo)*, 48, 465, 1999.

45. Moriya, Y., Ito, K., and Murai, S., "Effects of experimental osteoporosis on alveolar bone loss in rats," *J. Oral Sci.*, 40, 171, 1998.

46. Hunziker, J., Wronski, T.J., and Miller, S.C., "Mandibular bone formation rates in aged ovariectomized rats treated with anti-resorptive agents alone and in combination with intermittent parathyroid hormone," *J. Dent. Res.*, 79, 1431, 2000.

47. Straub, B., Muller, M., Schrader, M., et al., "Osteoporosis and mild metabolic acidosis in the rat after orchiectomy and their prevention: should prophylactic therapy be administered to patients with androgen deprivation?" *J. Urol.*, 165, 1783, 2001.

48. Lugero, G.G., de Falco Caparbo, V., Guzzo, M.L., et al., "Histomorphometric evaluation of titanium implants in osteoporotic rabbit," *Implant. Dent.*, 9, 303, 2000.

49. Hansen, V.B., Forman, A., Lundgaard, A., et al., "Effects of oophorectomy on functional properties of resistance arteries isolated from the cancellous bone of the rabbit femur," *J. Orthop. Res.*, 19, 391, 2001.

50. Dannucci, G.A., Martin, R.B., and Patterson-Buckendahl, P., "Ovariectomy and trabecular bone remodeling in the dog," *Calcif. Tissue Int.*, 40, 194, 1987.

51. Malluche, H.H., Faugere, M.C., Friedler, R.M., and Fanti, P., "1,25-Dihydroxyvitamin D3 corrects bone loss but suppresses bone remodeling in ovariohysterectomized beagle dogs," *Endocrinology*, 122, 1998, 1988.

52. Faugere, M.C., Friedler, R.M., Fanti, P., and Malluche, H.H., "Bone changes occurring early after cessation of ovarian function in beagle dogs: a histomorphometric study employing sequential biopsies," *J. Bone Miner. Res.*, 5, 263, 1990.

53. Shen, V., Dempster, D.W., Birchman, R., et al., "Lack of changes in histomorphometric, bone mass, and biochemical parameters in ovariohysterectomized dogs," *Bone*, 13, 311, 1992.

54. Fukuda, S. and Iida, H., "Effects of orchidectomy on bone metabolism in beagle dogs," *J. Vet. Med. Sci.*, 62, 69, 2000.

55. Newman, E., Turner, A.S., and Wark, J.D., "The potential of sheep for the study of osteopenia: current status and comparison with other animal models," *Bone*, 16, 277S, 1995.

56. Scholz-Ahrens, K.E., Delling, G., Jungblut, P.W., et al., "Effect of ovariectomy on bone histology and plasma parameters of bone metabolism in nulliparous and multiparous sows," *Z. Ernaehrungswiss.*, 35, 13, 1996.

57. Mosekilde, L., Weisbrode, S.E., Safron, J.A., et al., "Calcium-restricted ovariectomized Sinclair S-1 minipigs: an animal model of osteopenia and trabecular plate perforation," *Bone*, 14, 379, 1993.

58. Lill, C.A., Fluegel, A.K., and Schneider, E., "Sheep model for fracture treatment in osteoporotic bone: a pilot study about different induction regimens," *J. Orthop. Trauma*, 14, 565, 2000.

59. Hornby, S.B., Ford, S.L., Mase, C.A., and Evans, G.P., "Skeletal changes in the ovariectomized ewe and subsequent response to treatment with 17 oestradiol," *Bone*, 17, 389S, 1995.

60. Torricelli, P., Fini, M., Giavaresi, G., et al., "Isolation and characterization of osteoblast cultures from normal and osteopenic sheep for biomaterials evaluation," *J. Biomed. Mater. Res.*, 52, 177, 2000.

61. Thorndike, E.A. and Turner, A.S., "In search of an animal model for postmenopausal diseases," *Front. Biosci.*, 16, 17, 1998.

62. Johnson, R.B., Gilbert, J.A., Cooper, R.C., et al., "Alveolar bone loss one year following ovariectomy in sheep," *J. Periodontol.*, 68, 864, 1997.

63. Jerome, C.P. and Peterson, P.E., "Nonhuman primate models in skeletal research," *Bone*, 29, 1, 2001.

64. Hotchkiss, C.E. and Brommage, R., "Changes in bone turnover during the menstrual cycle in cynomolgus monkeys," *Calcif. Tissue Int.*, 66, 224, 2000.

65. Colman, R.J., Kemnitz, J.W., Lane, M.A., et al., "Skeletal effects of aging and menopausal status in female rhesus macaques," *J. Clin. Endocrinol. Metab.*, 84, 4144, 1999.

66. Chen, Y., Shimizu, M., Sato, K., et al., "Effects of aging on bone mineral content and bone biomarkers in female cynomolgus monkeys," *Exp. Anim.*, 49, 163, 2000.

67. Jerome, C.P., Turner, C.H., and Lees, C.J., "Decreased bone mass and strength in ovariectomized cynomolgus monkeys (*Macaca fascicularis*)," *Calcif. Tissue Int.*, 60, 265, 1997.

68. Adams, M.R., Williams, J.K., Clarkson, T.B., et al., "Effects of oestrogens and progestogens on coronary atherosclerosis and osteoporosis of monkeys," *Baillieres Clin. Obstet. Gynaecol.*, 5, 915, 1991.

69. Mann, D.R., Gould, K.G., and Collins, D.C., "A potential primate model for bone loss resulting from medical oophorectomy or menopause," *J. Clin. Endocrinol. Metabol.*, 71, 105, 1990.

70. Mann, D.R., Rudman, C.G., Akinbami, M.A., and Gould, K.G., "Preservation of bone mass in hypogonadal female monkeys with recombinant human growth hormone administration," *J. Clin. Endocrinol. Metabol.*, 74, 1263, 1992.

71. Stroup, G.B., Hoffman, S.J., Vasko-Moser, J.A., et al., "Changes in bone turnover following gonadotropin-releasing hormone (GnRH) agonist administration and estrogen treatment in cynomolgus monkeys: a short-term model for evaluation of antiresorptive therapy," *Bone*, 28, 532, 2001.

72. Kapadia, R.D., Stroup, G.B., Badger, A.M., et al., "Applications of micro-CT and MR microscopy to study pre-clinical models of osteoporosis and osteoarthritis," *Technol. Health Care*, 6, 361, 1998.

73. Mackey, M.S., Stevens, M.L., Ebert, D.C., et al., "The ferret as a small animal model with BMU-based remodeling for skeletal research," *Bone*, 17, 191S, 1995.

74. Patschan, D., Loddenkemper, K., and Buttgereit, F., "Molecular mechanisms of glucocorticoid-induced osteoporosis," *Bone*, 29, 498, 2001.

75. Weinstein, R.S., Jilka, R.L., Parfitt, A.M., and Manolagas, S.C., "Inhibition of osteoblastogenesis and promotion of apoptosis of osteoblasts and osteocytes by glucocorticoids. Potential mechanisms of their deleterious effects on bone," *J. Clin. Invest.*, 15, 274, 1998.

76. Ortoft, G., Andreassen, T.T., and Oxlund, H., "Growth hormone increases cortical and cancellous bone mass in young growing rats with glucocorticoid-induced osteopenia," *J. Bone Miner. Res.*, 14, 710, 1999.

77. Cvetkovic, M., Mann, G.N., Romero, D.F., et al., "The deleterious effects of long-term cyclosporin A, cyclosporin C, and FK506 on bone mineral metabolism *in vivo*," *Transplantation*, 57, 1231, 1994.

78. Grardel, B., Sutter, B., Flautre, B., et al., "Effects of glucocorticoids on skeletal growth in rabbits evaluated by dual-photon absorptiometry, microscopic connectivity and vertebral compressive strength," *Osteoporos. Int.*, 4, 204, 1994.

79. Waters, R.V., Gamradt, S.C., Asnis, P., et al., "Systemic corticosteroids inhibit bone healing in a rabbit ulnar osteotomy model," *Acta Orthop. Scand.*, 71, 316, 2000.

80. Fisher, D.E., "The role of fat embolism in the etiology of corticosteroid-induced avascular necrosis: clinical and experimental results," *Clin. Orthop.*, 130, 68, 1978.

81. Warman, M. and Boskey, A.L., "Effect of high levels of corticosteroids on the lipids of the long bones of the mature rabbit," *Metab. Bone Dis. Relat. Res.*, 4, 319, 1983.

82. Wang, G.J., Chung, K.C., and Shen, W.J., "Lipid clearing agents in steroid-induced osteoporosis," *J. Formos. Med. Assoc.,* 94, 589, 1995.

83. Southard, T.E., Southard, K.A., Krizan, K.E., et al., "Mandibular bone density and fractal dimension in rabbits with induced osteoporosis," *Oral Surg. Oral Med. Oral Pathol. Oral Radiol. Endod.,* 89, 244, 2000.

84. Fujimoto, T., Niimi, A., Sawai, T., and Ueda, M., "Effects of steroid-induced osteoporosis on osseointegration of titanium implants," *Int. J. Oral Maxillofac. Implants,* 13, 183, 1998.

85. Akkas, N., Yeni, Y.N., Turan, B., et al., "Effect of medication on biomechanical properties of rabbit bones: heparin induced osteoporosis," *Clin. Rheumatol.,* 16, 585, 1997.

86. Lyles, K.W., Jackson, T.W., Nesbitt, T., and Quarles, L.D., "Salmon calcitonin reduces vertebral bone loss in glucocorticoid treated beagles," *Am. J. Physiol.,* 264, E938, 1993.

87. Chavassieux, P., Pastoureau, P., Chapuy, M.C., et al., "Glucocorticoid-induced inhibition of osteoblastic bone formation in ewes: a biochemical and histomorphometric study," *Osteoporos. Int.,* 3, 97, 1993.

88. Takata, S. and Yasui, N., "Disuse osteoporosis," *J. Med. Invest.,* 48, 147, 2001.

89. Zeng, Q.Q., Jee, W.S., Bigornia, A.E., et al., "Time responses of cancellous and cortical bones to sciatic neurectomy in growing female rats," *Bone,* 19, 13, 1996.

90. Orsatti, M.B., Fucci, L.L., Valenti, J.L., and Puche, R.C., "Effect of bicarbonate feeding on immobilization osteoporosis in the rat," *Calcif. Tissue Res.,* 21, 195, 1976.

91. Shaker, J.L., Fallon, M.D., Goldfarb, S., et al., "WR-2721 reduces bone loss after hindlimb tenotomy in rats," *J. Bone Miner. Res.,* 4, 885, 1989.

92. Uhthoff, H.K., Sekaly, G., and Jaworski, Z.F., "Effect of long-term nontraumatic immobilization on metaphyseal spongiosa in young adult and old beagle dogs," *Clin. Orthop.,* 192, 278, 1985.

93. Jee, W.S., Li, X.J., and Ke, H.Z., "Skeletal adaptations to mechanical usage in the rat," *Cell Mater.,* 1S, 131, 1991.

94. Klein, L., Player, J.S., Heiple, K.G., et al., "Isotopic evidence for resorption of soft tissues and bone in immobilized dogs," *J. Bone Joint Surg. Am.,* 64, 225, 1982.

95. Thomas, T., Skerry, T.M., Vico, L., et al., "Ineffectiveness of calcitonin on a local-disuse osteoporosis in the sheep: a histomorphometric study," *Calcif. Tissue Int.,* 57, 224, 1995.

96. Thomas, T., Vico, L., Skerry, T.M., et al., "Architectural modifications and cellular response during disuse-related bone loss in calcaneus of the sheep," *J. Appl. Physiol.,* 80, 198, 1996.

97. Grynpas, M.D., Kasra, M., Renlund, R., and Pritzker, K.P., "The effect of pamidronate in a new model of immobilization in the dog," *Bone,* 17, 225S, 1995.

98. Ellsasser, J.C., Moyer, C.F., Lesker, P.A., and Simmons, D.J., "Effect of low doses of disodium ethane-1-hydroxy-1,1-diphosphonate on disuse osteoporosis in the denervated cat tail," *Clin. Orthop.,* 91, 235, 1973.

99. Kawano, S., Kanda, K., Ohmori, S., et al., "Effect of estrogen on the development of disuse atrophy of bone and muscle induced by tail-suspension in rats," *Environ. Med.,* 41, 89, 1997.

100. Chappard, D., Chennebault, A., Moreau, M., et al., "Texture analysis of X-ray radiographs is a more reliable descriptor of bone loss than mineral content in a rat model of localized disuse induced by the *Clostridium botulinum* toxin," *Bone,* 28, 72, 2001.

101. Young, D.R. and Schneider, V.S., "Radiographic evidence of disuse osteoporosis in the monkey (*M. nemestrina*)," *Calcif. Tissue Int.,* 33, 631, 1981.

102. Young, D.R., Niklowitz, W.J., Brown, R.J., and Jee, W.S., "Immobilization-associated osteoporosis in primates," *Bone,* 7, 109, 1986.

103. Zorbas, Y.G., Naexu, K.A., and Federenko, Y.F., "Mechanisms of osteoporosis development during prolonged restriction of motor activity in dog," *Rev. Esp. Fisiol.,* 50, 47, 1994.

104. Little, D.G., Cornell, M.S., Briody, J., et al., "Intravenous pamidronate reduces osteoporosis and improves formation of the regenerate during distraction osteogenesis. A study in immature rabbits," *J. Bone Joint Surg. Br.,* 83, 1069, 2001.

105. Kawata, T., Fujita, T., Tokimasa, C., et al., "Suspension 'hypokinesia/hypodynamia' may decrease bone mass by stimulating osteoclast production in ovariectomized mice," *J. Nutr. Sci. Vitaminol. (Tokyo),* 44, 581, 1998.

106. Morey, E.R. and Baylink, D.J., "Inhibition of bone formation during spaceflight," *Science,* 201, 1138, 1978.

107. Rantakokko, J., Uusitalo, H., Jamsa, T., et al., "Expression profiles of mRNAs for osteoblast and osteoclast proteins as indicators of bone loss in mouse immobilization osteopenia model," *J. Bone Miner. Res.*, 14, 1934, 1999.

108. Anderson, J.E., Lentz, D.L., and Johnson, R.B., "Recovery from disuse osteopenia coincident to restoration of muscle strength in mdx mice," *Bone*, 14, 625, 1993.

109. Tuukkanen, J., Wallmark, B., and Jalovaara, P., "Changes induced in growing rat by immobilization and remobilization," *Bone,* 12, 113, 1991.

110. Sievanen, H., Kannus, P., and Jarvinen, T.L., "Immobilization distorts allometry of rat femur: implications for disuse osteoporosis," *Calcif. Tissue Int.*, 60, 387, 1997.

111. Kannus, P., Järvinen, T.L.N., and Sievänen, H., "Effects of immobilization, three forms of remobilization and subsequent deconditioning on bone mineral content and density in rat femora," *J. Bone Miner. Res.,* 11, 1339, 1996.

112. Rubin, C., Xu, G., and Judex, S., "The anabolic activity of bone tissue, suppressed by disuse, is normalized by brief exposure to extremely low-magnitude mechanical stimuli," *FASEB J.,* 15, 2225, 2001.

113. Brighton, C.T., Tadduni, G.T., Goll, S.R., and Pollack, S.R., "Treatment of denervation/disuse osteoporosis in the rat with a capacitively coupled electrical signal: effects on bone formation and bone resorption," *J. Orthop. Res.*, 6, 676, 1988.

114. Muths, E. and Reichman, O.J., "Kangaroo rat bone compared to white rat bone after short-term disuse and exercise," *Comp. Biochem. Physiol. A Physiol.,* 114, 355, 1996.

115. Smith, R.L., Thomas, K.D., Schurman, D.J., et al., "Rabbit knee immobilization: bone remodeling precedes cartilage degradation," *J. Orthop. Res.*, 10, 88, 1992.

116. Lindgren, J.U., DeLuca, H.F., and Mazess, R.B., "Effects of 1,25(OH)2D3 on bone tissue in the rabbit: studies on fracture healing, disuse osteoporosis, and prednisone osteoporosis," *Calcif. Tissue Int.,* 36, 591, 1984.

117. Dhem, A., Ars-Piret, N., and Waterschoot, M.P., "The effects of nandrolone decanoate on rarefying bone tissue," *Curr. Med. Res. Opin.*, 6, 606, 1980.

118. Rubin, C., Turner, A.S., Bain, S., et al., "Anabolism — low mechanical signals strengthen long bones," *Nature (London)*, 412, 603, 2001.

119. Rubin, C., Sun, Y.Q., Hadjiargyrou, M., and McLeod, K., "Increased expression of matrix metalloproteinase-1 in osteocytes precedes bone resorption as stimulated by disuse: evidence for autoregulation of the cell's mechanical environment?" *J. Orthop. Res.,* 17, 354, 1999.

120. Gross, T.S., Akeno, N., Clemens, T.L., et al., "Selected Contribution: Osteocytes upregulate HIF-1alpha in response to acute disuse and oxygen deprivation," *J. Appl. Physiol.*, 90, 2514, 2001.

121. Milicic, M. and Jowsey, J., "Effect of fluoride on disuse osteoporosis in the cat," *J. Bone Joint Surg. Am.,* 50, 701, 1968.

122. Minne, H.W., Pfeilschifter, J., Scharla, S., et al., "Inflammation-mediated osteopenia in the rat: a new animal model for pathologic loss of bone mass," *Endocrinology,* 115, 50, 1984.

123. Hoshino, K., Hanyu, T., Arai, K., and Takahashi, H.E., "Mineral density and histomorphometric assessment of bone changes in the proximal tibia early after induction of type II collagen-induced arthritis in growing and mature rats," *J. Bone Miner. Metab.*, 19, 76, 2001.

124. Enokida, M., Yamasaki, D., Okano, T., et al., "Bone mass changes of tibial and vertebral bones in young and adult rats with collagen-induced arthritis," *Bone*, 28, 87, 2001.

125. Moran, E.L., Fornasier, T.L., and Bogoch, T.R., "Pamidronate prevents bone loss associated with carrageenan arthritis by reducing resorptive activity but not recruitment of osteoclasts," *J. Orthop. Res.*, 18, 873, 2000.

126. Fountos, G., Kounadi, E., Tzaphlidou, M., et al., "The effects of inflammation-mediated osteoporosis (IMO) on the skeletal Ca/P ratio and on the structure of rabbit bone and skin collagen," *Appl. Radiat. Isot.*, 49, 657, 1998.

127. Bunger, C., Bunger, E.H., Harving, S., et al., "Growth disturbances in experimental juvenile arthritis of the dog knee." *Clin. Rheumatol.,* 3, 181, 1984.

128. Yoshitake, H., Rittling, S.R., Denhardt, D.T., and Noda, M., "Osteopontin-deficient mice are resistant to ovariectomy-induced bone resorption," *Proc. Natl. Acad. Sci. U.S.A.,* 6, 96, 8156, 1999.

129. Simonet, W.S., Lacey, D.L., Dunstan, C.R., et al., "Osteoprotegerin: a novel secreted protein involved in the regulation of bone density," *Cell,* 89, 309, 1997.

130. Bucay, N., Sarosi, I., Dunstan, C.R., et al., "Osteoprotegerin-deficient mice develop early onset osteoporosis and arterial calcification," *Genes Dev.,* 12, 1260, 1998.

131. Mizuno, A., Amizuka, N., Irie, K., et al., "Severe osteoporosis in mice lacking osteoclastogenesis inhibitory factor/osteoprotegerin," *Biochem. Biophys. Res. Commun.,* 247, 610, 1998.

132. Min, H., Morony, S., Sarosi, I., et al., "Osteoprotegerin reverses osteoporosis by inhibiting endosteal osteoclasts and prevents vascular calcification by blocking a process resembling osteoclastogenesis," *J. Exp. Med.,* 192, 463, 2000.

133. Li, B., Boast, S., de los Santos, K., et al., "Mice deficient in Abl are osteoporotic and have defects in osteoblast maturation," *Nat. Genet.,* 24, 304, 2000.

134. Xu, T., Bianco, P., Fisher, L.W., et al., "Targeted disruption of the biglycan gene leads to an osteoporosis-like phenotype in mice," *Nat. Genet.,* 20, 78, 1998.

135. Delany, A.M., Amling, M., Priemel, M., et al., "Osteopenia and decreased bone formation in osteonectin-deficient mice," *J. Clin. Invest.,* 105, 915, 2000.

136. Ducy, P., Amling, M., Takeda, S., et al., "Leptin inhibits bone formation through a hypothalamic relay: a central control of bone mass," *Cell,* 100, 197, 2000.

137. Ogata, N., Chikazu, D., Kubota, N., et al., "Insulin receptor substrate-1 in osteoblast is indispensable for maintaining bone turnover," *J. Clin. Invest.,* 105, 935, 2000.

138. Kuro-o, M., Matsumura, Y., Aizawa, H., et al., "Mutation of the mouse klotho gene leads to a syndrome resembling ageing," *Nature* (*London*), 390, 45, 1997.

139. Rosen, C.J., Beamer, W.G., and Donahue, L.R., "Defining the genetics of osteoporosis: using the mouse to understand man," *Osteoporos. Int.,* 12, 803, 2001.

140. Takeda, T., Hosokawa, M., and Higuchi, K., "Senescence-Accelerated Mouse (SAM): a novel murine model of accelerated senescence," *J. Am. Geriatr. Soc.,* 39, 911, 1991.

141. Matsushita, M., Tsuboyama, T., Kasai, R., et al., "Age-related changes in bone mass in the Senescence-Accelerated Mouse (SAM): SAM-R/3 and SAM-P/6 as new murine models for senile osteoporosis," *Am. J. Pathol.,* 125, 276, 1986.

142. Delmas, P.D., Vergnaud, P., Arlot, M.E., et al., "The anabolic effect of human PTH (1-34) on bone formation is blunted when bone resorption is inhibited by the bisphosphonate tiludronate — is activated resorption a prerequisite for the *in vivo* effect of PTH on formation in a remodeling system?" *Bone,* 16, 603, 1995.

143. Champ, J.E., Binkley, N., Havighurst, T., et al., "The effect of advancing age on bone mineral content of female rhesus monkeys," *Bone,* 19, 485, 1996.

144. Black, A., Tilmont, E.M., Handy, A.M., et al., "A nonhuman primate model of age-related bone loss: a longitudinal study in male and premenopausal female rhesus monkeys," *Bone,* 28, 295, 2001.

145. Kaymakci, B. and Wark, J.D., "Precise accurate mineral measurements of excised sheep bones using X-ray densitometry," *Bone Miner.,* 25, 231, 1994.

146. Cadossi, R. and Cane, V., "Pathways of transmission of ultrasound energy through the distal metaphysis of the second phalanx of pigs: an *in vitro* study," *Osteoporos. Int.,* 6, 196, 1996.

147. Kawagoe, K., Saito, M., Shibuya, T., et al., "Augmentation of cancellous screw fixation with hydroxyapatite composite resin (CAP) *in vivo,*" *J. Biomed. Mater. Res.,* 53, 678, 2000.

148. Lippuner, K., Vogel, R., Tepic, S., et al., "Effect of animal species and age on plate-induced vascular damage in cortical bone," *Arch. Orthop. Trauma Surg.,* 111, 78, 1992.

149. Schnitzer, T., Bone, H.G., Crepaldi, G., et al., "Therapeutic equivalence of alendronate 70 mg once-weekly and alendronate 10 mg daily in the treatment of osteoporosis. Alendronate Once-Weekly Study Group," *Aging* (*Milan*), 12, 1, 2000.

150. Peter, C.P., Guy, J., Shea, M., et al., "Long term safety of the aminobisphosphonate alendronate in adult dogs. I. General safety and biomechanical properties of bone," *J. Pharmacol. Exp. Ther.,* 276, 271, 1996.

151. Okazaki, A., Matsuzawa, T., Perkin, C.J., and Barker, M.H., "Intravenous single and repeated dose toxicity studies of cimadronate (YM175), a novel bisphosphonate, in beagle dogs," *Toxicol. Sci.,* 20, 27, 1995.

152. Pienkowski, D., Doers, T.M., Monier-Faugere, M.C., et al., "Calcitonin alters bone quality in beagle dogs," *J. Bone Miner. Res.,* 12, 1936, 1997.

153. Lafage, M.H., Balena, R., Battle, M.A., et al., "Comparison of alendronate and sodium fluoride effects on cancellous and cortical bone in minipigs. A one-year study," *J. Clin. Invest.,* 95, 2127, 1995.

154. Boivin, G., Deloffre, P., Perrat, B., et al., "Strontium distribution and interactions with bone mineral in monkey iliac bone after strontium salt (S 12911) administration," *Bone Miner. Res.,* 11, 1302, 1996.

6 Radiology of Osteoporotic Bone

Leon Lenchik and Bryon Dickerson

CONTENTS

I. INTRODUCTION

The recent proliferation of radiologic techniques capable of *quantitative* measurement of bone mass has revolutionized the field of osteoporosis. At the same time *qualitative* approaches to the radiologic evaluation of osteoporotic bone have been all but forgotten. By "qualitative" we mean techniques

0-8493-1033-4/02/$0.00+$1.50

where the image rather than the number provides the essential information. In considering conventional radiography (plain films), computed tomography (CT), magnetic resonance (MR) imaging, and skeletal scintigraphy (bone scans), our primary aim is to place the qualitative aspects of these techniques into proper perspective.

II. ROLE OF RADIOLOGY

The role of radiology in the assessment of osteoporotic bone can be considered from either a clinical or a research perspective.

In clinical practice, the overwhelming goal is to make the diagnosis of osteoporosis prior to the first fracture. This is justified by the abundant data that show the risk of subsequent fractures increasing dramatically after the first fracture.[1] In that regard, qualitative radiologic examinations have the same limitation as clinical history and physical examination: they allow diagnosis of osteoporosis in its advanced stages, usually in the setting of a fracture caused by minimal trauma. In contrast, bone densitometry allows diagnosis of osteoporosis prior to fracture by providing accurate, quantitative measurement of bone mass.[2-7] The clinical utility of bone densitometry is well established and is discussed in detail in other chapters.

Despite their apparent limitation in the early diagnosis of osteoporosis, the utility of qualitative radiologic examinations in the overall management of patients with osteoporosis cannot be ignored. Conventional radiography should be used to refer patients for bone densitometry, to help confirm the presence of fracture, and occasionally to aid in the differential diagnosis of low bone mass.

Many reputable organizations, including the World Health Organization (WHO) and the International Osteoporosis Foundation (IOF), advocate using the radiographic finding of osteopenia as an indication for bone densitometry.[3,4] This recommendation is driven in part by the need to identify patients with false-positive findings on radiographs. In reality, the rate of false-positive findings on radiographs is much less of a problem than that of false negatives. Therefore, a better reason to confirm radiographic osteopenia with densitometry relates to pharmacologic intervention. Clinical decisions regarding what patients are candidates for therapy are often inappropriate in the absence of densitometric data. To be convinced of this fact we must realize that antifracture efficacy of antiresorptive agents has been proved only in subjects recruited based on the presence of fracture or based on the presence of low bone mineral density (BMD) determined with bone densitometry.[8-15] Because measurement of BMD before starting therapy reduces the number of patients who would otherwise receive therapy unnecessarily, patients with radiographic osteopenia should be referred for densitometry.

Another role of conventional radiographs in the care of patients with osteoporosis relates to differential diagnosis. Findings on plain films may help in the differential diagnosis of conditions associated with low bone mass. For example, a patient who presents with osteoporosis based on a bone densitometry examination may be found on plain films to have multiple lytic lesions indicative of multiple myeloma. Conventional radiographs are sometimes obtained as an adjunct to bone densitometry to exclude such patients and, together with laboratory evaluation, to help determine the etiology of osteoporosis. For this reason, we discuss imaging findings in patients with secondary causes of osteoporosis later in this chapter.

However, the main role of conventional radiography relates to fractures. Certainly, the practice of orthopaedic surgery depends on accurate diagnosis, classification, and follow-up of fractures and would not be possible without conventional radiography. The broad topic of radiographic diagnosis of osteoporotic fractures is beyond the scope of this text.

Having considered the role of radiology in the evaluation of a patient with osteoporosis, it is important to mention its role in a research environment. For a researcher studying osteoporotic bone, the issue of bone strength is usually paramount. Although material properties of bone in general and BMD in particular are important determinants of strength, they are not the only components of whole bone strength.[16] There is increasing interest in the research community in defining both the structural and microarchitectural determinants of bone strength. Conventional radiography, CT, and MR imaging are used to measure the size of bones and to characterize their shape as well as to assess trabecular architecture.[17] In this research, quantitative information is derived from these qualitative techniques. The importance of such research cannot be overstated. Increasing understanding of how bone structure contributes to bone strength may lead to radiologic measurements of bone structure becoming a routine part of clinical practice. Some clinicians are already obtaining measurements of the hip axis length using dual X-ray absorptiometry (DXA).

Unfortunately, the role of radiologic examinations is determined by the availability of particular radiologic equipment. In the developing countries, where access to quantitative densitometry is limited, it may be appropriate to diagnose osteoporosis from visual inspection of conventional radiographs. Such an approach has low sensitivity, but high specificity. Although the approach is not ideal for quantifying the severity of disease or determining the need for therapy, it is preferable to clinical evaluation alone. Before the use of bone densitometry became so widespread, some authors proposed using radiologic indices to help characterize osteoporosis on plain films.[18-21] Because these indices may still have a role in research in developing countries, we discuss them in the next section.

Clearly, qualitative radiologic assessment has many important roles in both research and clinical practice. We now describe in more detail various techniques used for such assessment.

III. RADIOLOGIC TECHNIQUES

A. CLINICAL APPLICATIONS OF RADIOLOGIC TECHNIQUES

Several radiologic techniques may be used in the evaluation of patients with osteoporosis including conventional radiography (plain films), CT, MR imaging, and skeletal scintigraphy (bone scans). Potential use of these techniques for research purposes merits separate consideration.

1. Conventional Radiography

Of all the available techniques, conventional radiographs are used most widely because of their versatility and low cost.

On radiographic film, bones appear white because the absorption of X-rays is greater in bone than in soft tissue. X-ray absorption by tissue is determined in part by the atomic number. The high atomic number of calcium results in relatively high absorption of X-rays by calcium-containing tissues such as bone. In contrast, decreased calcium content in bones of patients with osteoporosis generally results in decreased attenuation of X-rays and thus increased lucency on X-ray film. When bones appear more lucent (i.e., less white), the finding is termed *osteopenia*.

To understand why the finding of osteopenia on plain films may not indicate that the patient has osteoporosis, various factors that affect the quality of a radiographic image must be considered. These factors include exposure time and voltage, film-focus distance, bone thickness and mineral content, soft tissue composition, X-ray scatter, film and screen properties, and film processing. Because the finding of osteopenia is technique dependent, a poorly trained technologist might produce radiographs where osteoporotic patients appear normal or normal patients appear osteoporotic.

Further limiting the use of plain films in the diagnosis of osteoporosis is the subjectivity of the radiologic interpretation.[22] Early in the course of osteoporosis there is poor agreement among readers regarding the radiographic finding of osteopenia and what one radiologist calls *osteopenia*, another may call *normal*.[22]

Last, in the absence of fractures, conventional radiographs have low sensitivity for the diagnosis of osteoporosis.[23-25] Bone loss of approximately 30 to 50% is required before it is detected on radiographs.[23-25] Consequently, plain-film results are normal in many patients who have osteoporosis on the basis of bone densitometry (Figure 6.1A and B).

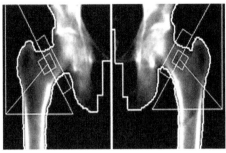

Region	BMD (g/cm²)	Young-Adult T-Score	Age-Matched Z-Score
Total			
Left	0.690	-2.6	-0.3
Right	0.672	-2.7	-0.4
Mean	0.681	-2.7	-0.4
Difference	0.019	0.2	0.2

A

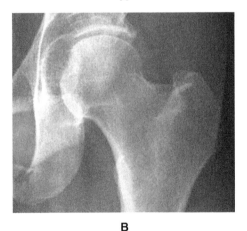

B

FIGURE 6.1 Osteoporosis. (A) DXA scan of the hips in an 83-year-old Caucasian woman shows mean total hip T-score = −2.7, consistent with WHO criteria for osteoporosis. (B) AP radiograph of the left hip, in the same woman, shows preserved radiodensity and trabecular pattern. With no evidence for osteoporosis, this is a false-negative radiograph.

2. Computed Tomography

In patients with osteoporosis, CT scanning is especially valuable for the diagnosis of occult fractures and for classification of complex fractures.

The physical principles that explain the appearance of bones on CT scans are similar to those of conventional radiographs. During the acquisition of CT scans, X rays penetrate tissue from multiple directions, their respective attenuations are discriminated using a computer, and a cross-sectional image is produced. Such presentation of density information eliminates superimposed structures and results in improved contrast resolution when compared with plain films.[26] For this reason, CT scans are more sensitive than plain films in the evaluation of soft tissues and in the detection of subtle bony erosions.[26]

In the evaluation of osseous structures, obtaining thin sections (i.e., 1 to 2 mm collimation) and reconstructing the data in sagittal and coronal planes is often helpful. CT scans are usually obtained to evaluate regions where bony anatomy is complex such as the spine and pelvis. For

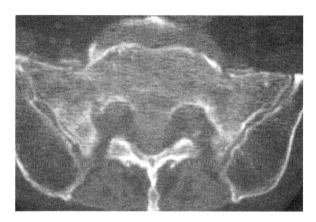

FIGURE 6.2 Occult sacral insufficiency fracture. CT scan of the sacrum in an elderly woman with back pain shows bilateral cortical disruption in the sacral ala, indicating fracture. The conventional radiographs in the same woman were normal.

example, CT scanning is ideal for detecting radiographically occult fractures of the sacrum (Figure 6.2).

3. Magnetic Resonance Imaging

The primary value of MR imaging in patients with osteoporosis is to exclude malignancy underlying a fracture.

The physical principles of MR imaging are quite different from those of conventional radiographs and CT. To begin with, there is no ionizing radiation. More importantly, MR images depend less on tissue density and more on hydrogen content of tissues. MR imaging allows far better contrast resolution than CT; differentiation of fluid, fat, cartilage, muscle, tendon, and ligament is superior.[27] In addition, MR images are especially sensitive to subtle abnormalities of the bone marrow.[27] Another advantage of MR is direct multiplanar imaging in any plane. The main disadvantage of MR is its high cost.

Compared with other radiologic methods, MR imaging is technically more demanding. Dedicated coils are used for particular skeletal sites to optimize the signal-to-noise ratio. Different pulse sequences are selected to optimize either the spatial or contrast resolution. Each pulse sequence, in turn, has specific imaging parameters including plane and axis designation, scan timing (TR, TE, TI, flip angle), scan range (field of view, slice thickness and spacing), and acquisition timing (number of excitations, frequency direction). Ideally, all of these technical parameters are tailored to a particular clinical question.

Bone and soft tissue neoplasms, infection, bone infarcts, as well as ligament, tendon, and muscle injuries are well depicted with MR imaging. In general, fluid, edema, and inflammation are low signal (i.e., dark) on T1-weighted images and high signal (i.e., bright) on T2-weighted images, whereas cortical bone is dark on both T1- and T2-weighted images.

In patients with osteoporosis with fracture, MR images after administration of intravenous gadolinium may show enhancing soft tissue mass indicating an underlying malignancy (Figure 6.3 A and B). In any patient with normal plain films but a high index of suspicion for fracture, MR imaging is valuable. In fact, the choice among CT, MR, and bone scan in the workup of radiographically occult fractures is often determined by clinician and radiologist preferences. The authors' preference is to use MR imaging in most of these cases (Figure 6.4). This is because, after a fracture has been excluded, MR images may determine other causes of the patient's symptoms such as muscle or ligament tear, osteonecrosis, or infection (Figure 6.5).

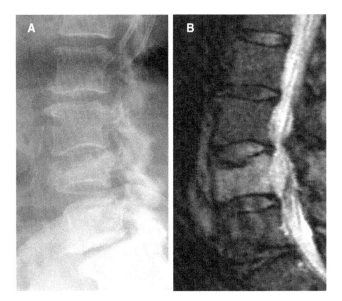

FIGURE 6.3 Lymphoma. (A) Lateral radiograph of the lumbar spine in a 55-year-old woman with back pain shows a compression fracture of L4 vertebra. (B) Sagittal MR image (T1-weighted, with intravenous gadolinium) in the same woman shows enhancement of the entire vertebra and of the epidural extension. Biopsy revealed lymphoma.

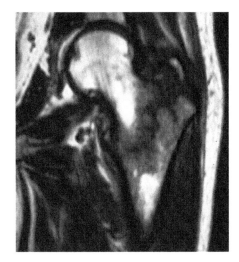

FIGURE 6.4 Occult intertrochanteric fracture. Coronal MR image (T1-weighted) shows a low-signal intensity intertrochanteric fracture line. The conventional radiographs in the same woman were normal.

4. Skeletal Scintigraphy

Bone scanning uses a physiologic marker (methylene diphosphonate, MDP) to detect abnormalities in bone metabolism. Either the entire body or specific parts may be imaged. Bone scanning is more sensitive to bone turnover than conventional radiographs and CT.[28] However, bone scans are generally used in combination with plain films, owing to their high spatial resolution. In patients with osteoporosis, bone scans may be obtained to detect coexistent metastatic disease and evaluate its extent, to assess for occult fractures, and to exclude osteomyelitis (Figure 6.6).

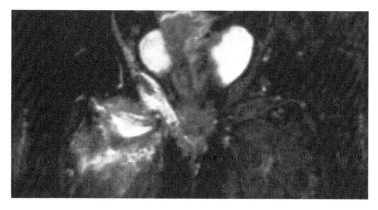

FIGURE 6.5 Adductor strain. Coronal MR image (STIR), in a patient with suspected hip fracture after a fall, shows high-signal intensity within the adductor muscle group indicating a strain.

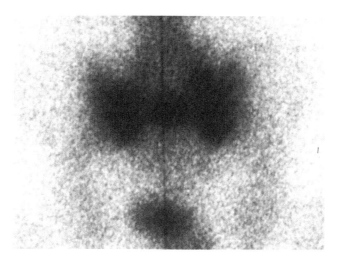

FIGURE 6.6 Occult sacral insufficiency fracture. Bone scan of the pelvis shows intense radiopharmaceutical uptake in the sacrum in an H-shaped pattern, indicating bilateral sacral insufficiency fractures. The conventional radiographs of the sacrum were normal.

B. RESEARCH APPLICATIONS OF RADIOLOGIC TECHNIQUES

The research applications of the above techniques will be discussed in three broad categories: (1) radiologic indices, (2) cortical measurement, and (3) assessment of trabecular architecture.

1. Radiologic Indices

Prior to the proliferation of bone densitometry, various approaches to the evaluation of conventional radiographs in patients with osteoporosis were proposed.

In the evaluation of spine radiographs, the Saville index grades the severity of osteoporosis as follows: Grade 0 — normal bone density; Grade 1 — minimal loss of bone density with end plates becoming prominent; Grade 2 — prominent vertical trabecula and thinning of vertebral end plates; Grade 3 — vertebral end plates are less visible; Grade 4 — ghostlike vertebrae, with bone density equal to soft tissue and no discernible trabecular pattern.[18]

In the evaluation of hip radiographs, the Singh index is most widely used: Grade 6 — all normal trabecular groups are visible; Grade 5 — secondary compressive group is not visible; Grade 4 — secondary tensile group is not visible; Grade 3 — principal tensile group is visible in the upper but not lower portion; Grade 2 — principal tensile group is not visible; and Grade 1 — no principal trabecular groups are visible.[19]

In addition to the above indices, which are based on qualitative assessment of the image, other indices based on quantitative measurements have been proposed.[20,21] These indices are best considered *radiogrammetry*, which is discussed in the next section.

2. Cortical Measurement

Radiogrammetry refers to measurement of cortical thickness in any tubular bone, usually the metacarpals.[29-35] A conventional radiograph of the long bone is obtained, the cortical thickness on either side of the medullary space is measured, and the results usually expressed as combined cortical thickness (CCT) or cortical area (CA).[29-35] In normal individuals, the CCT of the second metacarpal is at least 50% of the width of the shaft. Because radiogrammetry is a densitometric technique, its clinical utility should be judged on the basis of its ability to predict fractures. Metacarpal radiogrammetry was predictive of incident hip fractures in at least one large epidemiologic study of elderly women (the Study of Osteoporotic Fractures).[36]

In the clinical setting, radiogrammetry has recently reappeared in a slightly modified form. Digital X-ray radiogrammetry (DXR) involves scanning a radiograph of the forearm with a high-resolution scanner and having the digital image analyzed. Based on the cortical thickness of metacarpals, radius, and ulna, a BMD-equivalent DXR bone density is then calculated.[37-39]

In the research setting, radiogrammetry is useful for studying changes in cortical bone but has several potential limitations.[29-35] Measurement errors may occur due to variable soft tissue thickness and variations in radiographic technique. Moreover, the technique does not measure intracortical resorption of bone and may not measure endosteal resorption, the types of resorption indicative of high bone turnover.

3. Trabecular Architecture

In the research environment, plain films, CT scans, and MR images have been used to evaluate the architecture of trabecular bone.[17] Texture analysis has been used to evaluate trabecular structure on conventional radiographs and CT scans.[40-43] These studies suggest that trabecular texture parameters may reflect the anisotropy of trabecular structures.[40-43] Chevalier et al.[44] have used high-resolution CT images of the lumbar spine to calculate a "trabecular fragmentation index." This is based on ratio of length of trabecular network and number of discontinuities found in a particular image. An alternative approach to the thresholding method has been termed the ridge/valley detection method.[45]

There has also been research on using fractal analysis to evaluate trabecular architecture.[46-49] Such analysis assumes that the trabecular network may be characterized as an object with a characteristic fractal dimension. For example, Caligiuri et al.[49] reported that fractal analysis provided better discrimination than BMD between women with and without fractures based on spine radiographs. Unfortunately, the relationships of fractal analysis to bone density and to mechanical properties are highly dependent on the method used to perform fractal analysis.[47] Certainly, application of fractal analysis to the evaluation of trabecular structure warrants further study.

Clearly, deriving structural parameters from a two-dimensional radiograph and even a high-resolution CT image is technically challenging.[50] Invariably, techniques that assess microstructure are dependent on excellent image quality.[50] On conventional radiographs, there is also the problem of overprojection of trabecular structures whereas on CT scans, the problem relates to slice thickness and radiation dose.[50] Because most structural parameters (e.g., trabecular connectivity) cannot be determined from two-dimensional information alone, three-dimensional assessment is essential. At present, such information is difficult to obtain *in vivo*. In contrast, microCT has been used *in vitro* and *in vivo* in small animals and allows fairly precise analysis of the trabecular architecture.[51,52]

Perhaps someday such research into the radiologic assessment of trabecular structure will help improve the care of patients with osteoporosis.

IV. INDICATIONS FOR RADIOLOGY

The main indications for radiologic evaluation of patients with osteoporosis are the presence or suspicion of fracture or unexplained loss of height. The evaluation usually begins with conventional radiographs but may ultimately require CT, MR, or scintigraphy. Some centers still obtain conventional radiographs as a routine adjunct to bone densitometry. Although this was common practice at the time when quality of DXA images was poor, and did not allow identification of artifacts, it is no longer necessary with modern DXA equipment. However, plain films should be obtained whenever significant pathology (e.g., fractures or tumors) is suspected on a DXA image.

V. TERMS AND DEFINITIONS

Osteoporosis has been defined in many different ways. The clinical definition requires the presence of a fragility fracture, the histologic definition requires normally mineralized bone to be present in reduced quantity, and the densitometric definition requires BMD measurement at least 2.5 standard deviations below the young adult mean.[53,54] Perhaps the most widely used definition describes osteoporosis as "a systemic skeletal disease characterized by low bone mass and microarchitectural deterioration of bone tissue, with a consequent increase in bone fragility and susceptibility to fracture."[54] Having different definitions for the same disease has led to some confusion in the interpretation of conventional radiographs.

Contributing to the confusion is the fact that many metabolic bone disorders, including osteomalacia and osteoporosis, often present with the finding of decreased radiographic density. When interpreting conventional radiographs, terms such as osteopenia, osteoporosis, deossification, demineralization, osteolysis, and rarefaction are often used interchangeably. Ideally, all radiologists would use the term *osteopenia* as a generic descriptor, regardless of causality. The term *osteopenia* is preferred to the term *osteoporosis* largely because it is difficult to distinguish between the various causes of decreased radiographic bone density and because there are specific pathogenic implications attached to the term *osteoporosis*.

Using the term *osteopenia* as a generic descriptor is complicated by the fact that the WHO uses the same term for BMD measurement between 1.0 and 2.5 standard deviations below the young adult mean. The WHO criteria were intended for quantitative bone mass measurements. Because radiologic interpretation of bone radiographs is qualitative, perhaps the term *osteopenia* should be avoided when interpreting radiographs. The problem with that approach is that radiologists and other health-care providers have been using the term *osteopenia* for the interpretation of X-ray films long before the WHO criteria were published. For this reason, it would have been more appropriate for the WHO to choose another term.

Because of the various definitions and potential confusions about terminology, it is important to alert the referring clinicians that the terms *osteopenia* and *osteoporosis* have different meanings in the interpretation of radiographs than they do in the interpretation of densitometry examinations: one is qualitative and subjective; the other is quantitative and objective.

VI. IMAGING FINDINGS

A. GENERAL

Although the gold standard for the diagnosis of osteoporosis is bone densitometry, with early osteoporosis, plain films are commonly normal.[55-59] With more advanced disease, the most common

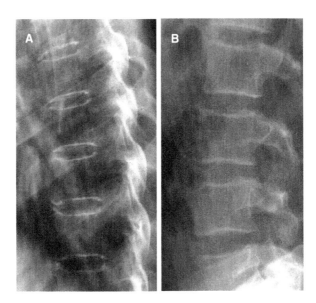

FIGURE 6.7 Spinal osteoporosis. (A) Lateral radiograph of the thoracic spine shows generalized osteopenia along with thinning and accentuation of cortical rim. (B) Lateral radiograph of the lumbar spine shows prominent vertical, weight-bearing trabeculae giving rise to a striated or corduroy appearance.

finding is generalized osteopenia.[55-59] Osteopenia is usually accompanied by cortical thinning and change in the trabecular pattern.[55-59] The latter is due to selective resorption of smaller, non-weight-bearing trabeculae. As the smaller trabeculae are resorbed and disappear from view, the larger weight-bearing trabeculae hypertrophy and become more evident and more sharply defined.[55-59] In contrast to that of osteomalacia the bone surfaces in patients with osteoporosis are well defined, with sharp margins. Commonly, radiographs of patients with osteoporosis show fractures, especially of the vertebrae, proximal femur, distal radius, and proximal humerus.

B. SPINE

On radiographs of the spine the diagnosis of osteoporosis may be suggested based on osteopenia, changes in trabecular pattern, and vertebral fractures.[55-59] In general, osteopenia is more noticeable in the central portion of the vertebral body. In fact, as the trabeculae in the central portion become more lucent, the cortex of superior and inferior vertebral margins appears denser (Figure 6.7A). Change in the trabecular pattern involves preferential loss of horizontal trabeculae and hypertrophy of vertical trabeculae (Figure 6.7B). This gives rise to a striated or corduroy appearance that may mimic hemangioma. If necessary, MR imaging should be used to confirm the diagnosis of hemangioma by showing high signal on T1-weighted images.

   Vertebral fractures and deformities are typically classified as wedge, crush, or biconcave (Figure 6.8).[60] The midthoracic, lower thoracic, and upper lumbar vertebral bodies are more severely affected. Multiple wedging of the vertebral bodies leads to a kyphosis of the thoracic spine. Unfortunately, the nomenclature for describing vertebral fracture is not standardized.[60] Also lacking in standardization are the diagnostic criteria.[61-64] Fractures may be detected based on qualitative assessment of the X-ray image or based on actual measurements of vertebral dimensions (i.e., morphometry). At our center, we use the qualitative approach except for equivocal cases where we use a difference of more than 4 mm or more than 20% between the anterior, middle, or posterior height of the vertebrae to indicate a fracture. For research, we use both semiquantitative and quantitative approaches to vertebral characterization. We grade fractures as mild, moderate, or severe based on vertebral height reduction of 20 to 30%, 30 to 40%, or >40%, respectively (Figure 6.9A and B).

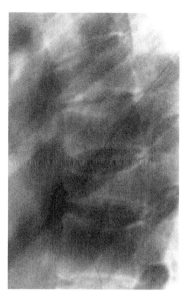

FIGURE 6.8 Advanced osteoporosis. Lateral radiograph of the thoracic spine shows generalized osteopenia, a wedge fracture, and a biconcave fracture.

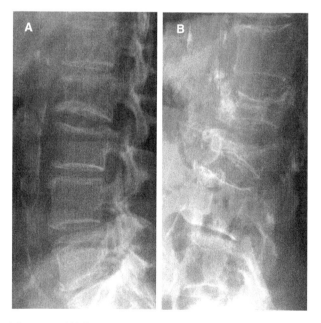

FIGURE 6.9 Vertebral fractures. (A) Lateral radiograph of the lumbar spine shows generalized osteopenia and a mild inferior end plate fracture of L2 vertebra. (B) Lateral radiograph of the lumbar spine shows generalized osteopenia and two severe crush fractures.

There are serious pitfalls in the evaluation of spine radiographs for the presence of fractures. For example, poor technique where lateral projection is really an oblique projection may lead to the vertebrae appearing as fractured. Similar "pseudofractures" may be seen on the lateral projection in patients with scoliosis. In addition, it is important to recognize other abnormalities in vertebral shape that may mimic a fracture. Examples include "butterfly" vertebrae (congenital anomaly),

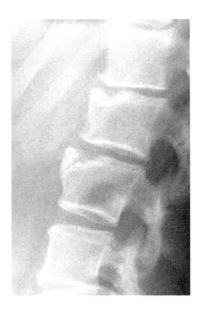

FIGURE 6.10 Limbus vertebrae. Lateral radiograph of the lumbar spine shows deformity of the anterior superior corner of L2 and L3 vertebrae. This is typical appearance for a limbus vertebra, a developmental anomaly.

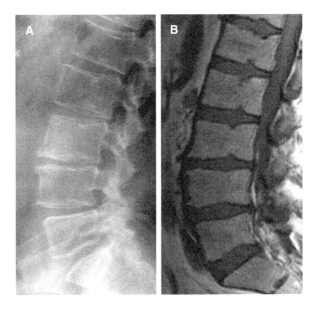

FIGURE 6.11 Schmorl's nodes. (A) Lateral radiograph of the lumbar spine shows central irregularity of the vertebral end plates indicating Schmorl's nodes. (B) Sagittal MR image (T1-weighted) in the same individual confirms multiple Schmorl's nodes.

"cupid's bow" (developmental variant), limbus vertebra (developmental variant), Schmorl's nodes (vertebral osteochondrosis or Scheurmann's disease), and "H-shaped" vertebrae (sickle cell disease or Gaucher's disease) (Figures 6.10, 6.11A and B, 6.12).

Despite the difficulties inherent in vertebral fracture assessment, their diagnosis is essential for appropriate clinical management. Part of the reason for this is that having a vertebral deformity is

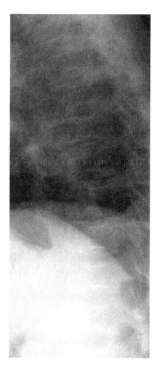

FIGURE 6.12 Sickle cell disease. Lateral radiograph of the thoracolumbar spine shows H-shaped deformity of the vertebral end plates typical of sickle cell disease.

a very strong risk factor for subsequent fractures, both at new vertebral sites, proximal femur, and at other sites susceptible to osteoporosis.[1] Another reason is that as many as two thirds of these fractures do not manifest as acute painful events.[1] Therefore, careful scrutiny of all pertinent radiographs (including lateral chest radiographs) and DXA scan images for the presence of vertebral fracture should be encouraged (Figure 6.13).

Critical to the evaluation of vertebral fractures on imaging studies is the fact that not all vertebral fractures are due to osteoporosis. In particular, antecedent trauma, infection, and tumor must be excluded (Figure 6.14A and B). In many cases, MR imaging is useful for differentiating osteoporotic fractures from pathologic fractures by showing contrast enhancement of bone marrow and adjacent soft tissues in pathologic fractures (see Figure 6.3). However, early after fracture there may be enhancement even in the absence of tumor. MR imaging is also useful in determining the chronicity of fracture; those that retain high signal on T2-weighted sequences are still healing, whereas those that show normal marrow signal are healed (Figure 6.15A and B).

C. PROXIMAL FEMUR

The diagnosis of osteoporosis may be suggested based on radiographs of the hip that show osteopenia, changes in trabecular pattern, and fractures.[55-59] Singh et al.[19] first characterized the five trabecular groups of the proximal femur: (1) principal compressive group, (2) secondary compressive group, (3) greater trochanter group, (4) principal tensile group, and (5) secondary tensile group. As already discussed in the Radiologic Indices Section, these trabecular groups can be used as a semiquantitative estimate of trabecular bone loss at the hip (Figure 6.16A and B).

The diagnosis of hip fracture on imaging studies is less difficult than that of vertebral fracture. Both intracapsular and extracapsular fractures are usually seen on conventional radiographs (Figure 6.17A and B). However, in suspected cases of fracture where the plain films are normal, bone scan, CT, or MR can provide the correct diagnosis (see Figure 6.4).

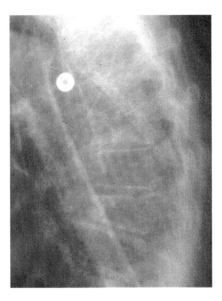

FIGURE 6.13 Asymptomatic vertebral fracture. Lateral view from a chest X-ray obtained for chest pain shows two anterior wedge fractures. Even although these fractures were not symptomatic, it is essential to describe these fractures in an X-ray report because they contribute substantially to the future risk of spine and hip fractures, and as such should impact the long-term clinical management of this patient.

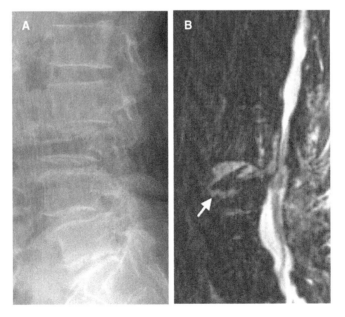

FIGURE 6.14 Discitis and vertebral osteomyelitis. (A) Lateral radiograph of the lumbar spine shows a compression fracture of L3 vertebra, the superior end plate is indistinct. (B) Sagittal MR image (T2-weighted, with fat saturation) in the same individual shows high signal intensity extending from L2–L3 intervertebral disc into the L3 vertebra and the epidural space. Biopsy and microbiology revealed discitis/osteomyelitis.

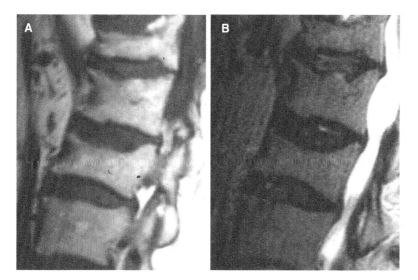

FIGURE 6.15 Vertebral fractures on MR imaging. (A) Sagittal MR image (T1-weighted) shows multiple compression fractures; (B) sagittal MR image (T2-weighted, with fat saturation) in the same individual shows the same chronic compression fractures. Note that on both pulse sequences the signal intensity of marrow in the fractured and nonfractured adjacent vertebrae is the same, indicating that these are chronic (i.e., healed) fractures.

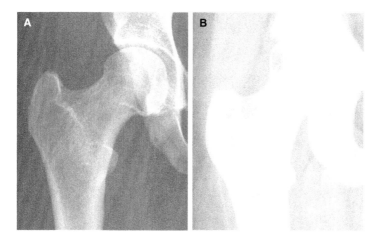

FIGURE 6.16 Proximal femur osteoporosis. (A) AP radiograph of a hip in a woman with normal DXA results shows normal radiodensity and trabecular pattern. (B) In contrast, AP radiograph of a hip in another woman with a total hip T-score of –2.8 shows generalized osteopenia along with decreased visualization of tensile trabecular groups and prominence of principal compressive trabecular group.

D. APPENDICULAR SITES

At skeletal sites rich in cortical bone such as the metacarpals and metatarsals, the plain film findings of osteoporosis are somewhat different from those at the spine or hip.[55-59] Typically, there is endosteal, periosteal, or intracortical thinning. Intracortical thinning occurs from bone resorption within Haversian channels. Intracortical bone resorption appears on radiographs as longitudinal

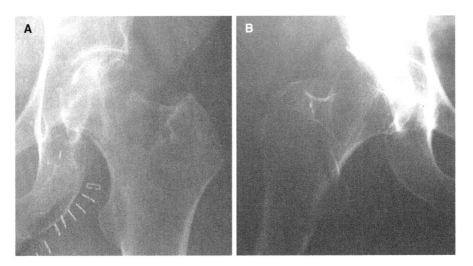

FIGURE 6.17 Hip fractures. (A) AP radiograph of left hip shows a subcapital fracture. (B) AP radiograph of right hip shows an intertrochanteric fracture.

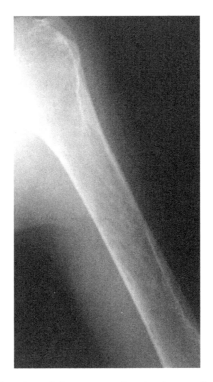

FIGURE 6.18 Intracortical and endosteal bone resorption in the proximal humerus of a woman with osteoporosis.

striation or tunneling, which may mimic a nutrient foramen (Figure 6.18). The principal feature of advanced disease is progressive widening of the medullary canal due to endosteal resorption, the so-called "trabeculization" of the cortex (Figure 6.19A and B). In contrast, periosteal resorption may indicate that secondary causes for osteoporosis may be present (e.g., hyperparathyroidism).

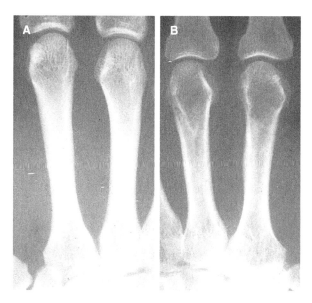

FIGURE 6.19 Metacarpal osteoporosis. (A) Normal cortical thickness of the metacarpals. (B) In contrast, note marked thinning of the cortices in a woman with osteoporosis.

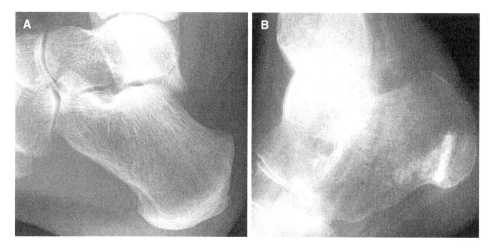

FIGURE 6.20 Calcaneal osteoporosis. (A) Normal trabecular pattern and cortical thickness of the calcaneus. (B) In contrast, note marked thinning of the cortices and loss of trabecular pattern in a woman with osteoporosis. The dense sclerotic line in the posterior aspect of the calcaneus is an insufficiency fracture.

Patients with osteoporosis involving appendicular sites rich in trabecular bone, such as the calcaneus and the distal radius, present with plain film findings similar to what has been described in the spine.[55-59] At the calcaneus, there is loss of non-weight-bearing trabeculae, accentuation of weight-bearing trabeculae, and thinning of the cortex (Figure 6.20A and B). At the distal radius, thin cortices are the dominant findings prior to a Colles' fracture (Figure 6.21A and B).

VII. APPROACH TO RADIOLOGIC INTERPRETATION

When evaluating imaging studies in patients with suspected osteoporosis, the following questions are important:

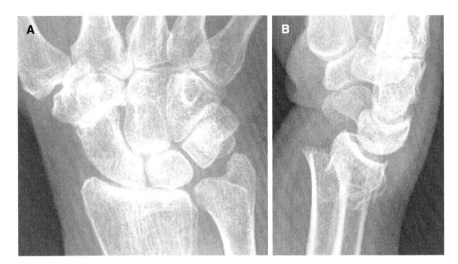

FIGURE 6.21 Wrist osteoporosis. (A) Cortical thinning of the distal radius and ulna and the carpal bones in a woman with osteoporosis. (B) Colles' fracture of the distal radius in another woman with osteoporosis.

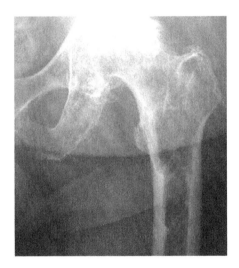

FIGURE 6.22 Multiple myeloma. AP radiograph of left hip shows generalized osteopenia. In addition there are multiple focal lytic lesions in the proximal femur indicating multiple myeloma. Osteoarthritis of the hip joint is also visible.

1. *What is the anatomic distribution of the findings?* In other words, are the findings generalized, regional, or focal? By definition, generalized osteoporosis involves the entire skeleton. However, the spine, pelvis, and ribs (i.e., axial skeleton) are often most severely affected. In contrast, regional osteoporosis usually affects some portion of the appendicular skeleton. The list of differential considerations for generalized osteoporosis should also include osteomalacia, hyperparathyroidism, and multiple myeloma. Findings that suggest osteomalacia rather than osteoporosis include indistinct trabeculae and poorly defined interfaces between cortical and trabecular bone.[59] The finding of bone resorption at characteristic sites accurately differentiates patients with hyperparathyroidism from patients with primary osteoporosis.[59] Differentiation from myeloma is possible when multiple lytic lesions are seen (Figure 6.22). The causes of regional osteoporosis include immobilization and disuse, reflex sympathetic dystrophy syndrome (RSDS), transient regional osteoporosis, and

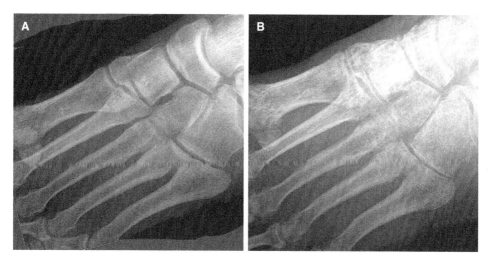

FIGURE 6.23 Osteoporosis of disuse. (A) Oblique radiograph of the foot obtained at the time of calcaneus fracture shows normal mineralization of bones. (B) Radiograph of the same foot 5 months later, after internal fixation of the fracture, shows patchy osteopenia caused by disuse.

inflammatory arthritis. The main causes of focal osteoporosis are tumors and infection. Because the ultimate goal is to keep the patient from suffering an osteoporotic fracture, it is important to note whether weight-bearing or non-weight-bearing bones are affected.

2. *Are the dominant findings in cortical or trabecular bone?* It is common to use the term primary osteoporosis for conditions in which low bone mass is attributed to menopause (type I) or aging (type II) and the term *secondary osteoporosis* for conditions in which low bone mass is attributed to identifiable factors other than aging and menopause.[53,54] Generally, postmenopausal osteoporosis (type I) typically affects trabecular bone more than cortical bone. The spine is more affected than the hip, and spine fractures are more common than hip fractures.[53,54] In contrast, senile osteoporosis (type II) typically affects both trabecular bone and cortical bone. Both the spine and the hip are affected and both spine and hip fractures are common.[53,54] There are some causes of secondary osteoporosis (e.g., hyperparathyroidism) where greater loss of cortical bone than trabecular bone is typical.

3. *Can the osteopenia be characterized as high turnover or low turnover?* Certainly, this question is best answered with biochemical markers. However, some patients with rapid bone loss (e.g., osteoporosis of disuse) have characteristic X-ray findings. These include patchy areas of trabecular lucency, intracortical striations, or lucent metaphyseal bands (Figure 6.23A and B).[59]

4. *Is there evidence of past or present fractures?* This information is critical to clinicians in terms of diagnosis, prognosis, and patient management. It cannot be overemphasized that for the clinical diagnosis of osteoporosis, the presence of a fragility fracture is sufficient, regardless of the bone densitometry results. Bone densitometry may be useful in patients with fracture to assess disease severity or to serve as a basis for monitoring that therapy, but for diagnosis it is not essential. In terms of prognosis, any fracture significantly increases the risk of subsequent fractures. Thus, the recognition of a fracture helps clinicians and their patients be better informed about the overall fracture risk. In terms of patient management, the presence of fracture is often the difference between medical therapy alone vs. medical therapy, surgery, and physical rehabilitation.

VIII. SECONDARY CAUSES OF OSTEOPOROSIS

In adults, causes of secondary osteoporosis include endocrine (hypogonadism, hyperadrenocorticism, thyrotoxicosis, hyperparathyroidism, acromegaly, hyperprolactinemia, pregnancy, diabetes

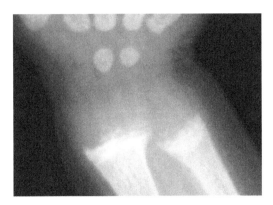

FIGURE 6.24 Rickets. AP radiograph of the wrist in a boy with rickets shows widening, fraying, and cupping of the metaphyses of the distal radius and ulna.

mellitus type 1), congenital (osteogenesis imperfecta, Ehlers–Danlos syndrome, homocystinuria, mastocytosis, ochronosis, Gaucher's disease), nutritional (alcoholism, malabsorbtion, malnutrition, calcium deficiency, vitamin D deficiency), and drug related (glucocorticoids, phenytoin, phenobarbital, heparin, gonadotropin-releasing hormone antagonists).[53,54]

Because radiologic evaluation may help differentiate primary osteoporosis from some forms of secondary osteoporosis, further discussion of rickets, osteomalacia, hyperparathyroidism, renal osteodystrophy, hyperthyroidism, hypercorticism, and acromegaly is appropriate.

A. RICKETS AND OSTEOMALACIA

Rickets and osteomalacia describe a group of disorders characterized by incomplete mineralization of normal osteoid tissue.[65-67] Rickets is a disorder of growing bone in which there is hypomineralization of the growth plate. Osteomalacia occurs after the cessation of growth. The growth plate is not involved but there is hypomineralization of the trabecular and cortical bone. Abnormalities in vitamin D metabolism often result in rickets and osteomalacia.[65-67]

The most common radiologic finding in patients with rickets is generalized osteopenia.[68,69] Other findings are apparent at the growth plates and include increased lucency, widening, elongation, irregularity (fraying), and cupping of the metaphyses (Figure 6.24).[68,69] The most involved parts of the skeleton are the costochondral junctions of the middle ribs (rachitic rosary), the distal femur, both ends of the tibia, the distal radius and ulna, and the proximal humerus.[68,69] The differential diagnosis includes hypophosphatasia and metaphyseal chondrodysplasia (Schmid type).[68,69] The most common complication of rickets is skeletal deformity.[68,69] In neonates, posterior flattening and squaring of the skull (i.e., craniotabes) may be seen. In early childhood, bowing deformities of arms and legs are common (Figure 6.25). In older children, scoliosis, vertebral end plate deformities, basilar invagination of the skull, triradiate deformity of the pelvis, and slipped capital femoral epiphysis may be seen.

In patients with osteomalacia, the most common radiologic finding is also generalized osteopenia.[68,69] The presence of indistinct bony trabeculae and Looser zones suggests the diagnosis (Figure 6.26A and B).[68,69] Looser zones are insufficiency-type stress fractures that occur in a bilateral and symmetric distribution.[68,69] The characteristic sites include the inner margins of the femoral neck, the proximal ulna, the axillary margin of the scapula, the pubic rami, and the ribs.[68,69] The most common complications of osteomalacia are skeletal deformity (vertebrae and skull) and fractures (vertebral bodies and long bones).[70]

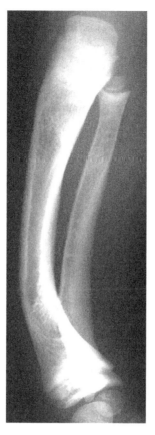

FIGURE 6.25 Rickets. Lateral radiograph of the leg shows generalized osteopenia and anterior bowing of the tibia.

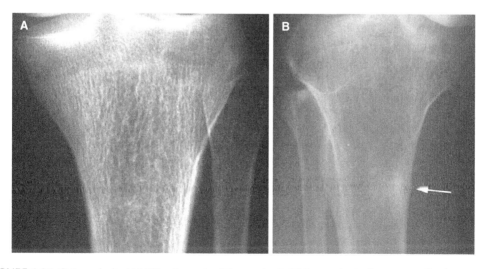

FIGURE 6.26 Osteomalacia. (A) AP radiograph of the proximal tibial metaphysis shows generalized osteopenia and indistinct bony trabecula characteristic of osteomalacia. (B) AP radiograph of the proximal tibia in another patient with osteomalacia shows an insufficiency fracture (Looser zone) of the medial cortex of the tibia.

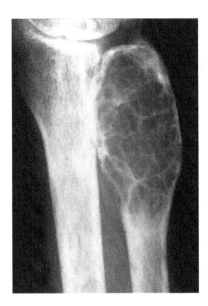

FIGURE 6.27 Brown tumor. Oblique radiograph of the wrist in a patient with hyperparathyroidism shows a well-defined, expansile lesion of the distal ulna, indicating a Brown tumor.

B. PRIMARY HYPERPARATHYROIDISM

Primary hyperparathyroidism may be caused by a single parathyroid adenoma (80%), hyperplasia (15 to 20%), or, rarely, carcinoma (<0.5%). Primary hyperparathyroidism is characterized by incompletely regulated excessive secretion of parathyroid hormone.[71-73] Secondary hyperparathyroidism is usually caused by chronic renal insufficiency.

The most common radiologic finding in patients with hyperparathyroidism is generalized osteopenia.[72] Other findings include bone resorption, bone sclerosis, focal lytic or sclerotic lesions (e.g., brown tumors; see Figure 6.27), chondrocalcinosis, soft-tissue calcification, and vascular calcification.[72]

The most characteristic finding is bone resorption. It may be classified as subchondral, trabecular, endosteal, intracortical, subperiosteal, subligamentous, and subtendinous.[72] Subperiosteal resorption is most often seen in the hands and feet (Figure 6.28). The radial aspects of the middle phalanges and the tufts of distal phalanges are most commonly affected (i.e., acro-osteolysis). Trabecular resorption is most often seen in the diploic space of the skull ("salt and pepper" appearance) (Figure 6.29). Subligamentous and subtendinous resorption is most often seen at the inferior margin of the clavicle, at the insertion of the plantar aponeurosis and Achilles tendon on the calcaneus, at the ischial tuberosities of the pelvis, at the tuberosities of the humerus, and at the femoral trochanters. Subchondral resorption may be seen in the sacroiliac joints, sternoclavicular joints, acromioclavicular joints, symphysis pubis, and discovertebral junction (Figure 6.30). Erosions may involve the bare areas of the interphalangeal joints, the proximal medial aspect of long bones, and the lamina dura of the mandible.

Radiologic findings that are more common in secondary than in primary hyperparathyroidism include osseous sclerosis and soft-tissue calcification.[72] In contrast, chondrocalcinosis (e.g., menisci, triangular fibrocartilage, pubic symphysis) is more common in primary than in secondary hyperparathyroidism.[72]

Musculoskeletal complications of hyperparathyroidism include laxity, avulsion, and rupture of tendons and ligaments. Tendon rupture is most common in the quadriceps and patellar tendons and is best demonstrated with MR imaging.

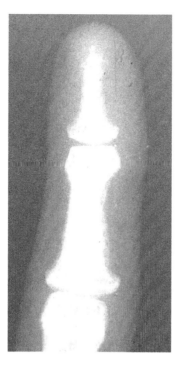

FIGURE 6.28 Hyperparathyroidism. AP radiograph of a finger in a woman with primary hyperparathyroidism shows subperiosteal bone resorption along the radial aspect of the middle phalanx and bone resorption in the tuft of the distal phalanx (acro-osteolysis). Bone resorption in these locations is characteristic of hyperparathyroidism.

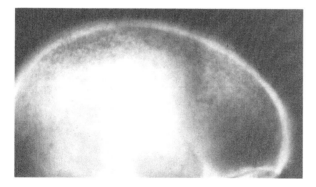

FIGURE 6.29 Hyperparathyroidism. Lateral radiograph of the skull in a man with hyperparathyroidism shows trabecular resorption of the diploic space ("salt and pepper" appearance).

Differential diagnosis of imaging findings in patients with hyperparathyroidism is as follows. Subperiosteal resorption involving a single bone more commonly indicates neoplasm or osteomyelitis. Both severe osteoporosis and multiple myeloma may lead to endosteal resorption. Osseous sclerosis has a broad differential diagnosis, including metastatic disease, radiation-induced bone disease, hypoparathyroidism, myelofibrosis, mastocytosis, sickle cell disease, osteopetrosis, melorheostosis, and Paget's disease. Chondrocalcinosis may be seen with pyrophosphate arthropathy or hemochromatosis. The differential diagnosis for brown tumors includes other focal lytic lesions, such as giant cell tumor and fibrous dysplasia.

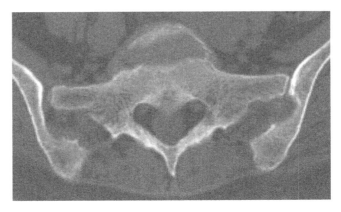

FIGURE 6.30 Hyperparathyroidism. CT scan of the sacroiliac joints shows bilateral subchondral and subligamentous erosions.

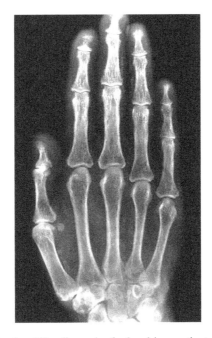

FIGURE 6.31 Renal osteodystrophy. AP radiograph of a hand in a patient with chronic renal failure shows generalized osteopenia, indistinct trabecular pattern, subperiosteal bone resorption along the radial aspect of the middle phalanges, acro-osteolysis, and vascular calcifications. These findings are typical of advanced renal osteodystrophy.

C. RENAL OSTEODYSTROPHY

The term *renal osteodystrophy* includes all of the disorders of bone and mineral metabolism associated with chronic renal insufficiency. It combines features of secondary hyperparathyroidism, rickets, osteomalacia, and osteoporosis.[74-76] In children, the findings of rickets dominate, whereas in adults the findings of secondary hyperparathyroidism dominate. Renal osteodystrophy is a spectrum ranging from primarily high-turnover bone disease (i.e., secondary hyperparathyroidism) to low-turnover bone disease (i.e., osteomalacia).[74-76]

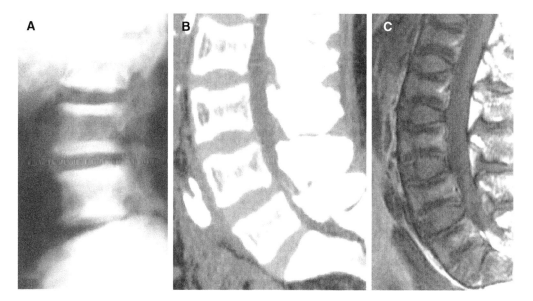

FIGURE 6.32 Rugger jersey spine. (A) Lateral radiograph of the spine in a patient with renal failure shows horizontal, bandlike ("rugger jersey") sclerosis of the vertebral bodies. (B) Sagittal reconstruction of a spine CT scan in the same individual shows similar sclerosis of the vertebral bodies. (C) Sagittal MR image (T1-weighted) shows bandlike regions of low signal corresponding to the bony sclerosis seen on plain film and CT.

Radiologic findings in patients with renal osteodystrophy are a combination of those from rickets, osteomalacia, secondary hyperparathyroidism, and osteoporosis (Figure 6.31).[77-81] Sclerosis of the spine classically has a "rugger-jersey" appearance (Figure 6.32A, B, and C). Patients undergoing dialysis may present with additional findings.[77-81] Aluminum toxicity may lead to osteomalacia, which commonly results in fractures. Carpal and phalangeal cysts may develop, likely as a result of osseous deposits of amyloid (Figure 6.33A and B). Spondyloarthropathy is also likely due to amyloid deposition and may mimic that of infectious discitis or neuropathic arthropathy.

Radiologic findings of secondary hyperparathyroidism associated with renal osteodystrophy may mimic those of primary hyperparathyroidism.[77-81] Similarly, osteomalacia secondary to other causes should be included in the imaging differential diagnosis.[77-81]

The most common complications of renal osteodystrophy are fractures.[77-81] These may involve osteomalacic bone, osteoporotic bone, brown tumors, or amyloid deposits. Complications of dialysis include carpal tunnel syndrome, osteomyelitis, septic arthritis, and osteonecrosis. Complications of renal transplantation include osteonecrosis, tendonitis, tendon ruptures, and fractures.

D. HYPERTHYROIDISM

The most common causes of hyperthyroidism in adults are toxic diffuse goiter and toxic nodular goiter.[82] Excessive thyroid hormone results in stimulation of bone formation and bone resorption; however, bone resorption is dominant.[82]

On conventional radiographs, generalized osteopenia is the most common finding.[82] Other findings include accelerated skeletal maturation, kyphosis, insufficiency fractures, and thyroid acropachy.[82]

Thyroid acropachy is a rare complication that occurs after treatment for hyperthyroidism.[83] A dense periosteal reaction with a feathery contour, seen in an asymmetric distribution, most prominent along the radial margin of metacarpals and phalanges, is virtually diagnostic (Figure 6.34).

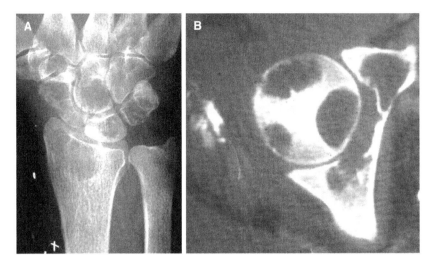

FIGURE 6.33 Amyloidosis. (A) AP radiograph of the wrist in a 70-year-old man undergoing dialysis shows multiple, well-defined lytic lesions in the carpal bones. (B) CT scan of the hip in another patient on dialysis shows lytic lesions in the femoral head and acetabulum, indicating amyloidosis.

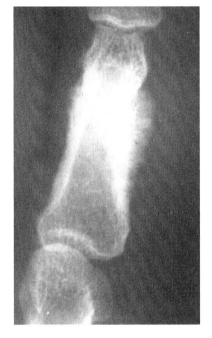

FIGURE 6.34 Thyroid acropachy. AP radiograph of the finger in a 45-year-old man with thyroid acropachy. Note the dense solid periosteal reaction with feathery contour (arrows) along the phalangeal shaft.

E. HYPERADRENOCORTISM

Excessive endogenous production of steroids resulting in Cushing's syndrome is usually due to bilateral adrenocortical hyperplasia and, less frequently, an adrenocortical adenoma or carcinoma.[84]

Whether due to endogenous or exogenous sources, excessive steroids result in demineralization of bone, particularly in the vertebrae, which are prone to fractures.[85] Marginal condensation of the

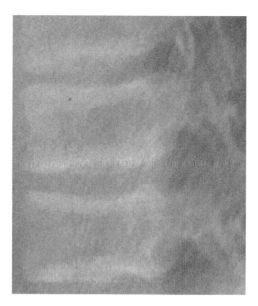

FIGURE 6.35 Glucocorticoid-induced osteoporosis. Lateral radiograph of the lumbar spine in a 40-year-old man receiving glucocorticoid therapy for asthma shows generalized osteopenia and "marginal condensation" subjacent to the end plates of vertebral bodies.

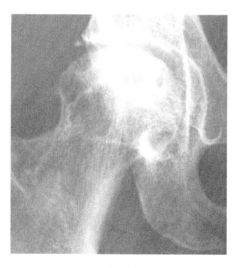

FIGURE 6.36 AVN of femoral head. AP radiograph of the hip shows subchondral sclerosis surrounding a region of lucency in the femoral head indicating AVN

end plates of compressed vertebrae is seen more commonly than in vertebral compressions due to other causes (Figure 6.35). It has been suggested that this finding is a manifestation of attempted repair with excess callus formation. Fractures of the proximal femur, ribs, pubic and ischial rami may also occur and show exuberant callus formation.

Occasionally, accurate diagnosis is facilitated by the presence of steroid-related complications such as osteonecrosis and osteomyelitis.[86,87] Ischemic necrosis of the head of the femur (Figure 6.36) and head of the humerus is especially common. The characteristic radiographic findings are an increase in radiodensity or sclerosis, sometimes known as "snow capping," collapse of bone with

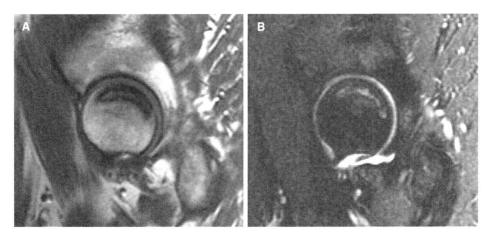

FIGURE 6.37 AVN of femoral head. (A) Sagittal MR image (T1-weighted) of the hip in a patient receiving glucocorticoid therapy shows a crescent-shaped black outline in the superior femoral head. (B) STIR of the same region shows the same black outline with central high signal (the double line sign). These findings are characteristic of the MR appearance of AVN.

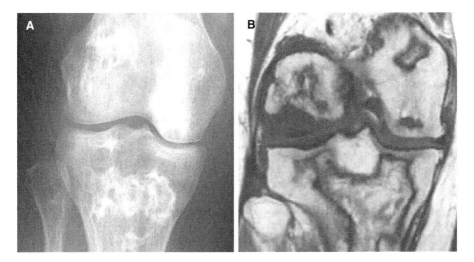

FIGURE 6.38 Bone infarcts. (A) AP radiograph of the knee in a patient receiving glucocorticoid therapy shows multiple serpentine areas of sclerosis characteristic of bone infarcts. (B) Coronal MR image (T1-weighted) of the knee in the same patient shows corresponding serpentine areas of low signal, characteristic of the MR appearance of osteonecrosis.

loss of volume, and linear subcortical radiolucencies (the "crescent sign").[86,87] On MR imaging, serpiginous regions of linear low signal intensity, often paralleled by linear high signal, are virtually diagnostic of osteonecrosis (Figure 6.37A and B).[86,87] In addition to involving the epiphyses, osteonecrosis commonly involves the shafts of long bones and may be seen in virtually any bone of the skeleton (Figure 6.38A and B). Although in its late stages osteonecrosis is apparent on conventional radiographs, early diagnosis requires the use of MR imaging.[86,87]

Nonskeletal findings of hyperadrenocorticism on imaging studies include excess subcutaneous, intra-abdominal, extrapleural, and epicardial fat accumulations as well as mediastinal widening.

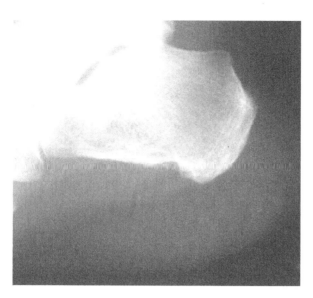

FIGURE 6.39 Acromegaly. Lateral radiograph of the foot in a 30-year-old man with acromegaly shows soft tissue thickening of the heel pad.

F. ACROMEGALY

Acromegaly is usually caused by a pituitary adenoma that produces excessive growth hormone stimulating bone formation and soft tissue proliferation.[88]

Imaging findings include soft tissue thickening in the heel pads and digits (Figure 6.39).[88] Bony enlargement is most common in the skull, vertebra, and phalangeal tufts (Figure 6.40).[88] Less common findings include enlargement of costochondral junctions, enlargement of the sella turcica and paranasal sinuses, intervertebral disk widening, posterior vertebral scalloping, spadelike phalangeal tufts, and arthropathy of large joints (Figure 6.41).[88]

Differential diagnosis of localized soft tissue thickening should include soft tissue edema, hemorrhage, or infection. Heel-pad thickening has been reported after long-term phenytoin therapy. Posterior vertebral scalloping may be seen in spinal neoplasms, neurofibromatosis, Marfan syndrome, Ehlers–Danlos syndrome, and achondroplasia.

IX. REGIONAL OSTEOPOROSIS

The causes of regional osteoporosis include reflex sympathetic dystrophy syndrome, transient regional osteoporosis, pregnancy-associated osteoporosis, immobilization, and disuse.[89-95] Affected patients are at risk for insufficiency fractures. The pathophysiology of regional osteoporosis is discussed in detail in other chapters.

The most common radiographic finding in patients with regional osteoporosis is osteopenia, which may be uniform, bundlike, or patchy (Figure 6.42).[96-99] In early stages, when conventional radiographs are normal, marrow edema on MR images (Figure 6.43) and increased radiopharmaceutical uptake on bone scan (Figure 6.44) may be observed.[96-99]

X. SUMMARY

Increased availability of bone densitometry has resulted in a fundamental shift in the approach to osteoporosis. Clinicians now view osteoporosis not as a disease of fractures, but as a disease of fracture risk. Because low bone mass is such a crucial (and quantifiable) component of this risk,

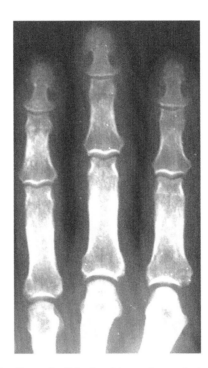

FIGURE 6.40 Acromegaly. AP radiograph of the hand in another patient with acromegaly shows spadelike enlargement of the phalangeal tufts associated with soft tissue overgrowth.

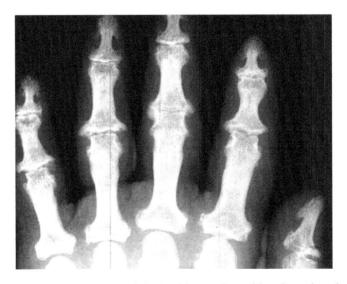

FIGURE 6.41 Acromegaly. AP radiograph of the hand in a patient with arthropathy related to acromegaly shows joint-space narrowing and osteophytes involving the interphalangeal joints of the digits.

densitometry has become essential to patient care. Despite the shift toward densitometry, and in some cases because of it, qualitative radiology continues to play an important role in the evaluation of osteoporotic bone. In this chapter we discussed conventional radiography, CT, MR imaging, and skeletal scintigraphy by focusing on the role of these techniques in clinical and research settings as well as on the imaging findings of osteoporosis and their differential diagnosis.

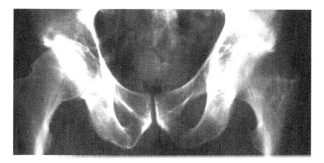

FIGURE 6.42 Transient osteoporosis. Frontal radiograph of the pelvis in a patient with a 3-month history of left hip pain shows relative osteopenia of the left proximal femur when compared to the right. Patient's symptoms resolved without complications.

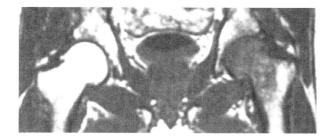

FIGURE 6.43 Transient osteoporosis. Coronal MR image (T1-weighted) in a patient with left hip pain shows relative low signal in left proximal femur when compared to normal marrow signal of the right, indicating bone marrow edema. Conventional radiographs were normal and patient's symptoms and MR finding resolved.

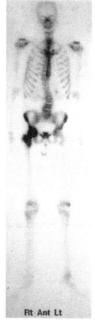

FIGURE 6.44 Transient osteoporosis. Bone scan in a woman with a 2-month history of right hip pain shows intense radiopharmaceutical uptake in the right proximal femur. Because the patient's symptoms resolved without complications, the findings were attributed to transient regional osteoporosis.

REFERENCES

1. Klotzbuecher, C.M., Ross, P.D., Landsman, P.B., et al., "Patients with prior fractures have an increased risk of future fractures: a summary of the literature and statistical synthesis," *J. Bone Miner. Res.,* 4, 721, 2000.

2. Kanis, J.A., Melton, L.J., III, Christiansen, C., et al., "The diagnosis of osteoporosis," *J. Bone Miner. Res.,* 9, 1137, 1994.

3. Genant, H.K., Cooper, C., Poor, G., et al., "Interim report and recommendations of the World Health Organization task-force for osteoporosis," *J. Bone Miner. Res.,* 10, 259, 1999.

4. Kanis, J.A. and Gluer, C.C., "An update on the diagnosis and assessment of osteoporosis with densitometry. Committee of Scientific Advisors, International Osteoporosis Foundation," *Osteoporos. Int.,* 11, 192, 2000.

5. Genant, H.K., Engelke, K., and Fuerst, T., "Noninvasive assessment of bone mineral and structure: state of the art," *J. Bone Miner. Res.,* 11, 707, 1996.

6. Lenchik, L., Rochmis, P., and Sartoris, D.J., "Optimized interpretation and reporting of dual X-ray absorptiometry (DXA) scans," *Am. J. Roentgenol.,* 171, 1509, 1998.

7. Marshall, D., Johnell, O., and Wedel, H., "Meta-analysis of how well measures of bone mineral density predict occurrence of osteoporotic fractures," *Br. Med. J.,* 312, 1254, 1996.

8. Black, D.M., Cummings, S.R., Karpf, D.B., et al., "Randomized trial of effect of alendronate on risk of fracture in women with existing vertebral fractures," *Lancet,* 348, 1535, 1996.

9. Cummings, S.R., Black, D.M., Thompson, D.E., et al., "Effect of alendronate on risk of fracture in women with low bone density but without vertebral fractures: results from the Fracture Intervention Trial," *J. Am. Med. Assoc.,* 280, 2077, 1998.

10. Ettinger, B., Black, D.M., Mitlak, B.H., et al., "Reduction of vertebral fracture risk in postmenopausal women with osteoporosis treated with raloxifene: results from a 3-year randomized clinical trial. Multiple Outcomes of Raloxifene Evaluation," *J. Am. Med. Assoc.,* 282, 637, 1999.

11. Harris, S.T., Watts, N.B., Genant, H.K., et al., "Effects of risedronate treatment on vertebral and nonvertebral fractures in women with postmenopausal osteoporosis," *J. Am. Med. Assoc.,* 282, 1344, 1999.

12. McClung, M.R., Geusens, P., Miller, P.D., et al., "Effect of risedronate on the risk of hip fracture in elderly women. Hip Intervention Program Study Group," *N. Engl. J. Med.,* 344, 333, 2001.

13. Chesnut, C.H., III, Silverman, S., Andriano, K., et al., "A randomized trial of nasal spray salmon calcitonin in postmenopausal women with established osteoporosis: the prevent recurrence of osteoporotic fractures study. PROOF Study Group," *Am. J. Med.,* 109, 267, 2000.

14. McClung, M.R., "Therapy for fracture prevention," *J. Am. Med. Assoc.,* 282, 687, 1999.

15. Eastell, R., "Treatment of postmenopausal osteoporosis," *N. Engl. J. Med.,* 338, 736, 1998.

16. Beck, T.J., "On measuring bone to predict osteoporotic fracture: moving beyond statistical inference," *Radiology,* 199, 612, 1996.

17. Genant, H.K., Gordon, C., Jiang, Y., et al., "Advanced imaging of the macrostructure and microstructure of bone," *Horm. Res.,* 54, S24, 2000.

18. Saville, P.D., "A quantitative approach to simple radiographic diagnosis of osteoporosis: its application to the osteoporosis of rheumatoid arthritis," *Arthritis Rheum.,* 10, 416, 1967.

19. Singh, M., Nagrath, A.R., and Maini, P.S., "Changes in trabecular pattern of the upper end of the femur as an index of osteoporosis," *J. Bone Joint Surg.,* 52A, 457, 1970.

20. Bloom, R.A., "A comparative estimation of the combined cortical thickness of various bone sites," *Skeletal Radiol.,* 5, 167, 1980.

21. Nielsen, S.P., "The metacarpal index revisited: a brief overview," *J. Clin. Densitom.,* 4, 199, 2001.

22. Jergas, M., Uffmann, M., Escher, H., et al., "Interobserver variation in the detection of osteopenia by radiography and comparison with dual X-ray absorptiometry of the lumbar spine," *Skeletal Radiol.,* 23, 195, 1994.

23. Finsen, V. and Anda, S., "Accuracy of visually estimated bone mineralization in routine radiographs of the lower extremity," *Skeletal Radiol.,* 17, 270, 1988.

24. Haller, J., Andre, M.P., Resnick, D., et al., "Detection of thoracolumbar vertebral body destruction with lateral spine radiography. Part II. Clinical investigation with computed tomography," *Invest. Radiol.,* 25, 523, 1990.

25. Haller, J., Andre, M.P., Resnick, D., et al., "Detection of thoracolumbar vertebral body destruction with lateral spine radiography. Part I: Investigation in cadavers," *Invest. Radiol.*, 25, 517, 1990.

26. Genant, H.K., Cann, C.E., Chafetz, N.I., and Helms, C.A., "Advances in computed tomography of the musculoskeletal system," *Radiol. Clin. North Am.*, 19, 645, 1981.

27. Moon, K.L., Jr., Genant, H.K., Davis, P.L., et al., "Nuclear magnetic resonance imaging in orthopaedics: principles and applications," *J. Orthop. Res.*, 1, 101, 1983.

28. Ryan, P.J. and Fogelman, I., "Bone scintigraphy in metabolic bone disease," *Semin. Nucl. Med.*, 3, 291, 1997.

29. Meema, H.E. and Meindok, H., "Advantages of peripheral radiogrametry over dual-photon absorptiometry of the spine in the assessment of prevalence of osteoporotic vertebral fractures in women," *J. Bone Miner. Res.*, 7, 897, 1992.

30. Crespo, R., Revilla, M., Usabiago, J., et al., "Metacarpal radiogrammetry by computed radiography in postmenopausal women with Colles' fracture and vertebral crush fracture syndrome," *Calcif. Tissue Int.*, 62, 470, 1998.

31. Aguado, F., Revilla, M., Villa, L.F., and Rico, H., "Cortical bone resorption in osteoporosis," *Calcif. Tissue Int.*, 60, 323, 1997.

32. Maggio, D., Pacifici, R., Cherubini, A., et al., "Age-related cortical bone loss at the metacarpal," *Calcif. Tissue Int.*, 60, 94, 1997.

33. Lazenby, R.A., "Bias and agreement for radiogrammetric estimates of cortical bone geometry," *Invest. Radiol.*, 32, 12, 1997.

34. Horsman, A. and Simpson, M., "The measurement of sequential changes in cortical bone geometry," *Br. J. Radiol.*, 48, 471, 1975.

35. Geusens, P., Dequeker, J., Verstraeten, A., and Nijs, J., "Age-, sex-, and menopause-related changes of vertebral and peripheral bone: population study using dual and single photon absorptiometry and radiogrammetry," *J. Nucl. Med.*, 27, 1540, 1986.

36. Jergas, M., San Valentin, R., Black, D., et al., "Radiogrammetry of the metacarpals predicts future hip fractures," *J. Bone Miner. Res.*, 10, S371, 1995.

37. Jorgensen, J.T., Andersen, P.B., Rosholm, A., and Bjarnason, N.H., "Digital X-ray radiogrammetry: a new appendicular bone densitometric method with high precision," *Clin. Physiol.*, 20, 330, 2000.

38. Nielsen, S.P. and Hyldstrup, L., "Metacarpal index by digital X-ray radiogrammetry: normative reference values and comparison with dual X-ray absorptiometry," *J. Clin. Densitom.*, 4, 299, 2001.

39. Hyldstrup, L., Jorgensen, J.T., Sorensen, T.K., and Baeksgaard, L., "Response of cortical bone to antiresorptive treatment," *Calcif. Tissue Int.*, 68, 135, 2001.

40. Geraets, W.G.M., Van Der Stelt, P.F., Netelenbos, C.J., et al., "A new method for automatic recognition of the radiographic trabecular pattern," *J. Bone Miner. Res.*, 5, 227, 1990.

41. Caligiuri, P., Giger, M.L., Favus, M.J., et al., "Computerized radiographic analysis of osteoporosis: preliminary evaluation," *Radiology*, 186, 471, 1993.

42. Ouyang, X., Majumdar, S., Link, T.M., et al., "Morphometric texture analysis of spinal trabecular bone structure assessed using orthogonal radiographic projections," *Med. Phys.*, 25, 2037, 1998.

43. Link, T., Majumdar, S., Konermann, W., et al., "Texture analysis of direct magnification radiographs of vertebral specimens: correlation with bone mineral density and biomechanical properties," *Acad. Radiol.*, 4, 167, 1997.

44. Chevalier, F., Laval-Jeantet, A.M., Laval-Jeantet, M., and Bergot, C., "CT image analysis of the vertebral trabecular network *in vivo*," *Calcif. Tissue Int.*, 51, 8, 1992.

45. Haralick, R.M., "Ridges and valleys on digital images," *Comp. Vision Graph. Image Proc.*, 22, 28, 1983.

46. Majumdar, S., Weinstein, R.S., and Prasad, R.R., "Application of fractal geometry techniques to the study of trabecular bone," *Med. Phys.*, 20, 1611, 1993.

47. Majumdar, S., Lin, J., Link, T., et al., "Fractal analysis of radiographs: assessment of trabecular bone structure and prediction of elastic modulus and strength," *Med. Phys.*, 26, 1330, 1999.

48. Samarabandu, J., Acharya, R., Hausmann, E., et al., "Analysis of bone X-rays using morphologic fractals," *IEEE Trans. Med. Imag.*, 12, 466, 1993.

49. Caligiuri, P., Giger, M.L., and Favus, M., "Multifractal radiographic analysis of osteoporosis," *Med. Phys.*, 21, 503, 1994.

50. Laib, A. and Rüegsegger, P., "Comparison of structure extraction methods for *in vivo* trabecular bone measurements," *Comput. Med. Imag. Graph.*, 23, 69, 1999.

51. Ito, M., Nakamura, T., Matsumoto, T., et al., "Analysis of trabecular microarchitecture of human iliac bone using microcomputed tomography in patients with hip arthrosis with or without vertebral fracture," *Bone*, 23, 163, 1998.

52. Barbier, A., Martel, C., de Vernejoul, M.C., et al., "The visualization and evaluation of bone architecture in the rat using three-dimensional X-ray microcomputed tomography," *J. Bone Miner. Metab.*, 17, 37, 1999.

53. Hodgson, S.F., Watts, N.B., Bilezikian, J.P., et al., "American Association of Clinical Endocrinologists 2001 Medical Guidelines for Clinical Practice for the Prevention and Management of Postmenopausal Osteoporosis," *Endocr. Pract.*, 7, 293, 2001.

54. Anonymous, "Consensus Development Conference: diagnosis, prophylaxis, and treatment of osteoporosis," *Am. J. Med.*, 94, 646, 1993.

55. Mankin, H.J., "Metabolic bone disease," *J. Bone Joint Surg.*, 76A, 760, 1994.

56. Reynolds, W.A. and Karo, J.J., "Radiologic diagnosis of metabolic bone disease," *Orthop. Clin. North Am.*, 3, 521, 1972.

57. Steinbach, H.L., "The roentgen appearance of osteoporosis," *Radiol. Clin. North Am.*, 2, 191, 1964.

58. Mayo-Smith, W. and Rosenthal, D.I., "Radiographic appearance of osteopenia," *Radiol. Clin. North Am.*, 29, 37, 1991.

59. Pitt, M., "Osteopenic bone disease," *Orthop. Clin. North Am.*, 14, 65, 1983.

60. Faciszewski, T. and McKiernan, F., "Calling all vertebral fractures, classification of vertebral compression fractures: a consensus for comparison of treatment and outcome," *J. Bone Miner. Res.*, 17, 185, 2002.

61. Ismail, A.A., Cooper, C., Felsenberg, D., et al., "Number and type of vertebral deformities: epidemiologic characteristics and relation to back pain and height loss. European Vertebral Osteoporosis Study Group," *Osteoporos. Int.*, 9, 206, 1999.

62. O'Neill, T.W., "The prevalence of vertebral deformity in European men and women: the European vertebral osteoporosis study," *J. Bone Miner. Res.*, 11, 1010, 1996.

63. Black, D.M., Palermo, L., Nevitt, M.C., et al., "Defining incident vertebral deformity: a prospective comparison of several approaches. The Study of Osteoporotic Fractures Research Group," *J. Bone Miner. Res.*, 14, 90, 1999.

64. Genant, H.K., Jergas, M., Palermo, L., et al., "Comparison of semiquantitative visual and quantitative morphometric assessment of prevalent and incident vertebral fractures in osteoporosis. The Study of Osteoporotic Fractures Research Group," *J. Bone Miner. Res.*, 11, 984, 1996.

65. Finch, P.J., Ang, L., Eastwood, J.B., et al., "Clinical and histologic spectrum of osteomalacia among Asians in South London," *Q. J. Med.*, 83, 439, 1992.

66. Gloriex, F.H., "Rickets, the continuing challenge," *N. Engl. J. Med.*, 325, 1875, 1991.

67. Mankin, H.J., "Rickets, osteomalacia, and renal osteodystrophy: an update," *Orthop. Clin. North Am.*, 21, 81, 1990.

68. Pitt, M.J., "Rickets and osteomalacia are still around," *Radiol. Clin. North Am.*, 29, 97, 1991.

69. Steinbach, H.L. and Noetzli, M., "Roentgen appearance of the skeleton in osteomalacia and rickets," *Am. J. Roentgenol.*, 1964. 91, 955,

70. Reginato, A.J., Falasca, G.F., Pappu, R., et al., "Musculoskeletal manifestations of osteomalacia: report of 26 cases and literature review," *Semin. Arthritis Rheum.*, 28, 287, 1999.

71. Consensus Development Conference Panel, "Diagnosis and management of asymptomatic primary hyperparathyroidism," *Ann. Intern. Med.*, 114, 593, 1991.

72. Genant, H.K., Heck, L.L., Lanzl, L.H., et al., "Primary hyperparathyroidism: a comprehensive study of clinical, biochemical, and radiographic manifestations," *Radiology*, 109, 513, 1973.

73. Silverberg, S.J., Gartenberg, F., Jacobs, T.P., et al., "Longitudinal measurements of bone density and biochemical indices in untreated primary hyperparathyroidism," *J. Clin. Endocrinol. Metab.*, 80, 723, 1995.

74. Parfitt, A.M., "The hyperparathyroidism of chronic renal failure: a disorder of growth," *Kidney Int.*, 52, 3, 1997.

75. Sherrard, D.J., Hercz, G., Pei, Y., et al., "The spectrum of bone disease in end-stage renal failure: an evolving disorder," *Kidney Int.*, 43, 436, 1993.

76. Rodino, M.A. and Shane, E., "Osteoporosis after transplantation," *Am. J. Med.*, 104, 459, 1998.

77. Greenfield, G.B., "Roentgen appearance of bone and soft tissue changes in chronic renal disease," *Am. J. Roentgenol.,* 116, 749, 1972.

78. Olmastroni, M., Seracini, D., Lavoratti, G., et al., "Magnetic resonance imaging of renal osteodystrophy in children," *Pediatr. Radiol.,* 27, 865, 1997.

79. Resnick, D., "Abnormalities of bone and soft tissue following renal transplantation," *Semin. Roentgenol.,* 13, 329, 1978.

80. Shapiro, R., "Radiologic aspects of renal osteodystrophy," *Radiol. Clin. North Am.,* 10, 557, 1972.

81. Tigges, S., Nance, E.P., Carpenter, W.A., et al., "Renal osteodystrophy: imaging findings that mimic those of other disorders," *Am. J. Roentgenol.,* 165, 143, 1995.

82. Wietersen, F.K. and Balow, R.M., "The radiologic aspects of thyroid disease," *Radiol. Clin. North Am.,* 5, 255, 1967.

83. Scanlon, G.T. and Clemett, A.R., "Thyroid acropachy," *Radiology,* 83, 1039, 1964.

84. Sissons, H.A., "The osteoporosis of Cushing's syndrome," *J. Bone Joint Surg.,* 38B, 418, 1956.

85. Rosenberg, E.F., "Rheumatoid arthritis: osteoporosis and fractures related to steroid therapy," *Acta Med. Scand.,* 162, S211, 1958.

86. Cruess, R.L., Ross, D., and Crawshaw, E., "The etiology of steroid-induced avascular necrosis of bone," *Clin. Orthop.,* 113, 178, 1975.

87. Mitchell, D.G., Rao, V.M., Dalinka, M.K., et al., "Femoral head avascular necrosis: correlation of MR imaging, radiographic staging, radionuclide imaging, and clinical findings," *Radiology,* 162, 709, 1987.

88. Lang, E.K. and Bessler, W.T., "The roentgenologic features of acromegaly," *Am. J. Roentgenol.,* 86, 321, 1961.

89. Arnstein, A.R., "Regional osteoporosis," *Orthop. Clin. North Am.,* 3, 585, 1972.

90. Dunne, F., Walters, B., Marshall, T., et al., "Pregnancy associated osteoporosis," *Clin. Endocrinol.,* 39, 487, 1993.

91. Kozin, F., McCarty, D.J., Simms, J., et al., "The reflex sympathetic dystrophy syndrome. I. Clinical and histologic studies: evidence for bilaterality, response to corticosteroids and articular involvement," *Am. J. Med.,* 60, 321, 1976.

92. McCord, W.C., Nies, K.M., Campion, D.S., et al., "Regional migratory osteoporosis: a denervation disease," *Arthritis Rheum.,* 21, 834, 1978.

93. Naides, S.J., Resnick, D., and Zvaifler, N.J., "Idiopathic regional osteoporosis: a clinical spectrum," *J. Rheumatol.,* 12, 763, 1985.

94. Smith, R., Athanasou, N.A., Ostlere, S.J., et al., "Pregnancy associated osteoporosis," *Q. J. Med.,* 88, 865, 1995.

95. Smith, R. and Phillips, A.J., "Osteoporosis during pregnancy and its management," *Scand. J. Rheumatol. Suppl.,* 107, 66, 1998.

96. Genant, H.K., Kozin, F., Bekerman, C., et al., "The reflex sympathetic dystrophy syndrome: a comprehensive analysis using fine-detail radiography, photon absorptiometry and bone and joint scintigraphy," *Radiology,* 117, 21, 1975.

97. Lequesne, M., Kerboull, M., Bensasson, M., et al., "Partial transient osteoporosis," *Skeletal Radiol.,* 2, 1, 1977.

98. Van de Berg, B.E., Malghem, J.J., Labaisse, M.A., et al., "MR imaging of avascular necrosis and transient marrow edema of the femoral head," *Radiographics,* 13, 501, 1993.

99. Wilson, A.J., Murphy, W.A., Hardy, D.C., et al., "Transient osteoporosis: transient bone marrow edema?" *Radiology,* 167, 757, 1988.

7 Densitometry and Morphometry of Osteoporotic Bone

Giuseppe Guglielmi and Daniele Diacinti

CONTENTS

I. INTRODUCTION

Measurement of bone mineral content of the axial and appendicular skeleton constitutes an important aspect of the detection and follow-up of metabolic bone disease, particularly osteoporosis.

Osteoporosis is a systemic skeletal disease characterized by low bone mass and microarchitectural deterioration of bone tissue, with a consequent increase in bone fragility and susceptibility to fracture. Although the occurrence of fractures depends on a variety of factors, bone mineral density (BMD) is the most important determinant. Early diagnosis of osteoporosis, fracture risk prediction, and assessment of efficacy of treatment therefore are of great interest. Simple bone radiographs remain an important cornerstone in detection and differential diagnosis of osteopenia, but are not sufficient to diagnose early bone loss because losses of up to 20 to 40% of bone mass may occur before a noticeable change is detected. Over the past several years, a number of noninvasive techniques have been developed to evaluate bone mass more sensitively at a number of skeletal sites and relate the measurements to age-matched control subjects. The purpose of this chapter is to review basic methodology and developments in radiology such as dual X-ray absorptiometry (DXA) and quantitative computed tomography (QCT), which are widely used in clinical practice. Results from recent studies using new applications of ultrasound techniques in the detection and

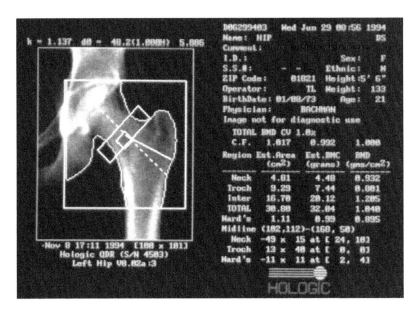

FIGURE 7.1 DXA at the hip site showing ROIs analyzed: femoral neck (oblong box), Ward's area (box), and trochanter.

assessment of bone structure and strength and morphometric evaluation of osteoporotic vertebral fracture are also discussed.

II. DUAL X-RAY ABSORPTIOMETRY

In the last decade, dual-photon absorptiometry (DPA) has been replaced by DXA. This technique is based on the same principle as DPA but uses an X-ray tube instead of a radionuclide source. The concept has existed since the 1960s, but it was not until 1987 that DXA was made commercially available.[1,2] The use of an X-ray system results in shorter scan time, greater accuracy and precision, and the lack of radionuclide decay. Additional technical improvements such as internal calibration have helped to improve the accuracy and precision.[3,4] The usual locations for DXA measurements are the lumbar spine, proximal femur, radius, and whole body (Figures 7.1 and 7.2). Because of the high resolution of DXA scanners, anatomic details of the examined region are depicted clearly. The digital image resulting from the measurement allows a gross survey of the examined region. Bone density measurements are provided as bone mineral content (BMC) in g/cm of bone length or as BMD in g/cm^2. The elaborate software of DXA devices allows for an automated identification of regions of interest with distinct compositions such as the femoral neck or the ultradistal radius. At the lumbar spine, every vertebral body can be measured separately and fractured vertebrae can be excluded from the analysis. Due to osteophytes, aortic calcifications, degenerative joint disease, and intervertebral space narrowing, the measured BMD may be increased artificially in the posterior-anterior (PA) measurement of the lumbar spine; furthermore, the area measurement includes substantial portions of cortical bone, thereby reducing sensitivity for the distinction between osteoporotic and healthy subjects.[5] As a consequence, it is necessary to obtain a lateral conventional radiograph of the spine at least once before the first DXA measurement of a patient, to estimate the magnitude of degenerative changes present and to take those into consideration when interpreting the results. On the other hand, lateral scanning of the lumbar spine by DXA enables the radiologist to evaluate the vertebral bodies with an almost exclusive measurement of trabecular bone.

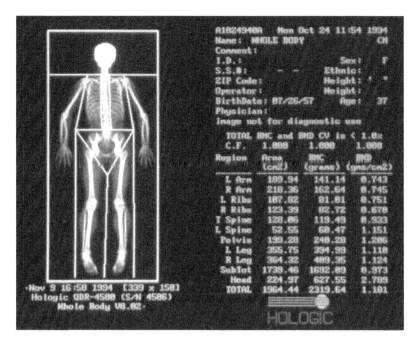

FIGURE 7.2 DXA of the whole body with regional areas of analysis (head, chest, pelvis, arms, and legs). With appropriate software programs information on whole and regional body composition (muscle and fat mass) can be obtained.

Problems that arise from superimposition of vertebral posterior elements are largely avoided. Improvement has occurred in discriminating age-related bone loss and in distinguishing normal women from women with osteoporosis with lateral DXA, which indicates the superior sensitivity of this method compared to PA scanning (Figure 7.3). The correlation between lateral DXA and QCT, which measures the vertebral body, has been found to be stronger than that of PA-DXA and QCT.[6] This method can reduce the error intrinsic in the PA examination of the lumbar spine. The currently used generation of DXA scanners permits rotation of the X-ray tube with a C-arm so that lateral spine measurements can be done with the patient remaining in a supine position after the PA investigation. Using DXA for obtaining lateral images of the lumbar spine offers the additional advantage that the scanning beam, in contrast to conventional cone beam radiography, is always parallel to the vertebral end plates. This allows an improved definition of vertebral dimensions for a morphometric analysis.

At the proximal femur, the clinically most important sites are probably the intertrochanteric region and Ward's triangle, because they consist mostly of trabecular bone, having only small cortical contributions at the anterior and posterior femoral aspect.

The advanced generation of scanners uses a fan beam and multidetector arrays, decreasing the examination time by a factor of 4 to 10. A total body examination now requires less than 2 min. This advance reduces movement artifacts, improves the patient's comfort, and enhances patient throughput. Radiation dose for these investigations is very low: for a PA lumbar spine measurement it is about 1 μSv for standard resolution examinations. Consequently, no expensive shielding of the exam room is necessary, a factor that contributes to the moderate costs of this modality. DXA has taken the place of the DPA with a distribution of over 3000 systems worldwide, thereby reaching great acceptance in clinical medicine and research. Low radiation dose, availability, and ease of use have made DXA the most widely used technique for measurements of bone density in clinical trials and epidemiologic studies.[7-13]

A. Peripheral QCT

Special-purpose peripheral QCT (pQCT) scanners have been employed for measurements of BMC and BMD of peripheral skeleton. Peripheral QCT allows for a true volumetric measurement of appendicular bone without superimposition of other tissues and provides exact three-dimensional localization of the target volume. Ease of use, the possibility of separately assessing cortical and trabecular bone, and measuring BMD, BMC, and axial area make the method an interesting alternative to the techniques of single photon absorptiometry (SPA) and single X-ray absorptiometry (SXA). With the commonly used clinical pQCT scanner, measurements in the distal radius are performed at only one site with a single axial slice of 2.5 mm thickness located at 4% of the ulnar length from the distal radial cortical end plate.[26-28]

For *in vitro* studies, the accuracy of the method was calculated to be about 2%.[29,30] The short-term *in vivo* precision of the clinical pQCT has been measured using groups of healthy young volunteers, and the average absolute precision errors ranges from 1.8 to 3.4 mg/cm^3 for the trabecular and from 3.8 to 8.5 mg/cm^3 for the total region.[31] The relationship between pQCT parameters and aging in healthy subjects was evaluated in several studies. Grampp et al.[31] found only small annual BMD changes in healthy volunteers of −0.30% in total, −0.25% in trabecular, and 0.19% in cortical BMD. Schneider et al.[32] found annual decreases of 0.5% in the trabecular BMD of healthy women and 1.9% in women with osteoporosis. Butz et al.[33] found changes of 0.9% in the trabecular and 1.1% in the total BMD. Guglielmi et al.[34] showed a linear decline with aging by an overall slope of −1.28 and −0.55 mg/cm^3/year for total and trabecular BMD measurements. pQCT measurements of BMD at the radius were found to be successful in distinguishing between patients with and without osteoporosis, and in monitoring subjects during clinical studies. Different from other methods, pQCT as a method capable of three-dimensional imaging inherently bears the capability of providing information related to the architecture of bone. In addition, it allows determination of the material property by estimation of the bone mass per volume unit. It may hence be applied to noninvasive estimation of bone mechanical properties at the organ level, beyond the possibilities of standard densitometry.[35] Excellent results have been obtained, correlating pQCT-assessed mechanical parameters, such as the second moment of inertia and its derivatives, with ultimate failure load.[36,37]

B. Volumetric QCT

While the use of standard QCT has centered on two-dimensional characterization of vertebral trabecular bone, there is interest in developing three dimensional, or vQCT, techniques to improve spinal measurements and to extend QCT assessments to the proximal femur. These three-dimensional techniques encompass the entire object of interest with stacked slices or spiral CT scans, and can use anatomic landmarks to automatically relevant projections. Not only can vQCT determine BMC or BMD of the entire bone or sub region, such as a vertebral body or femoral neck, it can also provide separate analysis of the trabecular or cortical components. Because a true and highly accurate volumetric rendering is provided, important geometric and biomechanically relevant assessments can be derived such as cross-sectional moment of inertia and finite-element analysis.[38-43]

IV. QUANTITATIVE ULTRASOUND

During the past few years a number of different approaches for the assessment of skeletal status by means of quantitative ultrasound (QUS) have been developed. The attractiveness of QUS as an alternative or complementary technique to BMD measurements lies in its low cost, portability, ease of use, and the lack of exposure to ionizing radiation. These benefits combined with clinical results showing good diagnostic sensitivity for fracture discrimination have encouraged further basic investigation and commercial development. Currently available systems measure ultrasound parameters primarily in trabecular bone (calcaneus, patella), cortical bone (tibia), or integral bone (hand phalanges). QUS measurement methods take into account either ultrasound velocity or speed of sound (SOS) or broadband ultrasound attenuation (BUA), or both. Ultrasound velocity is considered mainly related to bone density and elasticity and BUA is related to bone density and trabecular structure.

Measurements of the peripheral skeleton with QUS are rapid and inexpensive and may be useful in population screening. Many studies increasingly confirm the predictive value of various types of peripheral densitometry for all types of fracture and more recently for QUS parameters. The parameters measured with QUS are influenced not only by bone density but also by bone structure (trabecular number, connectivity, and orientation) and composition. It has been shown that osteoporosis involves a deterioration in both bone architecture and bone mass. The QUS technique reflects structural characteristics of bone and therefore it may provide additional information independent of those of current X-ray-based measures of bone density.[44-48]

A. INVESTIGATION OF QUS IN VITRO

Many researchers have found a close correlation between the mechanically and ultrasonically determined elastic modulus of human and bovine cancellous bone.[49,50] Njeh et al.[51] and Bouxsein et al.[52] have reported a significant correlation ($r = 0.82$ and 0.71, respectively) between ultrasound velocity and ultimate strength of the human calcaneus. Moreover, Bouxsein et al.[52] found that both calcaneal BMD and BUA were highly correlated with femoral failure load ($r = 0.63$ and 0.51, respectively). Nicholson et al.[53] reported a higher correlation among calcaneal BMD, BUA, and bone velocity with femoral strength ($r = 0.75$, 0.69, and 0.63). However, they found that femoral BMD was a significantly better predictor of femoral strength than calcaneal ultrasound. The consensus is that in vitro QUS parameters (velocity and BUA) are good predictors of mechanical properties, especially stiffness and strength.

The relationship between QUS and physical density has also been investigated in vitro. McCloskey et al.[54] reported measurements of BUA and physical density on samples of calcaneus obtained from cadavers and concluded that there was a high correlation ($r = 0.85$). McKelvie et al.[55] obtained a similar correlation ($r = 0.83$) between BUA and physical density of the calcaneus. Laugier et al.,[56] using an imaging system that allowed site-matched BMD measurement and acoustic measurement, found higher correlations. They found a correlation coefficient of 0.87 between BUA and BMD, 0.94 between bone velocity and BMD, and 0.92 between BUA and bone velocity. Evans and Tavakoli[57] found a poor correlation ($r = 0.33$) between BUA and physical density, but a highly significant correlation ($r = 0.85$) between velocity and physical density of bovine femur. It has been suggested by Langton et al.[50] that the high correlation between BUA and physical density in the human as compared to the bovine samples could be due to smaller structural variation in the human calcaneus. When a large density range is used, BUA exhibits a nonlinear relationship with density, but is linear within the clinically relevant density. In a study on the bones of pig phalanges, Cadossi and Canè[58] demonstrated that macroscopic morphologic changes in bone tissue induce alterations in ultrasound transmission. Recently, De Terlizzi et al.[59] have investigated the influence of bone tissue density and elasticity on U.S. propagation in specimens excised from phalanges of pig and they have shown that ultrasound technique gives separate information on bone density and elasticity that X-ray-based densitometric methods do not provide.

Structure is one of the qualities of bone that ultrasound is purported to measure as opposed to density only as measured by DXA. Structure can be defined in terms of connectivity, porosity, and anisotropy. Evidence has come from QUS anisotropy, histomorphometric and others, but the evidence is not conclusive.[60-63] Rho et al.[64] have used fractal dimension to characterize bone connectivity. They found that after adjusting for density, significant correlation was found between the elastic modulus and BUA or fractal dimension. The clinical significance of the structure information is being debated since the biologic variation in a unidirection is limited. However, it is believed that structure information in conjunction with density should improve fracture prediction.

B. Investigation of QUS in Vivo

There has been a tendency to correlate QUS with the established ionizing radiation measurements of BMD. The correlation coefficients have ranged from 0.34 to 0.83.[65-69] These correlations, although significant, are weak. It has been argued that this is because QUS is dependent on other aspects of bone in addition to density. The interpretation of the correlations between QUS and absorptiometry techniques is complicated by many factors, including measurement site assessed by BUA and bone densitometry techniques, effects of different ultrasound systems used, the different modes of interaction of ultrasound and photon-based techniques, age range or population group studied, and precision and accuracy. On the other hand, the relationship between QUS and density could be a dynamic relationship rather than a simple linear regression. It is generally accepted that ultrasound and DXA interact differently with bone, and a high correlation between them should not be expected. Therefore, simple linear regression is not really an appropriate way of relating these two modalities. Attention is now directed toward diagnostic accuracy of ultrasound rather than simple correlation with BMD using statistical techniques such as ROC analysis z-scores, odds ratios, and relative risk.

Numerous cross-sectional studies of ultrasound normative data have been reported,[65-70] all showing that QUS parameters are inversely correlated with age, showing a significant decrease in both BUA and SOS, especially after menopause. Typical rates of change are 0.5 to 1.0 dB/MHz (0.5 to 1.0%) per year for BUA and 1 to 5 m/s (0.1 to 0.3%) per year for SOS at the heel, patella, and tibia. However, there are substantial differences between different devices. The first longitudinal study was performed by Schott et al.[65] on 140 healthy postmenopausal women measured at the calcaneus. The decrease that they observed over 2 years was −1.0% + 4.3% for BUA and −0.8% + 0.6% for SOS. The decrease in SOS was significantly larger soon after postmenopause compared to later in life. A similar trend was observed for BUA, but this did not reach statistical significance. Similar results have been found by Krieg et al.[66] in institutionalized elderly women.

Cross-sectional patient studies have demonstrated that QUS can discriminate normal from osteoporotic subjects as well as traditional bone densitometry techniques.[67-70] Recent studies have demonstrated that ultrasound velocity discriminates between fracture and control groups.[71-74] Velocity measured at the calcaneus has similar diagnostic sensitivity to spine BMD and femoral neck BMD for distinguishing patients with vertebral fractures from controls.[75] However, Gonnelli et al.[76] observed that although SOS was an independent predictor of vertebral fracture, BMD was a slightly better predictor. The first prospective study of hip fractures measuring QUS and BMD reported by Hans et al.[77] observed that velocity measured at the calcaneus had the same diagnostic sensitivity as femoral neck BMD in predicting hip fractures. The increased risk associated with a decrease of 1 standard deviation was estimated as 2.0 for both ultrasound velocity and femoral BMD. Guglielmi et al.[78] and Benitez et al.[79] have shown that hand phalangeal ultrasound velocity reflects age-related bone loss and differentiates between healthy and osteoporotic subjects. In a large multicenter study including more than 10,000 subjects, Wuster et al.[80] have demonstrated that ultrasound investigation at the hand phalanges is a valid methodology for osteoporosis assessment. Recently, Frost et al.[81] have shown that QUS and BMD are equally strongly associated with risk factors for osteoporosis.

V. DIAGNOSIS OF OSTEOPOROTIC VERTEBRAL FRACTURE BY MORPHOMETRY

A. Definition of Vertebral Fracture

Vertebral fractures are the most common of all osteoporotic fractures, especially in Caucasian women and men in Europe and the United States,[82-87] and represent a frequently used end point in clinical trials and epidemiologic studies on osteoporosis investigating the effectiveness of different therapeutic regimens.[88-93] However, the epidemiologic data are unreliable for various reasons. First, most vertebral fractures occur in the absence of specific trauma, are asymptomatic, and, therefore, elude clinical diagnosis. Second, the lack of a "gold standard" definition of vertebral fractures on radiographs has given rise to different ways of defining them. Third, osteoporotic vertebral fractures really are deformities of vertebral bodies without the visible discontinuity of bone architecture that accompanies fractures of long bones. The deformities resulting from the loss of anterior, middle, and posterior heights of vertebral bodies results in typical patterns, anterior wedging, biconcavity and crushing, respectively. In everyday clinical practice, the spinal radiograph is still the standard tool used to identify vertebral fractures. The assessment by radiologists of conventional radiographs of the thoracic and lumbar spine in lateral and anterior-posterior (AP) projections generally is uncomplicated, allowing the classification of severe vertebral fractures. However, osteoporotic vertebral fractures often appear as such mild vertebral deformities that the radiologic visual approach may cause disagreement about whether a vertebra is fractured.[94] Because there is no "gold standard" of deformity it may sometimes be difficult to discriminate the osteoporotic vertebral fracture from a normal variant in vertebral shape or from a vertebral deformation that may have occurred long ago.[95,96] Furthermore, there is variation in vertebral size and shape at different levels of the spine. In fact the anterior and posterior vertebral height increases from T3 to L2, but for L3–L5 the posterior height is lower than the anterior height.[97] Vertebral size also varies between individuals: large people tend to have larger vertebrae.[98]

An effort to reduce the high subjectivity with poor reproducibility in qualitative readings of the spine radiographs was introduced more than a decade ago: vertebral morphometry based on vertebral body height measurements.[99-102] For the diagnosis of vertebral fractures it is necessary to compare the vertebral heights calculated with the normal respective values of the reference population, a sample of premenopausal or postmenopausal women.[103-105] Some studies demonstrated that vertebral heights significantly change with age in healthy women, showing rates of loss of 1.2 to 1.5 mm/year.[107-110] Age-related decrease of vertebral heights influences the definition of normal range of vertebral shape. In fact a deformity that may be in excess of 2 standard deviations from the mean in younger subjects may be well within this limit 20 years later.[101] There is still disagreement in establishing a threshold of height reduction that would allow unequivocal discrimination between vertebral fractures, deformities, and normal shape.[96] Therefore, to define vertebral fractures, various morphometric algorithms have been developed that use different cutoff levels of the vertebral height ratios in respect to the normal range for that vertebral level.[111-113] These methods mainly focus on the identification of vertebral fracture assessing the vertebral height ratio of each vertebra. Nevertheless, the number of vertebral fractures may not be representative of the severity of spinal osteoporosis, especially in the case of the biconcavity fractures, which represent deformations of only the end plate. Some methods have also been developed that calculate spine indices for estimating the severity of spinal deformity and for assessing progression of vertebral deformation during follow-up.[114-116]

There are two techniques, morphometric X-ray radiography (MRX) and morphometric X-ray absorptiometry (MXA), used to perform quantitative vertebral morphometry.

B. MORPHOMETRIC X-RAY RADIOGRAPHY

MRX was introduced as early as 1960 by Barnett and Nordin,[117] to measure the vertebral heights on conventional lateral radiographs of the thoracic and lumbar spine. Before performing the measurement of vertebral heights a reader has to identify the vertebral levels; to make this easier, T12 and L1 should be seen on both the lateral thoracic and lumbar radiographs. The vertebral bodies should be marked so that they can be more easily identified in other reading sessions or when compared with follow-up radiographs. The measurement of vertebral heights is performed by so-called point digitization of radiographs. On the lateral radiographs, each vertebra from T4 to L5 (or L4, because of highly variable shape of L5) is marked with six points, which are digitized with a cursor on a translucent digitizer with a resolution of 0.1 mm.[118] With six-point digitization, which is the most widely used technique, the four corner points of each vertebral body are marked and an additional point in the middle of both the upper and lower end plates. The manual point placement for the performance of vertebral height measurements is performed according to Hurxthal,[119] who excluded the uncinate process at the posterior-superior border of thoracic vertebrae from vertebral height measurement and extensively discussed the projection geometry of vertebral bodies. When the outer contours of the end plate are not superimposed (incorrect patient positioning or severe scoliosis), the middle points are chosen in the center between the upper and the lower contour. Furthermore, Schmorl's nodes and osteophytes should be ignored for placement of the vertebral points. The x and y coordinates of each point are stored in the computer, and the software automatically calculates the posterior, middle, and anterior vertebral heights, their ratios, and other morphometric indices.[120]

C. MORPHOMETRIC X-RAY ABSORPTIOMETRY

To overcome some of the limitations of MRX a new method, MXA, has been developed by two major manufacturers of DXA equipment: Hologic, Inc. (Waltham, MA) and Lunar Corporation (Madison, WI).[121,122] In Hologic systems, two views of the thoracic and lumbar spine are acquired: a PA scan and a lateral scan. The PA spine image is acquired to visualize spinal anatomy such as scoliosis, and to determine the centerline of the spine. This information is used in subsequent lateral scans to maintain a constant distance between the center of the spine and the X-ray tube (for all subjects at all visits) regardless of patient position or degree of scoliosis, thus eliminating the geometric distortion.[123] Each lateral scan covers a distance extended to a maximum of 46 cm, imaging the vertebrae from L4 to T4. The Lunar Expert XL scanner determines the starting position of the lateral morphometry scan by positioning a laser spot 1 cm above the iliac crest.[124] The Lunar Expert scanner was the first bone densitometer to feature a full-fledged C-arm design, which was introduced in the QDR-4500A by Hologic (Figures 7.5 and 7.6). The scanner arm can be rotated 90°, so that lateral scans can be obtained with the patient in the supine position. The QDR-4500A has four scan modes available to acquire lateral scans of the spine.[125] One mode uses a single-energy X-ray beam with very short scan time (12 s). However, the analysis may be affected by soft tissue artifacts in the image caused by the prominent imaging of lung structures. These artifacts are absent from the other three — fast (F), array (A), and high definition (HD) — that use a dual-energy beam.

In the new DXA scanners, Delphy (Hologic, Inc.) and Prodigy (Lunar Corp.), the image resolution of the lateral spine has been improved by a factor of 2, achieved by doubling the number of detectors and by even finer collimation of the X-ray beam. The improved image resolution allows a better vertebral morphometry.[126] After the scan, the program automatically identifies vertebral levels and indicates the vertebral centers. The six-point placement for the determination of the vertebral heights is semiautomated. The operator uses a mouse pointing device to specify the 13 locations of the anterior inferior corner of the vertebrae L4 to T4. Then the MXA software computes the positions of the remaining five vertebral points. To guide the operator during image analysis of follow-up scans the vertebral end plate markers from the previous scan are superimposed on the current scan improving long-term precision. After the analysis is finished, a final report is displayed. It gives information on the measured vertebral body heights and their ratios, and includes an assessment of the patient's fracture status based on normative data and different models for fracture assessment using quantitative morphometry.[127]

D. COMPARISON OF MRX AND MXA

Both techniques have a good precision: the coefficients of variability (CV%) of MRX and MXA are similar, ranging from 1.2 to 3.4% (CV intraoperator) and from 1.9 to 5.3% (CV interoperator) by various authors.[94,102,121,128] For MXA, the precision obtained with two systems, Hologic and Lunar, is similar.[128] One of the major advantages of MXA over conventional radiography is the

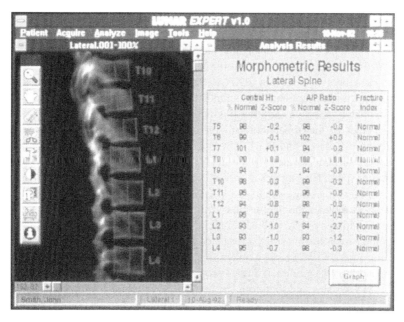

FIGURE 7.5 MXA image of lateral thoracolumbar spine scan showing morphometric measurements and results for each vertebral body from T10 to L4.

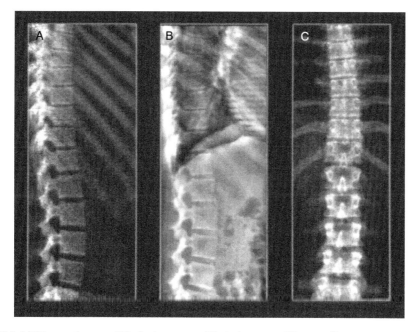

FIGURE 7.6 MXA scan images: (A) single energy; (B) dual energy; (C) centerline scan.

reduced radiation dose applied to the patient. In fact, the effective dose equivalent of conventional radiographs of the lumbar and thoracic spine in the lateral projection totals 800 to 1200 µSv and, by contrast, in MXA is <10 µSv.[129,130] A further advantage of MXA over MXR when using the scanning fan-beam geometry of DXA devices is the absence of distortion and magnification effects inherent in the standard X-ray technique.[131] Ideally, end plates are always parallel in MXA because of the line-by-line exposure and the simultaneous movement of X-ray source and detector along the spine. While MXA is able to assess the entire spine in a single image, in conventional radiography, radiographs of the lumbar and thoracic spine have to be taken separately, so the identification of the vertebral levels to perform MRX may be difficult at times.

The principal source of error for MXA is the relatively limited spatial resolution (0.5 to 1 lp/mm) compared with conventional radiographs that, using a fast screen, provide a spatial resolution of approximately 5 lp/mm. Another limitation of the MXA is the limited visualization in the single-energy images of the upper thoracic spine (T4 and T5) and thoracolumbar junction as a result of overlying soft tissue and bony (ribs, shoulder blade) structures. This limitation at times makes it extremely difficult to identify the intervertebral spaces. Dual-energy images are able to visualize the entire spine, but may result in very noisy images that do not allow a clear distinction of anatomic structures. In obese patients the MXA images may be very noisy because the increased soft tissue thickness reduces the photon flux significantly.

Studies that compared MXA with MRX found excellent agreement with qualitative and quantitative radiographic assessment using fan-beam dual-energy DXA images, particularly for moderate and severe deformities.[132,133] The poor image quality of MXA limits the diagnostic value of this technique compared to MRX. In fact, a large proportion of vertebrae are not visualized sufficiently for analysis on MXA scans and therefore the number of vertebral fractures identified is reduced, particularly in the upper thoracic spine. However, because of some distinct advantages, such as a substantially reduced effective dose to the patient and acquisition of a single image of the thoracic and lumbar spine, MXA is a potentially useful technique to identify prevalent vertebral fractures.

VI. CONCLUSION

Quantitative morphometry is unable to distinguish osteoporotic vertebral fractures by vertebral deformities due to other factors, such as degenerative spine and disc disease. This limitation is a characteristic of any method of quantitative morphometry, but the limited spatial resolution of the DXA images in MXA may increase this problem. Instead, MRX with its superior image quality has the potential for qualitative reading of the radiographs to aid the differential diagnosis. In fact, although it is recognized that the visual interpretation of radiographs is subjective, it is also true that an expert eye can better distinguish between true fractures and vertebral anomalies compared to quantitative morphometry. Therefore, for assessment of vertebral deformities visual semiquantitative approaches based on standardized criteria were developed.[134-136] The radiologists or experienced clinicians assign numeric scores to vertebral deformities, according to their type and their severity without making measurements of vertebral heights. These methods can provide reasonable reproducibility, sensitivity, and specificity, and excellent agreement on the diagnosis of prevalent and incident vertebral fractures may be achieved among trained observers using a semiquantitative method.[137]

In conclusion, a combination of semiquantitative visual and quantitative morphometric methods might be the best approach to fracture definition, as suggested by National Osteoporosis Foundation Working Group on Vertebral Fractures and by the International Osteoporosis Foundation.

REFERENCES

1. Cameron, J.R. and Sorenson, J., "Measurement of bone mineral *in vivo*: an improved method," *Science*, 142, 230, 1963.
2. Kellie, S.E., "Measurement of bone density with dual energy X-ray absorptiometry (DEXA)," *J. Am. Med. Assoc.*, 267, 286, 1992.
3. Wahner, H.W. and Fogelman, I., *The Evaluation of Osteoporosis: Dual Energy X-Ray Absorptiometry in the Clinical Practice*, Martin Dunitz, London, 1994.

4. Mazess, R., Chesnut, C.H., McClung, M., and Genant, H.K., "Enhanced precision with dual energy X-ray absorptiometry," *Calcif. Tissue Int.*, 51, 14, 1992.
5. Rupich, R.C., Griffin, M.G., Pacifici, R., et al., "Lateral dual-energy radiography: artifact error from rib and pelvic bone," *J. Bone Miner. Res.*, 7, 97, 1992.
6. Guglielmi, G., Grimston, S.K., Fischer, K.C., et al., "Osteoporosis: diagnosis with lateral and postero-anterior dual X-ray absorptiometry compared with quantitative CT," *Radiology*, 192, 845, 1994.
7. Reginster, J.Y., Deroisy, R., Zegels, B., et al., "Long-term performance *in vitro* and *in vivo* of dual energy X-ray absorptiometry," *Clin. Rheumatol.*, 14, 180, 1995.
8. Genant, H.K., Grampp, S., Glüer, C.C., et al., "Universal standardization for dual X-ray absorptiometry: patient and phantom cross-calibration results," *J. Bone Miner. Res.*, 9, 1503, 1994.
9. Genant, H.K., Glüer, C.C., Faulkner, K., et al., "Acronysm in bone densitometry," *Radiology*, 184, 878, 1992.
10. Guglielmi, G., Glüer, C.C., Majumdar, S., et al., "Current methods and advances in bone densitometry," *Eur. Radiol.*, 5, 129, 1995.
11. Adams, J.E., "Single and dual energy X-ray absorptiometry," *Eur. Radiol.*, 7, 20, 1997.
12. Grampp, S., Genant, H.K., Mathur, A., et al., "Comparison of noninvasive bone mineral measurements in assessing age-related loss, fracture discrimination, and diagnostic classification," *J. Bone Miner. Res.*, 12, 697, 1997.
13. Guglielmi, G., Genant, H.K., and Passariello, R., "Bone densitometry: an update," *Eur. Radiol.*, 7, 1, 1997.
14. Rüegsegger, P., Elasser, U., Anliker, M., et al., "Quantification of bone mineralization using computed tomography," *Radiology*, 121, 93, 1976.
15. Genant, H.K., Cann, C.E., Ettinger, B., et al., "Quantitative computed tomography of vertebral spongiosa: a sensitive method for detecting early bone loss after oophorectomy," *Ann. Intern. Med.*, 97, 699, 1982.
16. Pacifici, R., Susman, N., Carr, P.L., et al., "Single and dual energy tomography analysis of spinal trabecular bone: a comparative study in normal and osteoporotic women," *J. Clin. Endocrinol. Metab.*, 64, 209, 1987.
17. Glüer, C.C., Reiser, U.J., Davis, C.A., et al., "Vertebral mineral determination by quantitative computed tomography (QCT): accuracy of single and dual energy measurements," *J. Comput. Assist. Tomogr.*, 12, 242, 1988.
18. Block, J.E., Smith, R., Glüer, C.C., et al., "Models of spinal trabecular bone loss as determined by quantitative computed tomography," *J. Bone Miner. Res.*, 4, 249, 1989.
19. Steiger, P., Block, J.E., Steiger, S., et al., "Spinal bone mineral density by quantitative computed tomography: effect of region of interest, vertebral level, and technique," *Radiology*, 175, 537, 1990.
20. Guglielmi, G., Giannatempo, G.M., Blunt, B.A., et al., "Spinal bone mineral density by quantitative computed tomography in a normal Italian population," *Eur. Radiol.*, 5, 269, 1995.
21. Boden, S.D., Goodenough, D.J., Stockam, C.D., et al., "Precise measurement of vertebra bone density using computed tomography without the use of an external reference phantom," *J. Digit. Imag.*, 2, 31, 1989.
22. Goodsitt, M.M., "Conversion relations for quantitative CT bone mineral density measured with solid and liquid calibration standards," *Bone Miner.*, 19, 145, 1992.
23. Faulkner, K.G., Glüer, C.C., Grampp, S., et al., "Cross calibration of liquid and solid QCT calibration standards: corrections to UCSF normative data," *Osteoporos. Int.*, 3, 36, 1993
24. Glüer, C.C., Engelke, K., Jergas, M., et al., "Changes in calibration standards for quantitative computed tomography: reccomendations for clinical practice," *Osteoporos. Int.*, 3, 288, 1993.
25. Guglielmi, G., "Quantitative computed tomography (QCT) and dual X-ray absorptiometry (DXA) in the diagnosis of osteoporosis," *Eur. J. Radiol.*, 20, 185, 1995.
26. Schneider, P. and Borner, W., "Periphere quantitative Computer Tomographie zur Knochenmineral-messung mit einem neuen speziellen QCT Scanner, " *RoFo.*, 154, 292, 1991.
27. Rüegsegger, P., Durand, E., and Dambacher, M.A., "Localization of regional forearm bone loss from high resolution computed tomographic images," *Osteoporos. Int.*, 1, 76, 1991.
28. Rüegsegger, P., Durand, E., and Dambacher, M.A., "Differential effects of aging and disease on trabecular and compact bone density of the radius," *Bone*, 12, 99, 1991.

29. Takada, M., Engelke, K., Hagiwara, S., et al., "Accuracy and precision study *in vitro* for peripheral quantitative computed tomography," *Osteoporos. Int.*, 6, 307, 1996.
30. Guglielmi, G., Cammisa, M., De Serio, A., et al., "Long term *in vitro* precision of single slice peripheral quantitative computed tomography (pQCT): multicenter comparison," *Technol. Health Care*, 5, 375, 1997.
31. Grampp, S., Lang, P., Jergas, M., et al., "Assessment of the skeletal status by quantitative peripheral computed tomography: short-term precision *in vivo* and comparison to dual X-ray absorptiometry," *J. Bone Miner. Res.*, 10, 1566, 1995.
32. Schneider, P., Butz, S., Allolio, B., et al., "Multicenter German reference database for peripheral quantitative computer tomography," *Technol. Health Care*, 3, 69, 1995.
33. Butz, S., Wuster, C., Scheidt-Nave, C., et al., "Forearm BMD as measured by peripheral quantitative computed tomography (pQCT) in a German reference population," *Osteoporos. Int.*, 4, 179, 1994.
34. Guglielmi, G., De Serio, A., Fusilli, S., et al., "Age-related changes assessed by peripheral QCT in healthy Italian women," *Eur. Radiol.*, 10, 609, 2000.
35. Ferretti, J.L., Capozza, R.F., Mondelo, N., et al., "Interrelationship between densitometric properties of rat femora: inferences concerning mechanical regulation of bone modeling," *J. Bone Miner. Res.*, 8, 1389, 1993.
36. Ferretti, J.L., Gaffuri, O., Capozza, R.F., et al., "Dexamethasone effects on mechanical, geometric and densitometric properties of rat femur diaphyses by peripheral computerized tomography and bending tests," *Bone*, 16, 119, 1995.
37. Augat, P., Reeb, H., and Claes, L.E., "Prediction of fracture load at different skeletal sites by geometric properties of the cortical shell," *J. Bone Miner. Res.*, 11, 1356, 1996.
38. Lang, T.F., Li, J., Harris, S.T., et al., "Assessment of vertebral bone mineral density using volumetric quantitative CT," *J. Comput. Assist. Tomogr.*, 23, 130, 1999.
39. Lang, T.F., Augat, P., Lane, N.E., and Genant, H.K., "Trochanteric hip fracture: strong association with spinal trabecular bone mineral density measured with quantitative CT," *Radiology*, 209, 525, 1998.
40. Genant, H.K., Gordon, C., Jiang, Y., et al., "Advanced imaging of bone macro and micro structure," *Bone*, 25, 149, 1999.
41. Jiang, Y., Zhao, J., Augat, P., et al., "Trabecular bone mineral and calculated structure of human bone specimens scanned by peripheral quantitative computed tomography: relation to biomechanical properties," *J. Bone Miner. Res.*, 13, 1783, 1998.
42. Müller, R., Hildebrand, T., Hauselmann, H.J., and Rüegsegger, P., "*In vivo* reproducibility of three-dimensional structural properties of noninvasive bone biopsies using 3D-pQCT," *J. Bone Miner. Res.*, 11, 1745, 1996.
43. Link, T.M., Majumdar, S., Grampp, S., et al., "Imaging of trabecular bone structure in osteoporosis," *Eur. Radiol.*, 9, 1781, 1999.
44. Hans, D., Schott, A.M., and Meunier, P.J., "Ultrasonic assessment of bone: a review," *Eur. J. Med.*, 2, 157, 1993.
45. Kaufman, J.J. and Einhorn, T.A., "Ultrasound assessment of bone," *J. Bone Miner. Res.*, 8, 517, 1993.
46. Glüer, C.C., for the International Quantitative Ultrasound Consensus Group, "Quantitative ultrasound techniques for the assessment of osteoporosis: expert agreement of current status," *J. Bone Miner. Res.*, 12, 1280, 1997.
47. Njeh, C.F., Boivin, C.M., and Langton, C.M., "The role of ultrasound in the assessment of osteoporosis: a review," *Osteoporos. Int.*, 7, 7, 1997.
48. Njeh, C.F., Hans, D., Fuerst, T., et al., *Quantitative Ultrasound: Assessment of Osteoporosis and Bone Status*, Martin Dunitz, London, 1999.
49. Turner, C.H. and Eich, M., "Ultrasonic velocity as a predictor of strength in bovine cancellous bone," *Calcif. Tissue Int.*, 49, 116, 1991.
50. Langton, C.M., Njeh, C.F., Hodgskinson, R., et al., "Prediction of mechanical properties of the human calcaneus by broadband ultrasonic attenuation," *Bone*, 18, 495, 1996.
51. Njeh, C.F., Hodgskinson, R., Currey, J.D., et al., "Orthogonal relationships between ultrasonic velocity and material properties of bovine cancellous bone," *Med. Eng. Phys.*, 18, 373, 1996.
52. Bouxsein, M.L., Courtney, A.C., and Hayes, W.C., "Ultrasound and densitometry of the calcaneus correlate with the failure loads of cadaveric femurs," *Calcif. Tissue Int.*, 56, 99, 1995.

53. Nicholson, P.H.F., Lowet, G., Cheng, X.G., et al., "Assessment of the strength of the proximal femur *in vitro*: relationship with ultrasonic measurements of the calcaneus," *Bone*, 20, 219, 1997.

54. McCloskey, E.V., Murray, S.A., Charlesworth, D., et al., "Assessment of broadband attenuation in the os calcis *in vitro*," *Clin. Sci.*, 78, 221, 1990.

55. McKelvie, M.L., Fordham, J., Clifford, C., et al., "*In vitro* comparison of quantitative computed tomography and broadband ultrasonic attenuation of trabecular bone," *Bone*, 10, 101, 1989.

56. Laugier, P., Droin, P., Laval-Jeantet, A.M., et al., "*In vitro* assessment of the relationship between acoustic properties and bone mass density of the calcaneus by comparison of ultrasound parametric imaging and quantitative computed tomography," *Bone*, 20, 157, 1997.

57. Evans, J.A. and Tavakoli, M.B., "Ultrasonic attenuation and velocity in bone," *Phys. Med. Biol.*, 35, 1387, 1990.

58. Cadossi, R. and Canè, V., "Pathways of transmission of ultrasound energy through the distal metaphysis of the second phalanx of pigs: an *in vitro* study," *Osteoporos. Int.*, 6, 196, 1996.

59. De Terlizzi, F., Battista, S., Cavani, F., et al., "Influence of bone tissue density and elasticity on ultrasound propagation: an *in vitro* study," *J. Bone Miner. Res.*, 15, 2458, 2000.

60. Glüer, C.C., Wu, C.Y., Jergas, M., et al., "Three quantitative ultrasound parameters reflect bone structure," *Calcif. Tissue Int.*, 55, 46, 1994.

61. Kotzki, P.O., Buyck, D., Hans, D., et al., "Influence of fat on ultrasound measurements of the os calcis," *Calcif. Tissue Int.*, 54, 91, 1994.

62. Miller, C.G., Herd, R.J., Ramalingam, T., et al., "Ultrasonic velocity measurements through the calcaneus: which velocity should be measured?" *Osteoporos. Int.*, 3, 31, 1993.

63. Strelitzki, R., Clarke, A.J., and Evans, J.A., "The measurement of the velocity of ultrasound in fixed trabecular bone using broadband pulses and single-frequency tone bursts," *Phys. Med. Biol.*, 41, 743, 1996.

64. Rho, J.Y., Flaitz, D., Swarnakar, V., et al., "The characterization of broadband ultrasound attenuation and fractal analysis by biomechanical properties," *Bone*, 20, 497, 1997.

65. Schott, A.M., Hans, D., Garnero, A., et al., "Age-related changes in os calcis ultrasonic indices: a 2-year prospective study," *Osteoporos. Int.*, 5, 478, 1995.

66. Krieg, M.A., Thiebaud, D., and Burckhardt, P., "Quantitative ultrasound of bone in institutionalized elderly women: a cross sectional and longitudinal study," *Osteoporos. Int.*, 6, 189, 1996.

67. Rosenthall, L., Tenehouse, A., and Caminis, J., "A correlative study of ultrasound calcaneal and dual-energy X-ray absorptiometry bone measurements of the lumbar spine and femur in 1000 women," *Eur. J. Nucl. Med.*, 22, 402, 1995.

68. Van Daele, P.L., Burger, H., Algra, D., et al., "Age-associated changes in ultrasound measurements of the calcaneus in men and women: the Rotterdam Study," *J. Bone Miner. Res.*, 9, 1751, 1994.

69. Gregg, E.W., Kriska, A.M., Salamone, L.M., et al., "The epidemiology of quantitative ultrasound: a review of the relationships with bone mass, osteoporosis and fracture risk," *Osteoporos. Int.*, 7, 89, 1997.

70. Hans, D., Schott, A.M., Arlot, M.E., et al., "Influence of anthropometric parameters of the os calcis," *Osteoporos. Int.*, 5, 371, 1995.

71. Ross, P., Huang, C., Davis, J., et al., "Predicting vertebral deformity using bone densitometry at various skeletal sites and calcaneus ultrasound," *Bone*, 16, 325, 1995.

72. Glüer, C.C. and Hans, D., "How to use ultrasound for risk assessment: a need for defining strategies," *Osteoporos. Int.*, 9, 193, 1999.

73. Pluijm, S.M.F., Graafmans, W.C., Bouter, L.M., and Lips, P., "Ultrasound measurements for the prediction of osteoporotic fractures in elderly people," *Osteoporos. Int.*, 9, 550, 1999.

74. Frost, M.L., Blake, G.M., and Fogelman, I., "Can the WHO criteria for diagnosing osteoporosis be applied to calcaneal quantitative ultrasound?" *Osteoporos. Int.*, 7, 390, 2000.

75. Schott, A.M., Weill-Engerer, S., Hans, D., et al., "Ultrasound discriminates patients with hip fracture equally well as dual energy X-ray absorptiometry and independently of bone mineral density," *J. Bone Miner. Res.*, 10, 243, 1995.

76. Gonnelli, S.V., Cepollaro, C., Agnusdei, D., et al., "Diagnostic value of ultrasound analysis and bone densitometry as predictors of vertebral deformity in postmenopausal women," *Osteoporos. Int.*, 5, 413, 1995.

77. Hans, D., Dargent-Molina, P., Schott, A.M., et al., "Ultrasonographic heel measurements to predict hip fracture in elderly women: the EPIDOS perspective study," *Lancet*, 348, 511, 1996.
78. Guglielmi, G., Cammisa, M., De Serio, A., et al., "Phalangeal U.S. velocity discriminates between normal and vertebrally fractured subjects," *Eur. Radiol.*, 9, 1632, 1999.
79. Benitez, C.L., Schneider, D.L., Barrett-Connor, E., and Sartoris, J., "Hand ultrasound for osteoporosis screening in postmenopausal women," *Osteoporos. Int.*, 11, 203, 2000.
80. Wuster, C., Albanese, C., De Aloysio, D., et al., "Phalangeal osteosonogrammetry study: age-related changes, diagnostic sensitivity, and discrimination power," *J. Bone Miner. Res.*, 15, 1603, 2000.
81. Frost, M.L., Blake, G.M., and Fogelman, I., "Quantitative ultrasound and bone mineral density are equally strongly associated with risk factors for osteoporosis," *J. Bone Miner. Res.*, 16, 406, 2001.
82. Melton, L.J., III, "Epidemiology of spinal osteoporosis," *Spine*, 22, 2S, 1997.
83. Cooper, C., "Epidemiology of vertebral fractures in western populations," *Spine*, 8, 1, 1995.
84. Wasnich, R.D., "Vertebral fracture epidemiology," *Bone,* 18, 179, 1996.
85. Davies, K.M., Stegman, M.R., Heaney, R.P., and Recker, R.R., "Prevalence and severity of vertebral fracture: the Saunders County Bone Quality Study," *Osteoporos. Int.,* 6, 160, 1996.
86. O'Neill, T.W., Felsenberg, D., Varlow, J., et al., "The prevalence of vertebral deformity in European men and women: the European Vertebral Osteoporosis Study," *J. Bone Miner. Res.*, 11, 1010, 1996.
87. Samelson, E.J., Hannan, M.T., Felson, D.T., et al., "Risk factors for incidence of vertebral fracture in men and women: 25-year follow-up results from the Framingham Osteoporosis Study," *J. Bone Miner. Res.,* 14, S147, 1999.
88. "National Osteoporosis Foundation Working Group on Vertebral Fractures: report assessing vertebral fractures," *J. Bone Miner. Res.*, 10, 518, 1995.
89. Kanis, J.A., Delmas, P., Burckhardt, P., et al., "Guidelines for diagnosis and management of osteoporosis. The European Foundation for Osteoporosis and Bone Disease," *Osteoporos. Int.*, 7, 390, 1997.
90. Liberman, U.A., Weiss, S.R., Broll, J., et al., "Effect of oral alendronate on bone mineral density and the incidence of fractures in postmenopausal osteoporosis," *N. Engl. J. Med.,* 333, 1437, 1995.
91. Nevitt, M.C., Ross, P.D., Palermo, L., et al., "Association of prevalent vertebral fractures, bone density, and alendronate treatment with incident vertebral fractures: effect of number and spinal location of fractures," *Bone*, 25, 613, 1999.
92. Cummings, S.R., Black, D.M., Thompson, D.E., et al., "Effect of alendronate on risk of fracture in women with low bone density but without vertebral fractures: results from the Fracture Interventional Trial," *J. Am. Med. Assoc.*, 280, 2077, 1998.
93. Hochberg, M.C., Ross, P.D., Black, D., et al., "Larger increases in bone mineral density during alendronate therapy are associated with a lower risk of new vertebral fractures in women with postmenopausal osteoporosis. Fracture Inteventional Trial Research Group," *Arthritis Rheum.*, 42, 1246, 1999.
94. Hedlund, L.R. and Gallagher, J.C., "Vertebral morphometry in diagnosis of spinal fractures," *Bone Miner.*, 5, 59, 1988.
95. Kleerokoper, M. and Nelson, D.A., "Vertebral fracture or vertebral deformity?" *Calcif. Tissue Int.*, 50, 5, 1992.
96. Ziegler, R., Scheidt-Nave, C., and Leidig-Bruckner, G., "What is a vertebral fracture?" *Bone*, 18, 169, 1996.
97. Johnell, O., O'Neill, T., Felsenberg, D., et al., "Anthropometric measurements and vertebral deformities. European Vertebral Osteoporosis Study (EVOS) Group," *Am. J. Epidemiol.*, 146, 287, 1997.
98. Davies, K.M., Recker, R.R., and Heaney, R.P., "Normal vertebral dimensions and normal variation in serial measurements of vertebrae," *J. Bone Miner. Res.*, 4, 341, 1989.
99. Gallagher, J.C., Hedlund, L.R., Stoner, S., and Meeger, C., "Vertebral morphometry: normative data," *Bone Miner.*, 4, 189, 1988.
100. Ross, P.D., Yhee, Y.K., He, Y.-F., et al., "A new method for vertebral fracture diagnosis," *J. Bone Miner. Res.*, 8, 167, 1993.
101. Evans, S.F., Nicholson, P.H.F., Haddaway, M.J., and Davie, M.W.J., "Vertebral morphometry in women aged 50–81 years," *Bone Miner.*, 21, 29, 1993.
102. Diacinti, D., Acca, M., and Tomei, E., "Metodica di radiologia digitale per la valutazione dell'osteoporosi vertebrale," *Radiol. Med.*, 91, 1, 1995.

103. Hermann, A.P., Brixen, K., Andresen, J., and Mosekilde, L., "Reference values for vertebral heights in Scandinavian females and males," *Acta Radiol.*, 34, 48, 1993.

104. Black, D.M., Cummings, S.R., Stone, K., et al., "A new approach to defining normal vertebral dimensions," *J. Bone Miner. Res.*, 6, 883, 1991.

105. Melton, L.J., III, Lane, A.W., Cooper, C., et al., "Prevalence and incidence of vertebral deformities," *Osteoporos. Int.*, 3, 113, 1993.

106. O'Neill, T.W., Varlow, J., Felsenberg, D., et al., "Variation in vertebral height ratios in population studies," *J. Bone Miner. Res.*, 9, 1895, 1994.

107. Cline, M.G., Meredith, K.E., Boyer, J.T., and Burrows, B., "Decline in height with age in adults in a general population sample: estimating maximum height and distinguishing birth cohort effect from actual loss of stature with aging," *Hum. Biol.*, 61, 415, 1989.

108. Nicholson, P.H.F., Haddaway, M.J., Davie, M.W.J., and Evans, S.F., "Vertebral deformity, bone mineral density, back pain and height loss in unscreened women over 50 years," *Osteoporos. Int.*, 3, 300, 1993.

109. Burger, H., Van Daele, P.L.A., Gashuis, K., et al., "Vertebral deformities and functional impairment in men and women," *J. Bone Miner. Res.*, 12, 152, 1997.

110. Diacinti, D., Acca, M., D'Erasmo, E., et al., "Aging changes in vertebral morphometry," *Calcif. Tissue Int.*, 57, 426, 1995.

111. Eastell, R., Cedel, S.L., Wahner, H., et al., "Classification of vertebral fractures," *J. Bone Miner. Res.*, 6, 207, 1991.

112. Smith-Bindman, R., Cummings, S.R., Steiger, P., and Genant, H.K., "A comparison of morphometric definitions of vertebral fracture," *J. Bone Miner. Res.*, 6, 25, 1991.

113. McCloskey, E.V., Spector, T.D., Eyres, K.S., et al., "The assessment of vertebral deformity: a method for use in population studies and clinical trials," *Osteoporos. Int.*, 3, 138, 1993.

114. Minne, H.W., Leidig, C., Wuster, C.H.R., et al., "A newly developed spine deformity index (SDI) to quantitative vertebral crush fractures in patients with osteoporosis," *Bone Miner.*, 3, 335, 1998.

115. Smith-Bindman, R., Steiger, P., Cummings, S.R., and Genant, H.K., "The index of radiographic area (IRA): a new approach to estimating the severity of vertebral deformity," *Bone Miner.*, 15, 137, 1991.

116. Mazzuoli, G.F., Diacinti, D., Acca, M., et al., "Relationship between spine bone mineral density and vertebral body heights," *Calcif. Tissue Int.*, 62, 486, 1998.

117. Barnett, E. and Nordin, B.E.C., "Radiographic diagnosis of osteoporosis: new approach," *Clin. Radiol.*, 11, 166, 1960.

118. Jergas, M. and San Valentin, R., "Techniques for the assessment of vertebral dimensions in quantitative morphometry," in *Vertebral Fracture in Osteoporosis*, Genant, H.K., Jergas, M., and van Kuijk, C., Eds., University of California Osteoporosis Research Group, San Francisco, 1995, 163.

119. Hurxthal, L.M., "Measurement of vertebral heights," *Am. J. Roentgenol.*, 103, 635, 1968.

120. Banks, L.M., van Kuijk, C., and Genant, H.K., "Radiographic technique for assessing osteoporotic vertebral fracture," in *Vertebral Fracture in Osteoporosis*, Genant, H.K., Jergas, M., and van Kuijk, C., Eds., University of California Osteoporosis Research Group, San Francisco, 1995, 131.

121. Steiger, P. and Wahner, H., "Instruments using fan-beam geometry, " in *The Evaluation of Osteoporosis. Dual Energy X-Ray Absorptiometry in Clinical Practice*, Wahner, H. and Fogelman, I., Eds., Martin Dunitz, London, 1994, 281.

122. Adams, J.E., "Single and dual energy X-ray absorptiometry," in *Bone Densitometry and Osteoporosis*, Genant, H.K., Guglielmi, G., and Jergas, M., Eds., Springer-Verlag, Heidelberg, 1998, 305.

123. Blake, J.M., Jagathesan, T., Herd, R.J.M., and Fogelman, I., "Dual X-ray absorptiometry of the lumbar spine: the precision of paired anteroposterior/lateral studies," *Br. J. Radiol.*, 67, 624, 1994.

124. Harvey, S.B., Hutchinson, K.M., Rennie, E.C., et al., "Comparison of the precision of two vertebral morphometry programs for the Lunar Expert-XL imaging densitometer," *Br. J. Radiol.*, 71, 388, 1998.

125. Blake, G.M., Rea, J.A., and Fogelman, I., "Vertebral morphometry studies using dual-energy X-ray absorptiometry," *Semin. Nucl. Med.*, 27, 276, 1997.

126. Rea, J.A., Steiger, P., Blake, G., and Fogelman, I., "Optimizing data acquisition and analysis of morphometric X-ray absorptiometry," *Osteoporos. Int.*, 8, 177, 1998.

127. Rea, J.A., Chen, M.B., Li, J., et al., "Morphometry X-ray absorptiometry and morphometric radiography of the spine: a comparison of analysis precision in normal and osteoporotic subjects," *Osteoporos. Int.*, 9, 536, 1999.

128. Crabtree, N., Wright, J., Walgrove, A., et al., "Vertebral Morphometry: repeat scan precision using the Lunar Expert-XL and the Hologic 4500A. A study for the 'WISDOM' RCT of hormone replacement therapy," *Osteoporos. Int.*, 11, 537, 2000.

129. Lewis, M.K. and Blake, G.M., "Patient dose in morphometric X-ray absorptiometry," *Osteoporos. Int.*, 5, 281, 1995.

130. Njeh, C.F., Fuerst, T., Hans, D., et al., "Radiation exposure in bone mineral density assessment," *Appl. Radiat. Isot.*, 50, 215, 1999.

131. Kalender, W.A. and Eidloth, H., "Determination of geometric parameters and osteoporosis indices for lumbar vertebrae from lateral QCT localizer radiographs," *Osteoporos. Int.*, 1, 197, 1991.

132. Rea, J.A., Chen, M.B., Li, J., et al., "Morphometry X-ray absorptiometry and morphometric radiography of the spine: a comparison of prevalent vertebral deformity identification," *J. Bone Miner. Res.*, 15, 564, 2000.

133. Ferrar, L., Jiang, G., Barrington, N.A., and Eastell, R., "Identification of vertebral deformities in women: comparison of radiologic assessment and quantitative morphometry using morphometric radiography and morphometric X-ray absorptiometry," *J. Bone Miner. Res.*, 15, 575, 2000.

134. Nielsen, V.A.H., Podenphant, J., Martens, S., et al., "Precision in assessment of osteoporosis from spine radiographs," *Eur. J. Radiol.*, 13, 11, 1991.

135. Genant, H.K., Wu, C.Y., van Kuijk, C., and Nevitt, M., "Vertebral fracture assessment using a semiquantitative technique," *J. Bone Miner. Res.*, 8, 1137, 1993.

136. Black, D.M., Palermo, L., Nevitt, M.C., et al., "Comparison of methods for defining prevalent vertebral deformities: the study of osteoporotic fractures," *J. Bone Miner. Res.*, 10, 890, 1995.

137. Genant, H.K., Jergas, M., Palermo, L., et al., "Comparison of semiquantitative visual and quantitative morphometric assessment of prevalent and incident vertebral fractures in osteoporosis," *J. Bone Miner. Res.*, 11, 984, 1996.

8 Noninvasive Analysis of Bone Mass, Structure, and Strength

José Luis Ferretti, Gustavo R. Cointry, and Ricardo F. Capozza

CONTENTS

I. INTRODUCTION

The aim of this minireview is not just to comment on the many partial approaches to a noninvasive assessment of bone strength making use of the standard densitometric techniques that have been already reported, or to compare them with the less numerous attempts made employing other available methodologies. In fact, this would have been practically impossible because very few suitable, comparative studies that have been specifically performed with that purpose were reported.

Instead, a general background, some elementary guidelines, and a comprehensive set of basic references are offered about what appear to be the most reasonable ways to face the problem, despite the regrettable lack of resources we have at hand to solve it. It is expected that (1) this will help many readers criticize and even improve the reference elements they currently manage to diagnose osteoporosis; and (2) it will also encourage the research of new developments in this extremely interesting and important field.

0-8493-1033-4/02/$0.00+$1.50
© 2003 by CRC Press LLC

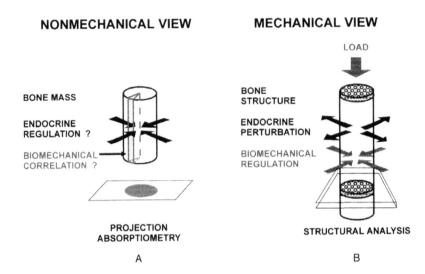

FIGURE 8.1 Conceptual contrasts between the nonmechanical view of bone physiology (A), which regards the skeleton as a metabolically controlled mass, the quality of which could be assessed by the absorptiometric measurement of its projected shadow, and the mechanical view (B), which considers the bones as structures under directional, biomechanical control disturbed by the endocrine-metabolic systems, the quality of which must be determined by assessing its cross-sectional properties, size, and shape.[65]

II. BONE CALCIFICATION, BONE MASS, BONE STIFFNESS, BONE STRENGTH

The clinical assessment of bone strength (and fracture risk) has always been a difficult challenge, and the problem is still far from solved.[1] The reason for that deficiency seems to be a matter of focus and target. The problem concerns not only how or how well to measure, but also essentially what to measure, and how to interpret the data.

During the last two decades the focus was (and it still is, rather unfortunately) set only on bone mineralization. This is explainable because of the wide acceptance and good standardization achieved by the densitometric techniques as noninvasive resources to measure bone mineral mass in the last two decades, while no successful attempts to assess some among the many other relevant bone properties were known until recently. As a result, the skeleton was (and still is) incorrectly assimilated to "an amount of mineral" resulting from a *metabolically controlled* balance between formation and destruction, that normally grows up to reach some peak value and then declines slower or sooner in different instances, *in parallel with* gains, savings and losses of structural strength (Figure 8.1A). This interpretation, although apparently correct, is actually incomplete and misleading.[2,3]

To avoid starting as iconoclasts, we must reckon that this concept is not completely wrong. In fact, good (sometimes quite good) correlations have been reported between bone mineralization and strength in densitometric studies, in many different instances.[4-14] However, late rather than early, the true situation was revealed. On the one hand, wide overlaps have been long reported between densitometric data of fractured and nonfractured individuals.[15,16] On the other hand, unexpectedly to many, some large, well-controlled studies of the effects of fluoride, calcitonin, raloxifene, and bisphosphonates on bone-weakening diseases showed a lack of proportionality (and even of parallelism, too) between the evolution of bone mineral "mass" and that of the fracture incidence rate.[17-20]

The first reaction was to deny, or at least relativize, the ability of bone densitometry to detect individuals at risk of fracture and to monitor therapeutic effects on bone strength.[2,17-23] Perhaps we should not go so far, but it seems as though the situation should be clarified to some degree. A glance at the general biology of the skeleton may help understand this question.

Think about nature, some 100 million years ago, trying to manage how to develop internal, supporting structures stiff enough to avoid excessive buckling-derived stress of the constitutive material (elastic behavior), and sufficiently tough to properly resist their separation into fragments under customary usage (plastic behavior). These determinants of whole-bone strength were obvious prerequisites to "leave the water" and eventually drag, walk, or run on Earth, climb trees or mountains, go back to water to swim, or fly.[24,25] In addition, a gender-specific adaptability of that structure for fighting for food and mates in males, and for breeding and delivering in females, also had to be handled.

All seems to indicate that the best available biological resource has always been to calcify collagen fibers.[24-29] Thus, supposedly every mechanism for promoting collagen calcification should have been tried, and some among these should have been eventually selected for survival. Not too bad a resource, indeed. In fact, stiffness (linear to calcification in all the skeletons) confers strength to the structure within a wide domain of values (think about girders constructed of different kinds of wood) and certainly within the normal or osteoporotic bone stiffness/strength range.[24,25,27,30-35]

However, stiffness also confers *brittleness* to the structure as it grows upward (consider glass or marble structures),[24-28,32] also within the normal bone stiffness/strength range. It seems to have been naturally impossible to achieve acceptable levels of both stiffness and strength of that basic, fibrous bony structure by just making it more and more densely calcified. Conceivably, a fracture should have always interrupted the process (and also the species' survival) well before any chance of positive selection could have been achieved.

Nevertheless, it also seems as if an optimal (not maximal) degree of calcification of bony tissues had already been developed long ago for all vertebrates. In fact, matrix calcification shows relatively constant values for different skeletal regions in the same or different individuals, either within the same or even between different vertebrate species, although it may increase somewhat (hence increasing the bone matrix brittleness) with the age of the subject.[36-42] Anyway, once the bone tissue is fully mineralized, the bone mineral content cannot be further changed in normal (not osteomalacic) conditions. Therefore, the only way to change the mineral content of a whole bone is the addition of new mineralized bone tissue through bone modeling, or the elimination of some of the old mineralized bone tissue through imbalanced ("disuse" type[43]) bone remodeling (Figure 8.2).

Therefore, some other mechanism(s), purportedly related to calcified bone mass additions and losses rather than to bone matrix calcification itself, must have been selected to solve the supporting problem of the skeletons. The concept that mineralization alone does not suffice to explain bone strength is not new. More than two decades ago it was stated that "it is much easier to demonstrate correlation between a particular characteristic of (cortical) bone and its mechanical behavior than to positively identify a direct cause-and-effect relationship between a single parameter and the (material) properties of bone."[36]

For every kind of structural problem, nature always seems to have selected the same type of solution: "If no further resources are at hand at this level of structural complexity, then let's go to a higher one." A higher level of complexity of any structure (an abstract concept) is achieved as soon as the circumstantial observer realizes that its properties "as a whole" represent more than the sum of the properties of its "separate parts" (which are automatically regarded as the "immediately lower" structural level).

In the case of bones, the resource selected for achieving the new level of complexity seemed to have been to render the calcified structure *anisotropic*, i.e., able to resist or respond to the environmental loads distinctly according to the *direction* in which it is deformed.[27,32,36,44] This seems to have been achieved by just arranging the spatial *distribution* of its significant elements as needed. Bone anisotropy was thus developed (and can also be described) chiefly at two different levels of complexity, namely, the *tissue* level (comprising no less than seven sublevels of bone "material" complexity) and the *organ* level.[44,45]

The tissue level (bone "material" properties) concerns the spatial disposition of crystals on the fibers, fibers within the lamellae, lamellae within the osteons, and osteons within the complex material

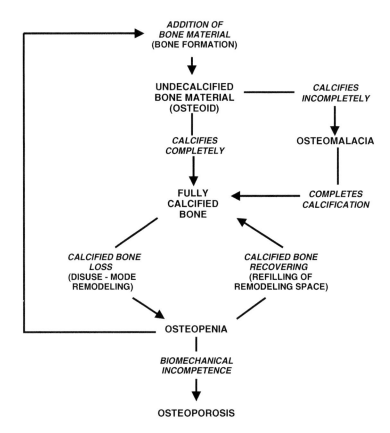

FIGURE 8.2 Mechanisms of the possible pathways for the processes of bone "calcification" and "decalcification." The mass of bone mineral can be *increased* because of either the calcification of the preexisting osteoid or the addition of newly formed bone. Bone mineral can be *decreased* only through unbalanced bone destruction, a process that has been proposed to be called *disuse-mode* remodeling.[43,65] The goals of either mechanical or pharmacologic interventions are grossly restricted to the eventually induced changes in one or more of those three mechanisms. The effects of any treatment on bone strength are restrained to only the *mechanically meaningful* changes induced in bone mass, chiefly concerning the distribution of the (ideally normal) mineralized tissue.

(bone microstructure),[34,45-56] as well as the distribution of cement lines[57] and microcracks or microdamage derived from mechanical usage[40,41,57,58] within the "solid" calcified matrix. Importantly, none of these factors is directly related to the quantitative degree of bone matrix mineralization.[59]

In addition to that source of complexity, the organ level (bone "structural" properties) concerns, among other things:

1. The spatial orientation and structural continuity of that composite material in the trabecular network in cancellous bone[60,61]
2. The more or less peripheral distribution of the compact shells with reference to critical, bending or torsional bone axes in long bones[62,63]
3. Generally speaking, the bone size and shape (bone architecture, geometry, or design)

As a result of that specific micro- and macroarrangement of the structure, both the calcified bone tissue and the whole bones show maximal *stiffness* and *toughness* (and secondarily maximal strength, as well) in the direction of the loads produced by customary usage in the corresponding skeletal regions.[44,64,65] Concerning the "solid" bone tissue, this property is known as *intrinsic* or

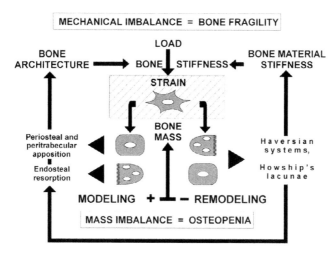

FIGURE 8.3 Schematic representation of the bone mechanostat,[64] the only feedback mechanism known for any bone property, that cybernetically controls bone *stiffness* through the directional modulation of bone modeling and remodeling as determined by the osteocyte-mediated sensing of the *strains* produced by the customary usage of the skeleton. Importantly, the resulting mass (lower) and stiffness balances (upper) are mutually independent, because the system does not control bone mass directly. In fact, no biological mechanism is known to control bone mass cybernetically.

material stiffness (or "elastic modulus," a property that seems to differ from cortical to trabecular bone "raw" material).[66,67] For the whole bones, this corresponds to their *structural* stiffness, or just the "bone(-organ) stiffness."[36,68] This stiffness is usually kept just high enough to withstand the everyday bone or bone tissue deformation under customary mechanical usage but sufficiently low to avoid microdamage or damage (and hence fracture),[43,64,65] *regardless of the degree of matrix calcification.*[69] Any further deformation will provoke microdamage and determine the initiation and progress of microcracks, thus affecting the plastic behavior of bone (bone toughness), a property that seems not to be critically dependent on bone mineralization.[59]

These facts are far from trivial. Bone deformability is the only skeletal property that is known to be homeostatically controlled anyway. The feedback system in question (the bone "mechanostat")[43,64] biomechanically senses the strains provoked by usage and gravity (presumably osteocytes do that) and directionally modulates bone modeling and remodeling (effected by osteoblasts and clasts through cell-to-cell messages sent by the osteocytes) accordingly.[70] As a result, *independent* balances of bone mass and strength are obtained (Figure 8.3).[15]

The endocrine-metabolic environment disturbs rather than controls the bone equilibrium and in no way contributes to the efficiency of the bone mechanostat (Figure 8.4). No hormone is known to homeostatically control any bone or skeletal property or function, while (disuse excepted) systemic disturbances are the cause of most of the known osteoporoses.

This further explains why the amount of calcium or calcified material within the bones is not a direct, independent determinant of their stiffness, toughness, or ultimate strength. Bone "mass" is just a surrogate of the two actual determinants of bone strength, i.e., the intrinsic stiffness and the spatial distribution of the mineralized tissue as determined by the mechanostat.[29] Bone *shape* can also account significantly for the whole-bone strength as shown by the femoral neck angle and length,[71-77] again regardless of bone calcification or mass (Figure 8.5).

In any case, the amount of mineralized tissue (bone "mass") may be actually relevant to bone strength, whether or not related to bone *size*. This could explain a good part of the acceptable correlations often found between the densitometric determinations of bone "mass" (unavoidably related to bone size)[78] and bone strength or fracture incidence.[4-14] Nevertheless, bone size is usually related to body size and to muscle mass and strength.[79-86] Therefore, the mineralized bone mass

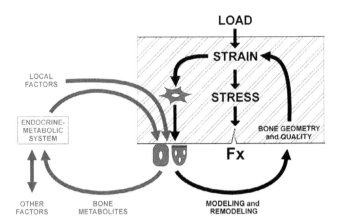

FIGURE 8.4 Schematic representation of how the biomechanical, cybernetic control of bone stiffness (bone mechanostat, right) is disturbed by the environmental (i.e., nondirectional) messages coming from the endocrine-metabolic and paracrine systems that control the mineral equilibrium of the internal *milieu* (left) by sharing the same receptors (osteoblasts and osteoclasts). Osteocytes could presumably be affected, too. Endocrine-metabolic disturbances are the cause of most of the known types of osteoporosis.

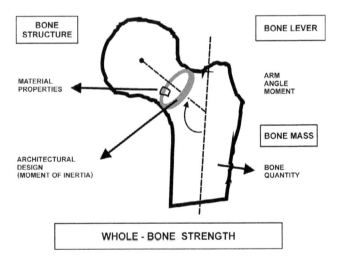

FIGURE 8.5 Determination of the strength of a bone by its material properties and macroarchitectural design. Bone mass is meaningful only concerning bone size, otherwise it could be regarded as a surrogate indicator.

data of individuals of different sizes should not be compared before some anthropometric and/or biomechanical adjustments are statistically performed. The problem becomes especially important concerning some gender-related differences,[79,82,87] because of the influence of the above-mentioned endocrine-metabolic factors.

III. WHAT TO MEASURE, AND HOW?

Aiming to guide the discussion on this matter following an integral vision of bone biomechanics, Figure 8.6 shows the way bone strength is biologically determined by both bone material and geometric properties.[29,89] Bone material properties concern bone matrix mineralization and microstructure (tissue level) and geometric properties comprise the amount ("mass") and spatial distribution of that matrix (organ level). In addition, muscle strength is also regarded in the scheme as

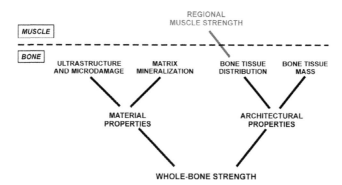

FIGURE 8.6 Synoptic representation of the determination of bone strength[29,89] as discussed in the text, showing the meaningful influence of the regional muscle strength as a strong determinant of the macro-architecture of the bone tissues under the cybernetic control of the bone mechanostat.

the chief biomechanical determinant (well over the influence of gravity in most of cases) of the architectural design of bone structure.[81,84-86,90]

The question of whole-bone anisotropy practically rules out any attempt to correlate results from different skeletal regions,[91,92] despite the high statistical significance they may show.[93] The analysis of this matter will be obviated in this chapter, for the following reasons:

1. The regional determination of bone strength is highly specific to the particular biomechanical environment;[94] hence, the mechanical translation of the same indicators should change in different skeletal sites.
2. The therapeutic effects on bone mass and strength (that are not necessarily interdependent)[17-20,92] should also be distinctly affected by different treatments and biomechanical environments in different skeletal regions.
3. The biomechanical impact of the induced changes in bone mass and strength (that are not necessarily interdependent) will also depend on the previous integrity of the bone structure in each skeletal region.

Therefore, the strength of bones should be evaluated regarding all the four determinants of bone "material" and "geometric" properties (see Figure 8.6) as well as in proportion to the strength of the regional muscles as chief biomechanical inductor.[80-86] This new concept may sound strange to many, but it expresses the only visible way to approach a true evaluation of bone strength from the clinical point of view.[43,83]

Accordingly, the following sections will deal with (1) the noninvasive measurements of the four biomechanically relevant bone properties in the skeletal regions of interest, and (2) the way that information should be interpreted and combined. The noninvasive analysis of muscle properties and the muscle–bone interactions concerning the diagnosis of osteopenias and osteoporoses are dealt with in a separate chapter.

A. NONINVASIVE MEASUREMENT OF BONE MECHANICAL PROPERTIES

Theoretically at least, there should always be some suitable formula for calculation of the strength of any region of the skeleton noninvasively, concerning any way of deformation, provided that the necessary data of all its four biological components (Figure 8.6) were available. This assumption seems to define the problem quite well, but it also poses a tremendous challenge. In fact, what kind of variables should we measure for each kind of property in each case, and how could we do that? Let's describe the state of the art concerning each of those four determinants.

1. Noninvasive Assessment of Bone Matrix Mineralization

The accurate measurement of the actual degree of mineralization of the ideally "solid" bone matrix is actually impossible, even by directly weighing a small piece of it, just because of the high concentration of tiny pores or ducts it contains for cells and vessels. It could rather be calculated by physicochemical analysis of its components. In so doing, we would find that the normal "solid" bone substance contains approximately:

- 58% of "pure," unmineralized matrix (water, ground substance, and fibers) with a density of 1.0 g/cm^3 (which affords 0.58 g/cm^3 to its density)
- 42% of "pure" mineral (hydroxyapatite) with a density of 3.2 g/cm^3 (which adds further 1.34 g/cm^3 to that density)

This gives a whole density of the composite bone matter of 0.58 + 1.34 = 1.92 g/cm^3, which is assumed to be the *true* density of the naturally mineralized, "solid" bone tissue.

Even the density of the whole bone including all hard substance, cells, vessels, marrow, etc. (i.e., the *apparent* or Archimedean bone density) could only be measured accurately by destructive methods. However, quantitative computed tomography (QCT, especially the "peripheral," high-resolution application, pQCT, produced by Norland/Stratec) is able to assess noninvasively the "volumetric *mineral* density" (vBMD) of either the whole bone slice studied or of the separate cortical, cortical-subcortical, or trabecular regions of it.[95-100]

Importantly, this measurement does not correspond to the apparent density of all the matter within the bone region studied, but only to the *density of the mineral fraction* of it. This is estimated by comparison of the absorption coefficients of the measured bone and that of a standardized phantom, which gives the bone mineral content (BMC) of the tissue.[98] The BMC is then divided by the known volume of the whole tomographic slice to obtain its vBMD. The vBMD of the *cortical* bone tissue assessed as a separate measurement could be regarded to vary in linear proportion with both the apparent density of the compact bone and the true density of the ideally solid mineralized matrix, provided that the (relatively small) space occupied by the pores could be considered irrelevant (and invariable) for comparison purposes.

This does not mean that QCT or pQCT is able to assess any material bone property directly. However, we could assume that the cortical vBMD measured by this technique would parallel the intrinsic stiffness of the "solid" bone material, provided that constancy of both the other micro-structural biological determinants of that property and the directionality of the bone deformation involved in the analysis could be assumed.[26,27,101,102] Thus, the vBMD data will by no means describe the "elastic modulus" of the "solid" bone tissue, although they would provide a useful reference of the mechanical ability of bone material that could be employed for proportional, comparative purposes in that case.[95-97,103]

2. Noninvasive Assessment of the Mineralization-Unrelated, Microstructural Determinants of Bone Matrix Stiffness/Strength (Bone Anisotropy at the Material or Tissue Level of Complexity)

Unfortunately, there is no practical way to assess this property noninvasively, and it could be assumed that this could not even be performed by any absorptiometric procedure, because the biological determinants involved are unrelated to the degree of bone tissue mineralization.

However, this would not imply that there will not be any chance to evaluate the bone material properties as a whole (that is, more completely than regarding only the matrix mineralization as QCT or pQCT do) by other techniques. The quantitative ultrasonometry (QUS) of the speed of sound (SOS; not the "broadband ultrasound attenuation," BUA) along (not across) cortical (not trabecular) bone with little interference of soft tissues (as on the internal face of the tibia, the external aspect of the radius, and the hand phallanxs) could provide some relevant information about the biomechanical behavior of that kind of tissue as a whole (i.e., regarding all the matrix mineralization and the microstructural factors of bone material quality together) (Figure 8.5).[35,104-108] This approach has still to be biomechanically validated, but it could be regarded as a promising technique for improving the resources currently at hand to evaluate this crucial aspect of bone strength noninvasively, eventually in a more integrated way than by QCT or pQCT.[107,109-112]

3. Noninvasive Determination of the Amount of Mineralized Bone Mass (and of the Bone Mineral Density)

It has been stressed already that the amount of mineralized bone mass would only be related to bone strength as a surrogate, size-related parameter.[78,89,113] However, there are a couple of reasons that strongly justify the inclusion of bone mass measurements in this chapter: (1) the wide diffusion and high popularity of the densitometric techniques developed for that purpose (single-photon absorptiometry, SPA; double-photon absorptiometry, DPA; and especially double-beam X-ray absorptiometry, DEXA), and (2) the high degree of standardization achieved concerning how the data provided by DEXA could be interpreted as supported by a great number of clinical evidences and agreements between many research groups, including World Health Organization (WHO) and National Institutes of Health (NIH) experts.[3-14] Also, the tomographic determination of bone "mass" will be discussed for reference purposes.

Of the early achievements reported employing SPA and DPA, the DEXA technology provides highly accurate and precise determinations of the bone mineral content (BMC) of the whole body and of well-standardized skeletal regions such as the lumbar spine (L2–L4 segment, assessed either in front or lateral projections), the hip (including the femoral neck, the Ward's triangle, and the greater trochanter as separate regions), and the distal radius. The BMC is assessed following a procedure similar to that employed by QCT, i.e., by comparison with standard phantoms. These differ for different manufacturers (Norland, Hologic, Lunar-USA), so that different results are obtained for the same measurements with different equipment, and some transformation algorithms must be applied for comparative purposes. The same limitations apply to the determination of BMC by QCT or pQCT (the latter is currently restricted to measuring only long bones, the head, and the cervical spine). In addition, the tomographic techniques are regionally restricted to analyze the bone slice studied.[98,99] Only DEXA is able to study wide regions of the skeleton, including the whole body.[83]

Importantly, neither the DEXA nor QCT-assessed BMCs represent the true mineralized bone mass or the amount of bone within the bone, but only the amount of mineral within the bone region. Therefore, the absorptiometric BMCs should be taken as indicators of the bone tissue mass only when bone tissue mineralization can be assumed to be normal (or at least constant, in comparative studies).

A further limitation of their clinical interpretation comes from the fact that BMCs are obviously size-related indicators, regardless of the technique employed in their determination. To overcome this inconvenience, two different kinds of procedures have been developed for DEXA and QCT/pQCT devices, respectively, giving rise to the absorptiometric concept of bone mineral density (BMD), with some particular characteristics in each case, as follows.

a. The Densitometric Approach: Bone Areal Mineral Density (the "Classic" BMD)

The DEXA-assessed BMC is usually related to the skeletal region in which it has been measured by just expressing its value per unit of the *projected area* of the corresponding bone(s). Obviously, the result is not a *volumetric* density but an "areal" or *projection* density, similar to population or hair densities, which is nevertheless called bone mineral *density* of the studied skeletal region. This calculation is frequently applied also to whole-body measurements, producing a BMD value that may be useful for metabolic analysis but that would have no clear clinical correlate in biomechanical

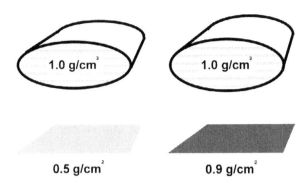

FIGURE 8.7 Projection absorptiometry captures only two of the three spatial axes describing the bone volume. Two bodies of the same volumetric or apparent (Archimedean) density will give different values of areal density, in linear proportion with the difference in length of the axis that is not captured by the determination. This shows how the areal BMD (DEXA) is affected by bone size.

terms. Some sophistication has recently been added to DEXA determinations in search of some biomechanical correlate, enabling the systems to estimate the bone "volume" and hence the "volumetric" BMD of the studied region from the obtained projection area, and even its cross-sectional moment of inertia (CSMI), with some obvious limitations. Extensive experimental and clinical validation is still needed for those attractive approaches.[75,78,114]

The areal BMD values can be reported in crude form or as percentiles, but they are more usually standardized for determined age ranges as *z-scores* ("scores" = deviations from the means in standard deviation units) or related to a proposed reference value for "normal" young individuals (*t-scores*) that should necessarily vary for anthropometrically or genetically different populations.[21] The universally accepted scale proposed by the WHO[3,5-8] establishes the following:

- *t*-score values over –1.0 indicate a "normal" condition.
- Those between –1.0 and –2.5 express an osteopenia.
- Those below –2.5 correspond to an osteoporosis.
- Osteoporosis is considered "established" when one or more fractures attributable to the diagnosed osteopenia have also taken place.

Anthropometrically, the expression of BMC as BMD captures only two of the three axes of bone volume (Figure 8.7), disregarding at least a part of the high influence of bone and body size on the measurement. Therefore, the DEXA-BMD is somewhat dependent on bone and body size, an important feature when the studied individuals differ anthropometrically or are of different genders.[3,5-8,78,83,115] Other inconveniences come, in the special case of the lumbar spine determinations, from the undesirable sum of an amount of mineral from the posterior processes of the vertebrae or the big vessels in the frontal projection, and from the increase in variance affecting the measurements in lateral projection.

Despite these problems, the DEXA-BMD has been shown to correlate fairly well with bone strength or fracture risk (of the same regions), especially when the studied bones work predominantly in compression (as do the vertebral bodies).[3,5-13,113] In this special circumstance the mere amount of mineralized tissue, or the bone size, accounts significantly for bone strength with relative independence from bone design.[116,117] In any case, the exclusive use of this indicator for predicting bone strength or fracture risk would be biomechanically inadequate because it completely disregards both bone geometry and *anisotropy*.[3,27,45,62,63,118,119] This pitfall becomes especially evident when the BMD values are applied to monitoring therapeutic effects on fracture incidence over time as related only to the bone mass changes, either in the same or (more evidently) in different skeletal regions.[17,18,20]

Those observations suggest that the WHO scale of *t*-scores[3,2-8,19] (as well as any kind of DEXA determination of bone mass) should be applied to the diagnosis of *osteopenia* (i.e., an *anthropometrically low bone mass*) rather than to that of *osteoporosis* (i.e., a biomechanically assessed condition of *increased bone fragility resulting from an osteopenia*, as the new NIH conception correctly points out).[3,43]

b.   The Tomographic Approach: The Volumetric BMD (vBMD)

On using QCT or pQCT the bone slice thickness is a known, pre-fixed condition and the cross-sectional area is easily measurable by the system.[95,98-100,120] This allows calculation of the volume of the slice or of selected regions of interest (ROIs). The BMC determined can thus be expressed per unit of that volume, actually as a volumetric BMD (vBMD), which would correspond to the apparent mineral density of the tissue in question, comprising the spaces that are not filled with solid bone. Obviously, this density will correspond only to the amount of tissue (bone plus pores, cells, vessels, marrow, etc.) comprised within the selected ROI within the bone slice, or eventually to the whole slice. The vBMD values cannot be extrapolated to a larger region of the bone or to different regions of the same bone, much less to different bones, although it could be proposed that the cortical vBMD values should not vary substantially between different skeletal regions of the same individual.

The vBMD will always express the amount of mineral per unit of tissue volume in the selected ROI, so that:

- When vBMD is determined in the whole-bone slice, it expresses the degree of concentration of mineral in the bone as an organ (in that region), regardless of the type of tissue. Therefore, this property could be regarded as representing closely the same thing as the DEXA-BMD.
- If the ROI comprises only *trabecular* bone, its vBMD will express the relative concentration of the trabecular network in the studied site, equivalent to the "apparent" density of that cancellous bone. If it can be assumed that intertrabecular connectivity is normal or unchanged in comparative studies, the trabecular vBMD can be regarded as an indirect indicator of the *structural* (not intrinsic or material) stiffness or strength of the trabecular network.[12]
- When the vBMD is calculated for an ROI containing only *cortical* bone, it should be more or less closely proportional to the true mineral density of the solid bone matrix, depending on the degree of intracortical porosity and provided that osteomalacia and bone displasia can be excluded. This value may be also proportional to the mechanical quality (stiffness, or elastic modulus) of the composite, calcified bone material as long as any variation in the other, microstructural determinants of that property (see Figure 8.6) could be neglected.[26,32,102] The bone material properties are thought to vary usually little within different bones of the same individual.[29] In any case, they may vary substantially within different sections of a given cortical bone ROI, according to their relative degree of porosity.[29] On selecting and fixing an adequate "lower" attenuation threshold for selecting the ROI (say, 0.8/cm for human pQCT studies), the relative degree of intracortical porosity of the comprised bone tissue could be estimated for comparative purposes (provided that osteomalacia could be previously excluded by other means). By varying the attenuation threshold, different "density-distribution" zones can also be defined (Figure 8.8).[122] These may be important for achieving a more descriptive evaluation of the biomechanical properties of the integrated cortical shell, especially in postmenopausal women. The cortical vBMD can also be used for calculation of some bone strength indices[90,95,98,99,123] as described below. When the cortical shell is thinner than 2 mm,[124] as often seen in the human distal radius in postmenopausal or elderly individuals, the cortical cross-sectional area tends to be overestimated because of the so-called

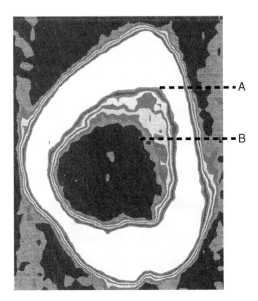

FIGURE 8.8 Scan obtained by pQCT of a tibial diaphysis from a premenopausal woman, in which only cortical bone is present. The zone indicated (A–B) shows how different density zones can be distinguished by selecting appropriate attenuation thresholds to describe the mechanical quality of the cortical shell with more detail.

partial-volume effect (relative abundance of pixels that are not filled with solid bone).[125] As a result, the determined vBMD value may tend artifactually to fall, giving place to systematic errors that would be proportional to the cortical thinness.

4. Noninvasive Determination of Bone Architecture (Bone Anisotropy at the Organ Level of Complexity)

The analysis of bone (macro) architecture differs for cortical and trabecular bone and accordingly with the type of strain (and hence strength) involved. In general terms, the amount of bone in the perpendicular cross section is by itself highly relevant to uniaxial compression strength determination.[68,89,113] For bending or torsional strains, however, the strength analysis concerns the cortical bone tissue *distribution* rather than the whole-bone mass.[27,45,62,63,113,118,119]

Bone size and shape are also architectural features that are relevant to bone strength in general terms. Tomographic or magnetic resonance imaging (MRI) techniques can measure the total ("blind") area of the bone cross section, which could be regarded as an unbiased estimator of the whole-bone size.[98,99] The DEXA technology can measure bone widths in the spine, hip, and radial region[77] and even some geometric features of the projected upper end of the femur, but unfortunately it is unable to study cortical and trabecular bone separately in any case. For that purpose, current approaches seem to be restricted to tomographic or MRI techniques.[1,126]

a. The Cortical Bone Problem

In vertebral bodies, cortical bone usually works in compression, so that its mass (or the cortical thickness) is highly relevant for the strain/strength analysis, and in any case the whole-bone strength will depend on the biomechanical condition of both the cortical shell and the trabecular network.[127,128] In long bones, which are normally deformed by usage either in compression, bending, or torsion, failure starts to occur only on the external surfaces, generally as a result of an insufficiency of tensile strength in every case.[24] Therefore, the cortical shell would be the only structure that protects long bones against fracture.

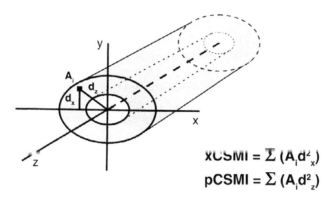

$$\text{xCSMI} = \Sigma \, (A_i d^2_x)$$
$$\text{pCSMI} = \Sigma \, (A_i d^2_z)$$

FIGURE 8.9 Schematic representation of the way the bending and torsional cross-sectional moments of inertia (xCSMI, pCSMI) are obtained by pQCT machines as the integral sum of the products of the area (A_i) of each of the selected pixels and the squared distance (d_x, d_z) to the corresponding, bending (x) or torsion (z) axes.[98] The more peripheral the disposition of the cortical shell with reference to the mechanically critical axis, the larger the corresponding CSMI.

Here again, for compression strength the cortical mass (i.e., the cross-sectional cortical bone area in tomographic slices)[129] is a first-order strength determinant, and the QCT analysis of cortical profiles seems to afford further precision to that approach.[130] However, for bending and torsional analysis, the external diameters of the shaft are also critically relevant, so that for bones with the same cross-sectional bone area but different external diameters, the wider ones will be the strongest.[24,25,27,68,82,113] In other words, the more *peripheral* the distribution of the available cortical bone mass in the shaft with reference to critical bending or torsional axes (regardless of the cortical thickness within a large extent), the stiffer and stronger the whole long bone will be concerning bending or torsion, respectively.

In architectural terms, there is a family of cross-sectional indicators that simultaneously capture both the cortical bone mass and its more or less peripheral distribution concerning specific reference axes. These are the CSMIs.[24,77,82,113] The ability of QCT/pQCT to study cross-sectional bone slices allows calculation not only of the cortical bone mass (cross-sectional area), but also of a number of CSMIs. They are determined as the integral sums of the products of the areas of all the pixels in the cortical ROI times their squared distances to the desired reference axes (Figure 8.9).[95,98,99] Thus, for bending analysis, *equatorial* or *Cartesian* CSMIs (xCSMI, yCSMI, etc.; generally known as *bending CSMIs*) can be calculated with respect to different bending axes (x, y, etc.); and for torsional analysis, a *polar* (pCSMI, or *torsional CSMI*) can be obtained with respect to the longitudinal bone axis (z) as indicated in the diagram.

The CSMIs seem to be reliable estimators of the architectural fitness of bones provided only that bending or torsion are relevant factors concerning the usual method of fracture. In fact, they have been shown to be more closely related to bone strength in diaphyseal than in metaphyseal bone regions, proposedly for that reason.[123,125,131,132]

The MRI analysis of cortical bone seems as promising as QCT or pQCT for these purposes.[1,126] Encouraging results are being reported with this powerful technology.

b.   The Trabecular Bone Problem

The mechanical role of trabecular bone seems to be mostly associated to the load transmission from the articular surfaces toward the inner aspect of cortical bone as a supporting frame for the articular cartilages.[65] In long-bone metaphyses this arrangement has to do with the pathogenesis of arthroses rather than with resistance to a traumatic fracture. Furthermore, whatever the mechanical role of trabecular bone and its eventual importance concerning fracture risk, this may vary for different skeletal regions, and even for the same site when the proportion between cortical and trabecular bone changes with age.

In the vertebral bodies, in which the collapse of the trabecular structure is clinically equivalent to a fracture, the trabecular network has been regarded as very relevant to bone integrity as the cortical shell, although the trabecular–cortical bone proportion varies widely with age.[120,127,128,133] In the distal radius, the trabecular BMC and vBMD seem to be slightly better discriminants between fractured and unfractured individuals than the cortical cross-sectional area, xCSMI, or pCSMI.[132]

Nevertheless, it seems reasonable to approach a separate, noninvasive evaluation of the strength of the trabecular network itself, which would obviously depend on both its material and architectural (mass/distribution) properties. In this regard, any absorptiometric determination of the trabecular mass (as the trabecular BMC provided by QCT or pQCT, or even the determination of BMC by DEXA in regions in which trabecular bone is highly predominant) would suffice to deal with the mass component of the cancellous bone strength in compression with acceptable accuracy.[9,95,98-100,113,134-137]

Combinations of vBMD indicators with some indicators of bone size such as the whole-bone cross-sectional area (QCT, pQCT, MRI) could also give reasonable approaches to noninvasive assessment of bone strength in compression, as discussed below. However, even in this case, bone mass will not represent a true indicator of bone strength, because its determination disregards the architectural properties of the trabecular network (whole-bone anisotropy) on which its strength also critically depends, especially in older persons, in pathologic conditions, and concerning bending or torsional strength analyses.[27,45,61-63,118,119] This inconvenience becomes important when it is necessary to evaluate the evolution of bone mass-dependent changes in bone strength.

Dealing with suitable indicators of the architectural properties of trabecular bone is actually a difficult challenge. Here the problem concerns not only the separate, quantitative analysis of trabecular bone mass (which is perfectly possible with QCT or pQCT,[95,98-100] but also the evaluation of some geometric properties of the network. Some recently developed, high-resolution pQCT scanners (Stratec, Germany; Scanco, Switzerland) provide an almost "histomorphometrical" definition of the trabecular image with that purpose, but unfortunately no equipment of this kind is currently available as a suitable, standardized device for noninvasive determinations in humans.

Among the architectural properties of the trabecular network, that most relevant to any biomechanical analysis seems to be the intertrabecular connectivity. Not too difficult to measure by bone histomorphometry (an invasive technique), the absorptiometric evaluation of this property has also been approached employing high-resolution QCT or pQCT.[138-141]

One of the most promising resources available from the scanners now on the market seems to be the so-called skeletonization of images of trabecular bone taken from vertebral bodies with spiral QCT[1,121,138,142,143] (ideally 2-mm thick) or from the distal radius with pQCT[144,145] or radiographic analysis.[146,147] This procedure requires separate computers to which the tomographic images have to be exported to render the traces of the trabecular network practically linear. After that, the geometric analysis of nodes and free ends could be easily performed employing a variety of techniques that may include fractal analyses.[148] The calculation of different kinds of proportions or associations between nodes and free ends of the network provides a number of "connectivity" indices.[139,144] Some of these indicators have already been shown to discriminate well between fractured and nonfractured individuals, yet they are still to be validated and standardized for clinical applications.

MRI scans provide almost histomorphometric description of the trabecular network, with promising results concerning the noninvasive evaluation of the cancellous bone strength with the aid of separate, dedicated computers.[89,121,149-151] Additionally, this technology is able to predict bone marrow characteristics. Results may be applicable to a biomechanical analysis of bone in the distal radius, spine, and femoral neck as soon as the corresponding correlates have been determined.

B. How to Interpret and Combine the Data

The double dependence of bone strength on the bone material and architectural properties (see Figure 8.6) points out the inability of any single bone measurement to describe fully the mechanical properties of bones. The above-mentioned partial possibilities of the currently available techniques and indicators are shown in the diagram. This means that, in addition to the pitfalls that every technique shows concerning accuracy, precision, and even ability to measure the right bone properties, the noninvasive measurement of bone strength also requires the development of a rationale for combining the available data into suitable formulae and duly interpreting the corresponding indices. Obviously, indicators of both bone material and geometric properties are needed to approach those formulae. This poses again the bone anisotropy problem, both at the tissue and organ levels of biological complexity.

Let's first discuss bone material properties. Until recently, it seemed that there should have been little or no trouble derived from bone anisotropy at the material or tissue level for the diagnosis of osteoporosis, because bone material properties were thought to vary relatively little, at least in adult persons. However, recent developments seem to indicate the opposite,[152-154] giving rise to a new concept that could affect our current understanding of osteoporosis, as discussed in a separate chapter. In any case, these conflicting concepts would *not* concern bone tissue anisotropy, which could be provisionally supposed to be unaffected in either case. The above proposal would undoubtedly simplify the problem because it would restrain the anisotropy question in practice to only one (the organ) level of complexity.

Nevertheless, this does not obviate the need to evaluate the bone material properties (even neglecting anisotropy) as valid components of the whole-bone strength assessment.[29,89,90,123] Therefore, we *actually need* some suitable indicators of bone material properties (at least one in each instance) to be included in the calculations for estimating any kind of whole-bone properties, even accepting that they may vary relatively little. For that purpose we may make use of only indirect indicators, such as the cortical vBMD, a tomographic indicator of the mineralization of the solid bone,[123] or eventually the ultrasonometric SOS of cortical bone, perhaps a more integral estimator of the bone tissue stiffness than the former.[104-107,109-112]

Concerning bone anisotropy at the organ level (bone geometric properties) the matter is far simpler and clearer than that. Bone architecture at the organ level seems to be "the" bone feature that has always been (and, of course, is still being) grossly changed by nature following an incredible large number of ways to adapt bone (macro)structure to the mechanical stimulation (strains) produced by the ecological environment (mechanical usage of the skeleton).[64,65]

We have a number of suitable indicators of the architectural fitness of the bone design, yet regrettably we do not have everything we need for analyzing every bone region and every possible instance and method of deformation or fracture. Among these indicators are the many available CSMIs (for bending or torsional analyses of cortical bone) and connectivity indices (for many kinds of analyses of trabecular bone), and also (restricted to compression strength analysis only) all the indicators of bone mass or size, i.e., the densitometric or tomographic BMCs (not the densitometric BMD), the tomographic or MRI-assessed cross-sectional bone areas, perimeters, and cortical thickness, and an indirect, nonselective estimator, the ultrasonometric BUA.

A critical matter in this concern is how to combine those or other indicators of bone material and geometric properties to obtain suitable indices of bone strength. Obviously, many kinds of combinations may apply with a reasonable chance of success.[79,106,130] The matter concerns the selection of true, mechanically meaningful indicators.

Perhaps the first approaches should conveniently consider cases that can be experimentally modeled in the simplest way. One of these instances is the bending or torsional strength analysis of tubular bones, in which the structural (whole-bone) stiffness should be directly proportional to both the elastic modulus (E) of cortical bone and the bending or torsional CSMIs.[31,68,113,123,155,156] Another approach may be to combine DEXA or pQCT data with the QUS-assessed SOS.[157]

In standardized, controlled conditions, such as those in which the three-point bending test of the geometrically quite homogeneous rat femur diaphysis is performed, we have found that the structural stiffness and strength (fracture load) correlated very closely with the product $E \times$ bending CSMI, with E mechanically calculated after the destructive test and the xCSMI taken noninvasively at the midshaft by pQCT. On replacing E in that formula by the pQCT-assessed vBMD of cortical bone we also obtained a very close correlation with the actual fracture load. This quite simple bone strength index (BSI = cortical vBMD $\times$ bending CSMI) predicted the mechanical behavior of that bone region, in those controlled conditions, significantly better than either the cortical vBMD or the CSMI alone, or the DEXA-assessed areal BMD of the mid-diaphyseal region of the same femurs.[123]

This does not mean that the same formula could be applied to different bone regions and/or methods of deformation or fracture with a similar perspective. Bone anisotropy (mostly at the organ level) forces the investigators to develop different approaches adapted to different situations, presumably facing a high specificity concerning bone region and method of deformation.

The pQCT machines can calculate automatically many similar indices, among them the so-called stress–strain index (SSI) related to torsional strength estimation,[90] for which the same preventions as those set for the SSI should apply. As an example of that, we have applied the above formula for the rat-femur-BSI to calculation of the same index at the human distal radius. This radial BSI discriminated fairly well between individuals with and without a Colles' fracture. However, this approach was not better than that provided by the BMC or the volumetric BMD of trabecular bone or the cross-sectional area or CSMI of cortical bone as single predictors.[132]

The matter is considerably more complex for skeletal regions in which trabecular bone plays a significant role as a structural strength determinant.[158] In these instances, both the material properties (intrinsic stiffness, etc.) of the solid tissue within the trabeculae and the architectural properties of the network (directionality, connectivity, etc.) should have to be dealt with to evaluate the contribution of cancellous tissue to the whole-bone strength. Perhaps the use of the vBMD of trabecular bone as an indicator of the structural strength of the network could be used in combination with some mass indicator, although connectivity would be neglected in this case. Good correlations between the product *trabecular vBMD $\times$ cross-sectional area* and the actual strength of vertebral bodies and femur proximal metaphyses have been reported.[159-162] Things sound far more complicated if a combination of trabecular and cortical bone indicators has to be employed, especially when age- and gender-related differences affect the proportion in which each type of tissue contributes to strength.[115,128]

Intuitively, any combination of independent, noninvasive indicators of different aspects of bone strength (ideally, those related to material and geometric properties) should offer a better approach to bone health or fracture risk than their use as separate predictors does. However, regrettably, there is not enough experimental evidence to support that assumption compellingly. Nevertheless, our current knowledge of bone biomechanics suggests that perhaps that kind of analysis would offer a valuable complement to the information provided by DEXA. Extensive research is strongly encouraged in this regard.

REFERENCES

1. Genant, H.K., Engelke, K., Fuerst, T., et al., "Noninvasive assessment of bone mineral and structure: state of the art," *J. Bone Miner. Res.,* 11, 707, 1996.
2. Kanis, J.A., "Prediction of fracture from low bone mineral density measurements overestimates risk," *Bone,* 26, 387, 2000.

3. NIH Consensus Development Panel on Osteoporosis Prevention, Diagnosis, and Therapy, "Osteoporosis prevention, diagnosis, and therapy," *J. Am. Med. Assoc.*, 285, 785, 2001.

4. Cummings, S.R., Black, D.M., Nevitt, M.C., et al., "Bone density at various sites for prediction of hip fractures," *Lancet*, 341, 72, 1993.

5. Kanis, J.A., Melton, J., Christiansen, C., et al., "The diagnosis of osteoporosis," *J. Bone Miner. Res.*, 9, 1137, 1994.

6. Kanis, J.A., "Assessment of fracture risk and its application to screening for postmenopausal osteoporosis: synopsis of a WHO report," *Osteoporos. Int.*, 4, 368, 1994.

7. Kanis, J.A., Devogelaer, J.P., and Gennari, C., "Practical guide for the use of bone mineral measurements in the assessment of treatment of osteoporosis: a position paper of the European Foundation for Osteoporosis and Bone Disease," *Osteoporos. Int.*, 6, 256, 1996.

8. Majumdar, S. and Genant, H.K., "WHO: Technical report. Assessment of fracture risk and its application to screening for postmenopausal osteoporosis: a report of a WHO study group," WHO, Geneva, 1994.

9. Tabensky, A.D., Williams, J., Deluca, V., et al., "Bone mass, areal, and volumetric bone density are equally accurate, sensitive, and specific surrogates of the breaking strength of the vertebral body: an *in vitro* study," *J. Bone Miner. Res.*, 11, 1981, 1996.

10. Lung, M., Felsanberg, D., Reeve, J., et al., "Bone density variation and its effects on risk of vertebral deformity in men and women studied in thirteen European centers: the EVOS Study," *J. Bone Miner. Res.*, 112, 1883, 1997.

11. Huang, C., Ross, P.D., and Wasnich, R.D., "Short-term and long-term fracture prediction by bone mass measurements: a prospective study," *J. Bone Miner. Res.*, 13, 107, 1998.

12. Melton, L.J., Atkinson, E.J., O'Connor, M.K., et al., "Bone density and fracture risk in men," *J. Bone Miner. Res.*, 13, 1915, 1998.

13. Miller, P.D., Zapalowski, C., Kulak, C.A.M., et al., "Bone densitometry: the best way to detect osteoporosis and to monitor therapy," *J. Clin. Endocrinol. Metab.*, 84, 1867, 1999.

14. Wasnich, R.D. and Miller, P.D., "Antifracture efficacy of antiresorptive agents are related to changes in bone density," *J. Clin. Endocrinol. Metab.*, 85, 231, 2000.

15. Beck, T.J., Looker, A.C., Ruff, C.B., et al., "Structural trends in the aging femoral neck and proximal shaft: analysis of the Third National Health and Nutrition Examination Survey dual-energy X-ray absorptiometry data," *J. Bone Miner. Res.*, 15, 2297, 2000.

16. Van der Linden, J.C., Homminga, J., Weinans, H., et al., "Mechanical consequences of bone loss in cancellous bone," *J. Bone Miner. Res.*, 16, 457, 2001.

17. Marshall, D., Johnell, O., and Wedel, H., "Meta-analysis of how well measures of bone mineral density predict occurrences of osteoporotic fractures," *Br. J. Med.*, 312, 1254, 1996.

18. Vilani, P., Bondino-Riquier, R., and Bouvenot, G., "Fragilité des données acquises de la science. L'example du fluor dans l'osteoporose," *Presse Med.*, 27, 361, 1998.

19. Sandor, T., Felsenberg, D., and Brown, E., "Comments on the hypotheses underlying fracture risk assessment in osteoporosis as proposed by the World Health Organization," *Calcif. Tissue Int.*, 64, 267, 1999.

20. Wilkin, T., "Changing concepts in osteoporosis," *Br. J. Med.*, 318, 862, 1999.

21. Aspray, T.J., Prentice, A., Cole, T.J., et al., "Low bone mineral content is common but osteoporotic fractures are rare in elderly rural Gambian women," *J. Bone Miner. Res.*, 11, 1019, 1996.

22. Webber, C.E., "Uncertainties in bone mineral density T scores," *Clin. Invest. Med.*, 21, 88, 1998.

23. Faulkner, K.G., "Bone matters: are density increases necessary to reduce fracture risk?" *J. Bone Miner. Res.*, 15, 183, 2000.

24. Wainwright, S.A., Biggs, W.D., Currey, J.E.D., et al., *Mechanical Design in Organisms*, Arnold, London, 1976.

25. Currey, J.D., "What should bones be designed to do?" *Calcif. Tissue Int.*, 36, S7, 1984.

26. Currey, J.D., "The mechanical consequences of variation in the mineral content of bone," *J. Biomech.*, 2, 1, 1969.

27. Currey, J.D., "The design of mineralized tissues for their mechanical functions," *J. Exp. Biol.*, 202, 3285, 1999.

28. Burstein, A.H., Zilka, J., Heiple, K., et al., "Contribution of collagen and mineral to the elastic-plastic properties of bone," *J. Bone Joint Surg.*, 57A, 956, 1975.

29. Martin, R.B., Burr, D.B., and Sharkey, N.A., *Skeletal Tissue Mechanics*, Springer, New York, 1998.
30. Jurist, J.M. and Foltz, A.S., "Human ulnar bending stiffness, mineral content, geometry and strength," *J. Biomech.,* 10, 455, 1977.
31. Ferretti, J.L., Capozza, R.F., Mondelo, N., et al., "Interrelationships between densitometrical, geometric and mechanical properties of rat femurs. Inferences concerning mechanical regulation of bone modeling," *J. Bone Miner. Res.,* 8, 1389, 1993.
32. Currey, J.D., "What determines the bending strength of compact bone?" *J. Exp. Biol.,* 202, 2495, 1999.
33. Keaveny, T.M., Wachtel, E.F., Ford, C.M., et al., "Differences between the tensile and compressive strengths of bovine tibial trabecular bone depend on modulus," *J. Biomech.,* 27, 1137, 1994.
34. Landis, W.J., "The strength of a calcified tissue depends in part on the molecular structure and organization of its constitutent mineral crystals in their organic matrix," *Bone,* 16, 533, 1995.
35. Fyhrie, D.P. and Vashishth, D., "Bone stiffness predicts strength similarly for human vertebral cancellous bone in compression and for cortical bone in tension," *Bone,* 26, 169, 2000.
36. Carter, D.R. and Spengler, D.M., "Mechanical properties and composition of cortical bone," *Clin. Orthop.,* 135, 192, 1978.
37. Currey, J.D., "Physical characteristics affecting the tensile failure properties of compact bone," *J. Biomech.,* 23, 837, 1990.
38. Grynpas, M., "Age- and disease-related changes in the mineral of bone," *Calcif. Tissue Int.,* 53, S57, 1993.
39. McAlden, R.W., McGeough, J.A., Barker, M.B., et al., "Age-related changes in the tensile properties of cortical bone," *J. Bone Joint Surg.,* 75A, 1193, 1993.
40. Parfitt, A.M., "Bone age, mineral density, and fatigue damage," *Calcif. Tissue Int.,* 53, S82, 1993.
41. Zioupos, P. and Currey, J.D., "Changes in the stiffness, strength, and toughness of human cortical bone with age," *Bone,* 22, 57, 1998.
42. Bailey, A.J., Sims, T.J., Ebbesen, E.N., et al., "Age-related changes in the biochemical properties of human cancellous bone collagen: relationship to bone strength," *Calcif. Tissue Int.,* 65, 203, 1999.
43. Frost, H.M., "Defining osteopenias and osteoporoses. Another view (with insights from a new paradigm)," *Bone,* 20, 385, 1997.
44. Frost, H.M., *Intermediary Organization of the Skeleton*, Vols. I and II, CRC Press, Boca Raton, FL, 1986.
45. Rho, J.Y., Kuhn-Spearing, L., and Zioupos, P., "Mechanical properties and the hierarchical structure of bone," *Med. Eng. Phys.,* 20, 992, 1998.
46. Portigliatti Barbos, M., Bianco, P., Ascenzi, A., et al., "Collagen orientation in compact bone: II. Distribution of lamellae in the whole of the human femoral shaft with reference to its mechanical properties," *Metab. Bone Dis. Relat. Res.,* 5, 309, 1984.
47. Ascenzi, A., Improta, S., Portigliatti Barbos, M., et al., "Distribution of lamellae in human femoral shafts deformed by bending with inferences on mechanical properties," *Bone,* 8, 319, 1987.
48. Martin, R.B. and Ishida, J., "The relative effects of collagen fiber orientation, porosity, density, and mineralization on bone strength," *J. Biomech.,* 22, 419, 1989.
49. Sasaki, N., "Orientation of bone mineral and its role in the anisotropic mechanical properties of bone. Transverse anisotropy," *J. Biomech.,* 22, 157, 1989.
50. Pidaparti, R.M.V. and Burr, D.B., "Collagen fiber orientation and geometry effects on the mechanical properties of secondary osteons," *J. Biomech.,* 25, 869, 1992.
51. Hasegawa, K., Turner, C.H., and Burr, D.B., "Contribution of collagen and mineral to the elastic anisotropy of bone," *Calcif. Tissue Int.,* 55, 381, 1994.
52. Claes, L.E., Wilke, H.J., and Kiefer, H., "Osteonal structure better predicts tensile strength of healing bone than volume fraction," *J. Biomech.,* 11, 1377, 1995.
53. Turner, C.H., Chandran, A., and Pidaparti, R.M.V., "The anisotropy of osteonal bone and its ultrastructural implications," *Bone,* 17, 85, 1995.
54. Bouxsein, M.L., Myers, E.R., and Hayes, W.C., "Biomechanics of age-related fractures," in *Osteoporosis*, Marcus, R., Feldman, D., and Kelsey, J., Eds., Academic Press, San Diego, CA, 1996, 373.
55. Ruggeri, S., Raspanti, M., Martini, D., et al., "Bone as a composite material: collagen fibers orientation and functional requirements," in *Recent Advances in Microscopy of Cells, Tissues and Organs*, Motta, P.M., Ed., A. Delfino, Rome, 1997, 167.

56. Weiner, S., Traub, W., and Wagner, H.D., "Lamellar bone: structure-function relations," *J. Struct. Biol.*, 126, 241, 1999.

57. Burr, D.B., Schlaffler, M.B., and Frederickson, R.G., "Composition of the cement line and its possible mechanical role as a local interface in human compact bone," *J. Biomech.*, 11, 939, 1988.

58. Schaffler, M.B., Choi, K., and Milgrom, C., "Aging and microdamage accumulation in human compact bone," *Bone*, 17, 521, 1995.

59. Wang, X.D., Masilamani, N.S., Mabrey, J.D., et al., "Changes in the fracture toughness of bone may not be reflected in its mineral density, porosity, and tensile properties," *Bone*, 23, 67, 1998.

60. Compston, J.E., "Connectivity of cancellous bone: assessment and mechanical implications," *Bone*, 15, 463, 1994.

61. Aaron, J.E., Shore, P.A., Shore, R.C., et al., "Trabecular architecture in women and men of similar bone mass with and without vertebral fracture: II. Three-dimensional histology," *Bone*, 27, 277, 2000.

62. Alho, A., Husby, T., and Hoiseth, A., "Bone mineral content and mechanical strength," *Clin. Orthop.*, 227, 292, 1988.

63. Beck, T.J., Ruff, C.B., Warden, K.E., et al., "Predicting femoral neck strength from bone mineral data," *Invest. Radiol.*, 25, 6, 1990.

64. Frost, H.M., "Bone 'mass' and the 'mechanostat': a proposal," *Anat. Rec.*, 219, 1, 1987.

65. Frost, H.M., *Introduction to a New Skeletal Physiology*, Vol. I, *Bone and Bones*, Pajaro Group, Pueblo, CO, 1995.

66. Rho, J.Y., Ashman, R.B., and Turner, C.H., "Young's modulus of trabecular and cortical bone material: ultrasonic and microtensile measurements," *J. Biomech.*, 26, 111, 1993.

67. Rice, J.C., Cowin, S.C., and Bowman, J.A., "On the dependence of the elasticity and strength of cancellous bone on apparent density," *J. Biomech.*, 155, 1988.

68. Baker, J.L. and Haugh, C.G., "Mechanical properties of bone: a review," *Trans. A.S.A.E.*, 678, 1979.

69. Burr, D.B. and Martin, R.B., "The effects of composition, structure and age on the torsional properties of the human radius," *J. Biomech.*, 16, 603, 1983.

70. Martin, R.B., "Toward a unifying theory of bone remodeling," *Bone*, 26, 1, 2000.

71. Beck, T.J., Ruff, C.B., and Bissessur, K., "Age-related changes in female femoral neck geometry: implications for bone strength," *Calcif. Tissue Int.*, 53, S41, 1993.

72. Faulkner, K.G., McClung, M., and Cummings, S.R., "Automated evaluation of hip axis length for predicting hip fracture," *J. Bone Miner. Res.*, 9, 1065, 1994.

73. Bhudhikanok, G.S., Wang, M.C., Eckert, K., et al., "Differences in bone mineral in young Asian and Caucasian American may reflect differences in bone size," *J. Bone Miner. Res.*, 11, 1545, 1996.

74. Cheng, X.G., Lowet, G., Boonen, S., et al., "Assessment of the strength of proximal femur *in vitro*: relationship to femoral bone mineral density and femoral geometry," *Bone*, 20, 213, 1997.

75. Duboeuf, F., Hans, D., Kotzki, P.O., et al., "Different morphometric and densitometric parameters predict cervical and throcanteric hip fracture: the EPIDOS Study," *J. Bone Miner. Res.*, 12, 1895, 1997.

76. Gnudi, S., Ripamonti, C., Gualtieri, G., et al., "Geometry of proximal femur in the prediction of hip fracture in osteoporotic women," *Br. J. Radiol.*, 72, 729, 1999.

77. Crabtree, N., Lunt, M., Holt, G., et al., "Hip geometry, bone mineral distribution, and bone strength in European men and women: the EPOS Study," *Bone*, 27, 151, 2000.

78. Carter, D.R., Bouxsein, M.L., and Marcus, R., "New approaches for interpreting projected bone densitometry data," *J. Bone Miner. Res.*, 7, 137, 1992.

79. Frost, H.M., "On the estrogen-bone relationship and postmenopausal bone loss: a new model," *J. Bone Miner. Res.*, 14, 1473, 1999.

80. Parfitt, A.M., "The two faces of growth: benefits and risks to bone integrity," *Osteoporos. Int.*, 4, 382, 1994.

81. Frost, H.M., Ferretti, J.L., and Jee, W.S.S., "Some roles of mechanical usage, muscle strength and the mechanostat in skeletal physiology, disease, and research," *Calcif. Tissue Int.*, 62, 1, 1997.

82. Ferretti, J.L., Capozza, R.F., Cointry, G.R., et al., "Gender-related differences in the relationships between densitometric values of whole-body bone mineral content and lean mass in humans between 2 and 87 years of age," *Bone*, 22, 683, 1998.

83. Ferretti, J.L., Schiessl, H., and Frost, H.M., "On new opportunities for absorptiometry," *J. Clin. Densitom.*, 1, 41, 1998.

84. Schönau, E., "The development of the skeletal system in children and the influence of muscular strength," *Horm. Res.,* 49, 27, 1998.
85. Rittweger, J. and Rauch, F., "What is new in musculo-skeletal interactions," *J. Musculoskel. Neuron. Interact.,* 1, 171, 200.
86. Rittweger, J., Beller, G., Ehrig, J., et al., "Bone-muscle strength indices for the human lower leg," *Bone,* 27, 319, 2000.
87. Gilsanz, V., Boechat, M.I., Gilsanz, R., et al., "Gender differences in vertebral sizes in adults: biomechanical implications," *Radiology,* 190, 678, 1994.
88. Orwoll, E., "Assessing bone density in men," *J. Bone Miner. Res.,* 15, 1867, 2000.
89. Ferretti, J.L., "Biomechanical properties of bone," in *Bone Densitometry and Osteoporosis,* Genant, H.K., Guglielmi, G., and Jergas, M., Eds., Springer, Berlin, 1998, 143.
90. Schiessl, H., Ferretti, J.L., Tysarczyk-Niemeyer, G., et al., "Noninvasive bone strength index as analyzed by peripheral quantitative computed tomography," in *Paediatric Osteology. New Developments in Diagnostics and Therapy,* Schönau, E., Ed., Elsevier, Amsterdam, 1996, 141.
91. Greenspan, S.L., Maitland-Ramsey, L., and Myers, E., "Classification of osteoporosis in the elderly is dependent on site-specific analysis," *Calcif. Tissue Int.,* 58, 409, 1996.
92. Roldán, E.J.A. and Ferretti, J.L., "How do anti-osteoporotic agents prevent fractures?" *Bone,* 26, 393, 2000.
93. Compston, J.E., "Pharmacologic interventions for the prevention of vertebral and nonvertebral fractures in women with postmenopausal osteoporosis: does site-specificity exist?" *Bone,* 27, 765, 2000.
94. Seeman, E., Duan, Y., Fong, C., et al., "Fracture site-specific deficits in bone size and volumetric density in men with spine or hip fractures," *J. Bone Miner. Res.,* 16, 120, 2001.
95. Ferretti, J.L., "Perspectives of pQCT technology associated to biomechanical studies in skeletal research employing rat models," *Bone,* 17, 353S, 1995.
96. Ferretti, J.L., "Effects of bisphosphonates on bone biomechanics," in *Bisphosphonate on Bones,* Bijvoet, O.L.M., et al., Eds., Elsevier, Amsterdam, 1995, 211.
97. Ferretti, J.L., Gaffuri, O.H., Capozza, R.F., et al., "Dexamethasone effects on structural, geometric and material properties of rat femur diaphyses as described by peripheral quantitative computed tomography (pQCT) and bending tests," *Bone,* 16, 119, 1995.
98. Ferretti, J.L., "Peripheral quantitative computed tomography for evaluating structural and mechanical properties of small bone," in *Mechanical Testing of Bone and the Bone–Implant Interface,* An, Y.H. and Draughn, R.A., Eds., CRC Press, Boca Raton, FL, 2000, 385.
99. Ferretti, J.L., Cointry, G.R., Capozza, R.F., et al., "Analysis of biomechanical effects on bone and on the bone-muscle interactions in small animal models," *J. Musculoskel. Neuron. Interact.,* 1, 263, 2001.
100. Gasser, J.A., "Assessing bone quantity by pQCT," *Bone,* 17, 145S, 1995.
101. Harp, J.H., Aronson, J., and Hollis, M., "Noninvasive determination of bone stiffness for distraction osteogenesis by quantitative computed tomography scans," *Clin. Orthop.,* 301, 42, 1994.
102. Les, C.M., Keyak, J.H., Stover, S.M., et al., "Estimation of material properties in the equine metacarpus with use of quantitative computed tomography," *J. Orthop. Res.,* 12, 822, 1994.
103. Capozza, R.F., Ferretti, J.L., Ma, Y.F., et al., "Tomographic (pQCT) and biomechanical effects of hPTH(1-38) on chronically immobilized or overloaded rat femurs," *Bone,* 17, 233S, 1995.
104. Brandenburger, G.H., "Clinical determination of bone quality: Is ultrasound an answer?" *Calcif. Tissue Int.,* 53, S151, 1993.
105. Glüer, C.C., "Quantitative ultrasound techniques for the assessment of osteoporosis; expert agreement on current status," *J. Bone Miner. Res.,* 12, 1280, 1997.
106. Gnudi, S., Gualtieri, G., and Malavolta, N., "Simultaneous densitometry and quantitative bone sonography in the estimation of osteoporotic fracture risk," *Br. J. Radiol.,* 71, 625, 1998.
107. Hans, D., Fuerst, T., Guglielmi, G., et al., "Quantitative ultrasound for assessing bone properties," in *Bone Densitometry and Osteoporosis,* Genant, H.K., Guglielmi, G., and Jergas, M., Eds., Springer, Berlin, 1998, 379.
108. Wüster, C., Albanese, C., De Aloysio, D., et al., "Phalangeal osteosonogrammetry study: age-related changes, diagnostic sensitivity, and discrimination power," *J. Bone Miner. Res.,* 15, 1603, 2000.
109. Rho, J.Y., Hobatho, M.C., and Ashman, R.B., "Relations of mechanical properties to density and CT numbers in human bone," *Med. Eng. Phys.,* 17, 347, 1995.

110. Strelitzki, R., Evans, J.A., and Clarke, A.J., "The influence of porosity and pore size on the ultrasonic properties of bone investigated using a phantom material," *Osteoporos. Int.*, 7, 370, 1997.

111. Hans, D., Srivastav, S.K., Singal, C., et al., "Does combining the results from multiple bone sites measured by a new quantitative ultrasound device improve discrimination of hip fracture?" *J. Bone Miner. Res.*, 14, 644, 1999.

112. Mehta, S.S., Öz, O.K., and Antich, P.P., "Bone elasticity and ultrasound velocity are affected by subtle changes in the organic matrix," *J. Bone Miner. Res.*, 13, 114, 1998.

113. Hayes, W.C., "Biomechanics of cortical and trabecular bone: implications for assessment of fracture risk," in *Basic Orthopaedic Biomechanics*, Mow, V.C. and Hayes, W.C., Eds., Raven Press, New York, 1991, 93.

114. Sievänen, H., Kannus, P., Nieminen, V., et al., "Estimation of various mechanical characteristics of human bones using dual energy X-ray absorptiometry: methodology and precision," *Bone*, 18, 17S, 1996.

115. Ortoft, G., Mosekilde, Li., Hasling, C., et al., "Estimation of vertebral body strength by dual photon absorptiometry in elderly individuals," *Bone*, 14, 667, 1993.

116. Ebbesen, E.N., Thomsen, J.S., Beck-Nielsen, H., et al., "Age- and gender-related differences in vertebral bone mass, density, and strength," *J. Bone Miner. Res.*, 14, 1394, 1999.

117. Duan, Y., Parfitt, A.M., and Seeman, E., "Vertebral bone mass, size, and volumetric density in women with spinal fractures." *J. Bone Miner. Res.*, 14, 1796, 1999.

118. Seeman, E., "From density to structure: growing up and growing old on the surfaces of bone," *J. Bone Miner. Res.*, 12, 509, 1997.

119. Seeman, E., "Bone size, mass, and volumetric density: the importance of structure in skeletal health," in *Osteoporosis in Men*, Orwoll, E.S., Ed., Academic Press, San Diego, CA, 1999, 87.

120. Ferretti, J.L., Capozza, R.F., Cointry, G.R., et al., "Densitometric and tomographic analysis of musculoskeletal interactions in humans," *J. Musculoskel. Neuron. Interact.*, 1, 18, 2000.

121. Lang, T.F., Keyak, J.H., Heitz, M.W., et al., "Volumetric quantitative computed tomography of the proximal femur: precision and relation to bone strength," *Bone*, 21, 101, 1997.

122. Roldán, E.J.A., Capiglioni, R., Capozza, R.F., et al., "Postmenopausal changes in the distribution of the volumetric vBMD of cortical bone. A pQCT study of the human leg," *J. Musculoskel. Neuron. Interact.*, 2, 157, 2001.

123. Ferretti, J.L., Capozza, R.F., and Zanchetta, J.R., "Mechanical validation of a tomographic (pQCT) index for noninvasive assessment of rat femur bending strength," *Bone*, 18, 97, 1996.

124. Louis, O., Willnecker, J., Soykens, S., et al., "Cortical thickness assessed by peripheral quantitative computed tomography. Accuracy evaluated on radius specimens," *Osteoporos. Int.*, 5, 446, 1995.

125. Augat, P., Gordon, C.L., Lang, T., et al., "Accuracy of cortical and trabecular bone measurements with peripheral quantitative computed tomography (pQCT)," *Phys. Med. Biol.*, 43, 2873, 1998.

126. Jergas, M.D., Majumdar, S., Keyak, J.H., et al., "Relationships between Young's modulus of elasticity, ash density, and MRI derived effective transverse relaxation T2 in tibial specimens," *J. Comput. Assist. Tomogr.*, 19, 472, 1995.

127. Mosekilde, Li., "Sex differences in age-related loss of vertebral trabecular bone mass and structure — biomechanical consequences," *Bone*, 10, 425, 1989.

128. Mosekilde, Li., Bentzen, S.M., Ortoft, G., et al., "The predictive value of quantitative computed tomography for vertebral body compressive strength and ash density," *Bone*, 10, 465, 1989.

129. Andresen, R., Werner, H.J., Schober, H.C., et al., "CT determination of bone mineral density and structural investigations on the axial skeleton for estimating the osteoporosis-related fracture risk by means of a risk score," *Br. J. Radiol.*, 72, 569, 1999.

130. Haidekker, M.A., Andresen, R., Evertsz, C.J.G., et al., "Evaluation of the cortical structure in high resolution CT images of lumbar vertebrae by analysing low bone mineral density clusters and cortical profiles," *Br. J. Radiol.*, 70, 1222, 1997.

131. Cheng, S., Toivanen, J.A., Suominen, H., et al., "Estimation of structural and geometric properties of cortical bone by computerized tomography in 78-year-old women," *J. Bone Miner. Res.*, 10, 139, 1995.

132. Schneider, P., Reiners, C., Cointry, G.R., et al., "Noninvasive (pQCT) assessment of bone quality and relative fracture risk at the distal radius in healthy and wrist-fractured individuals," *Osteoporos. Int.*, 12, 639, 2001.

133. Andresen, R., Werner, H.J., and Schober, H.C., "Contribution of the cortical shell of vertebrae to mechanical behaviour of the lumbar vertebrae with implications for predicting fracture risk," *Br. J. Radiol.*, 71, 759, 1998.

134. Bentzen, S.M., Hvid, I., and Jorgensen, J., "Mechanical strength of tibial trabecular bone evaluated by X-ray computed tomography," *J. Biomech.*, 20, 743, 1987.

135. Hayes, W.C., Piazza, S.J., and Zysset, P.K., "Biomechanics of fracture risk prediction of the hip and spine by quantitative computed tomography," *Radiol. Clin. North Am.* 29, 1, 1991.

136. Ebbesen, E.N., Thomsen, J.S., Beck-Nielsen, H., et al., "Lumbar vertebral body compressive strength evaluated by dual-energy X-ray absorptiometry, quantitative computed tomography, and ashing," *Bone,* 25, 713, 1999.

137. Haidekker, M.A., Andresen, R., and Werner, H.J., "Relationship between structural parameters, bone mineral density and fracture load in lumbar vertebrae, based on high-resolution computed tomography, quantitative computed tomography and compression tests," *Osteoporos. Int.,* 9, 433, 1999.

138. Chevallier, F., Laval-Jeantet, A.M., Laval-Jeantet, M., et al., "CT image analysis of the vertebral trabecular network *in vivo*," *Calcif. Tissue Int.,* 51, 8, 1992.

139. Cortet, B., Dubois, P., Boutry, N., et al., "Image analysis of the distal radius trabecular network using computed tomography," *Osteoporos. Int.,* 9, 410, 1999.

140. Dougherty, G., "Quantitative CT in the measurement of bone quantity and bone quality for assessing osteoporosis," *Med. Eng. Phys.,* 18, 557, 1996.

141. Engelke, K. and Kalender, W., "Beyond bone densitometry: assessment of bone architecture by X-ray computed tomography at various levels of resolution," in *Bone Densitometry and Osteoporosis,* Genant, H.K., Guglielmi, G., and Jergas, M., Eds., Springer, Berlin, 1998, 417.

142. Gordon, C.L., Lang, T.F., Augat, P., et al., "Image-based assessment of spinal trabecular bone structure from high-resolution CT images," *Osteoporos. Int.,* 8, 317, 1998.

143. Guglielmi, G., Lang, T.F., Cammisa, M., et al., "Quantitative computed tomography at the axial skeleton," in *Bone Densitometry and Osteoporosis,* Genant, H.K., Guglielmi, G., and Jergas, M., Eds., Springer, Berlin, 1998, 335.

144. Gordon, C.L., Webber, C.E., Adachi, J.D., et al., "*In vivo* assessment of trabecular bone structure at the distal radius from high-resolution computed tomography images," *Phys. Med. Biol.,* 41, 495, 1996.

145. Laib, A., Hildebrand, T., Häuselmann, H.J., et al., "Ridge number density: a new parameter for *in vivo* bone structure analysis," *Bone,* 21, 541, 1997.

146. Yates, J., Ross, P.D., Lydick, E., et al., "Radiographic absorptiometry in the diagnosis of osteoporosis," *Am. J. Med.,* 98, 41S, 1995.

147. Ross, P.D., "Radiographic absorptiometry for measuring bone mass," *Osteoporos. Int.,* 7, S103, 1997.

148. Pothuaud, L., Lespessailles, E., Harba, R., et al., "Fractal analysis of trabecular bone texture on radiographs: discriminant value in postmenopausal osteoporosis," *Osteoporos. Int.,* 8, 618, 1998.

149. Gordon, C.L., Webber, C.E., Christoforou, N., et al., "*In vivo* assessment of trabecular bone structure at the distal radius from high-resolution magnetic resonance images," *Med. Phys.,* 24, 585, 1997.

150. Majumdar, S., Genant, H.K., Grampp, S., et al., "Correlation of trabecular bone structure with age, bone mineral density, and ostreoporotic status: *in vivo* studies in the distal radius using high resolution magnetic resonance imaging," *J. Bone Miner. Res.,* 12, 111, 1997.

151. Majumdar, S. and Genant, H.K., "Applications of magnetic resonance imaging in the study of osteoporosis," in *Bone Densitometry and Osteoporosis,* Genant, H.K., Guglielmi, G., and Jergas, M., Eds., Springer, Berlin, 1989, 407.

152. Köwitz, J., Knippel, M., Schuhr, T., et al., "Alteration in the extent of collagen I hydroxylation, isolated from femoral heads of women with a femoral neck fracture caused by osteoporosis," *Calcif. Tissue Int.,* 60, 501, 1997.

153. Mori, S., Harruff, R., Ambrosius, W., et al., "Trabecular bone volume and microdamage accumulation in the femoral heads of women with and without femoral neck fractures," *Bone,* 21, 521, 1997.

154. Boskey, A.L., Wright, T.M., and Blank, R.D., "Collagen and bone strength," *J. Bone Miner. Res.,* 14, 330, 1999.

155. McCabe, F., Zhou, L.J., Steele, C.R., et al., "Noninvasive assessment of ulnar bending stiffness in women," *J. Bone Miner. Res.,* 6, 53, 1991.

156. Myburg, K.H., Zhou, L.J., Steele, C.R., et al., "*In vivo* assessment of forearm bone mass and ulnar bending striffness in healthy men," *J. Bone Miner. Res.,* 7, 1345, 1992.

157. Wu, C., Hans, D., He, B., et al., "Prediction of bone strength of distal forearm using radius bone mineral density and phalangeal speed of sound," *Bone,* 26, 529, 2000.
158. Vesterby, A., Mosekilde, Li., Gundersen, H.J.G., et al., "Biologically meaningful determinants of the *in vitro* strength in lumbar vertebrae," *Bone,* 12, 219, 1991.
159. Eriksson, S.A.V., Isberg, B.O., and Lindgren, U., "Prediction of vertebral strength by dual photon absorptiometry and quantitative computed tomography," *Calcif. Tissue Int.,* 44, 243, 1989.
160. Lotz, J.C. and Hayes, W.C., "Estimates of hip fracture risk from falls using quantitative computed tomography," *J. Bone Joint Surg.,* 72A, 689, 1990.
161. Cody, D.D., Goldstein, S.A., Flynn, M.J., et al., "Correlations between vertebral regional bone mineral density and whole bone fracture load," *Spine,* 16, 146, 1991.
162. Brinckmann, P., Biggemann, M., and Hilweg, D., "Prediction of the compressive strength of human lumbar vertebrae," *Spine,* 14, 606, 1989.

Part II

Osteoporotic Fractures

9 Osteoporotic Fractures — Epidemiology, Fall Cascade, Risk Factors, and Prevention

Jes Bruun Lauritzen

CONTENTS

I. EPIDEMIOLOGY

Osteoporotic fractures occur in sites where trabecular bone predominates compared to cortical bone, and they share common epidemiologic features concerning low-energy trauma, higher incidence in

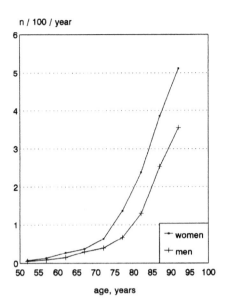

FIGURE 9.1 Age-specific incidence of hip fractures in women and men. (From Lauritzen, J.B., *Bone,* 18, 65S, 1996. With permission.)

women compared with men, and an exponential increase in age-specific incidence with aging.[1] The most common osteoporotic fractures are localized to the spine, distal radius, the hip, and the proximal humerus, but other types of fractures are also related to osteoporosis such as fractures of the pelvis, the femoral and tibial condyles including patella, and olecranon. Ankle fractures may to some extent show a different pattern in relation to osteoporosis.[2] The osteoporotic fractures of old age may also include fractures where cortical bone predominates, such as femoral, humeral, and tibial shaft fractures. The prevalence of osteoporosis can be defined as the percentage of the population with a bone mineral density of 2.5 standard deviations or more below the young normal mean. Using this definition, it has been estimated that one fourth of postmenopausal women are afflicted, corresponding to 26 million white women in the United States.[3]

In Figures 9.1 and 9.2, the age-specific incidence of fractures at the hip, radius, and humerus are given. The exponential pattern in age-specific incidence is obvious, except for the Colles' fracture, where 31% of these fractures in women in temperate geographic areas are sustained in icy and slippery weather. The Colles' fractures sustained in icy weather account for the plateau seen in age-specific incidence (Figure 9.2). In contrast, hip fractures do not have a statistical relationship to specific icy weather conditions, although there seems to be a seasonal variation in the rate of hip fractures. Only 12% of proximal humeral fractures are sustained in falls in icy weather.[4] A 60-year-old woman with an average life expectancy of 81 years has an estimated residual lifetime risk of radial, humeral, or hip fracture of 17, 8, and 14%, respectively.[5] A 60-year-old man with an average life expectancy of 77 years has an estimated risk of hip fracture of 6%. The residual lifetime risk of hip fracture for women surviving to the 25th percentile (88 years) is 33%, and for men (84 years) it is 15%.[5]

The age-specific incidence of hip fractures in older women has been variously reported ranging from an increasing tendency with time, to a constant level, or to a decreasing tendency with time.[6] Those who have accounted specifically for demographic changes do not show these marked changes.[5] The number of hip fractures occurring in the world in 1990 was estimated to be 1.7 million and is expected to reach 6.3 million by 2050, as a consequence of the increase in the elderly population.[7] There is a pronounced geographic variation in the incidence of hip fractures, with the highest rates in Caucasians in northern Europe followed by North America. The rates are intermediate in Asians and lowest in black populations.[8]

INCIDENCE OF RADIAL FRACTURE   INCIDENCE OF HUMERAL FRACTURE

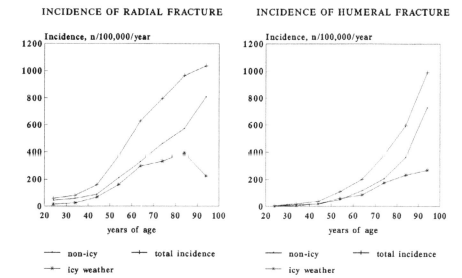

FIGURE 9.2 The age-specific incidences of distal radial or humeral fractures suffered in non-icy weather and icy weather among women, and the total age-specific incidence. (From Lauritzen, J.B. et al., *Osteoporos. Int.*, 3, 133, 1993. With permission.)

Hip fracture is the cause of the highest occupancy of hospital beds in Denmark.[6] In nursing homes the annual risk of hip fracture for women and men is 7 and 5%, respectively,[9] and elderly orthopaedic patients with falls or fracture share the same high risk of hip fracture. Among nursing home residents hip fractures constitute 50% of all fractures sustained, whereas clinically diagnosed vertebral fractures are infrequent, at least when one relates to hospital referral or contact.[10]

II. FALL CASCADE

Most fractures related to osteoporosis are due to falls: 92% of hip fractures, 96% of fractures in distal radius, 95% of proximal humeral fractures, 82% of foot and toe fractures, and 68% of fractures of the hand.[11] Of the clinically defined vertebral fractures in females only 10% are due to severe trauma, in contrast to one third in males.[12] In addition, perhaps only one third of these fractures in this population were clinically ascertained.[12]

The following conditions have been considered important for a fall to cause hip fracture: impact near the hip, protective reflexes, local soft tissue energy absorption, and bone strength.[13] These elements in the fall cascade are essential in the development of fractures (Figure 9.3). More than 90% of hip fractures are related to direct impact on the hip,[13-15] although only one fourth of impacts to the hip in elderly individuals lead to a hip fracture.[9] Rarely does a hip fracture occur without direct trauma.[16-18] Moreover, falls directly on the hip raise the odds ratio for a hip fracture about 20-fold.[19]

A. OCCURRENCE OF FALLS AND HIP FRACTURE

For people living in the community the annual rate of falls is 28 to 35% among those older than 65 years of age,[20-22] and 32 to 42% of subjects older than 75 years sustain at least one fall a year.[23,24] Among nursing home residents the occurrence of falls is 1.5 falls per resident per year, and more than 80% of nursing home residents experience at least one fall per year.[9]

Most falls do not cause major injuries,[25] but the risk of injuries after falls in elderly people is very high.[26] The annual incidence of falls on the hip among nursing home residents is 36 per 100

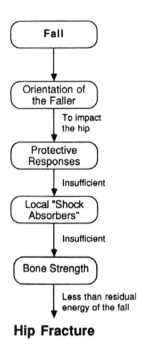

Hip Fracture

FIGURE 9.3 Fall cascade leading to fracture. (From Cummings, S.R. and Nevitt, M.C., *J. Gerontol.*, 44, M107, 1989. With permission.)

falls among women and 16 falls per 100 among men.[9] For cases of impact to the hip, the risk of fracture is about 0.25 in women and 0.33 in men in nursing homes.[9]

The incidence of hip fracture among nursing home residents is 6.8 and 5.3 per 100 per year among women and men, respectively.[9] The incidence among frequent fallers in nursing homes is about 14%. The risk of hip fracture among recurrent fallers in nursing homes treated for fall-related trauma in the emergency room is 41% within the next year. Orthopaedic in-patients older than 75 years of age have an annual risk of hip fracture of 4.1%, and those with dementia have a 6.5% risk. Those admitted due to fall have a risk of 5.6%, and those admitted with hip fracture have a risk of a subsequent new hip fracture of 4.7%. For those with a tendency to fall, the risk of a hip fracture is 6.6% per year and for those with visual impairment the risk is 6.2% per year.[27]

B. Force and Energy in Falls on the Hip

A fall from standing height is associated with a potential energy that may be sufficient to produce hip fracture even in young, healthy subjects.[28,29] For 82 patients who sustained a hip fracture, the potential energy has been estimated to be 442 joules (J).[19] However, this estimate, based on data from unprotected falls performed by a stuntwoman on a force platform, may be too high. In this case the energy was only 113 J, corresponding to an effective load acting on the hip of 35% of the body weight,[30] and a force of 3.5 kN (kilonewtons). These results suggest that susceptible subjects are far more likely to suffer a hip fracture in case of impact to the hip.

C. Protective Responses

Elderly people experience more traumas compared with young subjects. Reduced reaction time and degraded coordination are related to risk of fractures.[31] Many patients with hip fractures are admitted from nursing homes, and this group is characterized by disturbances in their neuromuscular functions.[32]

D. Energy Absorption

Energy absorption in soft tissue may be a more important factor than bone strength in relation to hip fractures.[28,33] Experimental studies have shown that energy absorption in soft tissue may account for up to 75% of the energy available in a fall.[34] This may partially explain why being overweight protects against hip fractures.

Women with hip fractures weigh on average 5 kg less compared with controls.[35,36] In addition, women with hip fractures seem to possess less soft tissue covering their hips compared with controls, even after adjustment for body mass index.[36] It has been suggested that body mass index is a surrogate for measuring the thickness of trochanteric soft tissue thickness.[37] For patients with Colles' fracture no significant difference in body weight is apparent, as overweight does not increase soft tissue mass around the wrist.

In one study, about 42% of recorded falls sustained within the home occurred in the bathroom.[38] However, impact attenuation of floor coverings has only a minor effect on the peak force from falls even when one compares terrazzo with a carpet floor covering.[39]

E. Bone Strength

To predict the risk of fracture of any structure, it is necessary to have information on both the imposed loads and the ultimate load-carrying capacity of the structure. Even though most falls in elderly people are low-energy falls, they differ from falls among young subjects. The fracture threshold for vertebral spine ranges from 2000 to 8000 N,[40] and for the distal radius the fracture threshold ranges from 200 to 280 N.[41]

The fracture threshold in the hip has been studied in cadavers and the results may differ according to setup and loading velocity. The loading angle to the neck seems important.[42] Depending on density the breaking strength in elderly cadaveric bone ranges from 1000 to 6000 N, with coefficients of determinations (r^2) between bone strength and density ranging from 0.7 to 0.9.[28,43] Bone strength can thus be estimated from bone mineral density.[43] However, bone density on its own is not a good clinical predictor of a later hip fracture as indicated by the major overlap in bone density among elderly fallers between hip fracture patients and controls.[44,45] In fact, the impact direction and impact site may be stronger predictors of hip fracture risk than femoral bone density,[46] whereas the potential energy available and the body mass index provide about the same level of predictability as density.

III. RISK FACTORS FOR FALLS AND FRACTURE

Risk factors for falls or fracture are listed in Table 9.1.[47] Myers et al.[48] categorized risk factors for falls into the following nine groups: general physical functioning, gait balance and physical performance, musculoskeletal and neuromuscular measures, demographic factors, sensory impairments, medical conditions, indicators of general health, medication use, and psychologic behavioral social and environmental factors.

Established intrinsic risk factors for falls include age, sex, race, previous fall or fracture, low body mass, medical comorbidities, musculoskeletal diseases, cognitive impairment, gait and balance disorders, sensory impairment, postural hypotension, use of certain medications including long- and median-acting benzodiazepines, sedative-hypnotic drugs, antidepressants, antihypertensive medications, antiarrhythmic drugs, diuretics, and antiseizure medications.[49]

Extrinsic risk factors include environmental hazards such as throw rugs, slippery and uneven surfaces, poor lightning, electrical cords, foot stools without handrails, slippery tub surfaces, and unsuitable footwear.[49]

Clinical series of patients with fractures, bone mineral density studies, case-control studies, and prospective studies have suggested a number of risk factors for osteoporotic fractures. Risk

TABLE 9.1
Risk Factors for Falls and Osteoporotic Fractures

Falls

Readily detectable impairment of balance, gait, or mobility
Polypharmacy — in particular, drugs acting on the central nervous system and drugs to lower blood pressure
Visual impairment
Impaired cognition or depression
Stroke or history of stroke; Parkinson's disease; or degenerative lower limb joint disease
Postural hypotension

Osteoporotic Fractures

Radiographic evidence of osteopenia
Loss of height associated with osteopenic vertebral deformity
Previous fragility fracture
Prolonged corticosteroid treatment
Chronic disorders associated with osteoporosis
History of premature menopause
History of maternal hip fracture
Low body mass index

Source: Cameron, S., *Br. Med. J.,* 322, 855, 2001. With permission.

---

factors for fracture are similar to those of falling, but additionally include low bone mineral density and fall characteristics such as frequency, direction of fall, and force of impact.[49] Other underlying causes are estrogen deficiency in women, vitamin D deficiency, inadequate calcium intake, high protein intake, corticosteroids, smoking, alcohol abuse, and sedentary lifestyle. The individual risk factor may be related to one or more steps in the fall cascade.

No general test for fall risk estimation is available, but postural sway test, Romberg test, measuring orthostatic hypotension, or muscle strength tests may give some valuable information. Tinetti et al.[50] proposed an index for chronic fallers. Dargent-Molina et al.[51] performed a prospective fall-risk measurement study including gait speed, tandem walk score, calf circumference, and visual acuity in addition to femoral bone mineral density (BMD) and calcaneal broadband ultrasound (BUA), and they found a relation to subsequent risk of hip fracture. Femoral BMD and calcaneal BUA and fall-risk score had approximately the same predictive ability.[51] A simple test has been suggested ("stop walking when talking"), which was a significant marker of later falls.[52]

The psychologic factor of fear of falling among elderly people is very prevalent and has been found to be an independent risk factor for activity restriction and secondary muscle atrophy and ultimately reduced health and quality of life.[53]

When one focuses on possible traditional modifiable risk factors related to hip fractures, about 10 to 16% of hip fractures are attributed to tobacco smoking, 11% are attributed to physical inactivity, 3% are related to excess alcohol consumption,[54] and about 25% are attributed to estrogen insufficiency in women.[55]

IV. PREVENTION OF OSTEOPOROTIC FRACTURES

A. PHYSICAL EXERCISE

Physical exercise is an important issue, as muscle mass and bone mass have a positive relationship. Unfortunately, no clear evidence is available concerning prevention of fractures. A randomized study with brisk walking found an increased risk of falling, but no increase in fractures.[56] Exercise has been shown in larger studies to improve balance and decrease risk of falling,[57] and the same has been seen after intervention with t'ai chi balance training.[58] Results suggest that a one-time physician-based exercise counseling session with minimal reinforcement, in a setting with high baseline levels of activity, does not further increase activity.[59] A randomized controlled physiotherapist-prescribed home-based program of strength and balance retraining exercises in women 80 years and older has been effective in reducing falls and injuries.[60,61] A randomized study with physical therapy rehabilitation for very frail nursing home residents provided modest mobility effects for these residents.[62] In another randomized study, improvements after home exercise in patients with hip fracture showed statistically significant changes in quadriceps strength and walking velocity.[63]

Running and swimming may not interfere significantly with bone density, as the loading is within the normal physiologic range far below submaximal stresses that increase muscle mass and subsequent bone mass. Isometric high load exercises or stimulation on special vibration platforms[64] can induce rather significant increases in bone mass. Swimming and running may have other positive health benefits. Physical activity, especially started early in life, is a safe and widely accepted way to affect bone strength and falling propensity,[65] but regular physical activity is also recommended for elderly people.

Concerning exercise for patients with vertebral fractures, specific physical back extension exercise programs without flexion seem to reduce the occurrence of subsequent vertebral fractures.[66] Several orthotic devices and braces, which increase lumbar lordosis and reduce thoracic kyphosis, may prove to be of benefit.

Immobilization leads to significant bone losses, and prevention of further decay may be needed during rehabilitation of patients with fractures or other medical diseases.

B. Nutrition

Nutrition is one of the environmental factors that is important for the development of healthy bone growth and maintenance of bone mass.[67] A concert of compounds are required to maintain a normal bone and calcium metabolism: calcium, phosphorus, protein, magnesium, zinc, copper, iron, fluoride, sodium, vitamins D, A, C, and K.[67] Other ingested compounds that influence bone metabolism are caffeine, which may reduce calcium intake further in subjects with low calcium intake, or plant-derived phytoestrogens (iproflavone), which may mimic estrogens, either as an estrogen agonist or antagonist.[68]

The system known as Dietary Reference Intakes (DRIs) for healthy populations delineates different levels of intakes including estimated average requirements (EAR), the recommended dietary allowance (RDA), the adequate intake (IA), and the tolerable upper limit level (UL).[69]

The best-documented evidence exists for calcium and vitamin D (see below), while the effects of other compounds have been difficult to quantitate. There is a positive association between body weight and BMD or hip fracture risk,[70] but low body mass may also be more likely to be linked to malnutrition in addition to undernutrition. In elderly women it has been shown that nutritional status correlates closely both with food intake and with disability[71] and hip fracture.[72] This may also explain why overweight seems to protect against osteoporosis and hip fractures. Other explanations are that a protective effect may be related to estrone production from androstendione in fat cells in postmenopausal women[73,74] or overweight induces greater stress on the skeleton, which stimulates bone strength.[75] Last, the soft tissue over the hip may passively protect against hip fractures.[30,33]

C. Drugs, Alcohol, Tobacco, Medication

The neuromuscular system may be influenced by the immediate effects of drugs and alcohol, and this may consequently increase the risk of falling. Current cigarette smoking is a risk factor, but no specific target intervention program has been instituted concerning osteoporosis, even though it is relevant for other reasons. The same matters for medications known to influence bone metabolism.

In a randomized study including withdrawal of psychotropic medication the rate of falls was reduced significantly, whereas the treatment arm with home-based exercise had a nonsignificant reduction in falls.[76]

It seems justified to modulate these risk factors whenever possible.

D. ADJUSTMENTS IN ENVIRONMENT

A trial of home hazard reduction with inspection, advice about repair, and group meetings with information about behavioral and physical aspects of fall risk demonstrated only a minimal, nonsignificant decrease in falls in the intervention group.[77] A prospective home dweller study including home safety inspection and simple home modifications found a 50% reduction in the number of falls during 1 year compared with the preceding period.[78]

One intervention study with home visits performed by occupational therapists and adjustments in the home environment has shown a statistically significant reduction in falls among frequent fallers.[79] Adjustments in the environment have also been performed as a part of multifaceted programs (see below).[80]

E. ESTROGEN

Numerous retrospective studies support the efficacy of estrogen in the prevention of postmenopausal osteoporosis and fractures.[55,81] Prospective studies measuring BMD confirm the bone loss-retarding effect of estrogen,[82-84] and on average estrogen increases BMD by 3% with 1 year of treatment.[85] Most studies have been performed in women with low risk of fracture. One randomized study among 47- to 75-year-old women did not show a statistically significant difference concerning new vertebral fractures mainly due to low power of the study.[86] In a much larger randomized study primarily focusing on coronary heart disease, estrogen did not show the expected statistically significant fracture reduction.[87] Estrogen, however, may protect against hip fractures on several levels: by improving bone strength, improving neuromuscular function, modifying fat deposition or improving the viscoelastic properties of soft tissue, and even a role in fall reduction has been proposed.

Related to estrogens are the selective estrogen receptor modulators (SERMs), of which raloxifene has been approved for clinical practice, based on a large clinical trial on reduction in vertebral fractures.[88] Tamoxifen, used in breast cancer therapy, has also been shown to increase BMD in the spine, but a randomized study in 1716 postmenopausal patients with breast cancer treated with adjuvant tamoxifen had significantly more trochanteric hip fractures (hazard ratio 2.1).[89]

Overall, estrogens possess a certain protective effect on all types of fractures, and their effects are linked to current use, which may be more difficult to obtain among very old women with a high fracture risk.[90]

F. VITAMIN D PLUS CALCIUM

Randomized nursing home studies with vitamin D_3[91] or vitamin D_3 + calcium[92] have shown a 20 to 30% reduction in hip fracture rate, probably partly due to a high prevalence of osteomalacia. A subgroup had bone density measurements and there was no marked change in density,[92] perhaps indicating that the rate of falls was reduced as well as the rate of hip fractures.

In a double-blind trial in 2578 persons 70 years of age and older who received 400 IU vitamin D_3 or placebo, 48 hip fractures occurred in the placebo group and 58 in the vitamin D_3 group ($p = 0.39$).[93] The participants in this study were in a healthier state compared to the nursing home residents mentioned above, and they were probably less calcium and vitamin D_3 depleted. In this study sunlight exposure was lower in the fracture population. A later randomized study with 500 mg calcium citrate malate and 700 IU vitamin D among home dwellers (176 men and 213 women) showed a rate of appendicular fractures of 12.8% in the placebo group compared with 5.9% in the treated group.[94] Bone densities did not differ between the two groups. The relative risk was 0.5 during this 3-year study.

The effect of calcium or vitamin D alone has produced conflicting results. Thus in a population of women over the age of 70 years in northern latitudes, primary and probably secondary prevention with calcium and vitamin D appears to be indicated as a cost-effective safe approach.[95]

G. Bisphosphonates

Common to all bisphosphonates is their potent capacity to inhibit bone resorption, and they are used to treat various diseases with high bone turnover as well as osteoporosis. There has been concern about a negative influence on bone healing and implants, but in dosages used for osteoporosis this does not seem to be the case.[96]

Among elderly women with low bone density the bisphosphonate alendronate has been shown in a randomized study to reduce the risk of nonvertebral fractures by 28%.[97] The rate of hip fractures was reduced by 50% in a 3-year intervention study among 1022 women with low BMD, and the number of hip fractures was 11 in the intervention group during the observation period (22 hip fractures in 1005 controls).[98] The antiresorptive effect of bisphosphonates can reduce the occurrence of spine fractures, but intermittent cyclical etidronate in postmenopausal women did not indicate any protection against hip fractures.[99] A later large observational case cohort study with etidronate indicates a significant risk reduction in an older population.[100] Risedronate has been shown in a randomized study among 2458 postmenopausal women to reduce both vertebral and nonvertebral fractures.[101]

H. Calcitonin

The skeletal effect of salmon calcitonin nasal spray therapy has been studied in a large 5-year double-masked randomized placebo-controlled study of 1255 postmenopausal women with established osteoporosis. The patients were randomized to either 100, 200, or 400 IU/day nasal salmon calcitonin. In the 200 IU group a statistically significant reduction in relative risk of new vertebral fractures (39%) was demonstrated.[102] Postfracture studies in patients with Colles'[103] or ankle[104] fractures have shown that calcitonin can reduce the postfracture bone loss to some extent.

I. Fluoride

Fluoride is one of the few orally active and bone-specific agents that can produce a substantial increase in spinal bone density in humans,[105] but unfortunately fluoride therapy seems to have an unfavorable benefit-to-risk profile, besides its established side effects. One side effect is the deleterious effect in cases with a nonobserved preexisting osteomalacia. Stress fractures are seen in patients with severe osteoporosis in fluoride therapy. One of the most serious fractures may be of the hip, where an increased risk has been observed,[106] although a revised analysis on dosage of fluoride, fracture, and density favored fluoride in the prevention of fracture.[107] Some strategies to reduce the benefit-to-risk profile have been suggested, i.e., cyclic, low dosage, slow-release, combination therapy, and avoiding calcium deficiency.[105]

J. Other Proposed Pharmacologic Approaches

Other possible candidates for prevention of fractures in the future may be androgens, anabolic steroids, fragments of parathyroid hormone (PTH), growth hormone (GH), insulin-like growth factor (IGF), and ipriflavone, but no evidence for fracture prevention is available yet.

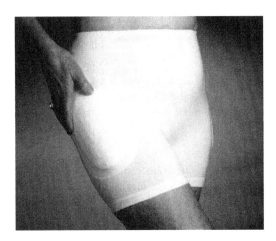

FIGURE 9.4. Hip protector (SAFEHIP).

K. HIP PROTECTORS

Various hip padding systems have emerged together with documentation.[108] There is an energy shunting type (horseshoe)[109] including the crash helmet type (Figure 9.4),[110,111] an energy absorptive type,[112-114] and an air bag type.[115] Laboratory experiments have suggested that some of the energy absorptive protectors may be insufficient to prevent hip fractures.[116-118]

V. EC REPORT ON OSTEOPOROSIS AND COCHRANE REVIEW

Based on several recent clinical and biomechanical studies hip protection has been recommended by the European Commission in the "Report on Osteoporosis in the European Community — Action for Prevention 1998":

> Any bone will break if the force is strong enough, but reducing the impact of the force may prevent fracture. Hip protectors have been developed to reduce the impact of trauma and protect the bone when a fall occurs from a standing position. Studies have demonstrated the protective value of protectors worn by vulnerable older women and men who have already sustained a fracture, particularly those in nursing homes.

In the Cochrane review on hip protectors from 1999,[119] the reviewers' conclusions were close to the European Commission report. The Cochrane review was based on four randomized trials, although they were categorized as *low to moderate quality*. Double blinding was not possible, and the reviewers did not comment on adjustment for rate of nonhip fractures, which may be relevant. Hip protectors are effective against hip fractures, and if the rate of nonhip fractures were to decrease in the intervention group, other preventive effects from the intention to treat might be operating, and this has not been observed. The Cochrane review states: "The generalizability of the results is beyond high-risk populations and ongoing trials may clarify this situation. Acceptability by users of the protectors remains a problem, due to discomfort and practicality." These statements correspond with the early clinical results with hip protectors. In a new meta-analysis the hip protector has been shown to prevent fractures of the pelvic rami (unpublished data).

Confirmed by the latest published randomized trial on hip protectors,[120] the related editorial written by L. Rubenstein[121] states that hip protectors are a breakthrough in fracture prevention.

TABLE 9.2
Randomized Clinical Studies in Nursing Homes with Hip Protectors[a]

Study	Follow-Up Months	Intervention No. Hip Fractures/ No. of Subjects	Control No. Hip Fractures/ No. of Subjects	Relative Risk	No. of Hip Fractures Avoided
Lauritzen et al.[9]	11	8/247	31/418	**0.44** 0.20–0.95 95% CL	10
Ekman et al.[124]	11	4/302	17/442	**0.34** 0.12–1.0 95% CL	8
Heikinheimo et al.[113]	12	1/36	5/36	**0.20**	4
Harada and Okuizumi[125]	19	0/30	4/24	**0.0**	5
Kannus et al.[120]	18	13/653	67/1148	**0.40** 0.2–0.8 95% CL	15

[a] Observed number of hip fractures occurring among nursing home residents in intervention and control group, and relative risk/hazard and estimated number of hip fractures avoided.

TABLE 9.3
Nonrandomized Observational Studies with Hip Protectors[a]

	Number of Hip Fractures	Number of Falls
Wortberg[112]		
10 months ($n = 28$)		
Falls with hip protector	0	16
Falls without hip protector	4	7
Parkkari[122]		
6 months ($n = 12$)		
Falls on hip protector	0	6
Users ($n = 12$)	0	
Nonusers ($n = 14$)	2	
Sandvig and Forsén[123]		
18 months ($n = 1070$)		
Falls recorded		2206 (46% protected)
Observed hip fractures	61	
Expected hip fractures	98	
Avoided hip fractures	37	

[a] Observed number of hip fractures associated with falls on hip protector during prospective observational studies among nursing home residents.

A. CLINICAL STUDIES

1. Nursing Homes

The effect of external hip protectors has been tested in five randomized controlled trials in nursing homes (Table 9.2), and three nonrandomized observational studies (Table 9.3).[112,122,123] The randomized

TABLE 9.4
**Effect of Hip Protectors among Elderly Home Dwellers Included
When Admitted to an Orthopaedic Department**

Risk Factors	Relative Risk	95% CL	No. of Hip Fractures Avoided
All	0.88	0.5–1.5	3
Men	0.33	0.04–2.7	4
Demented	0.42	0.21–2.4	8
Admitted with fall	0.71	0.37–1.4	6
Admitted with hip fracture	0.67	0.19–2.4	2
Fall tendency	0.48	0.09–2.5	4
Dizziness	0.89	0.4–2.0	1
Help coming out door	0.82	0.28–2.3	1
Visual impairment, distance	0.25	0.08–0.85	9*
Reduced vision	0.25	0.06–1.11	6

* $p < 0.05$.
Note: The number of hip fractures avoided in each risk group overlaps.
Source: Hindsø, K. and Lauritzen, J.B., *Osteoporos. Int.*, 8, 119, 1998. With permission.

studies showed a reduction in the rate of hip fractures between 0.0 and 0.44.[9,113,124,125] The Danish and Swedish randomized trials resulted in a reduction in relative risk during an 11-month period in nursing homes to 0.44[9] and 0.34.[124] These studies were based on an intention-to-treat analysis, and when treatment received is considered, i.e., the effect of a protector when in the use, then the protective effect is high. The recent Finnish study[120] presented results only for users of hip protectors, i.e., treatment received, and found a relative hazard of 0.4, while attempted estimation of intention to treat showed a relative hazard of about 0.67. The prospective observational study among 1070 Norwegian nursing home residents showed a reduction in hip fracture rate by 38% during 18 months, corresponding to 37 hip fractures avoided.[123] Pooling of data may not be appropriate due to cluster randomization and differences in data presentation concerning intention to treat vs. treatment received.

2. Home Dwellers

Trials with hip protectors among elderly subjects living at home are few, although some compliance studies have been performed. In our study,[126] the number of hip fractures avoided during an open intervention study among elderly (>74 years) orthopaedic patients was recorded in the intervention hospital ($n = 1006$) and compared with a control hospital ($n = 678$). The follow-up was 1 to 1.5 years. All elderly orthopaedic patients who received and accepted the hip protectors and did not return them were defined as users.

During follow-up, users reported 143 falls with impact on the hip protector, and no hip fractures occurred. Only two hip fractures occurred while the patients used their hip protectors, and in these cases no impact on the hip was reported.[126] Assuming each subject who had received a hip protector was a "user," the overall protective effect of the hip protectors was 12% and did not reach statistical significance.

The estimated number of hip fractures avoided in the elderly women and men with risk factors are given in Table 9.4. Only in patients with visual impairment did the prevention of hip fractures reach statistical significance. The confidence limits were rather wide due to the limited statistical power of the study. Based on actual and regular use of hip protectors (treatment received) the relative risk of hip fracture was overall 0.52 (intervention/controls, I/C: 187/678), and for those admitted due to falls or fractures (I/C: 711/459) or hip fractures (I/C: 60/244) the relative risk was,

TABLE 9.5
Compliance of Hip Protectors

Ref.	Late Compliance (%)	Comments
Lauritzen et al.[9]	24	Rate of users in registered falls over 11 months
Ekman et al.[124]	44	Registered user rate over 11 months
Sandvig and Forsén[123]	22	User rate at 18–22 months
Hindsø[127]	40	User rate after 2 years in those with primary acceptance

respectively, 0.52 (0.2 to 1.34, 95% confidence limits, CL), 0.43 (0.15 to 1.23, 95% CL) and 0.0 (0.0 to 1.0, 95% CL).[127]

B. COMPLIANCE

Based on a subgroup analysis in our early randomized nursing home study, hip protector wear compliance was 24%.[9] In this trial, the pads had to be retrieved and replaced in new sets of underwear for each change of underwear, and we believe this compromised compliance. The latest design of hip protectors is built into the undergarment (see Figure 9.4), which can be washed and dried easily. The hip protectors can be worn at night. In the more recent community-based trials the initial rate of acceptance was 57% (572/1006). At 3 months the compliance was 75%,[128] and at 2 years the compliance was 40%. The compliance rate has been reported between 24 and 91%,[9,112,113,122,124,125,128-130] reflecting a variety of compliance definitions ranging from primary acceptance to adherence in recorded falls. Compliance rate must therefore be described properly when compliance rates are compared. In Table 9.5 the user rate is given for four large clinical studies.

Although the majority of elderly users seem satisfied with the hip protectors, one third of those who stop complain of discomfort or practical problems.[128] Fear of falling increases compliance, and this fear is reduced with use of hip protectors. One third feel more confident when walking, with an additional 15% of elderly people using protectors spending more time outdoors.[131] Even though compliance may not reach 100%, the overall adherence of hip protectors has been high compared with other medical preventive modalities, and a 40% long-term compliance has been documented after 2 years.[127] Primary acceptance and adherence are important issues for the hip protection systems to work efficiently, and information and instructions including late follow-up may be needed.

C. COST-EFFECTIVENESS/COST-SAVINGS

Hip protectors are cost-saving among frail elderly subjects in the community or in nursing homes.[132] The cost-saving ratio may be about 1:3 for nursing home residents. For elderly home dwellers with risk factors for hip fracture, the cost-saving ratio may be 1:7. The ratio describes the relationship between costs spent for the intervention and money saved due to hip fractures avoided. Supporting all Danish women older than 70 years of age and men over 80 years with hip protectors has been estimated to be cost-saving.[132] At least for elderly people the hip protectors are cost-effective.[133] For clinical reasons, however, the preventive efforts should focus on frail elderly subjects with risk of falling and reduced bone strength. Several health systems offer hip protectors to nursing home residents and frail elderly subjects with a propensity to fall.

The effect of hip protectors in randomized clinical trials has shown a high efficacy among nursing home residents. The same effect and trend has been shown among frail elderly home dwellers, who have been introduced to hip protectors when admitted to an orthopaedic department.

TABLE 9.6
Recommended Preventive Actions against Osteoporotic Fractures

1. Maintaining physical activity; early active rehabilitation programs following injuries inducing accelerated bone loss
2. Securing a qualitatively and quantitatively sufficient diet
3. Adjustments and avoiding fall hazards in the home environment
4. Adjustment of medication interfering with neuromuscular status
5. Consider estrogen/estrogen-like therapy in postmenopausal women
6. Consider bisphophonates in subjects with vertebral fractures and low bone mass; some evidence for fluoride and calcitonin; not proven for PTH-fragments, IGF, GH, or iproflavone
7. Supplementation of vitamin D_3 and calcium among nursing home residents and elderly subjects
8. Use of hip protectors in elderly fall-prone subjects

Hip fracture has occurred even when wearing hip protectors, and the protectors have been said to induce hip fracture[134] if the undergarment with hip protectors is placed at knee level and subsequently initiates the fall. Even though a hip fracture may occur despite the use of hip protectors, i.e., an indirect trauma or spontaneous fracture, it is a rare occurrence.

The benefit of hip protectors in relation to prevention of periprosthetic hip fractures, luxation of hip arthroplasties, pressure sores, and chronic bursitis is yet to be outlined and studied further.

Pooling data from the Finnish and Danish studies shows the occurrence of fractures of the pelvic rami is also significantly reduced. The ratio between elderly patients admitted to the hospital with either hip fracture or fractures of the pelvic rami is 12:1 in our clinic.

Current evidence suggests protectors to be of benefit among nursing home residents and frail elderly home dwellers. Thus, it seems realistic to expect a reduction in the overall occurrence of hip fractures by 25 to 50% when a systematic intervention among frail elderly individuals in nursing homes, hospitals, and community is initiated.

D. MULTIFACTORIAL INTERVENTIONAL PROGRAMS

Multifactorial intervention trials have included home adjustments, medication adjustments, and exercise programs and have documented a decrease in falling after 1 year.[135] In the Prevention of Falls in the Elderly Trial among elderly patients presenting to emergency departments with fall-related injuries, the patients were randomized to an assessment and intervention of modifiable individual risk factors. The program included minimizing environmental hazards, reducing medication and multiple medication use, education in behavioral strategies to allow completion of tasks with minimal risk, learning techniques for rising from falls, and exercise programs.[80] The intervention decreased falls by 70%, and a similar trend was seen for fractures.[80]

In these multifaceted programs the specific effect from the various interventions may not be ruled out, but we expect to see more of these studies with inclusion of pharmacologic and non-pharmacologic approaches, where fractures are the end point.

VI. PREVENTIVE ACTIONS AGAINST OSTEOPOROTIC FRACTURES

The risk of falls and fractures is multifactorial, and prevention must also be multifactorial. Preventive actions against osteoporotic fractures should focus on several risk factors and not rely on a single factor. When the mechanisms of the development of these fractures are taken into consideration, intervention programs may then function effectively. Primary prevention targets basic lifestyle factors in the healthy and young population, whereas secondary prevention concerns subjects with risk factors for falls and osteoporosis, and tertiary prevention includes treatment and prevention of further disease, i.e., prevention of bone loss and falls and subsequent fractures.

Several newer studies indicate that the prevention of osteoporotic fractures is realistic, even in the elderly, definitely osteoporotic population, when the fundamental risk factors are modified. Proposed guidelines for prevention are outlined in Table 9.6.

REFERENCES

1. Melton, L.J., "Epidemiology of fractures," in *Osteoporosis: Etiology, Diagnosis and Management,* Riggs, B.L. and Melton, L.J., Eds., Raven Press, New York, 1995, 255.
2. Lauritzen, J.B. and Lund, B., "Risk of hip fractures after osteoporosis related fractures. 451 women with fracture of lumbar spine, olecranon, knee and ankle," *Acta Orthop. Scand.,* 64, 297, 1993.
3. Melton, L.J., "How many women have osteoporosis now?" *J. Bone Miner. Res.,* 10, 175, 1995.
4. Lauritzen, J.B., Schwarz, P., McNair, P., et al., "Radial and humeral fractures as predictors of subsequent hip, radial or humeral fractures in women, and their seasonal variation," *Osteoporos. Int.,* 3, 133, 1993.
5. Lauritzen, J.B., Schwarz, P., McNair, P., and Transbøl, I., "Changing incidence and residual lifetime risk of common osteoporosis-related fractures," *Osteoporos. Int.,* 3, 127, 1993.
6. Lauritzen, J.B., "Hip fractures. Epidemiology, risk factors, falls, energy absorption, hip protectors," *Dan. Med. Bull.,* 44, 155, 1997.
7. Cooper, C., Campion, G., and Melton, L.J., "Hip fractures in the elderly: a worldwide projection," *Osteoporos. Int.,* 2, 285, 1992.
8. Lau, E.M.C. and Leung, P.C., "The size of the problem," in *Management of Fractures in Severely Osteoporotic Bone,* Obrant, K., Ed., Springer, London, 2000, 3.
9. Lauritzen, J.B., Petersen, M.M., and Lund, B., "Effect of external hip protectors on hip fractures," *Lancet,* 341, 11, 1993.
10. Lauritzen, J.B., Petersen, M.M., and Lund, B., "Virkningen af eksterne hoftebeskyttere mod hoftebrud," *Ugeskr. Læger,* 155, 1523, 1993.
11. Cummings, S.R. and Nevitt, M.C., "Non-skeletal determinants of fractures: the potential importance of the mechanics of falls. Study of the osteoporotic fractures," *Osteoporos. Int.,* 4, 67, 1994.
12. Cooper, C., Atkinson, E.J., O'Fallon, W.M., and Melton, L.J., "Incidence of clinically diagnosed vertebral fractures: a population based study in Rochester Minnesota, 1985–1989," *J. Bone Miner. Res.,* 7, 221, 1992.
13. Cummings, S.R. and Nevitt, M.C., "A hypothesis: the causes of hip fractures," *J. Gerontol.,* 44, M107, 1989.
14. Lauritzen, J.B. and Askegaard, V., "Protection against hip fractures by energy absorption," *Dan. Med. Bull.,* 39, 91, 1998.
15. Hayes, W.C., Myers, E.R., Maitland, L.A., et al., "Relative risk of fall severity, body habitus and bone density in hip fracture among the elderly," *Trans. Orthop. Res. Soc.,* 16, 70, 1991.
16. Freeman, M.A.R., Todd, R.C., and Pirie, C.J., "The role of fatigue in the pathogenesis of senile femoral neck fractures," *J. Bone Joint Surg.,* 56B, 698, 1974.
17. Sloan, J. and Holloway, G., "Fractures neck of the femur: causes of the fall?" *Injury,* 12, 210, 1981.
18. Smith, L.D., "Hip fractures: the role of muscular contraction or intrinsic forces in the causation of fractures of the femoral neck," *J. Bone Joint Surg.,* 35B, 367, 1953.
19. Hayes, W.C., Myers, E.R., Morris, J.N., et al., "Impact near the hip dominates fracture risk in elderly nursing home residents who fall," *Calcif. Tissue Int.,* 52, 192, 1993.
20. Campbell, A.J., Reinken, J., Allan, B.C., and Martinez, G.S., "Falls in old age: a study of frequency and related clinical factors," *Age Ageing,* 10, 264, 1981.
21. Prudham, D. and Evans, J.G., "Factors associated with falls in the elderly: a community study," *Age Ageing,* 10, 141, 1981.
22. Blake, A.J., Morgan, K., Bendall, M.J., et al., "Falls by the elderly people at home: prevalence and associated factors," *Age Ageing,* 17, 365, 1988.
23. Tinetti, M.E., Speechley, M., and Ginter, S.F., "Risk factors for falls among elderly persons living in the community," *N. Engl. J. Med.,* 319, 1701, 1988.
24. Downton, J.H. and Andrews, K., "Prevalence, characteristics and factors associated with falls among the elderly living at home," *Age Clin. Exp. Res.,* 3, 219, 1991.

25. Berry, G., Fischer, R.H., and Lang, S., "Detrimental incidents, including falls, in an elderly institutional population," *J. Am. Geriatr. Soc.*, 29, 322, 1981.

26. Kiel, D.P., "Falls," *R. I. Med.*, 74, 75, 1991.

27. Hindsø, K. and Lauritzen, J.B., "Risk of subsequent hip fracture in elderly orthopaedic patients (abstr.)," *Osteoporos. Int.*, 8, 18, 1998.

28. Lotz, J.C. and Hayes, W.C., "The use of qunatitative computed tomography to estimate risk of fracture from falls," *J. Bone Joint Surg.*, 72A, 689, 1990.

29. Robinovitch, S.N., Hayes, W.C., and McMahon, T.A., "Prediction of femoral impact forces in falls on the hip," *ASME J. Biomech. Eng.*, 113, 336, 1991.

30. Askegaard, V. and Lauritzen, J.B., "Load on the hip in a stiff sideways fall," *Eur. J. Exp. Musculoskel. Res.*, 4, 111, 1995.

31. Adelsberg, A., Pitman, M., and Alexander, H., "Lower extremity fractures: relationship to reaction time and coordination time," *Arch. Phys. Med. Rehabil.*, 79, 737, 1989.

32. Stott, S. and Gary, D.H., "A prospective study of hip fracture patients," *N.Z. Med. J.*, 91, 165, 1980.

33. Lauritzen, J.B., McNair, P., and Lund, B., "Risk factors for hip fractures. A review," *Dan. Med. Bull.*, 40, 479, 1993.

34. Lauritzen, J.B. and Højgaard, L., "Estimate of hip fracture threshold adjusted for energy absorption in soft tissue," *J. Nucl. Med.*, 21, S48, 1994.

35. Elsasser, U., Hesp, R., Klenerman, L., and Wooton, R., "Deficit of trabecular and cortical bone in women with fracture of the femoral neck," *Clin. Sci.*, 59, 393, 1980.

36. Lauritzen, J.B., Petersen, M.M., Jensen, P.K., et al., "Body fat distribution and hip fractures (abstr.)," *Acta Orthop. Scand. Suppl.*, 63, 89, 1992.

37. Maitland, L.A., Myers, E.R., Hipp, J.A., et al., "Read my hips: measuring trochanteric soft tissue thickness," *Calcif. Tissue Int.*, 52, 85, 1993.

38. DeVito, C.A., Lambert, D.A., Sattin, R.W., et al., "Fall injuries among the elderly: community based surveillance," *J. Am. Geriatr. Soc.*, 36, 1029, 1988.

39. Maki, B.E. and Fernie, G.R., "Impact attenuation of floor coverings in simulated falling accidents," *Appl. Ergonom.*, 21, 107–114, 1990.

40. Mosekilde, Li., "Normal age-related changes in bone mass, structure and strength — consequences of the remodeling process," *Dan. Med. Bull.*, 1, 65, 1992.

41. Nicolic, V., Hancevic, J., Hudec, M., et al., "Absorption of the impact energy in the palmar soft tissues," *Anat. Embryol.*, 148, 215, 1975.

42. Pinella, T.P., Boardman, K.C., Bouxsein, M.L., et al., "Impact direction from a fall influences the failure load of the proximal femur as much as age-related bone loss," *Calcif. Tissue Int.*, 58, 231, 1996.

43. Courtney, A.C., Wachtel, E.F., Myers, E.R., and Hayes, W.C., "Age related reductions in the strength of the femur tested in fall loading configuration," *J. Bone Joint Surg.*, 77A, 387, 1995.

44. Cummings, S.R., Nevitt, M.C., Browner, W.S., Stone, K., Fox, K.M., Ensrud, K.E., et al., "Risk factors for hip fracture in white women," *N. Engl. J. Med.*, 332, 767, 1995.

45. Anonymous, "Bone density and risk of hip fracture in men and women; cross sectional analysis," *Br. Med. J.*, 315, 221, 1997.

46. Greenspan, S.L., Resnick, N.M., Maitland, L.A., et al., "Fall severity and bone mineral density as risk factors for hip fracture in ambulatory elderly," *J. Am. Med. Assoc.*, 271, 128, 1994.

47. Cameron, S., "Care of older people. Falls in late life and their consequences — implementing effective services," *Br. Med. J.*, 322, 855, 2001.

48. Myers, A., Young, Y., and Langlois, J.A., "Prevention of falls in the elderly," *Bone*, 18, 87S, 1996.

49. Wehren, L. and Magaziner, J., "Prevention of falls," in *Management of Fractures in Severely Osteoporotic Bone. Orthopaedic and Pharmacologic Strategies*, Obrant, K., Ed., Springer, London, 2000, 333.

50. Tinetti, M.E., Williams, T.F., and Mayewski, R., "Fall risk index for elderly patients based on number of chronic disabilities," *Am. J. Med.*, 80, 429, 2001.

51. Dargent-Molina, P., Haushesse, E., Favier, F., et al., "Fall related factors and risk of hip fracture: the EPIDOS prospective study," *Lancet*, 348, 145, 1996.

52. Lundin-Olsson, L., Nyberg, L., and Gustafson, Y., "Stop walking when talking as a predictor of falls in elderly people," *Lancet*, 349, 617, 1997.

53. Tennstedt, S., Howland, J., Lachman, M., et al., "A randomized, controlled trial of a group intervention to reduce fear of falling and associated activity restriction in older adults," *J. Gerontol.*, 53B, 384, 1998.

54. Høidrup, S., Grønbæk, M., Gottschau, A., et al., "Alcohol intake, beverage preference, and risk of hip fracture in men and women," *Am. J. Epidemiol.*, 149, 993, 1999.

55. Høidrup, S., Grønbæk, M., Pedersen, A.T., et al., "Hormone replacement therapy and hip fracture risk: effect modification by tobacco smoking, alcohol, physical activity, and body mass index," *Am. J. Epidemiol.*, 150, 1085, 1999.

56. Ebrahim, S., Thompson, P.W., Baskaran, V., and Evans, K., "Randomized placebo-controlled trial of brisk walking in the prevention of postmenopausal osteoporosis," *Age Ageing*, 26, 253, 1997.

57. Lord, S.R., Ward, J.A., Williams, P., and Strudwick, M., "The effect of a 12-months exercise trial on balance, strength, and falls in older women: a randomized controlled trial," *J. Am. Geriatr. Soc.*, 43, 1198, 1995.

58. Wolf, S.L., Barnhart, H.X., Kutner, N.G., et al., "Reducing frailty and falls in older persons: an investigation of t'ai chi and computerized balance training," *J. Am. Geriatr. Soc.*, 44, 489, 1996.

59. Norris, S.L., Grothaus, L.C., Buchner, D.M., and Pratt, M., "Effectiveness of physician-based assessment and counseling for exercise in a staff model HMO," *Prev. Med.*, 30, 513, 2000.

60. Campbell, A.J., Robertson, M.C., Gardner, M.M., et al., "Fall prevention over 2 years: a randomized controlled trial in women 80 years and older," *Age Ageing*, 28, 513, 1999.

61. Campbell, A.J., Robertson, M.C., Gardner, M.M., et al., "Randomised controlled trial of general practice programme of home based exercises to prevent falls in elderly," *Br. Med. J.*, 315, 1065, 1997.

62. Mukrow, C.D., Gerety, M.B., Kanten, D., et al., "A randomized trial of physical rehabilitation for very frail nursing home residents," *J. Am. Med. Assoc.*, 271, 519, 1994.

63. Sherrington, C. and Lord, S.R., "Home exercise to improve strength and walking velocity after hip fracture: a randomized controlled trial," *Arch. Phys. Med. Rehabil.*, 78, 208, 1997.

64. Hartard, M., Kleinmond, C., Schiessel, H., and Jeschke, D., "Recovery effects of Galileo 2000: a new device for training intervention (abstr.)," *Osteoporos. Int.*, 9, 24S, 1999.

65. Kannus, P. and Sievänen, H., "Physical activity," in *Management of Fractures in Severely Osteoporotic Bone*, Obrant, K., Ed., Springer, London, 2000, 383.

66. Sinaki, M. and Mikkelsen, B.A., "Postmenopausal spinal osteoporosis: flexion vs. extension exercises," *Arch. Phys. Med. Rehabil.*, 65, 593, 1984.

67. Ilich, J.Z. and Kerstetter, J.E., "Nutrition and bone health," in *Management of Fractures in Severely Osteoporotic Bone*, Obrant, K., Ed., Springer, London, 2000, 362.

68. Setchell, K.D., "Phytoestrogens: the biochemistry, physiology, and implications for human health of soya isoflavines," *Am. J. Clin. Nutr.*, 68, 1333S, 1998.

69. Standing Committee on the Scientific Evaluation of Dietary Reference Intakes, FNB, Institute of Medicine, "Dietary Reference Intakes for Calcium, Phosphorus, Magnesium, Vitamin D, and Fluoride," National Academy Press, Washington, D.C., 1997.

70. Kiel, D.P., Felson, D.T., Anderson, J.J., et al., "Hip fracture and the use of estrogens in postmenopausal women," *N. Engl. J. Med.*, 317, 1169, 1987.

71. Morgan, D.B., Newton, H.M.V., Schorah, C.J., et al., "Abnormal indices of nutrition in the elderly: a study of different clinical groups," *Age Ageing*, 15, 65, 1986.

72. Bonjour, J.P., Schurch, M.A., and Rizzoli, R., "Nutritional aspects of hip fractures," *Bone*, 18, 139S, 1996.

73. Grodin, J.M., Siitiri, P.K., and MacDonald, P.C., "Source of estrogen production in postmenopausal women," *J. Clin. Endocrinol. Metab.*, 36, 207, 1983.

74. Schindler, A.E., Ebert, A., and Friedrich, E., "Conversion of androstendione to estrone by human fat tissue," *J. Endocrinol. Metab.*, 35, 627, 1972.

75. Aloia, J.F., Cohn, S.H., Ostuni, J.A., et al., "Prevention and involutional bone loss by exercise," *Am. J. Med.*, 89, 356, 1978.

76. Campbell, A.J., Robertson, M.C., Gardner, M.M., et al., "Psychotropic medication withdrawal and a home-based exercise program to prevent falls: a randomized, controlled trial," *J. Am. Geriatr. Soc.*, 47, 850, 1999.

77. Hornbrook, M.C., Stevens, V.J., Wingfield, D.J., et al., "Preventing falls among community-dwelling older persons: results from a randomized trial," *Gerontologist*, 34, 16, 1994.

78. Thompson, P.G., "Preventing falls in the elderly at home: community-based program," *Med. J. Aust.,* 164, 530, 1996.

79. Cumming, R.G., Thomas, M., Szonyi, G., et al., "Home visits by an occupational therapist for assessment and modification of environmental hazards: a randomized trial of falls prevention," *J. Am. Geriatr. Soc.,* 147, 1397, 999.

80. Close, J., Ellis, M., Hooper, R., et al., "Prevention of falls in the elderly trial (PROFET): a randomised controlled trial," *Lancet,* 353, 93, 1999.

81. Kanis, J.A., Johnell, O., and Gulberg, B., "Evidence for efficacy of drugs affecting bone metabolism in preventing hip fractures," *Br. Med. J.,* 305, 1124, 1998.

82. Nachtigall, L.E., Nachtigall, R.H, Nachtigall, R.D., and Beckman, E.M., "Estrogen replacement therapy. A 10 year prospective study in relationship to osteoporosis," *Obstet. Gynecol.,* 53, 277, 1979.

83. Christiansen, C., Christiansen, M.S., McNair, P., et al., "Prevention of postmenopausal bone loss: controlled 2 year study in 315 normal females," *Eur. J. Clin. Invest.,* 10, 273, 1980.

84. Riis, B.J., Thomsen, K., Strøm,V., and Christiansen, C., "The effects of percutaneous estradiol and natural progesterone on postmenopausal bone loss," *Am. J. Obstet. Gynecol.,* 1156, 61, 1987.

85. Johnell, O., "Prevention of fractures in the elderly," *Acta Orthop. Scand.,* 66, 90, 1995.

86. Lufkin, E.G., Wahner, H.W., O'Fallon, W.M., et al., "Treatment of postmenopausal osteoporosis with transdermal estrogen," *Ann. Intern. Med.,* 117, 1, 1992.

87. Hulley, S., Grady, D., Bush, T., et al., "Randomized trial of estrogen plus progestin for secondary prevention of coronary heart disease in postmenopausal women. Heart and estrogen/progestin replacement study (HERS) research group," *J. Am. Med. Assoc.,* 280, 605, 1998.

88. Ettinger, B., Black, D.M., Mitlak, B.H., et al., "Reduction of vertebral fracture risk in postmenopausal women with osteoporosis treated with raloxifene," *J. Am. Med. Assoc.,* 282, 637, 1998.

89. Kristensen, B., Ejlertsen, B., Mouridsen, H.T., et al., "Femoral fractures in postmenopausal breast cancer patients treated with adjuvant tamoxifen," *Breast Cancer Res. Treatment,* 39, 321, 1996.

90. Obrant, K., "A personal algorithm for the prevention of fractures in orthopaedic practice," in *Management of Fractures in Severely Osteoporotic Bone,* Obrant, K., Ed., Springer, London, 2000, 565.

91. Heikinheimo, R.J., Inkovaara, J.A., Harju, E.J., et al., "Annual injection of vitamin D and fractures of aged bone," *Calcif. Tissue Int.,* 51, 105, 1992.

92. Chapuy, M.C., Arlot, M.E., Dubeouf, F., et al., "Vitamin D3 and calcium to prevent hip fractures in elderly women," *N. Engl. J. Med.,* 327, 1637, 1992.

93. Lips, P., Graafmans, W.C., Ooms, M.E., et al., "Vitamin D supplementation and fracture incidence in elderly persons. A randomized placebo-controlled trial," *Ann. Intern. Med.,* 124, 400, 1996.

94. Dawson-Hughes, B., Harris, S.S., Khall, E.A., and Dallal, G.E., "Effect of calcium and vitamin D supplementation on bone density in men and women 65 years of age or older," *N. Engl. J. Med.,* 337, 670, 1997.

95. Prince, R.L., "Calcium and vitamin D," in *Management of Fractures in Severely Osteoporotic Bone,* Obrant, K., Ed., Springer, London, 2000, 393.

96. Peter, C.P., Cook, W.O., Nunamaker, D.M., et al., "Effect of alendronate on fracture healing and bone remodeling in dogs," *J. Orthop. Res.,* 14, 74, 1996.

97. Liberman, V.A., Weiss, S.R., Bröll, J., et al., "Effect of oral alendronate on bone mineral density and the incidence of fractures in postmenopausal osteoporosis," *N. Engl. J. Med.,* 333, 1437, 1995.

98. Black, D.M., Cummings, S.R., Karpf, D.B., et al., "Randomised trial of effect of alendronate on risk of fracture in women with existing vertebral fractures," *Lancet,* 348, 1535, 1996.

99. Watts, N.B., Harris, S.T., Genant, H.K., et al., "Intermittent cyclical etidronate treatment of postmenopausal osteoporosis," *N. Engl. J. Med.,* 323, 73, 1990.

100. van Staa, T.P., Abenhaim, L., and Cooper, C., "Use of cyclical etidronate and prevention of nonvertebral fractures," *Br. J. Rheum.,* 37, 87, 1998.

101. Harris, S.T., Watts, N.B., Genant, H.K., et al., "Effects of risedronate treatment on vertebral and non-vertebral fractures in women with postmenopausal osteoporosis," *J. Am. Med. Assoc.,* 282, 1344, 1999.

102. Silverman, S.L., Chesnut, C., Adriano, K., et al., "Salmon calcitonin nasal spray reduces risk of vertebral fracture(s) in established osteoporosis and has continuous efficacy with prolonged treatment: accrued 5 year worldwide data of the PROOF study," *Bone,* 23, 174, 1998.

103. Crespo, R., Revilla, M., Crespo, E., et al., "Complementary medical treatment for Colles' fracture: a comparative, randomized, longitudinal study," *Calcif. Tissue Int.,* 60, 567, 1997.

104. Petersen, M.M., Lauritzen, J.B., Schwarz, P., and Lund, B., "The effect of nasal salmon calcitonin on postfracture osteopenia in patients with malleolar fracture — a randomized study," *Acta Orthop. Scand.,* 69, 347, 1998.

105. Lau, K.-H.W., "Fluoride therapy of established osteoporosis," in *Management of Fractures in Severely Osteoporotic Bone,* Obrant, K., Ed., Springer, London, 2000, 443.

106. Hedlund, L.R. and Gallagher, J.C., "Increased incidence of hip fracture in osteoporotic women treated with sodium fluoride," *J. Bone Miner. Res.,* 4, 223, 1989.

107. Riggs, B.L., O'Fallon, W.M., Lane, A., et al., "Clinical trial of fluoride therapy in postmenopausal osteoporotic women: extended observations and additional analysis," *J. Bone Miner. Res.,* 9, 265, 1994.

108. Lauritzen, J.B. and Hayes W.C., "Hip protectors," in *Management of Fractures in Severely Osteoporotic Bone,* Obrant, K., Ed., Springer, London, 2000, 353.

109. Hayes, W.C., Robinovitch, S.N., and McMahon, T.A., "Bone fracture prevention garment and method," U.S. patent, Washington, D.C., 1992.

110. Lauritzen, J.B. and Lund, B., "Impacts in patients with hip fractures and *in vitro* study of the padding effect: introduction of a hip protector (abstr.)," *Acta Orthop. Scand. Suppl.,* 61, 239, 1990.

111. Parkkari, J., Kannus, P., Heikkilä, J., et al., "Energy-shunting external hip protector attenuates the peak femoral impact force below the fracture threshold. An *in vitro* bimechanical study under typical falling conditions of the elderly," *J. Bone Miner. Res.,* 10, 1437l, 1995.

112. Wortberg, W.E., "Hüft-Fraktur-Bandage zur Verhinderung von Oberschenkelhals-brüchen bei älteren Menschen. Der Oberschenkelhalsbruch, ein biomechanisches Problem," *Z. Gerontol.,* 21, 173, 1988.

113. Heikinheimo, R., Pirkko, J., Heikki, A., and Mäki-Jokela, P., "To fall but not to break — safety pants," in *Proceeding of the 13th Triennial Congress of the International Ergonomics Association,* Tampere, Finland, 1997, 576.

114. Sellberg, M.S., Huston, J.C., and Kruger, D.H., "The development of a passive protective device for the elderly to prevent hip fractures from accidental falls," *Adv. Bioeng.,* 22, 505, 1992.

115. Charpentier, P.J., "A hip protector based on airbag technology *(abstr.),*" *Bone,* 18, 117S, 1996.

116. Hayes, W.C., Robinovitch, S.N., and McMahon, T.A., "Energy shunting hip padding system reduces femoral impact force from a simulated fall to below fracture threshold," in *Proceedings of the Third Injury Prevention through Biomechanics CDC Symposium,* 1993.

117. Robinovitch, S.N., Hayes, W.C., and McMahon, T.A., "Energy shunting hip padding system attenuates femoral impact force in a simulated fall," *J. Biomech. Eng.,* 117, 409, 1995.

118. Parkkari, J., Kannus, P., Poutala, J., and Vuori, I., "Force attenuation properties of various trochanteric padding materials under typical falling conditions of the elderly," *J. Bone Miner. Res.,* 9, 1391, 1994.

119. Parker, M.J., Gillespie, L.D., and Gillespie, W.J., "Hip protectors for preventing hip fractures in the elderly (Cochrane review)," the Cochrane Library, 1999, available at www.cochranelibrary.com.

120. Kannus, P., Parkkari, J., Niemi, S., et al., "Prevention of hip fracture in elderly people with use of a hip protector," *N. Engl. J. Med.,* 343, 1506, 2000.

121. Rubenstein, L., "Hip protectors — a breakthrough in fracture prevention. Editorial," *N. Engl. J. Med.,* 343, 1562, 2000.

122. Parkkari, J., "Hip fractures in the elderly. Epidemiology, injury mechanisms, and prevention with an external hip protector," *Acta Univ. Tamperensis,* 550, 1, 1997.

123. Sandvig, S. and Forsén, L., Eds., *Forebykning av Lårhalsbrudd ved Bruk av Hoftebeskytter. Et Helsetjenestetiltak,* Del 1, *Implementering og Gjennemføring,* Nordberg Trykk, Oslo, 2000.

124. Ekman, A., Mallmin, H., Michaelsson, K., and Ljunghal, S., "External hip protectors to prevent osteoporotic hip fractures," *Lancet,* 350, 563, 1997.

125. Harada, A. and Okuizumi, H., "Hip fracture prevention trial using hip protector in Japanese elderly (abstr.)," *Osteoporos. Int.,* 8, 121, 1998.

126. Hindsø, K. and Lauritzen, J.B., "Intervention study with hip protectors (abstr.)," *Osteoporos. Int.,* 8, 119, 1998.

127. Hindsø, K., Prevention of Hip Fractures Using External Hip Protectors. Risk Factors for Falls, Hip Fractures, and Mortality, and Evaluation of the Consequences of Fear of Falling among Older Orthopaedic Patients, Ph.D. thesis, University of Copenhagen, 1998.

128. Hindsø, K. and Lauritzen, J.B., "Behavioral attitude towards hip protectors in elderly orthopaedic patients (abstr.)," *Osteoporos. Int.,* 18, 119, 1998.

129. Villar, T., Hill, P., Inskip, H., et al., "Trochanteric hip protectors in the institutionalised elderly: a compliance study (abstr.)," *Osteoporos. Int. Suppl.*, 6, 111, 1996.

130. Ross, J.-E., Woodworth, G.W., and Wallace, R.B., "Compliance by elderly in wearing hip joint protectors (abstr.)," in *3rd International Conference on Injury Prevention and Control*, Melbourne, February 18–22, 1996, 298, 73.

131. Hindsø, K. and Lauritzen, J.B., "Effect of hip protectors on fear of falling (abstr.)," *Osteoporos. Int.*, 8, 119, 1998.

132. Lauritzen, J.B., Hindsø, K., and Singh, G., "Cost-effectiveness and external hip protectors (abstr.)," *Osteoporos. Int.*, 6, 130, 1997.

133. Kumar, B.A. and Parker, M.J., "Are hip protectors cost effective?" *Injury*, 31, 693, 2000.

134. Cameron, I. and Kurrle, S., "External hip protectors (letter)," *J. Am. Geriatr. Soc.*, 45, 1158, 1997.

135. Tinetti, M.E., Baker, D.I., McAvay, G., et al., "A multifactorial intervention to reduce the risk of falling among elderly people living in the community," *N. Engl. J. Med.*, 331, 821, 1994.

136. Lauritzen, J.B., "Hip fractures: incidence, risk factors, energy absorption, and prevention," *Bone*, 18, 65S, 1996.

10 Biochemical Markers in Osteoporotic Fractures in the Acute Phase and in the Healing Process

Masaaki Takahashi and Tsuyoshi Ohishi

CONTENTS

I. BIOCHEMICAL MARKERS OF BONE TURNOVER

One of the most important recent advances in osteoporosis has been the development of new biochemical markers of bone turnover or metabolism. New biochemical markers of bone turnover have proved to possess a good sensitivity and specificity to bone metabolism compared with the conventional biochemical markers. The investigations using newly developed biochemical markers of bone turnover have revealed many aspects of bone metabolism in physiologic and diseased conditions.[1-3] The integrity of bone is maintained through continuous remodeling by a combination of osteoclastic resorption and osteoblastic synthesis of bone. The imbalance of this coupling of bone remodeling results in bone loss and leads sequentially to fractures. Measuring bone resorption and formation markers provides the current information of the status of bone turnover. Table 10.1 shows the biochemical markers of bone turnover for bone formation and bone resorption that are currently used. Earlier markers, such as the total alkaline phosphatase and urinary hydroxyproline or urinary calcium, were of limited value. New biochemical markers of bone resorption, such as collagen cross-links, and of bone formation, such as bone-specific alkaline phosphatase and osteocalcin (OC), are better indicators of bone turnover. Collagen pyridinoline cross-links, products of collagen breakdown, can be used to assess bone resorption. Proteins released from osteoblasts, including osteocalcin, bone-specific alkaline phosphatase, and procollagen peptides, can be used to assess bone formation.

In the past decade, the bone markers for bone formation have been developed. Proteins released from osteoblasts, including OC (bone-specific) alkaline phosphatase, can be used to assess bone formation. OC, also called bone Gla protein, a 49 amino acid protein, is the most abundant noncollagenous protein in bone.[4] Although the complete biological function of osteocalcin is still unknown, OC is synthesized by osteoblasts and located only in bone. Evidence has shown that it reflects osteoblastic activity and bone formation.[5,6] Although newly synthesized OC is incorporated

---

TABLE 10.1
Biochemical Markers of Bone Turnover

Bone Formation

Osteocalcin (serum)
Alkaline phosphatase (serum)
  Total
  Bone-specific
Propeptides of type I collagen (serum)
  C-propeptide
  N-propeptide

Bone Resorption

Tartrate-resistant acid phosphatase (serum)
Hydroxyproline (urine)
Hydroxylysine glycosides (urine)
Collagen cross-links (urine and serum)
  Total pyridinoline, deoxypyridinoline
  Free pyridinoline, deoxypyridinoline
  Cross-linked N-telopeptide (NTx)
  Cross-linked C-telopeptide (CTx)
  Cross-linked C-telopeptide (ICTP) (serum)

---

into the bone matrix, part is released into the blood circulation.[7] Because circulating OC levels were initially measured using conventional radioimmunoassay (RIA), a variety of immunometric assays, using polyclonal or monoclonal antibodies, have been developed with better analytical sensitivity and specificity than conventional RIAs. However, those immunoassays have given discordant results in diverse clinical settings.[8,9] The discordance in results is caused by epitopic specificity and differential reactivity with circulating fragments of OC.[10,11] To overcome this problem, the two-site immunoassays for the measurement of the intact molecule of OC were developed.[12] However, the assays for intact OC have been found not to be superior to the conventional assays as was expected. It was reported that one third of circulating OC was intact OC, one third was a large N-terminal OC, and the rest were various smaller fragments.[13] The instability of intact OC is mainly caused by the cleavage of the C-terminal sequence of OC. Cleavage of the C-terminal sequences results in a large N-terminal midfragment. Intact OC turns out to be a large N-terminal midfragment.[13] Accordingly, intact molecules of OC *in vitro,* such as blood, serum, and plasma, are unstable.[14] Therefore, use of these assays requires control of temperature and time during storage and the avoidance of freezing and thawing. A two-site enzyme-immunoassay for detecting both a large N-terminal OC and intact OC was developed to be independent of an unstable C-terminal sequence.[15]

For many years, alkaline phosphatase (ALP) was the only bone formation marker for clinical utility. However, because it includes a large amount of a liver isozyme and a significant amount of isozyme from other tissues, its specificity to bone has been a problem. Therefore, in a disease with very high turnover of bone, e.g., Paget's disease, ALP can be a good index for bone formation, because it mostly originates from bone. However, it lacks the needed sensitivity in a disease with low turnover of bone, e.g., osteoporosis. To overcome this problem, an assay for bone-specific ALP has been developed to improve the specificity of ALP to bone. The assays for the purpose of measuring bone ALP include electrophoretic separation,[16] a heat-inactivation method,[17] precipitation of the sera with wheat germ lectin,[18] or immunoassay. Recently, several immunoassays using a specific antibody to bone ALP have been developed and are clinically available. An assay for measuring bone ALP with two monoclonal antibodies against two different epitopes of bone ALP has been used for evaluation of bone turnover.[19] There is extensive literature describing the bone

ALP molecule using this assay in various metabolic bone diseases. Also, more recently bone ALP EIA (enzyme immonoassay) was developed for measurement of bone ALP activity using a monoclonal antibody against bone ALP after immunoadsorption in microplate wells.[20,21]

Novel markers for collagen molecules have been developed to reflect bone formation. During the formation of type I collagen, which is a major component of bone matrix, the carboxy-terminal propeptide of type I collagen (PICP) is cleaved from procollagen molecules. In blood circulation, this propeptide represents bone formation because it is released during the synthesis of collagen.[22]

Pyridinoline (Pyr) is a trifunctional 3-hydroxypyridinium cross-link.[23,24] Deoxypyridinoline (Dpyr)[25] is minor analogue of Pyr. They are nonreducible cross-links and are believed to be physiologically essential to maintain the structure of the collagen fibril network in the matrix of the various tissues.[26] Pyr is distributed in most collagenous tissues, primarily in cartilage and bone; significant amounts of Dpyr are distributed more specifically in bone.[27] In the late 1980s, Pyr and Dpyr were proposed as bone resorption markers.[28] Since then, a number of studies have shown that urinary Pyr and Dpyr are more sensitive biochemical markers for bone resorption.[29] After newly synthesized collagen is incorporated into bone matrix, Pyr and Dpyr are formed following accretion into the extra cellular matrix through a series of enzymatic and nonenzymatic processes.[30] It is known that Pyr cross-links occur in type I collagen at two sites: carboxy-terminal telopeptide to helix and amino-terminal telopeptide to helix. During bone resorption, Pyr, Dpyr, and amino- and carboxy-terminal telopeptides of type I collagen including those cross-links are excreted into the circulation through collagen degradation. It has been reported that 40% are excreted into urine free of cross-links and 60% as the peptide-bound form.[31,32] Acid-hydrolysis makes the peptide-bound form free of cross-links. Therefore, after the hydrolysis of urine, the total amount of Pyr and Dpyr are measured by HPLC (free form + peptide-bound form). Without the hydrolysis of urine, free forms of Pyr and Dpyr are measured as an amount of amino acids (free form only) by high-performance liquid chromatography (HPLC) or by an immunoassay. Assays for measuring the cross-linked telopeptides of type I collagen have been developed. Amino-terminal cross-linked telopeptides (NTx)[33] and carboxy-terminal telopeptide of type I collagen (CTx)[34,35] have been assayed in urine or recently in serum. A serum assay for the carboxy-terminal cross-linked telopeptides (ICTP)[36] has also been developed. At the present time, collagen Pyr cross-links are the best biochemical markers for bone resorption. Collagen Pyr cross-links are currently measured by HPLC, or, more commonly, by commercially available kits, such as free Dpyr, NTx, and CTx immunoassays.

II. EVALUATION OF BONE TURNOVER IN VERTEBRAL FRACTURE AND HIP FRACTURE

Clinically recognized osteoporotic fractures include fractures of the hip, spine, and distal forearm that have resulted from minimal or moderate trauma (e.g., a fall from standing height or less) among peri- or postmenopausal women. There have been extensive publications indicating that bone turnover is increased in patients with osteoporotic fractures.

A cross-sectional comparison between 99 patients with fracture of the distal forearm and controls showed elevated OC levels in the patients.[37] A history of osteoporotic fractures of the hip, spine, or distal forearm was associated with the elevated Pyr and reduced bone formation as assessed by OC.[38] Biochemical indicators of bone resorption (calcium/creatinine urinary ratio, urinary free Pyr, and free Dpyr) were significantly higher in all patients with vertebral fractures or femoral neck fractures than those measured in control subjects.[39] Seibel et al.[40] reported that Pyr and Dpyr increased in vertebral osteoporosis compared with postmenopausal controls which were not age-matched, but ALP and OC did not change. Akesson et al.[41] studied bone turnover in elderly women with hip fracture using biochemical markers. Pyr and Dpyr significantly increased in the hip fracture group compared with young and age-matched elderly controls. OC significantly increased in elderly

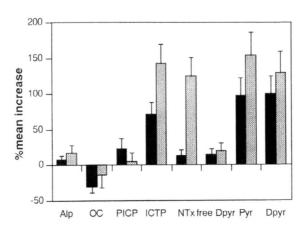

FIGURE 10.1 Percent mean increase of biochemical markers of bone turnover in patients with vertebral fractures and in patients with hip fractures. Percent mean increase was calculated against the values in postmenopausal controls. Solid columns are vertebral fractures, and dotted columns are hip fractures. Bars indicate SE. (From Takahashi, M. et al., *J. Endocrinol. Invest.*, 20, 112, 1997. With permission.)

controls compared with young controls, even though there was no significant difference in OC between the hip fracture group and young controls. ALP significantly increased in both the hip fracture group and the elderly control group compared with the young control group, but there was no difference between the hip fracture group and the elderly control group. In most studies, bone resorption markers have been reported to increase in patients with hip fracture. Bone resorption markers, serum tartrate-resistant acid phosphatase, urinary hydroxyproline, Pyr, and Dpyr all increased.[41-43] However, bone formation markers have been reported to increase, decrease, or not to change in hip fracture. It was reported that OC decreased, whereas ALP increased, did not change, or decreased. Chenung et al.[43] concluded that bone formation is reduced and bone resorption is increased in the patient with hip fracture by evaluating a combination of biochemical markers, including bone ALP, tartrate-resistant acid phosphatase, OC, and hydroxyproline.

The authors have studied the biochemical markers of bone turnover on the effect of menopause and osteoporosis by measuring them in healthy premenopausal and postmenopausal women, and in patients with vertebral osteoporotic fractures.[44] ALP, OC, PICP, Pyr, and Dpyr in the postmenopausal group were significantly higher than those in the premenopausal group. Bone resorption markers (ICTP, Pyr, and Dpyr) were much higher than bone formation markers (ALP, OC, and PICP) in the patients with vertebral fractures compared with healthy postmenopausal women, even though bone resorption markers were similar to bone formation markers in postmenopause. Therefore, it is likely that bone resorption markers increase more than bone formation markers in vertebral osteoporosis.

We have also evaluated the character and difference of bone turnover using the biochemical markers in vertebral fracture and hip fracture compared with healthy postmenopausal women.[45] Subjects were 44 healthy postmenopausal women, 30 patients with osteoporosis with vertebral fracture, and 31 patients with osteoporosis with hip fracture. To evaluate the changes in markers, we calculated a percent mean increase as a mean of (increase of a marker in patients against the values of markers in postmenopausal subjects) $\times$ 100 (percent). The percent mean increase of bone formation markers in postmenopausal patients with osteoporosis remained low (Figure 10.1). PICP increased a little or remained at the same levels as in the postmenopausal phase in patients with osteoporosis, but OC decreased in those patients. Because PICP is a cleavage of the carboxy-terminal extension peptides of type I procollagen, PICP is expected to reflect bone formation. It is reported that OC is produced by osteogenic cells, which are, in fact, osteoblasts and osteocytes.[46] Therefore, the difference between PICP and OC suggests that bone formation is at the same level at the postmenopausal phase whereas the activity of the osteogenic cells may decrease in osteoporosis. In comparison, the percent mean increase of bone resorption markers was high except for free Dpyr in patients with osteoporosis and NTx in vertebral fractures. Therefore, in osteoporosis, bone resorption exceeds formation, and bone formation and resorption are unbalanced. Free Dpyr increased in patients with osteoporosis only 20% over postmenopause, whereas Dpyr (total forms measured by HPLC) increased by 100%. Free Dpyr is measured in urine by EIA, but total Dpyr is measured by HPLC after hydrolysis of urine and expressed as a total amount of Dpyr including its peptide-bound form. The discrepancy between free Dpyr and total Dpyr suggests that Dpyr in urine did not increase as a free form but did increase as a peptide-bound form in patients with osteoporosis. This result was in accordance with the study by Garnero et al.[47] They reported that free Dpyr measured by both HPLC and ELISA did not change in patients with osteoporosis compared with premenopausal women, whereas total Pyr and total Dpyr did.[47] Generally, the patient with a hip fracture is regarded as more osteoporotic than the patient with a vertebral fracture. In our study, bone resorption markers were higher in hip fractures than in vertebral fractures. In contrast, bone formation markers, OC and PICP, were lower in hip fracture than in vertebral fracture. Therefore, bone formation is at lower levels in hip fracture than in vertebral fracture, but bone resorption increases more in hip fracture than in vertebral fracture. As a result, the imbalance between bone formation and resorption is more in hip fracture than in vertebral fracture. Lower bone mass in hip fracture than in vertebral fracture may be a result of this uncoupling between bone formation and resorption. Bone formation and resorption both increased and coupled in postmenopause, and bone resorption exceeded formation and uncoupled in osteoporosis.

We observed the different results from the previous findings in the comparison of biochemical markers of bone turnover between vertebral fracture and hip fracture. Bone resorption markers were higher in hip fracture than in vertebral fracture, which is in accordance with our previous studies. In contrast, bone formation markers tend to be lower in hip fracture than in postmenopausal controls. The former observations showed that bone formation markers in hip fracture were higher or similar compared with those in postmenopausal controls. These results indicate that uncoupling between bone formation and bone resorption is greater in hip fractures than in vertebral fractures.

The integrity of bone is maintained through continuous remodeling by a coupling of osteoclastic bone resorption and osteoblastic bone formation. The imbalance of this coupling of bone remodeling, which is called uncoupling, results in bone loss and leads sequentially to fractures. Measurement of both bone resorption markers and bone formation markers provides the indices for evaluating the status of bone turnover. An index that expresses coupling or uncoupling of bone resorption and formation was first proposed as an "uncoupling index" by Eastell et al.[48] Their index was calculated by calculating the z-scores of Pyr, Dpyr, and hydroxyproline and subtracting the OC z-score. We used their index to make an index of our own that expresses the uncoupling status of bone.[44] We later modified our former formula for the index and named it Uncoupling Status Index (USI).[45] If the number of markers used increases, we could estimate bone turnover more generally and accurately because each marker would have its own sensitivity and specificity to bone turnover. USI can also be generally used independently of the number of biochemical markers assayed. USI in postmenopause (+0.02), vertebral fractures (–2.88), and hip fracture (–5.60) can represent the imbalance of bone turnover in those groups. The coupling or uncoupling status of bone turnover could be easily evaluated by this simple index.

III. BIOCHEMICAL MARKERS IN THE ACUTE PHASE OF OSTEOPOROTIC FRACTURES

When we studied the biochemical markers of bone turnover in patients with osteoporosis, we chose the patients with vertebral fracture and hip fracture as the definite osteoporotic model. To avoid the effect of fracture itself on bone metabolism in the patients, we have previously set the collection period in vertebral fracture at more than 6 months from the latest fracture and in hip fracture within 3 days from the onset of fracture, before operation. However, it is not clear whether a fracture itself affects the concentrations of biochemical markers of bone metabolism or, if so, how soon after or for how long after the fractures. The ideal way to study this is to obtain samples before a fracture. This is not feasible, however, because it requires a huge amount of sampling and a long follow-up. A secondary way is to perform successive sampling immediately after a fracture to observe whether values change.

Most previous publications on longitudinal changes of biochemical markers of bone turnover after fractures have focused on the changes over a period of months. Few reports have looked for acute changes after fracture. Although a report of OC measurements within 22 hours of hip fracture[41] described a slight but significant correlation between OC and the time after fracture, the study was cross sectional. That report also studied the successive change of OC in 15 patients with hip fracture followed by daily measurements during the first postoperative week. In these patients, a decrease of the OC level and a decrease of all other measured variables were observed with time (the decrease was significant for all variables, reaching a nadir on days 2 and 3, and was most pronounced in cortisol and albumin). However, surgery was always performed within the first day after admittance. Therefore, surgery may have affected the change of those variables in the study. The Pyr and Dpyr excretion was not different between the day of admittance and day 6, when sampling was done. Obrant et al.[49] studied the change of OC in patients with diaphyseal fracture of the femur or tibiae, where hip fractures were not included. Seven patients were studied from the first day after fracture. Although the increase of OC with time became significant after the 60th day, they concluded that its increase in the first week was very slight. Roberts et al.[50] compared the concentrations of vitamin K_1 and OC before operation and 1 day after operation in patients with osteoarthritis of the hip and patients with femoral neck fracture. Both parameters were lower after the operation than before. Therefore, it seems surgery affects the concentration of serum vitamin K_1 and OC.

We studied 28 women with hip fracture, ages 64 to 94 years (mean, 80.3 years).[51] Their fractures were caused by low-energy trauma, such as a fall. They were immediately taken to an emergency room at a hospital. Serum and urine were collected from them on 3 successive days immediately after admission to the hospital (termed day 0). Most patients had surgery on day 2 after the sampling of that day. All had been ambulatory before the fracture. Exclusion criteria were hip fractures resulting from severe trauma, admission to the hospital >24 hours after the onset of fracture, blood transfusions or surgical procedures during the period of sample collection, past and present illnesses related to bone metabolism, and increased concentrations of serum creatinine. No subjects had been treated for osteoporosis and none received medications before or during the study that might have affected calcium metabolism. Serum OC was measured by RIA with a Yamasa OC kit (Chiba, Japan) with the use of polyclonal antibodies. Pyr and Dpyr in urine were measured by HPLC after hydrolysis according to an automated analysis described by Pratt et al.[52] ALP and OC did not change significantly during the 3 days (Figure 10.2). Pyr and Dpyr slightly but significantly increased on the third day ($p < 0.05$). Thus, biochemical markers of bone turnover were not affected for at least 48 hours after fracture. Therefore, the values of those measurements during the first 48 hours after fracture appear to reflect bone metabolism uninfluenced by the hip fracture itself.

IV. BIOCHEMICAL MARKERS IN THE HEALING PROCESS OF OSTEOPOROTIC FRACTURES

The process of fracture healing can be divided into three distinct stages: inflammatory (0 to 5 days), reparative (4 to 40 days), and remodeling (25 to 50 days).[53,54] The inflammatory stage involves hemorrhage from bone marrow and surrounding soft connective tissues and various inflammatory cell responses, followed by the formation of granulation tissues, which consists of abundant primitive mesenchymal cells at the fracture site. In the reparative stage, the fracture site is first surrounded by

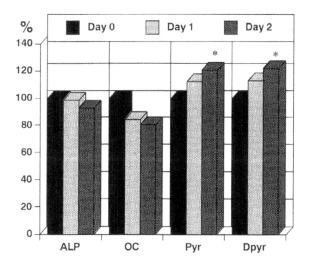

FIGURE 10.2 Changes of biochemical markers of bone turnover on the three successive days immediately after fracture in patients with hip fracture. Columns indicate the mean value. *By Wilcoxon signed-rank test, $p < 0.05$ vs. day 0. (From Takahashi, M. et al., *Clin. Chem.*, 44, 1583, 1998. With permission.)

cartilage callus, followed by the osseous callus, resulting in new bone formation. Once new bulky bone is formed at the fracture site, bone is remodeled into the original shape by osteoblastic bone formation and osteoclastic bone resorption according to Wolff's law in the remodeling stage. The changes of bone formation and bone resorption in the process of fracture healing are expected to be more dynamic than those changes occurring in the remodeling cycle alone because of aging.

Experimental animal models were developed for analyzing the sequences of gene or protein expressions involved in the process of fracture healing.[55] Because type I collagen constitutes about 90% of the organic matrix of bone and type III collagen is abundant in callus tissues, *de novo* synthetic and breakdown products of type I and type III collagen in sera and urine, as well as OC, can be measured in patients who sustained osteoporotic fractures. So far, PICP, bone ALP, and OC are measured as bone formation markers and direct measurement of urinary Pyr and Dpyr, urinary immunoreactive free Dpyr, NTx, ICTP, and CrossLaps (CTx) are currently available as bone resorption markers. Also, the amino-terminal extension peptide of type III procollagen (PIIINP) is measured as monitoring fracture callus formation and repair of soft connective tissues.

Is there any difference in the process of fracture healing between osteoporotic fractures and nonosteoporotic fractures? Walsh et al.[56] compared the fracture healing process between ovariec-tomized rats and normal rats using histologic and mechanical studies.[56] At 2 weeks, the differen-tiation in the callus formed in the ovariectomized rats appeared to lag behind that seen in the control rats, as seen by histologic study. Mechanical data from tensile and bending tests indicated ovariec-tomy impairs fracture healing. However, at 6 weeks the microscopic appearance of the callus was similar in the control and ovariectomized rats. These results indicate that the changes in biochemical parameters of bone metabolism after fracture in the patient with osteoporosis might differ from those in the patients without osteoporosis.

Joerring et al.[57] studied changes of type I and III collagen turnover after a Colles' fracture in 16 patients with osteoporosis. According to their results, significant increases were found of PIIINP and OC within 1 week and of PICP within 2 weeks. PICP and OC had leveled off by 9 months. Earlier increase of PIIINP compared with that of PICP could reflect callus formation around the fracture site of radius, and both PICP and OC reflected the new bone formation and remodeling stage in repair process. Åkesson et al.[58] compared levels of serum OC within 5 hours after a hip fracture to those 4.6 months after a fracture in the osteoporotic patients. Serum levels of OC

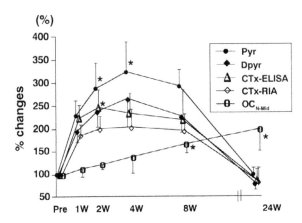

FIGURE 10.3 Changes of biochemical markers in the patients with trochanteric fractures (osteosynthesis group). Values are indicated as mean ± SE. Mean percent changes from initial values are plotted. *Compared with the initial values, $p < 0.05$. Values of Pyr, CTx-ELISA at week 2, Pyr at week 4, and OC_{N-Mid} at weeks 8 and 24 were statistically significant compared with initial values. (From Ohishi, T. et al., *Arch. Orthop. Trauma Surg.*, 118, 126–130, 1998. With permission.)

significantly increased 4.6 months after the fracture compared with levels immediately after the fracture, but they did not increase to the level of age-matched control. This study indicated that the ability to induce a fracture response during fracture healing was intact in elderly women who sustain a hip fracture although the bone formation was lower. McLaren et al.[59] reported the changes of bone resorption markers, urinary Pyr and Dpyr measured by HPLC, in 30 patients who sustained a femoral neck fracture. The levels of both Pyr and Dpyr in the patients with fractures were significantly higher than those in age-matched patients with osteoporosis without fractures, although urine sampling time was not clear. Ingle et al.[60] studied the serial changes in bone formation markers (bone ALP, OC, and procollagen type I N-terminal propeptide) and bone resorption markers (tartrate-resistant acid phosphatase, immunoreactive free Dpyr and NTx) after distal forearm fracture in 20 patients with osteoporosis. Both bone formation and resorption markers increased between 2 and 6 weeks by 13 to 52% compared to the baseline level, and bone resorption markers returned to baseline level at 52 weeks; however, bone formation markers were still elevated at 52 weeks. The loss of bone mineral density of the radius in the affected side was maximal at 6 weeks and had not returned to the baseline level by 52 weeks. The results confirmed that 1 year is not enough for complete recovery from the fracture, although it is not clear whether this prolonged increase of bone formation markers and decrease of bone mineral density is due to radius fracture alone or due to secondary systematic changes in the whole-body reaction, especially reflex sympathetic dystrophy or disuse atrophy. We examined serial changes in biochemical markers during fracture healing in 26 patients with osteoporosis.[61] The patients were divided into three groups; 9 underwent hip hemiarthroplasty for femoral neck fractures, 7 underwent osteosynthesis for trochanteric fractures, and 10 had spinal compression fractures. In the patients with osteosynthesis, bone resorption markers (urinary Pyr, Dpyr, and CTx) had their peak values between 2 and 4 weeks and returned to the baseline level at 24 weeks. Bone formation marker (N-mid OC) gradually increased after fracture and at the end of this study (24 weeks), it was still higher compared with the baseline level (Figure 10.3). In the endoprosthesis group, serial changes of bone resorption markers were similar to those observed in the osteosynthesis group, but serum levels of OC did not increase significantly (Figure 10.4). In the spinal fracture group, neither bone resorption nor bone formation markers changed significantly. Callus formation at the fracture site may be visible after osteosynthesis, while it is not expected after endoprosthesis. Therefore, the increase of OC in the osteosynthesis group might reflect the callus formation and subsequently the new bone formation. A prolonged increase of OC in our results was in good agreement with the results from Ingle et al.[60]

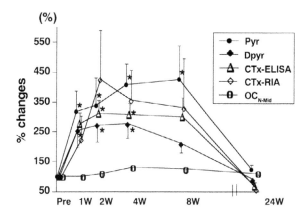

FIGURE 10.4 Changes of biochemical markers in the patients with femoral neck fractures (endoprosthesis group). Values are indicated as mean ± SE. Mean percent changes from initial values are plotted. *Compared with the initial values, $p < 0.05$. Values of Pyr, Dpyr at week 1, Pyr, Dpyr, CTx-ELISA at weeks 2 and 4, and Pyr at week 8 were statistically significant compared with initial values. (From Ohishi, T. et al., *Arch. Orthop. Trauma Surg.*, 118, 126, 1998. With permission.)

Biochemical markers of bone turnover are potentially useful for monitoring bone remodeling during fracture healing. At present, bone resorption and formation markers are employed to assess the disorders during fracture healing process and osteolysis after endoprosthesis, or to monitor during low-intensity ultrasound therapy for acceleration of the fracture healing. According to Joerring et al.,[62] the levels of PICP, ICTP, and PIIINP in the delayed healing group were considerably higher than those in the normal healing group at 2 weeks after the fracture in 16 patients with tibial fracture. In a study of 30 patients with tibial fracture, Emami et al.[63] reported that patients with delayed healing had lower levels of bone ALP between 4 and 7 weeks than did patients with normal healing. Biochemical markers could predict delayed union or pseudoarthrosis after fracture at an earlier stage. Antoniou et al.[64] measured levels of NTx in patients who underwent hip arthroplasty because of osteoarthritis to examine whether bone resorption markers could be used noninvasively to diagnose periprosthetic osteolysis. They found the patients with osteolysis after hip arthroplasty had significantly elevated levels of NTx compared with the control group for at least 1.5 years after the operation. Although their study is cross sectional and sample size is small, these findings showed a promising new approach by using the biochemical markers to the evaluation of osteolysis after joint replacement therapy.[65]

We should be careful interpreting values of biochemical parameters during fracture healing. It is still controversial whether levels of biochemical markers after fracture reflected sole fracture per se. First, patients with fractures were possibly forced to bed rest during a certain period. It is well known that bone resorption and bone formation markers could increase after bed rest.[66,67] Second, the operation procedure itself might modify the values of biochemical markers. An intramedullary reaming during the operation procedure of diaphyseal fracture or endoprosthesis led to acute bone necrosis, followed by elevation of bone resorption markers.[63,66] Third, a skin incision could affect the markers of collagen turnover, especially type III collagen.[69,70] An increase in serum PIIINP was found within the first week after abdominal surgery and its magnitude was related to the extent of the soft tissue operation. These results suggested that the increase of markers for collagen turnover after fracture operation was not only derived from bone remodeling process, but also from soft tissue repair. Fourth, skeletal injury including fracture or intramedullary nail placement affects the metabolism of other bone by producing a circulating osteogenic factor during the period of healing, according to Einhorn et al.[71] This study again suggested that biochemical markers for bone turnover not only reflected repair of sole fracture, but also whole-body collagen turnover.

REFERENCES

1. Calvo, M.S., Eyre, D.R., and Gundberg, C.M., "Molecular basis and clinical application of biological markers of bone turnover," *Endocr. Rev.,* 17, 333, 1996.
2. Garnero, P. and Delmas, P.D., "New developments in biochemical markers for osteoporosis," *Calcif. Tissue Int.,* 59, S2, 1996.
3. Christenson, R.H., "Biochemical markers of bone metabolism: an overview," *Clin. Biochem.,* 30, 573, 1997.
4. Hauschka, P.V., Lian, J.B., Cole, D.E., and Gundberg, C.M., "Osteocalcin and matrix Gla protein: vitamin K-dependent proteins in bone," *Physiol. Rev.,* 69, 990, 1989.
5. Epstein, S., "Serum and urinary markers of bone remodeling: assessment of bone turnover," *Endocr. Rev.,* 9, 437, 1988.
6. Lian, J.B. and Gundberg, C.M., "Osteocalcin biochemical considerations and clinical applications," *Clin. Orthop.,* 226, 267, 1988.
7. Price, P.A. and Nishimoto, S.K., "Radioimmunoassay for the vitamin-K dependent protein of bone and its discovery in plasma," *Proc. Natl. Acad. Sci. U.S.A.,* 77, 2234, 1980.
8. Tracy, R.P., Andrianorivo, A., Riggs, B.L., and Mann, K.G., "Comparison of monoclonal and polyclonal antibody-based immunoassays for osteocalcin: a study of sources of variation in assay results," *J. Bone Miner. Res.,* 5, 451, 1990.
9. Masters, P.W., Jones, R.G., Purves, D.A., et al., "Commercial assays for serum osteocalcin give clinically discordant results," *Clin. Chem.,* 40, 358, 1994.
10. Gundberg, C.M., Wilson, M.S., Gallop, P.M., and Parfitt, A.M., "Determination of osteocalcin in human serum: results with two kits compared with those by a well-characterized assay," *Clin. Chem.,* 31, 1720, 1985.
11. Gundberg, C.M. and Weinstein, R.S., "Multiple immunoreactive forms of osteocalcin in uremic serum," *J. Clin. Invest.,* 77, 1762, 1986.
12. Garnero, P., Grimaux, M., Demiaux, B., et al., "Measurement of serum osteocalcin with a human specific two-site immunoradiometric assay," *J. Bone Miner. Res.,* 7, 1389, 1992.
13. Garnero, P., Grimaux, M., Seguin, P., and Delmas, P.D., "Characterization of immunoreactive forms of human osteocalcin generated *in vivo* and *in vitro*," *J. Bone Miner. Res.,* 9, 255, 1994.
14. Takahashi, M., Kushida, K., Nagano, A., and Inoue, T., "Comparison of the analytical and clinical performance characteristics of an N-MID vs. an intact osteocalcin immunoradiometric assay," *Clin. Chim. Acta,* 294, 67, 2000.
15. Rosenquist, C., Qvist, P., Bjarnason, N., and Christiansen, C., "Measurement of a more stable region of osteocalcin in serum by ELISA with two monoclonal antibodies," *Clin. Chem.,* 10, 1439, 1995.
16. Behr, W. and Barnert, J., "Quantification of bone alkaline phosphatase in serum by precipitaion with wheat-germ lectin: a simplified method and its clinical plausibility," *Clin. Chem.,* 32, 1960, 1986.
17. Even, L.M., "Separation of alkaline phosphatase isoenzymes and evaluation of the clinical usefulness of this determination," *Am. J. Clin. Pathol.,* 61, 142, 1974.
18. Moss, D.W. and Whitby, L.G., "A simplified heat-inactivation method for investigating alkaline phosphatase isoenzymes in serum," *Clin. Chim. Acta,* 61, 63, 1975.
19. Garnero, P. and Delmas, P.D., "Assessment of the serum levels of bone alkaline phosphatase with a new immunoradiometric assay in patients with metabolic bone disease," *J. Clin. Endocr. Metab.,* 77, 1046, 1993.
20. Gomez, B.J., Ardakani, S., Ju, J., et al., "Monoclonal antibody assay for measuring bone specific alkaline phosphatase activity in serum," *Clin. Chem.,* 41, 1560, 1995.
21. Takahashi, M., Kushida, K., Hoshino, H., et al., "Comparison of bone and total alkaline phosphatase activity on bone turnover during menopause and in patients with established osteoporosis," *Clin. Endocrinol.,* 47, 177, 1997.
22. Eriksen, E.F., Charles, P., Melsen, F., et al., "Serum markers of type I collagen formation and degradation in metabolic bone disease: correlation with bone histomorphometry," *J. Bone Miner. Res.,* 8, 127, 1993.
23. Fujimoto, D., Akiba, K., and Nakamura, N., "Isolation and characterization of a fluorescent material in bovine Achilles tendon collagen," *Biochem. Biophys. Res. Commun.,* 76, 1124, 1977.

24. Robins, S.P., "Cross-linking of collagen. Isolation, structural characterization and glycosylation of pyridinoline," *Biochem. J.,* 215, 167, 1983.

25. Ogawa, T., Ono, T., Tsuda, M., and Kawanishi, Y., "A novel fluor in insoluble collagen: a cross-linking moiety in collagen molecule," *Biochem. Biophys. Res. Commun.,* 107, 1252, 1982.

26. Eyre, D.R., Wu, J.J., and Woods, P.E., "The cartilage collagens: structural and metabolic studies," *J. Rheumatol.,* 18, S49, 1991.

27. Eyre, D.R., Koob, T.J., and Van Ness, K.P., "Quantitation of hydroxypyridinium cross-links in collagen by high-performance liquid chromatography," *Anal. Biochem.,* 137, 380, 1984.

28. Black, D., Duncan, A., and Robins, S.P., "Quantitative analysis of the pyridinium cross-links of collagen in urine using ion-paired reversed-phase high-performance liquid chromatography," *Anal. Biochem.,* 169, 197, 1988.

29. Editorial, "Pyridinium cross-links as markers of bone resorption," *Lancet,* 340, 278, 1992.

30. Eyre, D.R., "Collagen cross-linking amino acids," *Meth. Enzymol.,* 144, 115, 1987.

31. Knott, L. and Bailey, A.J., "Collagen cross-links in mineralizing tissues: a review of their chemistry, function, and clinical relevance," *Bone,* 22, 181, 1998.

32. Takahashi, M., Suzuki, M., Naitou, K., et al., "Comparison of free and peptide-bound pyridinoline cross-links excretion in rheumatoid arthritis and osteoarthritis," *Rheumatology,* 38, 133, 1999.

33. Hanson, D.A., Weis, M.A.E., Bollen, A.M., et al., "A specific immunoassay for monitoring human bone resorption: quantitation of type I collagen cross-linked N-telopeptides in urine," *J. Bone Miner. Res.,* 7, 1251, 1992.

34. Bonde, M., Qvist, P., and Fledelius, C., "Immunoassay for quantifying type I collagen degradation products in urine evaluated," *Clin. Chem.,* 40, 2022, 1994.

35. Hoshino, H., Takahashi, M., Kushida, K., et al., "Urinary excretion of type 1 collagen degradation products in healthy women and osteoporotic patients with vertebral fracture and hip fracture," *Calcif. Tissue Int.,* 62, 36, 1998.

36. Risteli, J., Elomaa, I., Niemi, S., et al., "Radioimmunoassay for the pyridinoline cross-linked carboxy-terminal telopeptide of type I collagen: a new serum marker of bone collagen degradation," *Clin. Chem.,* 39, 635, 1993.

37. Mallmin, H., Ljunghall, S., and Larsson, K., "Biochemical markers of bone metabolism in patients with fracture of the distal forearm," *Clin. Orthop.,* 295, 259, 1993.

38. Melton, L.J., III, Khosla, S., Atkinson, E.J., et al., "Relationship of bone turnover to bone density and fractures," *J. Bone Miner. Res.,* 12, 1083, 1997.

39. Fiore, C.E., Pennisi, P., Gibilaro, M., et al., "Correlation of quantitative ultrasound of bone with biochemical markers of bone resorption in women with osteoporotic fractures," *J. Clin. Densitom.,* 2, 231, 1999.

40. Seibel, M.J., Cosman, F., Shen, V., et al., "Urinary hydroxypyridinium cross-links of collagen as markers of bone resorption and estrogen efficacy in postmenopausal osteoporosis," *J. Bone Miner. Res.,* 8, 881, 1993.

41. Akesson, K., Vergnaud, P., Gineyts, E., et al., "Impairment of bone turnover in elderly women with hip fracture," *Calcif. Tissue Int.,* 53, 162, 1993.

42. Chevalley, T., Rizzoli, R., Nydegger, V., et al., "Effects of calcium supplements on femoral bone mineral density and vertebral fracture rate in vitamin-D-replete elderly patients," *Osteoporos. Int.,* 4, 245, 1994.

43. Chenung, C.K., Panesar, N.S., Lau, E., et al., "Increased bone resorption and decreased bone formation in Chinese patients with hip fracture," *Calcif. Tissue Int.,* 56, 347, 1995.

44. Kushida, K., Takahashi, M., Kawana, K., and Inoue, T., "Comparison of markers for bone formation and resorption in premenopausal and postmenopausal subjects, and osteoporosis patients," *J. Clin. Endocrinol. Metab.,* 80, 2447, 1995.

45. Takahashi, M., Kushida, K., Hoshino, H., et al., "Evaluation of bone turnover in postmenopause, vertebral fracture, and hip fracture using biochemical markers for bone formation and resorption," *J. Endocrinol. Invest.,* 20, 112, 1997.

46. Kasai, R., Bianco, P., Robey, P.G., and Kahn, A.J., "Production and characterization of an antibody against the human bone GLA protein (BGP/osteocalcin) propeptide and its use in immunocytochemistry of bone cells," *Bone Miner.,* 25, 167, 1994.

47. Garnero, P., Gineyts, E., Arbault, P., et al., "Different effects of bisphosphonate and estrogen therapy on free and peptide-bound bone cross-links excretion," *J. Bone Miner. Res.*, 10, 641, 1995.

48. Eastell, R., Robins, S.P., Colwell, T., et al., "Evaluation of bone turnover in type I osteoporosis using biochemical markers specific for both bone formation and bone resorption," *Osteoporos. Int.*, 3, 255, 1993.

49. Obrant, K.J., Merle, B., Bejui, J., and Delmas, P.D., "Serum bone-Gla protein after fracture," *Clin. Orthop.*, 258, 300, 1990.

50. Roberts, N.B., Holding, J.D., Walsh, H.P.J., et al., "Serial changes in serum vitamin K1, triglyceride, cholesterol, osteocalcin and 25-hydroxyvitamin D3 in patients after hip replacement for fractured neck of femur or osteoarthritis," *Eur. J. Clin. Invest.*, 26, 24, 1996.

51. Takahashi, M., Kushida, K., Hoshino, H., et al., "Effect of fracture to biochemical markers and vitamin K in acute phase of patients with hip fracture," *Clin. Chem.*, 44, 1583, 1998.

52. Pratt, D.A., Daniloff, Y., Duncan, A., and Robins, S.P., "Automated analysis of the pyridinium cross-links of collagen in tissue and urine using solid-phase extraction and reversed-phase high-performance liquid chromatography," *Anal. Biochem.*, 15, 168, 1992.

53. Frost, H.M., "The biology of fracture healing," *Clin. Orthop.*, 248, 283, 1989.

54. Simmons, D., "Fracture healing perspectives," *Clin. Orthop.*, 200, 100, 1985.

55. Sandberg, M.M., Aro, H.T., and Vuorio, E.I., "Gene expression during bone repair," *Clin. Orthop.*, 289, 292, 1993.

56. Walsh, W.R., Sherman, P., Howlett, C.R., et al., "Fracture healing in rat osteopenia model," *Clin. Orthop.*, 342, 218, 1997.

57. Joerring, S., Jensen, L.T., Andersen, G.R., and Johansen, J.S., "Type I and III procollagen extension peptides in serum respond to fracture in humans," *Arch. Orthop. Trauma Surg.*, 111, 265, 1992.

58. Åkesson, K., Vergnaud, P., Delmas, P.D., and Obrant, K.J., "Serum osteocalcin increases during fracture healing in elderly women with hip fracture," *Bone*, 16, 427, 1995.

59. McLaren, A.M., Hordon, L.D., Bird, H.A., and Robins, S.P., "Urinary excretion of pyridinium cross-links of collagen in patients with osteoporosis and the effects of bone fracture," *Ann. Rheum. Dis.*, 51, 648, 1992.

60. Ingle, B.M., Hay, S.M., Bottjer, H.M., and Eastell, R., "Changes in bone mass and bone turnover following distal forearm fracture," *Osteoporos. Int.*, 10, 399, 1999.

61. Ohishi, T., Takahashi, M., Kushida, K., et al., "Changes of biochemical markers during fracture healing," *Arch. Orthop. Trauma Surg.*, 118, 126, 1998.

62. Joerring, S., Krogsgaard, M., Wilbek, H., and Jensen, L.T., "Collagen turnover after tibial fractures," *Arch. Orthop. Trauma Surg.*, 113, 334, 1994.

63. Emami, A., Larsson, A., Petren-Mallmin, M., and Larsson, S., "Serum bone markers after intramedullary fixed tibial fractures," *Clin. Orthop.*, 368, 220, 1999.

64. Antoniou, J., Huk, O., Zukor, D., et al., "Collagen cross-linked N-telopeptides as markers for evaluating particulate osteolysis: a preliminary study," *J. Orthop. Res.*, 18, 64, 2000.

65. Schneider, U., Breusch, S.J., Termath, S., et al., "Increased urinary cross-link levels in aseptic loosening of total hip arhtroplasty," *J. Arthroplasty*, 13, 687, 1998.

66. Pedersen, B.J., Schlemmer, A., Hassager, C., and Christiansen, C., "Changes in the carboxyl-terminal propeptide of type I procollagen and other markers of bone formation upon five days of bed rest," *Bone*, 17, 91, 1995.

67. Lueken, S.A., Arnaud, S.B., Taylor, A.K., and Baylink, D.J., "Changes in markers of bone formation and resorption in a bed rest model of weightlessness," *J. Bone Miner. Res.*, 8, 1433, 1993.

68. Joerring, S. and Jensen, L.T., "Changes in collagen metabolites in serum after cemented hip and knee arthroplasty," *Arch. Orthop. Trauma Surg.*, 112, 139, 1993.

69. Haukipuro, K., Melkko, J., Risteli, L., et al., "Connective tissue response to major surgery and postoperative infection, *Eur. J. Clin. Invest.*, 22, 333, 1992.

70. Haukipuro, K., Risteli, L., Kairaluoma, M.I., and Risteli, J., "Aminoterminal propeptide of type III procollagen in serum during wound healing in human beings," *Surgery*, 107, 388, 1990.

71. Einhorn, T.A., Simon, G., Devlin, V.J., et al., "The osteogenic response to distal skeletal injury," *J. Bone Joint Surg. Am.*, 72, 1374, 1990.

11 Osteopenias and Osteoporoses — Muscle–Bone Interactions, Absorptiometry, Safety Factors, and Fracture Risk

José Luis Ferretti and Harold M. Frost

CONTENTS

I. INTRODUCTION

The realization that muscle strength strongly influences postnatal bone health and the strength of load-bearing bones, plus a knowledge of how that occurs, has begun to affect conventional, "accepted wisdom" about the nature, pathogenesis, and diagnosis of osteoporoses and osteopenias, as well as their management in clinical settings and how they are studied in the clinic and laboratory. Great changes in these areas have begun, but they are far from complete. This chapter describes some causes of these changes for interested scientists and clinicians. To discuss these matters requires presenting an idea and defining some terms, and then summarizing some basic science

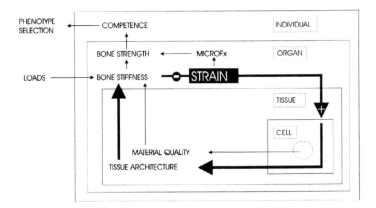

FIGURE 11.1 Schematic representation of the homeostatic system controlling bone stiffness as a function of bone architecture by modulating bone modeling and remodeling (bone "mechanostat"), regarding the different biological levels of structural complexity. The system compares bone stiffness to customary strains derived from the mechanical usage of the skeleton.

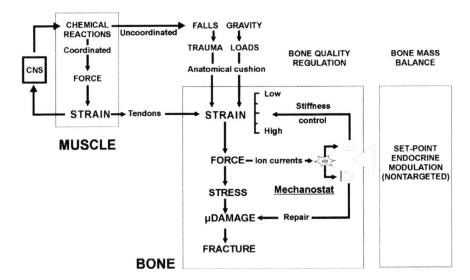

FIGURE 11.2 Didactic representation of the muscle–bone interactions showing the central role of the bone mechanostat and the modulation induced by the endocrine-metabolic environment.

developments in bone physiology that begin to affect the subjects in this chapter's title. This text shares some of that material with readers.

II. AN IDEA, SOME TERMS, AND ABSORPTIOMETRY

A. PROPOSITION 1

The following idea states the major purpose of our load-bearing bones: healthy load-bearing bones keep *voluntary* loads from causing *spontaneous* fracture (Figures 11.1 and 11.2) and/or bone pain, whether those loads are persistently subnormal, normal, or supranormal in size.[1] That would be the ultimate criterion of the health of such a bone, and achieving it could define "mechanical competence." It should be the chief goal of the biologic mechanisms of a bone and it would define the *relationship* between the strength of a bone and the size of the loads on it (Figure 11.3).

ETIOPATHOGENESIS OF OSTEOPOROSES
1 Primary, 2 Disuse, 3 Secondary, 4 Senile

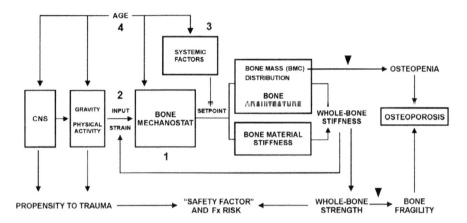

FIGURE 11.3 Interrelationships involved in the pathogenesis of all the osteopenic and osteoporotic conditions. The roles of the bone mechanostat and the interactions of mechanical stimulation, endocrine-metabolic factors, and age, as well as the rationale for the safety factor concept, are indicated. Osteoporoses are classified according to their pathogenetic relationship with the bone mechanostat condition (1, 2, 3) and the eventual influence of aging (4).

Thus, whereas mouse and horse femurs differ hugely in their strength, their health would depend on whether they satisfied Proposition 1 in the particular animals from which they came.

B. DEFINITIONS

Disorders: All statistical abnormalities or differences from the averages for otherwise comparable healthy subjects represent disorders, whether or not they also impair health.

Diseases: The subgroups of all disorders that impair health represent diseases. Thus, a person with one brown and one blue eye would have a disorder but not a disease; albinism should be harmless in Murmansk or Anchorage but a disease in equatorial Africa; and the inability to form bone is normal for sharks but a lethal disease for all mammals.

Osteopenia: Less bone mass (either with or without a consequent bone weakness) than the norm for otherwise comparable subjects (Figure 11.4 left). It need not also be a disease.

Osteoporosis: An osteopenia in which Proposition 1 is not satisfied, so voluntary activities instead of injuries cause spontaneous fractures and affected bones would not be healthy (Figure 11.3).

Bone quality: This seldom-defined term appears often in the osteoporosis literature. Here it would concern the ability of whole bones to satisfy Proposition 1.

C. THE ROLE OF NONINVASIVE ABSORPTIOMETRY

In the biomechanical and health domains the most important feature of whole bones is their strength *relative to the size of the voluntary loads on them.* No concurrent absorptiometric method can evaluate both the strength and the loads. Instead, those methods provide variably unreliable indicators of whole-bone strength (Figure 11.5). The currently popular dual energy X-ray absorptiometry (DEXA) uses different absorptions of X-rays with different energies to estimate the amount of mineral in a bone.[2-11] The values can be reported as bone mineral content (BMC) or bone mineral "density" (BMD), but the latter provides very unreliable indicators of whole-bone strength.[7,8,12,13] The same observation would apply to current ultrasound methods to assess bone "mass" as a broadband-ultrasound attenuation (BUA) measure.

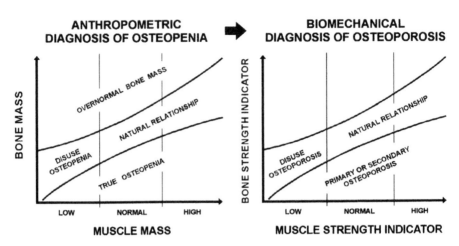

FIGURE 11.4 Muscle–bone relationships schematized from the anthropometric (left) and the biomechanical (right) points of view as required for achieving differential diagnoses of osteopenias (bone/muscle "mass/mass" relationships, left) and osteoporoses (bone/muscle "strength/strength" relationships, right).

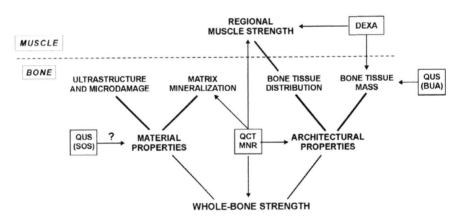

FIGURE 11.5 Musculoskeletal determinants of the strength of a whole bone, and major technologies that can assess some of them noninvasively, as referred to in the text.

However, standard or peripheral quantitative computed tomography (QCT, pQCT) can provide bone strength indices (BSIs) that evaluate whole-bone strength quite reliably by accounting for both the "mass"* and architectural contributions to whole-bone strength (Figure 11.5).[9,12-17] They see increasing use for that purpose in clinical work and in osteoporosis research. It may turn out that different BSIs would apply to diaphyseal and metaphyseal bone.

In time, magnetic resonance imaging (MRI) methods may replace the methods that depend on X-rays and ultrasound. Also, in the near future comparisons of muscle strength to whole-bone strength (Figures 11.4 and 11.5) should become the rule in most such work, once suitable normal reference values become available.

---

* When in quotes, bone "mass" in this chapter refers to its meaning in absorptiometry, not in physics.

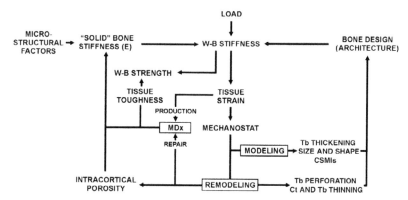

FIGURE 11.6 Biological interactions involved in the bone mechanostat, indicating the role of MDx as a disturbing factor in the determination of the stiffness (and/or strength) of a whole bone. Tb = trabecular; CT = cortical; W-B = whole bone.

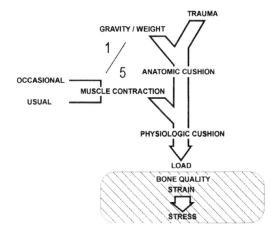

FIGURE 11.7 Mechanical components of the loads usually supported by the human skeleton, pointing out the significance of the regional muscle strength, proposed to be as much as five times more important than that coming from gravity.

III. SUMMARY OF PERTINENT FEATURES OF THE "UTAH PARADIGM"

A. THE "MUSCLE–BONE UNIT"

An elegant stratagem for designing a structure intended to carry loads without breaking would make the largest loads of the structure determine its strength (Figures 11.1 to 11.3 and 11.6). Apparently, human load-bearing bones do exactly that, and the Utah paradigm of skeletal physiology can explain how.[18-21]

Trauma excepted, the largest voluntary loads on bones come from muscle forces (Figure 11.7). Because of lever arm effects it takes well over 2 kg of muscle force on bones to move each kilogram of body weight around on Earth against the resistance of Earth's gravity.[22-24] Those forces cause bone strains that generate strain-dependent signals, which some cells can detect and monitor (Figures 11.1, 11.2, and 11.6).[23,24,26] As a result, a directional orientation of the cell-to-cell communication induces a local modulation of osteoblasts and osteoclasts affecting the two basic mechanisms of bone growth and turnover, namely, bone *modeling* and *remodeling*, causing adaptive changes in either or both bone *material quality* and bone *architecture*, which are the two biological

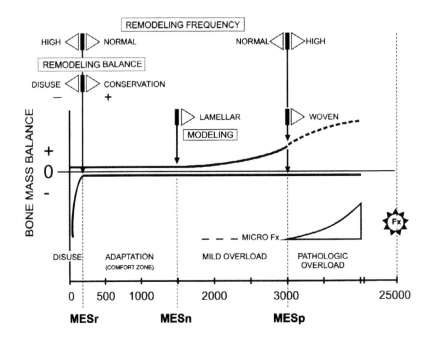

PEAK STRAIN VALUES, microstrains

FIGURE 11.8 Response of bone modeling and remodeling to the peak strains determined by the history of mechanical usage of a bone (expressed in microstrains, x), in terms of bone mass (or strength) balance (y). Approximate values of the significant threshold strains for triggering modeling (MESn), disuse-mode remodeling (MESr), and MDx (MESp) as described in the text are indicated.

determinants of bone strength (Figure 11.5). The mechanism involved in this homeostatic regulation of bone structure has been called bone *mechanostat* (Figures 11.1 to 11.3 and 11.6).[19]

Bone *modeling* comprises formation and resorption drifts that can increase the strength and "mass" of bone. When and where the strains on a bone exceed a threshold range (the MESm), that modeling turns on and strengthens the bone (Figure 11.8).

Basic multicellular unit (BMU)-based bone *remodeling* can turn bone over in small packets. It can work in disuse and conservative modes. "Disuse-mode" remodeling can remove bone when bone strains stay below another and lower threshold[25] but, curiously, that only affects bone next to marrow (i.e., hollow bones, and thus endocortical and trabecular bone). The resulting *disuse-pattern osteopenia* has reduced amounts of spongiosa, a thinned cortex, and an expanded marrow cavity, but the outside bone diameter does not decrease and may even increase slightly.[27-29] When bone strains lie below the MESr, disuse-mode remodeling begins to remove bone next to marrow; otherwise, conservation-mode remodeling tends to keep existing bone.[25] Presumably, disuse-mode remodeling causes all adult-acquired osteopenias on Earth and in astronauts living in microgravity situations in space.

For such reasons we can speak of a "muscle–bone unit" in which muscle strength strongly influences and may dominate the control of whole-bone strength after birth (Figures 11.2 and 11.5).[30] At present, that matter causes considerable discussion among skeletal physiologists.

In human females the rise in blood estrogen levels at puberty accompanies accumulation of bone next to marrow, and as estrogen levels fall at menopause disuse-mode remodeling begins to remove that bone.[10,16,25,31] The resulting disuse-pattern osteopenia makes affected bones weaker than before, but does not usually cause spontaneous fractures. Similar but slower phenomena accompany the rise and fall of androgens in pubertal and aging males.[26,31] In both situations the

MECHANOSTASIS

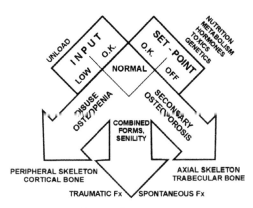

MECHANICAL FAILURE

FIGURE 11.9 Determination of bone weakness as a result of (1) a deficit in the mechanostat *input* because of a reduction in the mechanical usage of the skeleton ("disuse osteopenias," left), or (2) a displacement of the mechanostat *set point* because of a systemic disturbance ("symptomatic bone fragility," or "secondary osteopenias or osteoporoses," right). In addition, (3) different combinations of both etiologies can be observed in aging individuals ("senile" osteopenias or osteoporoses, center).

weaker bones are more likely to fracture from injuries such as falls, and those fractures usually affect the metaphyseal regions of extremity bones like the wrist and hip.[5]

B. Microdamage

Bone as a material is prone to fatigue damage called microdamage (MDx), which is caused by repeated strains.[23] Normally, remodeling BMUs can repair limited amounts of MDx by removing and replacing the damaged bone with new bone (see Figure 11.6). However, when strains exceed the highest threshold range, the bone operational MDx threshold (the MESp; see Figure 11.8), MDx begins to accumulate and can lead to spontaneous fractures.[32,33] Besides those fractures, excessive MDx accumulations cause stress fractures in athletes and special-forces trainees, and pseudofractures in osteomalacia.

In healthy subjects the MDx strain threshold lies above the modeling and remodeling thresholds but below the ultimate strength of bone as a material (Fx) (see Figure 11.8).[23] As a result the modeling threshold would normally make bones strong enough to prevent such fatigue failures. So, where E means typical peak bone strains from voluntary activities, and "<, <<, <<<" mean less than, much less than, and markedly less than, respectively,[32]

$$MESr < E < MESn \ll MESp \lll Fx$$

Because the modeling threshold lies well below the bone ultimate strength of load-bearing, bones normally have a *safety factor*. Didactically, the safety factor can be conceived of as the relationship between the *available* and the *needed* bone strength.

When expressed as a stress, the bone safety factor would equal the bone ultimate strength divided by its modeling threshold, and for healthy young human adults it would equal approximately 6.[33] In other words, healthy young adult bones would be about six times stronger than needed to carry the typical peak voluntary loads on them. How aging and disease might affect this safety factor is under study (Figures 11.3 and 11.9).

TABLE 11.1
Some Conditions That Can Cause Chronic
Muscle Weakness and Osteopenias
(and reduced whole-bone strength)[a]

Asthma	Emphysema	Pulmonary fibrosis
Renal failure	Hepatic failure	Cardiac failure
Malnutrition	Anemia	Polyarthritis
Metastatic cancer	Multiple sclerosis	Alzheimer's disease
Muscular dystrophy	Depression	Stroke
Organic brain syndrome	Huntington's chorea	Myelomeningocele
Lou Gehrig disease	Paralyses	Leukemia
Cystic fibrosis	Still's disease	Alcoholism
Drug addiction	Nursing home residence	Myasthenia gravis

[a] In causing an osteopenia the relative importance of the muscle weakness and the biomechanical-endocrinologic abnormalities accompanying some of these entries (see Figure 11.7) is still uncertain, as few past studies have compared the muscle and nonmechanical effects. The Utah paradigm suggests the muscle effects would dominate most biochemical-endocrinologic ones (see Figures 11.1 through 11.8).

C. OSTEOPOROTIC FRACTURES

Conventionally, these would include all fractures of extremity bones that accompany an osteopenia, plus all spontaneous fractures that accompany an osteopenia and that affect the spine and/or extremity bones (Figure 11.9).[31] However, many osteoporosis authorities designate as "fractures" some asymptomatic and probably gradual instead of sudden changes in vertebral body morphology (i.e., wedging, end-plate "cod-fishing") that can occur in some aging women and men. Many suspect such changes depend on excessive MDx.

IV. SYNTHESIS

Because load-bearing bones normally adapt their strength to the typical peak loads on them, persistent muscle weakness usually causes a disuse pattern osteopenia (Figures 11.2 to 11.4 and 11.9). Normally, muscle strength increases during growth, peaks in young adults, and then slowly declines so at 75 years of age less than half the young adult muscle strength usually remains.[22] This usually causes a corresponding disuse-pattern osteopenia (Figures 11.3 and 11.9). Persistent muscle weakness accompanies many chronic medical diseases, and Table 11.1 lists some examples. Presumably, the accompanying osteopenias stem more from the associated muscle weakness than from direct effects of those diseases on the biologic machinery of bone. Thus, age-related losses of muscle strength could cause most of the known human age-related loss of bone "mass" and of whole-bone strength.

Bones in the above osteopenias usually satisfy Proposition 1 so they would be healthy by that criterion. By the present definitions such osteopenias would be disorders but not diseases, and they have been called "physiologic osteopenias" (Figure 11.9 left).[1,34] Their fractures are always or nearly always caused by injuries such as falls, and they usually affect the metaphyseal regions of extremity bones like the wrist, hip, ankle, and humeral surgical neck (Figure 11.8).[5]

With the decline in estrogen levels after human female menopause, and the slower decline of androgen levels in aging men,[35] as well as other endocrine-metabolic disturbances, a disuse-pattern osteopenia takes place. In these instances, the physiologic proportionality between muscles and

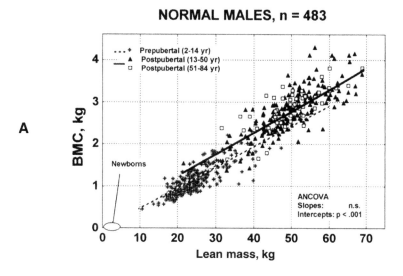

FIGURE 11.10 Densitometric muscle (lean, *x*)–bone (mineral, *y*) "mass/mass" relationships as assessed by DEXA[36] in the whole body of (A) normal pre- and postpubertal males and (B) normal prepubertal and pre- and postmenopausal females. The sex-hormone-related changes in the anthropometric proportionality between bones and muscles (compare Figure 11.4 left) as shifts in the interceptions of the corresponding curves are evident.

bones may vary (Figure 11.4).[36-39] These changes can be assessed from an anthropometric perspective by assessing muscle (lean) and bone (mineral) *masses* employing DEXA [Figures 11.4 (left), 11.10, and 11.11], eventually diagnosing a *secondary osteopenia*.[36-38] They could also be extrapolated to the biomechanical field by assessing the proportionality between muscle (cross sections) and bone (BSIs) *strengths* employing tomographic techniques (Figures 11.4 right and 11.12),[39] magnetic resonance or similar techniques, eventually diagnosing a *secondary osteoporosis*.

However, spontaneous fractures do occur in some disorders that associate with osteopenias, so by the Proposition 1 criterion they would be diseases as well. Examples include osteogenesis imperfecta in all of its variants[31,40] and idiopathic juvenile osteoporosis.[31,41] In those diseases the spontaneous fractures can affect both the spine and extremity bones.

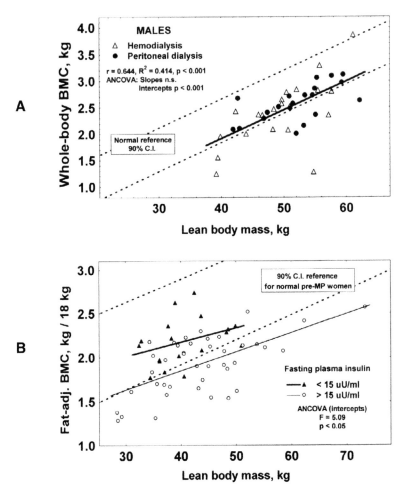

FIGURE 11.11 Densitometric muscle (lean, x)–bone (mineral, y) "mass/mass" relationships as assessed by DEXA in the whole body of (A) men affected by renal failure and undergoing chronic, stable peritoneal dialysis or hemodialysis[37] and (B) premenopausal women showing moderate (triangles) or severe (circles) normoglycemic hyperinsulinemia.[38] In both cases the systemic disturbance impaired the anthropometric bone–muscle proportionality (compare Figure 11.4 left) more than expected in normal individuals of the same gender and reproductive status. The 90% reference intervals for the normal population of the corresponding gender and reproductive status were taken from the data shown in Figure 11.10. (From Ferretti, J.L. et al., *Bone*, 22, 683, 1998. With permission.)

Other examples affect mostly postmenopausal women, but may also affect premenopausal women.[31] Curiously, spontaneous fractures in these women affect only the thoracic and lumbar vertebral bodies, and do not affect the pelvis or extremity bones (see Figure 11.8). Similar phenomena can affect some aging men.

Such disorders have been called "true osteoporoses" (see Figure 11.9 right) and would represent diseases according to the present definition of that term.[1,18,19,32-34]

V. COMMENTS AND CONCLUSION

A. ON RISK OF FRACTURE ANALYSES

Fractures from injuries and spontaneous fractures have different biologic and biomechanical pathogeneses. Fractures from injuries need not depend on some intrinsic bone disease, but spontaneous fractures should always depend on such a disease.

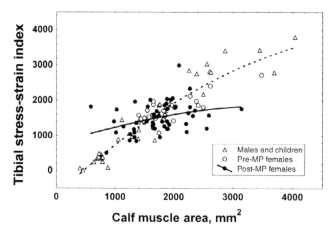

FIGURE 11.12 Correlations between tomographic (pQCT) indicators of bone strength (tibial SSI, y) [15,17] and muscle strength (cross-sectional area of the calf muscles, x) as assessed in calf scans of children, men, and premenopausal women (dashed curve) and of postmenopausal women.[39] The latter show a change in the bone–muscle proportionality that can be interpreted as a biomechanical impairment of bone structure as related to the assessed muscle strength (compare Figure 11.4 right) with reference to the premenopausal condition.

The main cause of osteoporotic extremity bone fractures is falls. Regardless of the severity of an accompanying osteopenia, *without falls such fractures do not occur.* In aging humans, falls increase due to impairments of muscle strength, neuromuscular coordination, balance, vision, and hearing (see Figures 11.6 and 11.7). It should follow that risk-of-fracture studies should account for those impairments, but up to this writing they have not.

Spontaneous fractures in true osteoporoses can only occur when one or some combination of three bone-biologic malfunctions occurs (see Figure 11.4):

1. Impaired MDx detection and repair
2. When modeling has failed to make bones strong enough to keep their strains below the operational bone MDx threshold
3. When disuse-mode remodeling has removed enough mechanically needed bone to let strains approach or exceed the MDx threshold

B. Do BMD and BMC Values and BUA Predict Fractures?

We suggest that this often-made claim is an exaggeration (see Figures 11.2 and 11.7). Currently, a typical risk-of-fracture study accounts for such data plus other so-called risk factors, and could lead to the conclusion that a given person has, say, a 23% chance of developing one or more "osteoporotic fractures" in the future. However, that depends on the observation that of 100 other people supposedly comparable to the person in question, experience found that 23% of them did develop one or more such fractures before they died. Unfortunately, such studies cannot tell in advance which persons would develop such fractures and which would not.

Granted, if the person in question does not fall, no wrist or hip fracture would occur, regardless of the severity of an accompanying osteopenia. It should follow that accounting for the causes of falls should improve the confidence and reliability of future risk-of-fracture analyses (see Figure 11.7), as should using more reliable indicators of whole-bone strength than the currently popular BMD values (see Figure 11.2). At present, this too causes discussion and dissension among skeletal physiologists.

C. On the WHO Criteria for Diagnosing Osteopenias and Osteoporoses

According to the World Health Organization (WHO) criteria, a person whose BMD value lies 2.5 standard deviations or more below age- or normal-for-young reference norms (which are called the *t*- and *z*-scores, respectively) would have an "osteoporosis," while lesser deviations would diagnose an "osteopenia."[42,43] Nevertheless, that stratagem would diagnose a person with a severe physiologic osteopenia as having an "osteoporosis" while a person with a mild true osteoporosis would be diagnosed as having an "osteopenia" (see Figure 11.9). Parfitt[44] recently commented on this matter and indicated that it must change. Like others, we agree.

D. Quo Vadis?

The above features supplement and in some ways challenge accepted wisdom about the varied disorders currently lumped under the "osteoporosis" umbrella. That incites discussion and some controversies, but in time it should lead to a better accepted wisdom and to improved diagnosis, management, and studies of those disorders.

GLOSSARY

Some terms used in the medical literature have imprecise or even multiple meanings; thus, the meanings of the terms as used in this chapter follow.

BMU: Basic multicellular unit of bone remodeling, a "packet" that has a sequence of activation–resorption–formation (ARF). Some like to call this mechanism a bone remodeling unit or BRU, which has a certain logic. In 4 or so months and in a biologically coupled ARF sequence, it turns over approximately 0.05 mm^3 of bone. When it makes less bone than it resorbs, this tends to remove bone permanently, usually only where bone touches marrow. Healthy adult humans may create and complete about 3 million new BMUs annually, but in disease and some other circumstances that number can be more than five times smaller or larger.

Bone "density": In absorptiometry this is an indicator of the *amount* of bone in the path of one or more X-ray beams. It does not signify density in terms of the true *mass of a unit volume* of bone.

Bone "mass": The amount of bone tissue in a bone or skeleton, preferably viewed as the whole-bone volume minus the volume of the soft tissues in the marrow cavity. In absorptiometry it does not mean mass as used in physics. When in quotes in this chapter it has the absorptiometric meaning.

Bone quality: Here, concerning the ability of bones to satisfy Proposition 1.

MESm, MESr: Minimum effective strains (or corresponding signals) for controlling the switching between on and off modeling (MESm), and for controlling the switching between disuse-mode and conservation-mode remodeling (MESr; see Figure 11.5). These are strain ranges instead of step functions, and the centers of those ranges can define their "set points." Currently, the set point of the MESm is thought to lie near 1000 to 1500 microstrain, and that of the MESr near 50 to 100 microstrain (1 microstrain = a deformation of 1 millionth (or 0.1%) of the bone or bone tissue length measured in unloaded conditions).

MESp: The operational microdamage threshold range of bone, currently thought to lie near 3000 microstrain (bone ultimate strength expressed as a strain lies near 25,000 microstrain; see Figure 11.5).

Modeling: Here, adjusting bone "mass," architecture, and strength by formation and resorption drifts.

Muscle strength: The maximum *momentary* contractile force of a muscle, which can be expressed in newtons. It differs from *endurance*, which concerns how long submaximal muscle forces can be exerted, as in marathon running. It differs from mechanical work or *energy*, which can be expressed in newton-meters, joules or kilowatt-hours. It differs from *power*, which concerns how rapidly muscles perform mechanical work and is usually expressed in newton-meters-seconds, joules-second or watts. Because bones seem to adapt their strength and stiffness to the typical peak momentary loads they carry, accounting for these distinctions can minimize errors in discussing mechanical usage effects on bone strength and "mass."

Strain: Deformation of a bone, including shortening, stretching, twisting (torque), bending, and in any combination. It causes resisting stresses. Biomechanicians often express strain in units of microstrain (see Figure 11.5). *A caveat:* while it has become customary to speak of strains as the primary signals that help control modeling and remodeling (see Figures 11.4 and 11.5), and to express the modeling and remodeling thresholds as corresponding strains (see Figure 11.5), strains also create other kinds of "primary signals" that then help control the adaptive biologic mechanisms of bone (see Figures 11.1 and 11.6).

ACKNOWLEDGMENTS

Dr. José Luis Ferretti received a grant from the Consejo de Investigaciones, National University of Rosario (CIUNR) and the Consejo Nacional de Investigaciones Científicas y Técnicas (CONICET), Argentina, for some of the research reported in this chapter. Collaboration with Dr. Gustavo R. Cointry and Dr. Ricardo F. Capozza (CEMFoC/CONICET) for this publication is gratefully acknowledged.

REFERENCES

1. Frost, H.M., *Osteoporoses: New Concepts and Some Implications for Future Diagnosis, Treatment and Research (Based on Insights from the Utah Paradigm),* Ernest Schering Research Foundation AG, Berlin, 1998, 7.
2. Ferretti, J.L., Spiaggi, E.P., Capozza, R., et al., "Interrelationships between geometric and mechanical properties of long bones from three rodent species with very different biomass: phylogenetic implications," *J. Bone Miner. Res.,* 7, 423, 1992.
3. Ferretti, J.L., Capozza, R.F., Mondelo, N., et al., "Interrelationships between densitometric, geometric, and mechanical properties of rat femora: inferences concerning mechanical regulation of bone modeling," *J. Bone Miner. Res.,* 8, 1389, 1993.
4. Ferretti, J.L., Gaffuri, O.H., Capozza, R.F., et al., "Dexamethasone effects on structural, geometric and material properties of rat femur diaphyses as described by peripheral quantitative computed tomography (pQCT) and bending tests," *Bone,* 16, 119, 1995.
5. Ferretti, J.L., Frost, H.M., Gasser, J.A., et al., "Perspectives on osteoporosis research: its focus and some insights of a new paradigm," *Calcif. Tissue Int.,* 57, 399, 1995.
6. Ferretti, J.L., "Perspectives of pQCT technology associated to biomechanical studies in skeletal research employing rat models," *Bone,* 17, 353, 1995.
7. Ferretti, J.L., Capozza, R.F., and Zanchetta, J.R., "Mechanical validation of a tomographic (pQCT) bone index for the noninvasive assessment of rat femur bending strength," *Bone,* 18, 97, 1996.
8. Ferretti, J.L., Frost, H.M., and Schiessl, H., "On new opportunities for absorptiometry," *J. Clin. Densitom.,* 1, 41, 1998.
9. Ferretti, J.L., "Peripheral quantitative computed tomography (pQCT) for evaluating structural and mechanical properties of small bone," in *Mechanical Testing of Bone and the Bone–Implant Interface,* An, Y.H. and Draughn, R.A., Eds., CRC Press, Boca Raton, FL, 2000, 385.
10. Ferretti, J.L., Cointry, G.R., Capozza, R.F., et al., "Analysis of biomechanical effects on bone and on the muscle–bone interactions in small animal models," *J. Musculoskel. Neuron. Interact.,* 1, 263, 2001.
11. Jiang, Y., Zhao, J., Rosen, C., et al., "Perspectives on bone mechanical properties and adaptive response to mechanical loading," *J. Clin. Densitom.,* 2, 422, 1999.

12. Augat, P., Reeb, H., and Claes, L., "Prediction of fracture load at different skeletal sites by geometric properties of the cortical shell," *J. Bone Miner. Res.*, 11, 1356, 1996.

13. Wilhelm, G., Felsenberg, D., Bogusch, G., et al., "Biomechanical examinations for validation of the Bone Strength-Strain Index SSI, calculated by peripheral quantitative computed tomography," in *Musculoskeletal Interactions,* Vol. II, Lyrithis, G.P., Ed., Hylonome Editions, Athens, 1999, 105.

14. Banu, M.J., Orhii, P.B., Mejia, W., et al., "Analysis of the effects of growth hormone, voluntary exercise, and food restriction on diaphyseal bone in female F344 rats," *Bone,* 25, 479, 1999.

15. Schiessl, H. and Willnecker, J., "New insights about the relationship between bone strength and muscle strength," in *Paediatric Osteology. Prevention of Osteoporosis — A Paediatric Task?* Schönau, E. and Matkovic, V., Eds., Excerpta Medica, Amsterdam, 1998, 33.

16. Schiessl, H., Frost, H.M., and Jee, W.S.S., "Estrogen-bone-muscle relationships," *Menopause Dig.,* 5, 10, 1998.

17. Schiessl, H. and Willnecker, J., "Muscle cross-sectional area and bone cross-sectional area in the lower leg measured with peripheral computed tomography," in *Musculoskeletal Interactions,* Vol. II, Lyritis, G.P., Ed., Hylonome Editions, Athens, 1999, 47.

18. Frost, H.M., "Why the ISMNI and the Utah paradigm? Their role in skeletal and extraskeletal disorders," *J. Musculoskel. Neuron. Interact.,* 1, 29, 2000.

19. Frost, H.M., "The Utah paradigm of skeletal physiology: an overview of its insights for bone, cartilage and collagenous tissue organs," *J. Bone Miner. Metab.,* 18, 305, 2000.

20. Jee, W.S.S., "Integrated bone tissue physiology: anatomy and physiology," in *Bone Mechanics Handbook*, 2nd ed., Cowin, S.C., Ed., CRC Press, Boca Raton, FL, 2001, 1.

21. Takahashi, H.E., *Spinal Disorders in Growth and Aging,* Springer-Verlag, Tokyo, 1995.

22. Burr, D.B., "Muscle strength, bone mass, and age-related bone loss," *J. Bone Miner. Res.,* 12, 1547, 1997.

23. Burr, D.B. and Milgrom, C., *Musculoskeletal Fatigue and Stress Fractures,* CRC Press, Boca Raton, FL, 2000.

24. Martin, R.B., Burr, D.B., and Sharkey, N.A., *Skeletal Tissue Mechanics,* Springer-Verlag, New York, 1998.

25. Frost, H.M., "On rho, a marrow mediator and estrogen: their roles in bone strength and "mass" in human females, osteopenias and osteoporoses (insights from a new paradigm)," *J. Bone Miner. Metab.,* 16, 113, 1998.

26. Marotti, G., "The osteocyte as a wiring transmission system," *J. Musculoskel. Neuron. Interact.,* 1, 133, 2000.

27. Garn, S., *The Earlier Gain and Later Loss of Cortical Bone,* Charles C Thomas, Springfield, IL, 1970.

28. Sedlin, E.D., "Uses of bone as a model system in the study of aging," in *Bone Dynamics,* Frost, H.M., Ed., Little-Brown, Boston, 1964, 655.

29. Smith, R.R. and Walker, R.R., "Femoral expansion in aging women: implications for osteoporosis and fractures," *Science,* 145, 156, 1964.

30. Frost, H.M., and Schönau, E., "The "muscle-bone unit" in children and adolescents," *J. Pediatr. Endocrinol. Metab.,* 13, 571, 2000.

31. Marcus, R., Feldman, D., and Kelsey, J., *Osteoporosis,* Academic Press, Orlando, FL, 1996.

32. Frost, H.M., "Does bone design intend to minimize fatigue failures? A case for the afirmative," *J. Bone Miner. Metab.,* 18, 278, 2000.

33. Frost, H.M., "From Wolff's law to the Utah paradigm: insights about bone physiology and its clinical applications," *Anat. Rec.,* 262, 398, 2001.

34. Frost, H.M., "On defining osteopenias and osteoporoses: problems! Another view (with insights from a new paradigm)," *Bone,* 20, 385, 1997.

35. Yao, W., Jee, W.S.S., Chen, J., et al., "Making rats rise to erect bipedal stance for feeding partially prevented orchidectomy-induced bone loss and added bone to intact rats," *J. Bone Miner. Res.,* 15, 1158, 2000.

36. Ferretti, J.L., Capozza, R.F., Cointry, G.R., et al., "Gender-related differences in the relationships between densitometric values of whole-body bone mineral content and lean mass in humans between 2 and 87 years of age," *Bone,* 22, 683, 1998.

37. Negri, A.L., Cointry, G.R., Salica, D., et al., "Bone/lean mass relationships in peritoneally-dialysed and haemodialysed men and women," *J. Bone Miner. Res.,* 16(Suppl. 1), S544, 2001.

38. Ulla, M.R., Stivala, M., Ghiglione, F., et al., "Altered relationships between mineral and lean masses in obese, euglycemic, hyperinsulinemic women," *J. Bone Miner. Res.,* 16(Suppl. 1), S402, 2001.

39. Ferretti, J.L., Roldán, E.J.A., Capozza, R.F., et al., "Muscle/bone interrelationships in the human leg. A pQCT study," *Bone,* 23, S510, 1998.

40. Shapiro, J.R., Primorac, D., and Rowe, D.W., "Osteogenesis imperfecta: current concepts," in *Principles of Bone Biology,* Bilezikian, J.P., Raisz, L.G., and Rodan, G.A., Eds., Academic Press, New York, 1996, 889.

41. Dimar, J.R., Campbell, M., Glassman, S.D., et al., "Idiopathic juvenile osteoporosis," *Am. J. Orthop.,* 24, 865, 1995.

42. Kanis, J.A., Melton, L.J., III, Christiansen, C., et al., "The diagnosis of osteoporosis," *J. Bone Miner. Res.,* 9, 1137, 1994.

43. Kanis, J.A., "Assessment of fracture risk and its application to screening for postmenopausal osteoporosis: synopsis of a WHO report," *Osteoporos. Int.,* 4, 368, 1994.

44. Parfitt, A.M., "Osteoporosis: 50 years of change, mostly in the right direction," in *Osteoporosis and Bone Biology,* Compston, J. and Ralston, S., Eds., International Medical Press, New York, 2000, 1.

12 Postfracture Osteopenia and Its Etiology

Joseph A. Spadaro and Walter H. Short

CONTENTS

I. INTRODUCTION

In his 1966 treatise, "Post Traumatic Osteopenia," Nilsson[1] points out that the earliest observations of bone loss following trauma were made by von Volkmann in 1862 and Sudeck in 1900, describing what was called "Sudeck's atrophy." The latter syndrome, now generally called reflex sympathetic dystrophy (RSD), was characterized by a prolonged, painful recovery from trauma and associated with a loss of bone mineral in the injured extremity. During the early development of radiography, the local bone density loss in RSD was large and more likely to be seen. More refined radiographic techniques, however, have since revealed that osteopenia following fracture or trauma is much more common. Furthermore, it became apparent as early as 1950 that loss of regional bone mass after fracture is quite rapid, while at the fracture location itself bone density may increase due to the formation of the callus. Observations continued and became more quantifiable with the development of single-photon (radionuclide) absorptiometry (SPA) and eventually dual-energy X-ray absorptiometry (DXA) and quantitative computed tomography (CT).[2] These noninvasive methods of

0-8493-1033-4/02/$0.00+$1.50

regional bone densitometry have enabled measurements to be made in thicker regions of the body such as the proximal femur and spine, as well as more precise longitudinal measurements with time.

There are several reasons scientists and clinicians are interested in postfracture or trauma-induced osteopenia. First, they are drawn to the fact that the loss is manifested rapidly, is quite large in relative magnitude, and in adults recovers only slowly at best. A loss of 10 to 20% within several weeks of injury is commonly reported. There are regional differences in the propensity of the skeleton to lose bone mass after trauma as well as differences among individuals, most of which are poorly understood. Second, there are clinically relevant matters. Reduced bone density is generally associated with a loss of strength and an increased likelihood of secondary fracture.[3-8] Pain and disability are possible. If the fracture occurs at a relatively young age, peak bone mass accumulation in the region may be reduced, leading to premature osteoporosis with age. Observation of local osteopenia months and years after a fracture can sometimes be misinterpreted as metabolic in origin. Finally, and most interesting, are the questions that postfracture osteopenia poses in terms of the regulation of bone mass and adaptive bone remodeling. If there is a strong component of "disuse" or mechanical unloading in this phenomenon, what is the mechanism? What additional factors are introduced by the fracture and associated soft tissue injury? What are the endocrine, neurologic, and vascular components? Why are loss and return rates asymmetric?

In this chapter, our aim is to present the nature and overview of regional postfracture osteopenia, gleaned from a number of reports published in the last 30 years since radiologic densitometry began to be widely available. While doing this, several mechanisms will be suggested and the evidence for them outlined. Some practical methodological and measurement issues and recommendations, based on the readings and experience, will also be discussed, along with some suggestions for future study. The important question of disuse osteopenia will be addressed only as it relates to the post-trauma condition, since disuse per se is covered specifically elsewhere in this book. Conditions that lead to recumbency and its after-effects (e.g., coma, spine fracture, or paralysis) and microgravity conditions in space travel, while certainly fascinating and important, are not discussed in any detail here.

II. BONE DENSITY CHANGES
AFTER UPPER EXTREMITY FRACTURE

A. COMPILATION OF DENSITY STUDIES

Densitometry of the upper extremity was easier to perform with early instrumentation and a number of excellent studies show the extent and time course of bone loss following fracture or trauma in that extremity. Table 12.1 lists ten postfracture or postsurgery bone density studies from 1974 to 2001. The fracture studies predominantly involved distal radius fracture with moderate trauma, such as a fall from standing height. All those listed used a comparison to the density in the contralateral, nonfractured arm and/or a baseline measurement in the ipsilateral arm. Cross-sectional studies without these internal controls that merely associate general bone density with fracture and control patient groups are much more numerous in the literature but were excluded here because they do not specifically distinguish bone loss due to fracture or treatment from bone loss that predisposes to fracture. Almost all the reports in Table 12.1 involved cast treatment for 4 to 6 weeks and time of observation varied from 1 to 128 months after fracture. The sites of measurement were the forearm (radius and ulna) and hand. The change in areal bone mineral density (BMD, g/cm^2) was generally the parameter measured and expressed here as an average percent change from baseline or contralateral control.

B. CHARACTERISTIC CHANGES WITH TIME

From Table 12.1 it is clear that there is a fairly wide distribution in the magnitude of bone loss, some of which is site dependent. In cases where the BMD measurement was over the fracture site,

TABLE 12.1
Postfracture Osteopenia Studies — Upper Extremity

Ref.	No. Cases	Median Age (years)	Fracture Site	Treatment	Densitometry Site(s)	Time Postfracture	Peak Change in BMD	Comments
Westlin, 1974[12]	19	64	Distal radius	Cast	SPA: distal radius, ulna	1, 2, 3, 4, 5, 6 mo	−18%	4 mo BMD max loss
Nilsson and Westlin, 1975[10]	74	62	Distal radius	Cast	SPA: distal radius + ulna	4 to 128 mo	−9% diaphysis; +20% ultradistal	Diaphyseal loss = 0 at 128 mo
Nilsson and Westlin, 1977[15]	69		Humerus or mid forearm	Cast	SPA: distal radius + ulna	40 to 66 mo	−15% ultradistal	Small loss after proximal humeral fx
Finsen and Benum, 1986[9]	20/29*	63/44*	Distal radius/forehand*	Cast ?	SPA: forearm/metacarpals*	31 mo (wrist)/12–24 mo (forehand)*	+39% distal radius −4% radius, −9% ulna/+8% metacarpal*; −2% wrist*	*Hand fx
Abbaszadegan et al., 1991[17]	31		Distal radius	Cast or ext. fixation	SPA: distal radius, ulna	9 wk	−11 to −21%	No difference by treatment; loss greater in severe fx
Bickerstaff et al., 1993[57]	33/44*	65/64*	Distal radius	Cast	SPA: metacarpals	2, 5, 8 mo	−6 to −10%/−14 to −23%*	Normal fx/*RSD fx
Houde et al., 1995[18]	8	48	None (hand surgery only)	Cast	SPA: distal radius, ulna	5, 10 wk	−4 to −8% ulna; −4.3 to −5.6% UD radius	Increase in BMD in untreated side at 5 wk only.
Ingle et al., 1999[14]	20	63	Distal radius	Cast	DXA, QUS: distal radius, ulna, carpal, digits	0, 1.5, 3, 6, 12 mo	−5% radius and ulna; −18% carpus; −9% hand	Formation and resorption markers increased
van der Poest Clement et al., 2000[13]	19/18*	65/66*	Distal forearm	Cast	DXA: forearm	0, 3, 6, 12 mo	−5% radius shaft; −11% distal	Untreated/*alendronate treated (bone markers decreased)
Spadaro and Short, 2001[11]	13/14*	47/50*	Distal radius	Cast	DXA: forearm	6–17 wk	−3 to −8%/−2 to −8%*	Fracture/*(nonfracture + carpal surgery)

Note: Studies of osteopenia after fracture of the upper extremities. The information included is from published reports in which changes in bone density (BMD) ipsilateral to the fracture were measured relative to the contralateral side or baseline. The percent changes in BMD are estimated average values over time and/or at different sites. Asterisks (*) refer to comments in the last column.

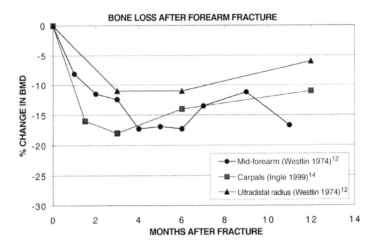

FIGURE 12.1 A composite graph of upper extremity bone density changes with time after distal forearm fracture taken from three representative studies. The average percent change in BMD was measured in the fractured arm relative to baseline or the equivalent site in the contralateral (nonfractured) arm. The rapid loss and slow return are evident. Data are for carpal BMD,[14] radius and ulna midshaft BMD,[12] and ultradistal radius BMD.[13]

either no change or an *increase* in density was found.[9-12] In general, maximum density losses seemed to be 3 to 9% in cortical sites and 8 to 20% in mostly trabecular bone sites, such as the carpal bone and the nonfractured ultradistal ulna. It is interesting to note that the density changes reported in the more recent papers, most of which used DXA, were more modest than losses reported earlier in which predominantly SPA was used. Figure 12.1 is a graphical representation of the data reported in three of the studies, which show the progression of loss after the fracture.[11-14] From this graph the chief features are evident, especially the rapid development of osteopenia, its typical magnitude, the relatively slow recovery, and the variation by site. Significant losses after forearm fracture are evident after 4 to 6 weeks, reach a maximum after 3 to 6 months and return to baseline in 1 to 2 years, although several authors report low density persisting for 5 to 12 years![12-14] Measurements in the bones of the hand and wrist by Ingle et al.[14] indicate the most extensive losses after distal radius fracture seem to occur in the carpal bones.

C. OTHER CONTRIBUTING FACTORS

Other observations may relate to the etiology of postfracture osteopenia in the upper extremity. Several studies have noted an increase in bone loss when the fractured distal radius was in the dominant arm.[11,12,16] Interestingly, Finsen and Benum[9] reported that after fractures in the hand (phalanges and metacarpals), an apparently opposite response was found. Bone density *increased* in several sites if the fractured hand was dominant, and *decreased* if the fractured hand was nondominant. One report indicated that the amount of bone loss in adults after fracture was marginally related to age at fracture.[17] Spadaro and Short[11] found the global forearm BMD loss at 4 months after a nondominant distal radius fracture was mildly correlated with patient age ($r = 0.45$). The findings of Nilsson and Westlin[10] also suggested a greater BMD loss in the mid-forearm with increasing age at fracture in women above 45 years ($r = 0.37$). From the latter long-term study, however, it was unclear whether younger women lost less bone or had a more complete subsequent restoration.

As for density changes at sites more remote from an upper extremity fracture, a variety of responses have been reported. Proximal humerus or midshaft fracture had little effect on the density of the radius and ulna ipsilaterally.[15] Ipsilaterally, distal radius fractures have been shown to lead to reduced density in the nonfractured ultradistal ulna and less in the radial and ulna midshaft,[9,11,13,14] but larger losses in the carpals and metacarpals.[14] Contralateral to the fracture, the effect of distal radius fractures seems to be uncertain. Westlin reported a 6% loss in the opposite distal radius, whereas more recently others have reported no difference.[9,12,13] However, after surgery and cast immobilization alone Houde et al.[18] observed a 7% increase in BMD in the contralateral (nonoperated) ultradistal radius. Data on this interesting question seem to be scarce and most researchers use the contralateral measurements as an attempt to control for the rather large intersubject and technical variations. It seems, nevertheless, that changes in bone density tend to be greater distal to the fracture and to decrease with increasing distance from it. A confounding factor in studying density changes at sites remote from the fracture is the possibility of preexisting generalized osteopenia in people who suffer a fracture of the forearm. Although this is well known in adults, a recent case/control study has also indicated that girls aged 3 to 15 years with recent distal forearm fractures have 3 to 6% lower bone density at all sites.[19]

D. Systemic Markers

Finally, some recent studies have correlated measurements of systemic markers for bone remodeling with bone density changes after distal forearm fracture. Ingle et al.[14] found that bone formation markers in the blood and urine became elevated rapidly (0 to 2 weeks), reached a maximum by 6 weeks (bone-specific alkaline phosphatase: +20%; osteocalcin: +20%; procollagen N-terminal peptides: +55%), and remained elevated (about 20%) at 1 year.[14] Resorption markers also appeared to be elevated after fracture, rising to a maximum between 1 and 4 weeks (tartrate resistant acid phosphatase: +22%; free pyridinoline: +18%; collagen N-telopeptides: +35%) and remained elevated at 1 year. The last two markers, however, had great variability and were not statistically different from control. These changes are consistent with activities during the phases of fracture healing and subsequent remodeling, but are also seen in subjects with osteoporosis. Van der Poest Clement et al.[13] found N-telopeptides and bone alkaline phosphatase decreasing with time after a distal forearm fracture. The latter may not be a contrary finding, however, due to the unavailability of controls or baseline readings.

III. BONE DENSITY CHANGES
AFTER LOWER EXTREMITY FRACTURES

A. Compilation of Density Studies

Studies of bone density changes following lower extremity fracture or osteotomy appeared predominantly after the advent of DXA technology that enabled accurate studies in thicker regions such as the femur, proximal tibia, as well as the more distal sites. Table 12.2 lists 14 studies in which density was assessed ipsilateral to the fracture with the contralateral (nonfractured) leg or ipsilateral leg baseline density as control. In this compilation, the fractures were predominantly of the tibia, but some were at the hip and ankle. Measurement sites were usually chosen to be accessible portions of the hip, femur, tibia, and calcaneus, excluding the fracture line. Areal BMD (g/cm^2) was the parameter, most often measured by DXA or SPA.[2] There was generally a surgical treatment involved with metallic implants and/or a fracture callus in the desired region of interest. Because of this, lower extremity densitometry studies following fracture present several problems of measurement not experienced in upper extremity series. There is also a much higher level of mechanical loading in these regions during normal ambulation and a sudden interruption by the injury and treatment for a longer period than for forearm injuries. Treatment regimes also varied and included graded levels of weight bearing with variable schedules.

B. Characteristic Changes with Time

From Table 12.2 it can be seen that while bone density loss was generally observed in all cases, the amount of loss varied considerably from study to study and by anatomical location. A number

TABLE 12.2
Postfracture Osteopenia Studies — Lower Extremity

Ref.	No. Cases	Median Age (years)	Fracture Site	Treatment	Densitometry Site(s)	Time Postfracture	Peak Change in BMD	Comments
van der Wiel et al., 1994[25]	16	60	Tibia	Cast ± surgery	DXA: proximal femur	0, 2, 4, 7, 13 mo	-2 to -15%	Contralateral: no significant change
Eyres and Kanis, 1995[20]	5/21/10	38/43/9	Tibial shaft	Cast or surgery	DXA: distal tibia	0–6 mo/8 yr/8 yr	-53%/-46%/0	Adult longitudinal/ adult/children
Finsen et al., 1988[26]	26	25	Femoral shaft	AO plate or IM nail	SPA: proximal tibia, distal femur	43 mo (mean)	-3 to -12%	—
Ingle et al., 1999[22]	14	63	Distal tibia/fibula	Not specified	DXA/US: distal tibia, hip, heel	0, 1.5, 3, 6, 12 mo	-12% (distal tibia); -3% hip, -2% (heel)	Bone remodeling markers increased 0–6 mo
Finsen, 1988[76]	20	67	Tibial osteotomy	Staples/cast	SPA: tibia, femur	1–24 mo	-4 to -10%	Max 52 wk. also femoral and contralateral loss
Karlsson et al., 1996[77]	102	77	Hip	Surgery	DXA: hip (custom)	0, 4, 12 mo	-4 to -7%	Total body fat +11%; total body lean mass -5%
van der Poest Clement et al., 1999[75]	11/19	63/81	Tibia, ankle	Cast ± surgery	DXA: hip	5 yr/9 yr	-4.7% troch.; -2.9% neck	5 and 9 yr same
Kannus et al., 1994[28]	34	38	Tibial shaft	Cast	DXA: tibia, femur, spine, forearm, calcaneus	9 yr	-11% (spine), -4 to -11% (knee region), -5% (calcaneus)	Loss larger in primarily nonunions

Finsen and Haave, 1987[27]	20	34	Tibial shaft	Cast/ walking cast	SPA: tibia, distal femur	2.5 yr	−3 to −8%	Could not find appropriate time of measurement
Ahl et al., 1988[78]	82	51	Ankle	Surgery/cast	SPA: calcaneous	17.5 mo	−4 to −8%	Loss greater for more severe fx; early vs. late weight bearing = same loss
Karlsson et al., 2000[24]	26	57	Tibial osteotomy	Int. fix./Cast	DXA: tibia, distal femur	0–15 mo	−10 to −35%	Tibial loss > femoral; irreversible at 15 mo
Andersson and Nilsson, 1979[23]	27	43	Tibial shaft	Cast ± pins	SPA: proximal tibia	0–24 mo	−25 to −45%	Stable loss −25%, functional brace = full cast
Sarangi et al., 1993[62]	60	32	Tibial shaft	Cast or surgery	DXA: distal tibia, calcaneous	4.5 mo	−49 to −45% (RSD); −24 to −34% (non-RSD)	RSD in 33% of cohort
Nilsson, 1966[1]	90	50	Tibial shaft	Cast	SPA: distal femur	1–14 yrs	−25%	—

Note: Studies of osteopenia after fracture of the lower extremities. The information included is from published reports in which changes in bone density (BMD) ipsilateral to the fracture were measured relative to the contralateral side or baseline. The percent changes in BMD are estimated average values over time and/or at different sites.

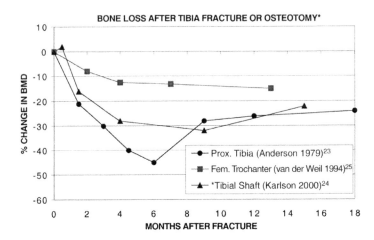

FIGURE 12.2 A composite graph of lower extremity bone density changes with time after tibial fracture or osteotomy using data taken from three representative studies. The average percent change in BMD was measured in the fractured arm relative to baseline or the equivalent site in the contralateral (nonfractured) arm. The rapid loss and slow return are similar to that for the upper extremity, while magnitudes are larger. Data are for femoral trochanter region BMD,[25] proximal tibial metaphysis BMD,[23] and proximal one third tibia shaft BMD.[24]

of authors report remarkable losses in the 25 to 50% range that, like the forearm, are achieved in 3 to 6 months and that persist substantially after a year or more with only a slow recovery. Eyers and Kanis[20] notably found persistence of such losses in the distal tibia for up to 8 years after tibial shaft fracture in adults. Cases followed at 15 to 38 years after lower extremity fracture have also shown smaller but persistently lower BMD in the femoral condyles and greater trochanter.[21] These authors found that in children, however, bone density showed almost complete recovery with time. A majority of the other studies in Table 12.2 reported losses in the 3 to 25% range in substantially similar locations. Although it is difficult to generalize from these data, it appears that losses at tibial sites generally exceed those at femoral sites after tibial fracture. Distal trabecular regions, such as the ultradistal ankle, tend to lose more density than cortical regions.[22] Figure 12.2 illustrates the time dependence of the density changes in the adult lower extremity sites after tibial fracture with data taken from three of the larger studies.[23-25] Similar to the upper extremity, postfracture losses are evident in a few weeks, continue well after remobilization begins, and then stabilize and recover slowly if at all.

C. Other Contributing Factors

Other specific observations may be worth noting in trying to understand the mechanisms. Tibial osteotomy and tibial fracture seem to generate the same responses in terms of magnitude and time course. Neither the type of internal fracture fixation nor the weight-bearing treatment program seems to make a difference.[24,26,27] However, people with primarily non-united fractures had twice the density loss as those whose fractures were primarily united.[28] Density and bone width over the fracture site itself are generally increased, as one would expect, and this increase tends to persist.[20] Global changes also have been recorded after lower extremity fracture. Lumbar BMD was reduced 9 to 12% in patients with fractures years after the fracture, although there were no differences from normal in the distal radius.[28] In two series of over 100 patients with hip fracture, a bone loss of 4.6% in the contralateral femoral neck was observed 1 year after fracture while fat mass (by DXA) increased by 4 to 11% and lean mass decreased by 6% during the same period.[29]

D. Systemic Markers

Systemic markers of bone metabolism have also been measured in conjunction with bone density studies after lower extremity fracture. Ingle et al.[22] found that bone *formation* markers in the blood and urine rapidly became elevated (0 to 2 weeks) after ankle fracture, reached a maximum by 6 weeks (bone-specific alkaline phosphatase: +19%; osteocalcin +35%; procollagen N-terminal peptides: +96%), and except for alkaline phosphatase, remained elevated (about 23 to 34%) at 1 year. These changes are quite similar to those reported for the upper extremity case, but somewhat larger in magnitude. In contrast, *resorption* markers (tartrate-resistant acid phosphatase, free pyridinoline, collagen N-telopeptides) did not show any significant elevation at the 1-year follow-up. In another series, serum alkaline phosphatase and serum phosphate levels were found by regression analysis to correlate well with the magnitude of bone loss in the ipsilateral proximal femur in the unloading phase following tibial fracture ($r = 0.67$ and 0.80, respectively).[25] Urinary hydroxyproline was also increased 26% during this phase and then returned to baseline 1 year after fracture. Dirschl et al.,[30] studying patients with hip fracture during the year after injury, found that low calcium and $1,25(OH)_2$vitamin D levels in the blood correlated with contralateral femoral and lumbar bone loss (2 to 5%). Therefore, despite some inconsistencies, there is reasonably good evidence that the postfracture condition is one of bone turnover and loss considerably higher than involutional levels.

IV. ETIOLOGY OF POSTFRACTURE OSTEOPENIA

A. Contribution of Immobilization/Disuse

Although it has been supposed that postfracture osteopenia is caused by the subsequently reduced loading and the disuse of the extremity, this is likely not the entire story. In human fracture studies, such as those described above, it is almost impossible to distinguish the responses of bone caused by the immobilization per se from those contributed to by the fracture trauma and repair because they are inevitably coupled. However, given their obvious importance, the effects of immobilization alone on bone in other situations such as nerve injury, paralysis, extended recumbency, tendon injury, and spaceflight are worth examining briefly. (A detailed discussion of immobilization/disuse osteopenia per se is covered elsewhere in this volume.) Briefly, there is a common pattern of rapid loss of bone density and slow return toward baseline, which seems similar to the fracture-induced density loss.[31-34] Radiologically, cortical bone lamellation or a double cortical line, scalloping of the cortices, and speckled or nonuniform areas of lucency have been described. Systemically, there is pronounced hypercalcuria, normal to high-normal serum calcium, elevated serum phosphorus and urinary hydroxyproline, and depressed parathyroid hormone (PTH) and $1,25(OH)_2$vitamin D. Bone metabolic and histologic changes seem to start with a rapid, unopposed, hyperresorption with a slow return of formation, reaching a new equilibrium at about 6 months from the start of immobilization.[34-36] This leaves a substantial decrease of trabecular bone volume. Cortical bone responds more slowly with thinning and porosity increasing after 3 to 6 months. The loss of bone is higher in adolescents than in adults, but has a greater capacity for recovery in the young. Weight-bearing bones are observed to lose more mass than non-weight-bearing bones.[34] Animal models of unloading tend to confirm these findings and also that bone already undergoing a high turnover rate is more subject to immobilization osteopenia than quiescent bone.[37-39]

From the above, it can be seen that the characteristics of immobilization osteopenia are fairly consistent with the observed temporal and spatial features of bone loss following fracture described earlier. In both fracture and nonfracture disuse situations, it is likely that a reduction in mechanical loading directly disrupts the cellular regulatory system that normally maintains bone mass equilibrium following the general scheme suggested by Frost.[40,41] An illustration of this is the study by Spadaro and Short[11] in which patients who suffered a distal radius fracture had very similar bone loss changes in the forearm to those with a similar immobilization following a carpal surgery with an intact forearm and therefore less trauma. Even with a fracture, the intact ipsilateral ulna showed similar bone density losses to those in the radius. The slower and incomplete restoration of bone density with increasing age at fracture may also be explained by a change in the adaptive response mechanism.[41,42] Microscopic observations also support a primarily disuse etiology. A study of biopsied bone from the proximal tibia in patients after tibial shaft fracture showed a huge increase in osteoid surface and osteoid volume compared to controls.[36] The abundant osteoid was not uniformly distributed but irregular in its location and the trabeculae were highly lamellar in appearance. Similarly, increased resorptive changes have been noted by Minaire et al.[35] in the iliac crests of patients after traumatic spinal cord lesions. These findings would suggest that after fracture, mechanical unloading leads to a high bone turnover state which occurs with an uncoupling of formation and resorption and consequent density loss. This has been described by Frost as the "regional acceleratory phenomenon."[43]

B. Trauma and Other Factors

Some more recent findings suggest that this picture may be oversimplified. In cosmonauts spending 1 to 6 months in the microgravity environment of the *Mir* space station, some trabecular bone loss in the distal tibia was observed, but none in the radius. Bone formation was depressed, but no dramatic increase in bone resorption markers were seen.[44] In rats immobilized by sciatic or femoral neurectomy, significant bone loss was observed only when a high turnover state was induced by estrogen or dietary calcium deficiency.[38] By analogy, fracture is also a source of high turnover factors as part of the fracture healing and remodeling sequences or by biochemical factors directly released by the traumatized tissues.[45,46]

The relative micromotion of the bone fragments after fracture or the presence of implant micromotion are stimulatory to bone formation in the fracture callus.[47] Interestingly, in studies of bone loss after hip fracture, it was found that the level of ambulation pre- or postfracture did not correlate well with the amount of bone loss.[30,32] Low serum levels of $1,25(OH)_2$vitamin D, however, were clearly associated with greater loss.[30] There are also hormonal and genetic components.[48-52] Bone density losses can also be mediated by changes in local blood and interstitial fluid flow, both of which are likely to occur following both trauma and immobilization.[53,54] An increase in blood flow and vascularity has been associated with local bone loss[55,56] and the exaggerated loss seen in algodystrophy.[57] Most of the current ideas on the microscopic and systemic consequences of disuse and fracture are being generated in animal models and the reader is referred to recent reviews.[31,58,59] Taken together, these observations suggest that osteopenia after fracture is not simply a result of immobilization or disuse and that a multifactorial etiology is involved.

Going a step farther, it is natural to expect that a complex etiology for postfracture osteopenia consisting of disuse (mechanical unloading) and trauma components will ultimately be explained at the cellular level. As for the mechanical unloading component, matrix–cell interactions and/or fluid shear effects are likely to hold the key.[31] Modulation of these unloading effects on bone cells by various systemic bone metabolic factors (e.g., PTH, estrogen, glutamate, growth hormone, $1,25(OH)_2$vitamin D) and paracrine factors (e.g., IGF-I, PTHrP, BMPs, TGF-β, RANKL, OPG, PG-E_2) are also likely.[31,37,51,59,60] In addition, similar factors and their modulators can be introduced or regulated by the cells at the fracture site and its subsequent healing. The trauma component may therefore influence bone metabolism and remodeling in parallel with the effects of mechanical unloading.[46]

C. Reflex Sympathetic Dystrophy (RSD) and Bone Loss

RSD or algodystrophy is a neurovascular complication of fracture characterized by pain, tenderness, swelling, stiffness, and patchy radiotranslucency of the bone.[57,61] Patients with evidence of this condition, which is often transient, typically have a severely increased postfracture osteopenia.

Following a distal radius fracture, patients with RSD have been found to have more than double the bone loss of non-RSD cases.[57] This effect results in trabecular bone loss of 25% and cortical bone loss of 15% at 7 weeks after the fracture. At 4 months after a tibial fracture, bone loss in the distal tibia was found to be 45% in patients with RSD as compared to 35% in those without RSD. Calcaneal BMD loss was 45% in RSD and 24% in normals.[62] No difference in time to union was evident. More important perhaps is the observation that recovery of bone loss is almost absent with patients with RSD, despite a resolution of symptoms.[57] One possible explanation for increased BMD loss and failure of recovery is the increased blood flow associated with RSD and disuse atrophy, which has been documented by ^{99}Tc-MDP bone scan. On the other hand, the increased pain and stiffness would lead to decreased use and load bearing and also could contribute to the bone loss. In any case, as many as 30% of people with upper or lower extremity fracture may show symptoms of RSD, even transiently. Persistent and markedly reduced bone density would be expected to increase secondary fracture risk and may signal the need for some type of intervention.

V. TREATMENT OF FRACTURE-INDUCED BONE LOSS

A. VARIOUS APPROACHES UNDER CONSIDERATION

As a consequence of the realization that postfracture osteopenia is responsible for a substantial and long-lasting bone loss and an increase in fracture risk, a number of ways to reverse this condition or prevent it are being explored. Assuming otherwise normal metabolic and endocrine function and adequate nutrition, both loading exercise and pharmacologic agents are possible avenues. Loading, especially in the early, more active phase of the remodeling process, would seem to be the most natural option[63] but meaningful loading or early ambulation may be difficult and unsafe in a fractured extremity and may not always be effective.[41] A new approach using a low-magnitude vibrational stimulus may have a place in this situation.[64] Bisphosphonates and estrogen response modulators are being more vigorously explored. In a controlled study following forearm fracture, a very positive response was recently obtained with alendronate.[13] Patients receiving 10 mg/day of alendronate for 1 year showed no substantial bone loss at all time periods and a slight increase in BMD in the ultradistal radius during the trial. Other agents are being studied in animal models and in the clinical setting.[65-70] Although the pharmacologic approach of using resorption inhibitors is very promising, it may be wise to examine the histologic responses to these agents, as the remodeling characteristics during the postfracture period are abnormal and the active fracture healing process is ongoing and may be adversely affected. In addition, although efficacy is commonly judged by restoration of bone density (BMD), the resulting cortical and trabecular structure may be abnormal and not actually functionally strong. In this case biomechanical and structural evaluation should be included with bone densitometry.

It is worth noting that treatment of postfracture osteopenia may not always be necessary, but is worth considering. Certain fractures have been found to be associated with subsequent fractures in the same region. Patients with fractures of the hip, tibia, femoral shaft, or hand are more likely to have fractures in the same side.[71] Radial fractures and hip fractures, in contrast, rarely refracture ipsilaterally at the same site. Younger patients may tend to recover bone mass spontaneously and rapidly and losses in some older patients may be modest and do not weaken bone very much. That said, it is becoming recognized that the existence of any low to moderate energy fracture should be a cause for suspicion of preexisting osteoporosis needing further evaluation. Only about 5 to 25% of patients with such fractures (including hip fractures) are currently being referred for medical evaluation or treatment.[72,73]

B. DENSITOMETRY MEASUREMENT ISSUES

Clinical densitometry and determination of the amount of localized postfracture bone loss may be difficult. The presence of the fracture callus likely confounds the interpretation with conventional bone densitometry techniques. Scans may be difficult to obtain because of a cast or fixation devices or because of difficulty in transport and positioning. A skilled technician, however, may be able to obtain BMD measurements using DXA, QCT, peripheral QCT (pQCT), or other methods, at ipsilateral locations not overlying the fracture itself and also the corresponding regions in the contralateral extremity for comparison.[2,74] Diagnostic BMD criteria for osteoporosis (e.g., *t*-scores below 2.5 vs. normative data) recommended by the World Health Organization for hip and spine in postmenopausal Caucasian women do not really apply to nonstandard sites and other populations.[3,73] More research on structural changes, methods of evaluation, and treatment specifically aimed at postfracture and immobilization-related osteopenia is clearly needed before such standards can be considered.

VI. SUMMARY

Fracture-induced osteopenia can occur rapidly and be substantial in magnitude with average localized losses from 5 to 50% a few months after injury (which may even become permanent). The rate and magnitude is far higher than involutional bone loss and varies substantially between individuals. Bone loss is greater in the young or when reflex sympathetic dystrophy is present. The mechanism of this degradation is still unclear. Measurement by current densitometry can be difficult in practice and confounded by preexisting generalized osteopenia and by the healing fracture. The characteristics of this form of secondary osteopenia suggest that the immobilization and disuse play a large role in its etiology, while hyperemia and chemical factors released by the fracture and its repair are also likely etiologic factors. Treatment with various agents and physical exercise is still evolving.

ACKNOWLEDGMENTS

We thank Stacey Leisenfelder and Mary Spadaro for their help with proofreading the manuscript and the Department of Orthopaedic Surgery for its support.

REFERENCES

1. Nilsson, B.E., "Post-traumatic osteopenia. A quantitative study of the bone mineral mass in the femur following fracture of the tibia in man using americium-241 as a photon source," *Acta Orthop. Scand.*, 37, 1S, 1966.
2. Mazess, R.B. and Barden, H.S., "Bone densitometry for diagnosis and monitoring osteoporosis," *Proc. Soc. Exp. Biol. Med.*, 191, 261, 1989.
3. Assessment of fracture risk and its application to screening for postmenopausal osteoporosis. Report of a WHO Study Group, *World Health Organ. Tech. Rep. Ser.*, 843, 1, 1994.
4. Kanis, J.A., Johnell, O., Oden, A., et al., "Risk of hip fracture according to the World Health Organization criteria for osteopenia and osteoporosis," *Bone*, 27, 585, 2000.
5. Mallmin, H., Ljunghall, S., and Naessen, T., "Colles' fracture associated with reduced bone mineral content. Photon densitometry in 74 patients with matched controls," *Acta Orthop. Scand.*, 63, 552, 1992.
6. Ross, P.D., Davis, J.W., Vogel, J.M., et al., "A critical review of bone mass and the risk of fractures in osteoporosis," *Calcif. Tissue Int.*, 46, 149, 1990.
7. Heaney, R.P., "Bone mass and osteoporotic fractures," *Calcif. Tissue Res.*, 47, 63, 1990.
8. Spadaro, J.A., Werner, F.W., Brenner, R.A., et al., "Cortical and trabecular bone contribute strength to the osteopenic distal radius," *J. Orthop. Res.*, 12, 211, 1994.
9. Finsen, V. and Benum, P., "Regional bone mineral density changes after Colles' and forehand fractures," *J. Hand Surg. [Br.]*, 11, 357, 1986.

10. Nilsson, B.E. and Westlin, N.E., "Long-term observations on the loss of bone mineral following Colles' fracture," *Acta Orthop. Scand.*, 46, 61, 1975.

11. Spadaro, J.A. and Short, W.H., "Bone loss in the immobilized forearm with and without fracture," in *Trans. Am. Soc. Bone Miner. Res.*, 23rd Annual Meeting, October 12–16, Phoenix, AZ, No. M342, 2001, 514.

12. Westlin, N.E., "Loss of bone mineral after Colles' fracture," *Clin. Orthop.*, 102, 194, 1974.

13. van der Poest Clement, E., Patka, P., Vandormael, K., et al., "The effect of alendronate on bone mass after distal forearm fracture," *J. Bone Miner. Res.*, 15, 586, 2000.

14. Ingle, B.M., Hay, S.M., Bottjer, H.M., et al., "Changes in bone mass and bone turnover following distal forearm fracture," *Osteoporos. Int.*, 10, 399, 1999.

15. Nilsson, B.E. and Westlin, N.E., "Bone mineral content in the forearm after fracture of the upper limb," *Calcif. Tissue Res.*, 22, 329, 1977.

16. Krolner, B., Tondevold, E., Toft, B., et al., "Bone mass of the axial and the appendicular skeleton in women with Colles' fracture: its relation to physical activity," *Clin. Physiol.*, 2, 147, 1982.

17. Abbaszadegan, H., Adolphson, P., Dalen, N., et al., "Bone mineral loss after Colles' fracture, " *Acta Orthop. Scand.*, 62, 156, 1991.

18. Houde, J.P., Schulz, L.A., Morgan, W.J., et al., "Bone mineral density changes in the forearm after immobilization," *Clin. Orthop.*, 317, 199, 1995.

19. Goulding, A., Cannan, R., Williams, S.M., et al., "Bone mineral density in girls with forearm fractures," *J. Bone Miner. Res.*, 13, 143, 1998.

20. Eyres, K.S. and Kanis, J.A., "Bone loss after tibial fracture. Evaluated by dual-energy X-ray absorptiometry," *J. Bone Joint Surg.*, 77B, 473, 1995.

21. Karlsson, M.K., Nilsson, B.E., and Obrant, K.J., "Bone mineral loss after lower extremity trauma. 62 cases followed for 15–38 years," *Acta Orthop. Scand.*, 64, 362, 1993.

22. Ingle, B.M., Hay, S.M., Bottjer, H.M., et al., "Changes in bone mass and bone turnover following ankle fracture," *Osteoporos. Int.*, 10, 408, 1999.

23. Andersson, S.M. and Nilsson, B.E., "Changes in bone mineral content following tibia shaft fractures," *Clin. Orthop.*, 144, 226, 1979.

24. Karlsson, M.K., Josefsson, P.O., Nordkvist, A., et al., "Bone loss following tibial osteotomy: a model for evaluating post-traumatic osteopenia," *Osteoporos. Int.*, 11, 261, 2000.

25. van der Wiel, H.E., Lips, P., Nauta, J., et al., "Loss of bone in the proximal part of the femur following unstable fractures of the leg," *J. Bone Joint Surg.*, 76A, 230, 1994.

26. Finsen, V., Svenningsen, S., Harnes, O.B., et al., "Osteopenia after plated and nailed femoral shaft fractures," *J. Orthop. Trauma*, 2, 13, 1988.

27. Finsen, V. and Haave, O., "Changes in bone-mass after tibial shaft fracture," *Acta Orthop. Scand.*, 58, 369, 1987.

28. Kannus, P., Jarvinen, M., Sievanen, H., et al., "Osteoporosis in men with a history of tibial fracture," *J. Bone Miner. Res.*, 9, 423, 1994.

29. Fox, K.M., Magaziner, J., Hawkes, W.G., et al., "Loss of bone density and lean body mass after hip fracture," *Osteoporos. Int.*, 11, 31, 2000.

30. Dirschl, D.R., Henderson, R.C., and Oakley, W.C., "Accelerated bone mineral loss following a hip fracture: a prospective longitudinal study," *Bone*, 21, 79, 1997.

31. Bikle, D.D. and Halloran, B.P., "The response of bone to unloading," *J. Bone Miner. Metab.*, 17, 233, 1999.

32. Ito, M., Matsumoto, T., Enomoto, H., et al., "Effect of non-weight bearing on tibial bone density measured by QCT in patients with hip surgery," *J. Bone Miner. Metab.*, 17, 45, 1999.

33. LeBlanc, A. and Schneider, V., "Can the adult skeleton recover lost bone?" *Exp. Gerontol.*, 26, 189, 1991.

34. Minaire, P., "Immobilization osteoporosis: a review," *Clin. Rheumatol.*, 8, 95, 1989.

35. Minaire, P., Meunier, P., Edouard, C., et al., "Quantitative histologic data on disuse osteoporosis," *Calcif. Tissue Res.*, 17, 57, 1974.

36. Obrant, K.J. and Nilsson, B.E., "Histomorphologic changes in the tibial epiphysis after diaphyseal fracture," *Clin. Orthop.*, 185, 270, 1984.

37. Kostenuik, P.J., Harris, J., Halloran, B.P., et al., "Skeletal unloading causes resistance of osteoprogenitor cells to parathyroid hormone and to insulin-like growth factor-I," *J. Bone Miner. Res.*, 14, 21, 1999.

38. Shen, V., Liang, X.G., Birchman, R., et al., "Short-term immobilization-induced cancellous bone loss is limited to regions undergoing high turnover and/or modeling in mature rats," *Bone*, 21, 71, 1997.

39. Weinreb, M., Rodan, G.A., and Thompson, D.D., "Osteopenia in the immobilized rat hind limb is associated with increased bone resorption and decreased bone formation," *Bone*, 10, 187, 1989.

40. Frost, H.M., "Bone 'mass' and the 'mechanostat': a proposal," *Anat. Rec.*, 219, 1, 1987.

41. Frost, H.M., "Why do bone strength and 'mass' in aging adults become unresponsive to vigorous exercise? Insights of the Utah paradigm," *J. Bone Miner. Metab.*, 17, 90, 1999.

42. Lanyon, L. and Skerry, T., "Postmenopausal osteoporosis as a failure of bone's adaptation to functional loading: a hypothesis," *J. Bone Miner. Res.*, 16, 1937, 2001.

43. Frost, H.M., "The regional acceleratory phenomenon: a review," *Henry Ford Hosp. Med. J.*, 31, 3, 1983.

44. Collet, P., Uebelhart, D., Vico, L., et al., "Effects of 1- and 6-month spaceflight on bone mass and biochemistry in two humans," *Bone*, 20, 547, 1997.

45. Yaoita, H., Orimo, H., Shirai, Y., et al., "Expression of bone morphogenetic proteins and rat distal-less homolog genes following rat femoral fracture," *J. Bone Miner. Metab.*, 18, 63, 2000.

46. Dubin, N.H., Monahan, L.K., Yu-Yahiro, J.A., et al., "Serum concentrations of steroids, parathyroid hormone, and calcitonin in postmenopausal women during the year following hip fracture: effect of location of fracture and age," *J. Gerontol. A. Biol. Sci. Med. Sci.*, 54, M467, 1999.

47. Spadaro, J.A., Mino, D.E., Chase, S.E., et al., "Mechanical factors in electrode-induced osteogenesis," *J. Orthop. Res.*, 4, 37, 1986.

48. Bauman, W.A., Spungen, A.M., Wang, J., et al., "Continuous loss of bone during chronic immobilization: a monozygotic twin study," *Osteoporos. Int.*, 10, 123, 1999.

49. Dehority, W., Halloran, B.P., Bikle, D.D., et al., "Bone and hormonal changes induced by skeletal unloading in the mature male rat," *Am. J. Physiol.*, 276, E62, 1999.

50. Kodama, Y., Dimai, H.P., Wergedal, J., et al., "Cortical tibial bone volume in two strains of mice: effects of sciatic neurectomy and genetic regulation of bone response to mechanical loading," *Bone*, 25, 183, 1999.

51. Ma, Y., Jee, W.S., Yuan, Z., et al., "Parathyroid hormone and mechanical usage have a synergistic effect in rat tibial diaphyseal cortical bone," *J. Bone Miner. Res.*, 14, 439, 1999.

52. Rantakokko, J., Uusitalo, H., Jamsa, T., et al., "Expression profiles of mRNAs for osteoblast and osteoclast proteins as indicators of bone loss in mouse immobilization osteopenia model," *J. Bone Miner. Res.*, 14, 1934, 1999.

53. Schoutens, A., Laurent, E., and Poortmans, J.R., "Effects of inactivity and exercise on bone," *Sports Med.*, 7, 71, 1989.

54. Hillsley, M.V. and Frangos, J.A., "Bone tissue engineering: the role of interstitial fluid flow," *Biotechnol. Bioeng.*, 43, 573, 1994.

55. Bergula, A.P., Huang, W., and Frangos, J.A., "Femoral vein ligation increases bone mass in the hindlimb suspended rat," *Bone*, 24, 171, 1999.

56. Gross, T.S., Damji, A.A., Judex, S., et al., "Bone hyperemia precedes disuse-induced intracortical bone resorption," *J. Appl. Physiol.*, 86, 230, 1999.

57. Bickerstaff, D.R., Charlesworth, D., and Kanis, J.A., "Changes in cortical and trabecular bone in algodystrophy," *Br. J. Rheumatol.*, 32, 46, 1993.

58. Jee, W.S. and Ma, Y., "Animal models of immobilization osteopenia," *Morphologie*, 83, 25, 1999.

59. Skerry, T.M., "Identification of novel signaling pathways during functional adaptation of the skeleton to mechanical loading: the role of glutamate as a paracrine signaling agent in the skeleton," *J. Bone Miner. Metab.*, 17, 66, 1999.

60. Hofbauer, L.C., Khosla, S., Dunstan, C.R., et al., "The roles of osteoprotegerin and osteoprotegerin ligand in the paracrine regulation of bone resorption," *J. Bone Miner. Res.*, 15, 2, 2000.

61. van der Laan, L., ter Laak, H.J., Gabreels-Festen, A., et al., "Complex regional pain syndrome type I (RSD): pathology of skeletal muscle and peripheral nerve," *Neurology*, 51, 20, 1998.

62. Sarangi, P.P., Ward, A.J., Smith, E.J., et al., "Algodystrophy and osteoporosis after tibial fractures," *J. Bone Joint Surg.*, 75B, 450, 1993.

63. Inman, C.L., Warren, G.L., Hogan, H.A., et al., "Mechanical loading attenuates bone loss due to immobilization and calcium deficiency," *J. Appl. Physiol.*, 87, 189, 1999.

64. Rubin, C., Xu, G., and Judex, S., "The anabolic activity of bone tissue, suppressed by disuse, is normalized by brief exposure to extremely low-magnitude mechanical stimuli," *FASEB J.*, 15, 2225, 2001.

65. Huuskonen, J., Arnala, I., Olkkonen, H., et al., "Pamidronate increases trabecular bone mineral density in immobilization osteopenia in male rats," *Ann. Chir. Gynaecol.*, 90, 37, 2001.

66. Mosekilde, L., Thomsen, J.S., Mackey, M.S., et al., "Treatment with risedronate or alendronate prevents hind-limb immobilization-induced loss of bone density and strength in adult female rats," *Bone*, 27, 639, 2000.

67. Sakai, A., Sakata, T., Ikeda, S., et al., "Intermittent administration of human parathyroid hormone (1-34) prevents immobilization-related bone loss by regulating bone marrow capacity for bone cells in ddY mice," *J. Bone Miner. Res.*, 14, 1691, 1999.

68. Sato, Y., Honda, Y., Kuno, H., et al., "Menatetrenone ameliorates osteopenia in disuse-affected limbs of vitamin D- and K-deficient stroke patients," *Bone*, 23, 291, 1998.

69. Watts, N.B., "Treatment of osteoporosis with bisphosphonates," *Rheum. Dis. Clin. North Am.*, 27, 197, 2001.

70. Petersen, M.M., Lauritzen, J.B., Schwarz, P., et al., "Effect of nasal salmon calcitonin on post-traumatic osteopenia following ankle fracture. A randomized double-blind placebo-controlled study in 24 patients," *Acta Orthop. Scand.*, 69, 347, 1998.

71. Finsen, V., Haave, O., and Benum, P., "Fracture interaction in the extremities: the possible relevance of post-traumatic osteopenia," *Clin. Orthop.*, 240, 244, 1989.

72. Freedman, K.B., Kaplan, F.S., Bilker, W.B., et al., "Treatment of osteoporosis: are physicians missing an opportunity?" *J. Bone Joint Surg.*, 82A, 1063, 2000.

73. NIH Consensus Conference, "Osteoporosis prevention, diagnosis, and therapy," *J. Am. Med. Assoc.*, 285, 785, 2001.

74. Mirsky, E.C. and Einhorn, T.A., "Bone densitometry in orthopaedic practice," *J. Bone Joint Surg. Am.*, 80, 1687, 1998.

75. van der Poest Clement, E., van der Wiel, H., Patka, P., et al., "Long-term consequences of fracture of the lower leg: cross-sectional study and long-term longitudinal follow-up of bone mineral density in the hip after fracture of lower leg," *Bone*, 24, 131, 1999.

76. Finsen, V., "Osteopenia after osteotomy of the tibia," *Calcif. Tissue Int.*, 42, 1, 1988.

77. Karlsson, M., Nilsson, J.A., Sernbo, I., et al., "Changes of bone mineral mass and soft tissue composition after hip fracture," *Bone*, 18, 19-22, 1996.

78. Ahl, T., Sjoberg, H.E., and Dalen, N., "Bone mineral content in the calcaneus after ankle fracture," *Acta Orthop. Scand.*, 59, 173, 1988.

13 Identification of Patients with a Fragility Fracture in a Fracture Clinic Setting

Earl R. Bogoch, Dagmar K. Gross, and Khalid Syed

CONTENTS

I. INTRODUCTION

Patients with undiagnosed osteoporosis may be referred to fracture clinics after sustaining fractures of the distal radius, proximal humerus, proximal femur, or vertebral body, occurring with minor trauma, as in a simple fall from standing height (*fragility fractures*). Patients presenting with fragility fractures require appropriate investigation and treatment of their osteoporosis to prevent future fractures. However, management is usually focused on care of the fracture and on patient rehabilitation, and there exist numerous impediments to the investigation and treatment of osteoporosis in this group of fracture clinic patients.

Treatment is especially important and valuable for this high-risk group of patients — those who have already experienced a fracture. The risk of future clinically serious fractures of the hip and the vertebrae is markedly increased in patients who have experienced the first fragility fracture.[1-7] The

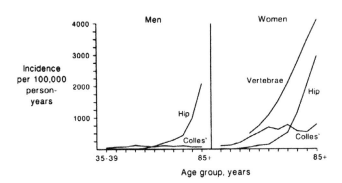

FIGURE 13.1 Incidence of fragility fractures with age. Note peak incidence of wrist fractures occurs earlier in life, whereas peak incidence of hip fractures occurs approximately 15 years later. (From Riggs, B.L. and Melton, L.J., III, *N. Engl. J. Med.,* 314, 1676, 1986. With permission.)

annual incidence of a second hip fracture in patients with a previous hip fracture was reported to be 15/1000 for men and 22/1000 for women over 60 years of age, much greater than the annual incidence of a first hip fracture in the general population (1.6/1000 for men and 3.6/1000 for women over 60).[5] Osteoporosis or osteopenia has been measured in one or more skeletal sites in 75 to 91% of patients with a distal radius fracture.[8-10] However, only 10 to 50% of patients with fragility fracture, almost exclusively female, are treated for osteoporosis following fracture.[11-19] Furthermore, the older the patient is at the time of wrist fracture, the less likely she is to be treated for osteoporosis.[18]

As the population ages, it becomes increasingly important for society to identify patients at high risk for hip and vertebral fractures and to prevent future fractures. It is estimated that in the United States, 32% of women and 17% of men sustain a fracture of the proximal femur by the age of 90.[20] By the early 1990s, more than 240,000 Americans[21] and 23,000 Canadians[22] presented annually with hip fractures, the majority of which are presumed to be due to osteoporosis. In the 4-year period from 1994/1995 to 1998/1999, there was a 53% increase in the number of hip fractures in Ontario, Canada.[23] Projections indicate that the incidence of hip fracture will more than double by the year 2040 in the United States[21] and increase nearly fourfold by 2041 in Canada.[22] Mortality after hip fracture remains high, in the region of 22 to 33% within 1 year of hip fracture, compared to 4.7% in matched controls, despite modern health care.[14,24-30] The death rate for men in the year following hip fracture remains nearly twice that for women.[22,25,27,28,31,32] Also, loss of independence occurs to a significant degree in patients who survive a hip fracture, with 22 to 27% of survivors requiring permanent admission to a chronic care facility in the year following the fracture.[24,33,34] Only 21 to 41% of survivors return to their prefracture levels of activities of daily living and social functioning.[30,32] Thus the orthopaedic and medical communities appear to be facing a crisis that could, in part, be mitigated by prevention of hip fracture in a high-risk population.

The fracture clinic is an ideal environment for identifying patients who are at risk for subsequent hip and vertebral fractures. The yield of screening for high-risk patients in fracture clinics is much higher than in undifferentiated populations or even in osteoporosis populations, such as female patients at a postmenopausal clinic. Data from fracture clinics in three Canadian hospitals indicate that visits for fragility fracture constituted 8.4% of all fracture clinic visits.[19] If a typically busy fracture clinic in a large, urban center has 10,000 patient visits per year, then 840 visits are for fragility fractures. Assuming that each patient with a fragility fracture visits the clinic three times, then a total of 280 patients present annually at a single fracture clinic. Furthermore, 56 to 70% of fragility fractures identified in clinic occur in the distal radius,[17,19,35] and most of these patients (75 to 91%) have osteoporosis or osteopenia.[10,14] Fracture of the wrist, usually a relatively low morbidity injury, is distributed with a peak incidence beginning in the middle decades of life, whereas hip fractures occur about 15 years later (Figure 13.1).[7,36,37] A Colles' fracture increases the relative risk of sustaining another fracture, such that 55 and 80% of patients are reported to experience a subsequent fracture within 10 and 20 years, respectively.[1,3] Thus, the wrist fracture may be considered to be a sentinel event, which brings to light undiagnosed osteoporosis and should make the patient and physician aware of the need for intervention to prevent subsequent hip fracture. The fragility fracture, a daily event in fracture clinics, presents an important public health opportunity.

II. CRITERIA FOR IDENTIFICATION OF PATIENTS AT RISK

All patients with a fragility fracture should be assessed for additional risk factors of osteoporosis and appropriately treated. The risk of fragility fracture is multifactorial, and patients who present with a fragility fracture in the clinic are likely to have at least one other established risk factor for osteoporosis and future fragility fractures.

Other than a previous fragility fracture, low bone mass is the single best indicator of increased risk for fragility fractures and osteoporosis.[22,38-40] Bone loss continues from age 40 throughout life and accelerates after 70 years of age in both women and men.[41,42] Patients with fragility fractures who are discovered to have low bone mass (osteopenia or osteoporosis) have the two most predictive factors for subsequent serious fractures. Such patients who are young and in generally satisfactory health can derive important benefits from treatment.

Established risk factors for osteoporosis and fragility fracture, other than low bone mass and a personal history of fragility fractures, as identified by the National Institutes of Health,[43] the National Osteoporosis Foundation,[44] the Osteoporosis Society of Canada,[45] and the Ontario Program for Optimal Therapeutics,[46] include the following:

1. Female sex
2. Advanced age (over 70 years)
3. History of fracture in first-degree relative
4. White race
5. Cigarette smoking
6. Low body weight (less than 57 kg, or 126 lbs)
7. Estrogen deficiency (ovarian status, early menopause)
8. Glucocorticosteroid use
9. Hypogonadism in men or in premenopausal women

The majority of patients presenting with fragility fractures in the clinic (70 to 77%) are postmenopausal women.[17,19] Gender is a principal factor predicting low bone mineral density (BMD).[17] Peri-menopausal women and women over 40 may also be at increased risk for osteoporosis,[15] as bone loss is accelerated during the transition time from perimenopause to postmenopause.[47]

Most patients who sustain vertebral collapse fractures are not referred for treatment in fracture clinics and are therefore not the principal target of screening programs in this setting. On the other hand, patients seen in the clinic who have back pain, progressive spinal deformity, or loss of height should be assessed for other risk factors listed above and should be investigated with radiographs to identify vertebral collapse fractures. If found, the same principles of investigation and treatment should apply to these individuals as well.

Men over 50 are also at increased risk for osteoporosis and fragility fractures, but are less likely than women to receive treatment.[13] Of men over 50 years of age, 19% have osteoporosis,[48] and up to 53% of men over age 65 have osteoporosis or osteopenia.[49] Bone loss has been found to accelerate with age, particularly in men.[41] Wrist fractures in men indicate a significantly increased risk of subsequent hip fracture,[4,7] and approximately one third of all hip fractures occur in men. Recent studies indicate that the risk factors identified above appear to be valid for men as well,[50,51] and men over age 60 who suffered hip fractures were found to have more risk factors for osteoporosis than age-matched women with hip fractures.[28] Coexisting medical conditions, such as hypogonadism, glucocorticosteroid treatment, renal disease, malabsorption, and alcoholism, contribute to osteoporosis in 40 to 60% of men affected.[52,53] Mortality after hip fracture is as much as twice as high in males when compared to females, and is greater in males than females at all ages over 50.[22,25,27,28,31,32,54] In this context, older men constitute an underinvestigated and undertreated patient group.

III. THE SCREENING ENVIRONMENT — THE FRACTURE CLINIC

In general, the fracture clinic is a high patient volume environment. A typical fracture clinic in an urban hospital in North America has a waiting area separated from a treatment area by a desk or office where administrative staff members greet the patients. In the treatment area, there are cubicles or curtained areas where orthopaedic surgeons, orthopaedic residents, physician's assistants, nurses, physical therapists, and orthopaedic technologists or cast technicians attend to the patients. Procedures, such as cast removal and application, wound care, and fracture reduction or pin removal under local anesthetic, may occur. Unless the fracture clinic has been newly designed and built, recently remodeled, or is generally superior, features of the environment may include lack of privacy, noise, delay, prolonged waiting times, and a sense of intense and rapidly paced clinical activity.

IV. BARRIERS TO EFFECTIVE IDENTIFICATION, INVESTIGATION, AND TREATMENT

Identification of patients with a fragility fracture for the purpose of investigation and treatment of underlying osteoporosis is necessary in order to prevent future fragility fractures. However, several barriers to the development of a successful screening program exist within contemporary fracture clinic and health-care environments.

A. ECONOMIC CONSIDERATIONS

Any formal screening program requires an economic evaluation of the cost of the program in relation to the projected savings in health-related costs of the outcome to be prevented. In the case of fragility fracture prevention, costs are incurred immediately, whereas cost savings are realized only after a decade or more. If each clinic requires a dedicated staff member for implementation of a screening program, then the cost of screening increases dramatically. A screening program only becomes economically practical on a broad scale if it can be incorporated into the normal functions of the fracture clinic. The screening tasks must be acknowledged, understood, and accepted by the patients and the support staff if screening is to be cost-effective. Thus, the design of a fragility fracture screening program must facilitate its application in clinic.

The costs of densitometry testing must also be considered when selecting the categories of patients who will undergo this investigation.

B. INTENSE CLINICAL ACTIVITY

There is often an intense, rapid level of activity in a hospital fracture clinic, and the administrative, nursing, and orthopaedic staff of fracture clinics can be overburdened. The addition of a successful osteoporosis screening, investigation, and management program poses a new challenge. Because of the large volume of musculoskeletal injuries and the limited service resources in some jurisdictions, large numbers of patients may require treatment in a given clinic. A major hospital clinic in a large urban center typically receives 10,000 or more patient visits per year. Unless administrative systems function efficiently, patients often endure prolonged waiting times. In this environment, clinic caregivers are already under pressure to provide the care for which the patient has been referred in a timely manner.

Experience with research projects in Ontario fracture clinics has demonstrated that, even after there is agreement, consensus, and a pledge of cooperation from clinic staff, the inclusion of osteoporosis care and investigation into fracture clinic protocols is often forgotten or neglected. This tendency of fracture clinics to revert to the basics of care — to treat the fracture but not the osteoporosis — results in an additional challenge for health services researchers in the development, testing and implementation of new screening programs. It is important to have a screening program in the fracture clinic that employs visual education materials to inform the patients that their fracture may be the consequence of osteoporosis, thereby resulting in self-identification of patients to clinic staff.

Because a fracture clinic may serve 50 or even 100 or more patients on a given day, a screening program should provide practical, workable and sustainable recommendations.

C. Training of Clinic Staff

The previous training, knowledge, and experience of orthopaedic surgeons and nursing staff in fracture clinics may also present an obstacle to the development of effective screening programs. Until recently, clinic staff have not received training in osteoporosis identification and treatment for prevention of future osteoporosis-associated fractures, although there has been an awareness of osteoporosis as a cause of fracture for decades. Information on osteoporosis is starting to be incorporated into orthopaedic training program curricula.

Accurate bone mineral densitometry has been widely available for only a decade, and effective osteoporosis treatments have also been established only in recent years. Furthermore, the recognition that a patient with osteoporosis who has experienced a fracture is at very high risk for future hip fracture, a risk that can be reduced by treatment, is recent knowledge, necessary for individual staff who care for patients with a fragility fracture in fracture clinics.

D. Current Orthopaedic Practice

Osteoporosis investigation and care is still not widely considered by orthopaedic surgeons to be a part of the normal scope of practice when evaluating a patient.[55] Opinion leaders in orthopaedic surgery are currently acknowledging this problem.[56,57] In addition, the working environment in a busy fracture clinic may lack privacy, which may interfere with taking the detailed medical history necessary for elucidating the various risk factors of osteoporosis.

E. The Primary Care Physician

As part of standard practice, the consulting orthopaedic surgeon will provide a note to the primary care physician, and it is reasonable for some orthopaedic specialists to expect that osteoporosis care will fall within the responsibility of the primary care physician. However, there is currently a "care gap," in that primary care physicians may be uncertain about adopting osteoporosis care, and they may be unaware of the significance of the fragility fracture. In a study of an intervention to promote osteoporosis follow-up care pursued in five hospital fracture clinics when primary care physicians received a letter from the orthopaedic surgeon in the fracture clinic identifying the osteoporosis risk and recommending investigation and treatment, there was a significant increase in osteoporosis investigation (i.e., ordered densitometry), from 36 to 65%. However, there was, unfortunately, no significant increase in osteoporosis treatment.[58] In a series of focus groups, 32 family physicians expressed uncertainty about whom to screen for osteoporosis, when to start BMD testing, frequency of BMD testing, and how soon to expect a change with treatment. They also expressed a need for information on combinations of drugs and on the efficacy and long-term safety of drugs and non-pharmacologic interventions.[59] Other studies have found that medication costs, adverse effects of medications, co-morbidities, polypharmacy, and mental health problems in elderly people interfere with treatment of osteoporosis.[55,60]

F. LACK OF AWARENESS AMONG PATIENTS

The public currently knows more than in previous years about osteoporosis in general, because of interest in the popular media. Still, most people with fractures do not associate their injury with osteoporosis. Recent studies indicate that 89 to 97% of older individuals are aware of osteoporosis, but only half of the men realized that osteoporosis could affect them.[17,56,61] Unfortunately, most people interviewed were unclear about what could be done to prevent the condition. Men in particular appear to have an inadequate knowledge of osteoporosis, do not appreciate the fact that they may be vulnerable to bone loss, and may not participate in activities that prevent osteoporosis.[62] It is even less well appreciated by the public that fractures of the wrist, shoulder, hip, and spine caused by a simple fall are indicators of osteoporosis, and that the risk of future fracture is very high and can be markedly reduced. In fact, only 20 to 50% of patients with a fragility fracture know 1 year after the fracture that they have osteoporosis.[15,17,19] As a result, even well-informed patients may not request information about osteoporosis or may be skeptical when treatment is recommended to them.

G. OTHER FACTORS

Other factors that may discourage osteoporosis follow-up and treatment include ethnicity, socio-economic status, and gender. Non-English-speaking patients who were interviewed in hospital clinics in Toronto, in Cantonese, Mandarin, Italian, Portuguese, Vietnamese, and Hindi, were found to have less knowledge of osteoporosis and were less likely to exercise and follow nutritional practices beneficial to bone health than their English-speaking counterparts. It is likely that special efforts will be needed to intervene successfully for these patients after they sustain a fragility fracture.[63] Also, a general lack of understanding among men that they could be affected by osteoporosis is likely to influence appropriate follow-up, treatment, and compliance for this patient group. The potential effects of ethnicity, socioeconomic status, and gender on osteoporosis follow-up and treatment will require further investigation.

V. SUPPORT FOR THE DEVELOPMENT
OF SCREENING PROGRAMS

The development of screening programs with practical, workable, and sustainable recommendations is still in its infancy. Fracture clinics and individual orthopaedic surgeons who wish to improve osteoporosis care in patients with fragility fractures seen in the fracture clinic may seek useful collaborations from other organizations that have a natural interest in osteoporosis. Health-care funding organizations, such as health maintenance organizations (HMOs), other managed care plans, and Canadian provincial Ministries of Health, have a long-term interest in the development of cost-effective strategies to prevent hip fractures. Several voluntary associations, as well as pharmaceutical companies, also have a strong interest in osteoporosis care and may provide concrete assistance in the development of fragility fracture screening programs in fracture clinics. Professional associations of orthopaedic surgeons, nurses, and orthopaedic technologists also have a useful role in educating their members about osteoporosis screening and prevention programs. All of the above organizations are natural potential allies in these efforts for groups developing screening programs.

The Osteoporosis Society of Canada and the Ontario Orthopaedic Association are collaborating in the development of information materials (posters, pamphlets, tear sheets) that link a fracture occurring with minor trauma to osteoporosis and emphasize an increased risk to patients presenting with fracture for subsequent, serious fractures. While some major orthopaedic and osteoporosis organizations currently do not provide this information on their Web sites, the American Academy of Orthopaedic Surgeons and the Canadian Orthopaedic Association have sponsored information sessions at their annual meetings to increase awareness of this issue among their members.

Major pharmaceutical companies active in the field of osteoporosis have made unrestricted grants for research and education in the field of osteoporosis, including programs based in fracture clinics, targeting the patient with a fragility fracture. Specialists in internal medicine involved in osteoporosis care are often willing to cooperate in studies.

VI. ADMINISTRATIVE MECHANISMS TO IDENTIFY THE PATIENT AT RISK

An important step in a screening program is for the fracture clinic team to identify patients with fragility fractures at risk for future hip and vertebral fractures. One approach to accomplish this goal is for the chart of every patient who attends the clinic to be screened by administrative staff at the fracture clinic desk, as a standard procedure in the registration process. Every female patient over 40 and male patient over 50 years of age, who is referred or presents with a diagnosis of fracture of the wrist (distal radius), shoulder (proximal humerus), vertebral body or hip (femoral neck, intertrochanteric), is "flagged" or identified with a special chart cover to serve as a reminder or stimulus to the clinical caregivers. This step at the registration desk should be inclusive, to collect as many potential fragility fractures as possible. Those fractures that are manifestly not fragility fractures, such as a distal radius fracture suffered in a motorcycle accident by a large, robust, young male, otherwise in good health, can be excluded in a subsequent step by the orthopaedic surgeon. While the patient passes through the clinic, nurses, orthopaedic technologists, and other staff should educate the patient whose chart has been "flagged." Orthopaedic surgeons can accept the responsibility to speak to the patient about osteoporosis and to start investigation, simple treatment, and referral. The appropriate response by the orthopaedic surgeon will depend on the clinical case history, the level of preparation of the orthopaedic surgeon, and the consulting resources available in the community. An environment of cooperation among clinic staff is necessary. A weekly tally of identified or referred patients, collected by a designated staff member, may be helpful to stimulate and record the progress of screening. Practically, up to three quarters of the estimated 280 patients presenting with a fragility fracture at a typical fracture clinic annually have distal radius fractures. Even if the fracture clinic program were to extend screening only to patients with Colles' fracture, a successful initiative with this patient group alone would represent a useful contribution to the prevention of hip fractures.

VII. DISPOSITION OF PATIENTS WITH FRAGILITY FRACTURES IDENTIFIED IN FRACTURE CLINICS

A. ORTHOPAEDIC SURGEON

When the orthopaedic surgeon has determined that the patient has had a fragility fracture of the wrist, proximal humerus, vertebral body, or proximal femur, sustained with minimal trauma, he or she must be prepared, in addition to the management of the fracture, to set in motion a course of events that will result in accurate diagnosis and appropriate treatment of osteoporosis. A minimum standard of response would include the following steps:

1. Notify the patient regarding the underlying weakness of the bones, the increased risk of future hip fracture, and the ability to reduce risk through treatment.
2. Recommend investigation, where indicated.
3. Advise the patient regarding the need for adequate calcium and vitamin D intake, and in most cases, commence supplementation.

4. Discuss "bone building drugs" with the patient.
5. Refer the patient to an environment appropriate for follow-up, such as the primary care physician or an osteoporosis clinic.

It is essential that the orthopaedic surgeon help the patient understand that the fracture is probably indicative of osteoporosis and puts the patient at risk for a future hip fracture, which can be prevented with treatment.

The orthopaedic surgeon should also consider whether bone mineral densitometry should be ordered. If a densitometry facility is available within the institution that houses the fracture clinic, the procedure can be scheduled to immediately precede the next fracture clinic visit. This does not require a separate visit by the patient for testing. The result can be conveniently discussed with the patient at the visit that follows. This may serve to reinforce the education of the patient regarding osteoporosis and facilitates referral to the osteoporosis clinic or to the family physician by clarifying the level of the BMD.

Densitometry testing for a formal diagnosis of osteoporosis may not be necessary for certain groups of patients with fragility fractures, such as the frail elderly person with a serious hip fracture, who should usually be immediately treated with calcium and vitamin D, and bisphosphonates. However, for other patients with a fragility fracture, a low BMD result will confirm the osteoporosis diagnosis for the patient, improve compliance with treatment programs, and provide a baseline to determine whether or not there is improvement with treatment.

One practical approach to female patients who present with fragility fractures and low bone mass diagnosed in the fracture clinic is to classify them as follows:

1. Perimenopausal: Women in this period of life who have fragility fractures may choose to undergo hormone replacement therapy (HRT), selective estrogen receptor modulator (SERM) therapy, and/or bisphosphonates, in addition to calcium and vitamin D supplementation. This decision must be made outside the fracture clinic, by the family physician, gynecologist, or osteoporosis consultant.
2. Active elderly: Women in this group, in addition to calcium and vitamin D, are usually best managed with bisphosphonate medication.
3. Frail elderly: In this group, calcium and vitamin D alone are known to provide benefit, and a 43% reduction in hip fractures has been observed in European nursing homes when a calcium–vitamin D regimen was initiated.[64] The decision to add antiresorptive therapy, such as bisphosphonates, is controversial, and is more likely to be administered in the patient living independently who does not suffer from cognitive impairment.

In randomized clinical trials in institutionalized elderly people, padded hip protectors have been shown to reduce the risk of hip fracture by more than half.[65,66] All patients, but particularly those in groups 2 and 3 above, can benefit from fall prevention programs.

It is recognized that appropriate investigation of patients will identify a minority of women and a high proportion of men who have secondary osteoporosis on the basis of renal, gastrointestinal, inflammatory, or other conditions that require management.

Osteoporosis in males is, as noted previously, a condition that is currently poorly managed. Alendronate has been shown to be an effective treatment for osteoporosis and prevention of fractures in men.[67-69] In view of the above, males who have fragility fractures and underlying osteoporosis should generally be referred to osteoporosis consultants or clinics.

B. OTHER FRACTURE CLINIC PERSONNEL

All members of the fracture clinic team that undertakes an osteoporosis initiative, both administrative and professional, play an important role in promoting osteoporosis care for the benefit of the patients and should be empowered to raise the issue and remind each other of the joint effort.

Orthopaedic technologists can contribute substantially to the implementation of screening programs. These health-care providers spend time with the patient, applying casts, orthoses, and other devices. In our experience, when armed with the relevant information, orthopaedic technologists are highly motivated and useful allies in the education of the patient.

Nursing professionals can raise the issue of osteoporosis with the patient, indicate some of the interventions available to the patient, and prompt the surgeon regarding the condition.

Administrative staff in the fracture clinic can undertake the responsibility to flag patient charts to ensure that osteoporosis care is not forgotten in the busy clinic. In addition, administrative staff can make available and distribute printed educational materials in the clinic.

C. ADDITIONAL SUPPORT INITIATIVES

Educational and information materials that serve multiple purposes should be provided in the fracture clinic. These materials should provide osteoporosis information for patients, specifically written for the patient who has experienced a fracture, to motivate them to seek treatment. The materials can also inform the motivated patient regarding sources of information about osteoporosis, such as Web sites and toll-free telephone numbers. For example, materials distributed in fracture clinics in Ontario provide the toll-free telephone number and Web site address of the Osteoporosis Society of Canada. This organization supplies a cadre of well-prepared volunteers who provide information to members of the public who use the contact information. The materials should additionally encourage patients to discuss their condition with the family physician. Finally, the presence of printed materials in the clinic may also serve to maintain awareness of osteoporosis among fracture clinic staff.

Organizations of orthopaedic surgeons and orthopaedic technologists, which decide to promote osteoporosis care in fracture clinics, can also support these initiatives by sending fax, e-mail, or letter communications to members, recommending the above courses of action.

In most cases, it is not realistic to expect fracture clinic staff to undertake thorough investigation and treatment of osteoporosis of each patient presenting with fragility fracture. The role of the fracture clinic team is more likely to be contributory in identifying the patient at risk and initiating first steps in education of the patient, investigation, and treatment while referring the patient to an environment where definitive management is likely to occur. In a well-organized, multispecialty medical institution or organization, the line of referral for patient care is usually clear. The orthopaedic surgeon plays a key role by referring the patient and forwarding information to the primary care physician or osteoporosis consultant by means of a report or a consultation request.

VIII. TRAUMATIC FRACTURES IN PATIENTS WITH UNDIAGNOSED OSTEOPOROSIS

Although the immediate need is for patients presenting with fragility fractures to fracture clinics to be identified and referred for investigation and treatment, the fracture clinic team needs to be aware of the possibility that patients who sustain fractures through severe or major trauma may also have underlying osteoporosis. In a defined population of women who sustained either "low" or "high" trauma fractures, BMD was significantly reduced at the femoral neck, trochanter, ultradistal radius, and midradius, regardless of the severity of trauma.[70] When compared with the general population, the age-adjusted odds ratios for osteoporosis at one or more scanned sites were 2.7 and 3.1 in the low and high trauma groups, respectively. Considering the results of this study, selected patients with traumatic fractures should also undergo densitometry and be considered for referral, particularly if they present with some of the other risk factors of osteoporosis outlined earlier.

IX. CONCLUSION

Recognition of the typical fragility fracture, particularly that of the wrist, as an indicator for osteoporosis, provides the orthopaedic surgeon, fracture clinic team, and greater health-care community with an opportunity to prevent future hip fractures in an easily identified, undertreated, high-risk population. Although the concept of screening programs for osteoporosis among this group has gained acceptance, the widespread development and implementation of practical guidelines for an effective, sustainable program remain a future goal.

ACKNOWLEDGMENT

The authors thank Victoria Elliot-Gibson for reviewing the manuscript.

REFERENCES

1. Hindsø, K. and Lauritzen, J.B., "Osteoporosis and Colles' fracture," *Ugeskr. Læger,* 163, 5503, 2001.
2. Black, D.M., Arden, N.K., Palermo, L., et al., "Prevalent vertebral deformities predict hip fractures and new vertebral deformities but not wrist fractures. Study of Osteoporotic Fractures Research Group," *J. Bone Miner. Res.,* 14, 821, 1999.
3. Cuddihy, M.T., Gabriel, S.E., Crowson, C.S., et al., "Forearm fractures as predictors of subsequent osteoporotic fractures," *Osteoporos. Int.,* 9, 469, 1999.
4. Mallmin, H., Ljunghall, S., Persson, I., et al., "Fracture of the distal forearm as a forecaster of subsequent hip fracture: a population-based cohort study with 24 years of follow-up," *Calcif. Tissue Int.,* 52, 269, 1993.
5. Schroder, H.M., Petersen, K.K., and Erlandsen, M., "Occurrence and incidence of the second hip fracture," *Clin. Orthop.,* 289, 166, 1993.
6. Ross, P.D., Davis, J., Epstein, R., and Wasnich, R., "Preexisting fractures and bone mass predict vertebral fracture incidence in women," *Ann. Intern. Med.,* 114, 919, 1991.
7. Owen, R.A., Melton, L.J., III, Ilstrup, D.M., et al., "Colles' fracture and subsequent hip fracture risk," *Clin. Orthop.,* 171, 37, 1982.
8. Masud, T., Jordan, D., and Hosking, D.J., "Distal forearm fracture history in an older community-dwelling population: the Nottingham Community Osteoporosis (NOCOS) study," *Age Ageing,* 30, 255, 2001.
9. Waern, E., Johnell, O., Jutberger, H., et al., "Patients with forearm fracture should be diagnosed for osteoporosis," *J. Bone Miner. Res.,* 16, S514, 2001.
10. Earnshaw, S.A., Cawte, S.A., Worley, A., and Hosking, D.J., "Colles' fracture of the wrist as an indicator of underlying osteoporosis in postmenopausal women: a prospective study of bone mineral density and bone turnover rate," *Osteoporos. Int.,* 8, 53, 1998.
11. Bellantonio, S., Fortinsky, R., and Prestwood, K., "How well are community-living women treated for osteoporosis after hip fracture?" *J. Am. Geriatr. Soc.,* 49, 1197, 2001.
12. Black, J.N., Follin, S.L., and McDermott, M.T., "Osteoporosis diagnosis and management following hip fracture," *J. Bone Miner. Res.,* 16, S214, 2001.
13. Castel, H., Bonneh, D.Y., Sherf, M., and Liel, Y., "Awareness of osteoporosis and compliance with management guidelines in patients with newly diagnosed low-impact fractures," *Osteoporos. Int.,* 12, 559, 2001.
14. Davidson, C.W., Merrilees, M.J., Wilkinson, T.J., et al., "Hip fracture mortality and morbidity — can we do better? *N.Z. Med. J.,* 114, 329, 2001.
15. Khan, S.A., de Geus, C., Holroyd, B., and Russell, A.S., "Osteoporosis follow-up after wrist fractures following minor trauma," *Arch. Intern. Med.,* 161, 1309, 2001.
16. Orwig, D.L., Wehren, L., Yu Yahiro, J., et al., "Treatment of osteoporosis following a hip fracture: sending results of bone densitometry to primary care physicians does not increase use of pharmacologic therapy," *J. Bone Miner. Res.,* 16, S220, 2001.

17. Smith, M.D., Ross, W., and Ahern, M.J., "Missing a therapeutic window of opportunity: an audit of patients attending a tertiary teaching hospital with potentially osteoporotic hip and wrist fractures," *J. Rheumatol.*, 28, 2504, 2001.

18. Freedman, K.B., Kaplan, F.S., Bilker, W.B., et al., "Treatment of osteoporosis: are physicians missing an opportunity?" *J. Bone Joint Surg.*, 82A, 1063, 2000.

19. Hajcsar, E.E., Hawker, G., and Bogoch, E.R., "Physician practice patterns with respect to investigation and treatment for osteoporosis in patients with fragility fracture," *Can. Med. Assoc. J.*, 163, 819, 2000.

20. Gallagher, J.C., Melton, L.J., Riggs, B.L., and Bergstrath, E., "Epidemiology of fractures of the proximal femur in Rochester, Minnesota," *Clin. Orthop.*, 150, 163, 1980.

21. Cummings, S.R., Rubin, S.M., and Black, D., "The future of hip fractures in the United States. Numbers, costs, and potential effects of postmenopausal estrogen," *Clin. Orthop.*, 252, 163, 1990.

22. Papadimitropoulos, E.A., Coyte, P.C., Josse, R.G., and Greenwood, C.E., "Current and projected rates of hip fracture in Canada," *Can. Med. Assoc. J.*, 158, 870, 1997.

23. Ontario Orthopaedic Association, Board Retreat Minutes, January 11–13, 2001.

24. Wiktorowicz, M.E., Goeree, R., Papaioannou, A., et al., "Economic implications of hip fracture: health service use, institutional care and cost in Canada," *Osteoporos. Int.*, 12, 271, 2001.

25. Cree, M., Soskolne, C.L., Belseck, E., et al., "Mortality and institutionalization following hip fracture," *J. Am. Geriatr. Soc.*, 48, 283, 2000.

26. Sanders, K.M., Nicholson, G.C., Ugoni, A.M., et al., "Health burden of hip and other fractures in Australia beyond 2000," *Med. J. Aust.*, 170, 467, 1999.

27. Walker, N., Norton, R., Vander Hoorn, S., et al., "Mortality after hip fracture: regional variations in New Zealand," *N.Z. Med. J.*, 112, 269, 1999.

28. Diamond, T.H., Thornley, S.W., Sekel, R., and Smerdely, P., "Hip fracture in elderly men: prognostic factors and outcomes," *Med. J. Aust.*, 167, 412, 1997.

29. Keene, G.S., Parker, M.J., and Pryor, G.A., "Mortality and morbidity after hip fractures," *Br. Med. J.*, 307, 1248, 1993.

30. Jette, A.M., Harris, B.A., Cleary, P.D., and Campion, E.W., "Functional recovery after hip fracture," *Arch. Phys. Med. Rehabil.*, 68, 735, 1987.

31. Forsen, L., Sogaard, A.J., Meyer, H.E., et al., "Survival after hip fracture: short- and long-term excess mortality according to age and gender," *Osteoporos. Int.*, 10, 73, 1999.

32. Poor, G., Atkinson, E.J., O'Fallon, W.M., and Melton, L.J., III, "Determinants of reduced survival following hip fractures in men," *Clin. Orthop.*, 319, 260, 1995.

33. Cooper, C., "The crippling consequences of fractures and their impact on quality of life," *Am. J. Med.*, 103, 12S, 1997.

34. Cumming, R.G., Klineberg, R., and Katelaris, A., "Cohort study of institutionalization after hip fracture," *Aust. J. Public Health*, 20, 579, 1996.

35. Siris, E.S., Miller, P.D., Barrett-Connor, E., et al., "Identification and fracture outcomes of undiagnosed low bone mineral density in postmenopausal women: results from the National Osteoporosis Risk Assessment," *J. Am. Med. Assoc.*, 286, 2815, 2001.

36. Riggs, B.L. and Melton, L.J., III, "Involutional osteoporosis," *N. Engl. J. Med.*, 314, 1676, 1986.

37. Gallagher, J.C., Melton, L.J., III, and Riggs, B.L., "Examination of prevalence rates of possible risk factors in a population with a fracture of the proximal femur," *Clin. Orthop.*, 153, 158, 1980.

38. Eastell, R., Reid, D.M., Compston, J., et al., "Secondary prevention of osteoporosis: when should a non-vertebral fracture be a trigger for action?" *Q. J. Med.*, 94, 575, 2001.

39. Mirsky, E.C. and Einhorn, T.A., "Bone densitometry in orthopaedic practice," *J. Bone Joint Surg.*, 80A, 1687, 1998.

40. Marshall, D., Johnell, O., and Wedel, H., "Meta-analysis of how well measures of bone mineral density predict occurrence of osteoporotic fractures," *Br. Med. J.*, 312, 1254, 1996.

41. Burger, H., de Laet, C.E., van Daele, P.L., et al., "Risk factors for increased bone loss in an elderly population: the Rotterdam Study," *Am. J. Epidemiol.*, 147, 871, 1998.

42. Kanis, J.A. and Adami, S., "Bone loss in the elderly," *Osteoporos. Int.*, 4, S59, 1994.

43. National Institutes of Health, Osteoporosis Prevention, Diagnosis, and Therapy, NIH Consensus Statement, March 27–29, 2000.

44. National Osteoporosis Foundation, *Physician's Guide to Prevention and Treatment of Osteoporosis*, Washington, D.C., 1998.

45. Osteoporosis Society of Canada, "Prevention and management of osteoporosis: consensus statements from the Scientific Advisory Board of the Osteoporosis Society of Canada," *Can. Med. Assoc. J.,* 155, S921, 1996.

46. Ontario Program for Optimal Therapeutics, "Ontario Guidelines for the Prevention and Treatment of Osteoporosis," Printer Publications Ontario, Queens Printer of Ontario, Toronto, 2000.

47. Guthrie, J.R., Ebeling, P.R., Hopper, J.L., et al., "A prospective study of bone loss in menopausal Australian-born women," *Osteoporos. Int.,* 8, 282, 1998.

48. Melton, L.J., III, Atkinson, E.J., O'Connor, M.K., et al., "Bone density and fracture risk in men," *J. Bone Miner. Res.,* 13, 1915, 1998.

49. Herron, C., Harrington, L., Mobbs, K., et al., "Evaluation of osteopenia and osteoporosis in five groups of men, aged 65–93 years," *J. Bone Miner. Res.,* 16, S516, 2001.

50. Krall, E.A., Anderson, J.J., Miller, D.R., et al., "Parental and individual histories of fracture are associated with osteoporosis in men," *J. Bone Miner. Res.,* 16, S517, 2001.

51. Olszynski, W.P., Polischuk, C.O., Drinkwater, D.T., et al., "Effect of cigarette smoking and alcohol consumption on bone mineral density in men — data from the Canadian Multicentre Osteoporosis Study (CaMos)," *J. Bone Miner. Res.,* 16, S517, 2001.

52. Prelevic, G.M., "Osteoporosis in men," *J. R. Soc. Med.,* 94, 620, 2001.

53. Kelepouris, N., Harper, K.D., Gannon, F., et al., "Severe osteoporosis in men," *Ann. Intern. Med.,* 123, 452, 1995.

54. Center, J.R., Nguyen, T.V., Schneider, D., et al., "Mortality after all major types of osteoporotic fracture in men and women: an observational study," *Lancet,* 353, 878, 1999.

55. Simonelli, C., Killeen, K., Mehle, S., and Swanson, L., "Barriers to osteoporosis identification and treatment among primary care physicians and orthopedic surgeons," *Mayo Clin. Proc.*, 77, 334, 2002.

56. Tosi, L.L. and Lane, J.M., "Osteoporosis prevention and the orthopaedic surgeon: when fracture care is not enough," *J. Bone Joint Surg.,* 80A, 1567, 1998.

57. Rosier, R.N., "Expanding the role of the orthopaedic surgeon in the treatment of osteoporosis," *Clin. Orthop. Rel. Res.*, 385, 57, 2001.

58. Rideout, R., Hawker, G.A., Mahomed, N., and Bogoch, E.R., "An intervention to increase investigation and treatment of osteoporosis in fragility fracture patients," presented at American Society for Bone and Mineral Research, 22nd Annual Meeting, Toronto, Ontario, 2000, S294.

59. Jaglal, S.B., Hawker, G., Carroll, J., et al., "Information needs of family physicians for the management of osteoporosis," *J. Bone Miner. Res.,* 16, S290, 2001.

60. McKercher, H.G., Crilly, R.G., and Kloseck, M., "Osteoporosis management in long-term care. Survey of Ontario physicians," *Can. Fam. Physician*, 46, 2228, 2000.

61. Juby, A.G. and Davis, P., "A prospective evaluation of the awareness, knowledge, risk factors and current treatment of osteoporosis in a cohort of elderly subjects," *Osteoporos. Int.,* 12, 617, 2001.

62. Sedlak, C.A., Doheny, M.O., and Estok, P.J., "Osteoporosis in older men: knowledge and health beliefs," *Orthop. Nurs.*, 19, 38, 2000.

63. Cheung, A., personal communication, University Health Network, University of Toronto, Toronto, Canada, 2002.

64. Chapuy, M.C., Arlto, M.E., Duboeuf, F., et al., "Vitamin D3 and calcium to prevent hip fractures in elderly women," *N. Engl. J. Med.,* 327, 1637, 1992.

65. Kannus, P., Parkkari, J., Niemi, S., et al., "Prevention of hip fracture in elderly people with use of a hip protector," *N. Engl. J. Med.,* 343, 1506, 2000.

66. Lauritzen, J.B., Petersen, M.M., and Lund, B., "Effect of external hip protectors on hip fractures," *Lancet,* 341, 11, 1993.

67. Diamond, T., Sambrook, P., Williamson, M., et al., "Guidelines for treatment of osteoporosis in men," *Aust. Fam. Physician,* 30, 787, 2001.

68. Ringe, J.D., Faber, H., and Dorst, A., "Alendronate treatment of established primary osteoporosis in men: results of a 2-year prospective study," *J. Clin. Endocrinol. Metab.,* 86, 5252, 2001.

69. Orwoll, E., Ettinger, M., Weiss, S., et al., "Alendronate for the treatment of osteoporosis in men," *N. Engl. J. Med.,* 343, 604, 2000.

70. Sanders, K.M., Pasco, J.A., Ugoni, A.M., et al., "The exclusion of high trauma fractures may underestimate the prevalence of bone fragility fractures in the community: the Geelong Osteoporosis Study," *J. Bone Miner. Res.,* 13, 1337, 1998.

Part III

Surgical Management of Osteoporotic Fractures

14 Reactions of Normal and Osteoporotic Bone to Fixation Devices

Ermanno Bonucci

CONTENTS

I. INTRODUCTION

The internal fixation of bone is carried out through a surgical operation in which one or more skeletal segments are stabilized by inserting artificial devices into the bone. The main aim of this procedure is to reconstitute the anatomic continuity and functional integrity of a bone, rather in the same way as a mechanic may weld the various parts of a damaged metal scaffolding together by using devices such as screws, nails, plates, and wires. This similarity, however, only goes so far, because the mechanic joins up various pieces of inorganic materials, whereas the surgeon connects bone, a living tissue, to completely different, extraneous, nonliving materials. So, after an initial phase when the fixation devices hold the bone segments together through a surgical assemblage (primary fixation) — and here the comparison with a mechanical welding is plausible — a second phase inevitably involves the reparative reaction of bone. This phase leads either to further stabilization (secondary fixation) of the devices used, if these are surrounded and permeated by new bone, or to their loosening, if bone resorption prevails at the interface. Most of the problems connected with internal fixation derive from the contact between inorganic, nonliving materials and bone — an organic, living material. The topic has been reviewed several times.[1-5]

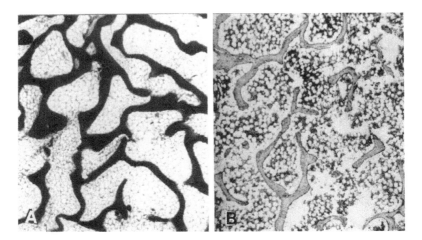

FIGURE 14.1 Needle biopsies of the iliac crest of (A) a young (24-year-old) and (B) an elderly (65-year-old) woman; the spongy bone consists of many, frequently connected trabeculae in (A) and of a few, often disconnected, trabeculae in (B). A, Von Kossa, original magnification ×20; B, Azure II–Methylene blue, original magnification ×30.

II. BONE AS A LIVING TISSUE

Even when it is highly mineralized, bone is not petrified in a perpetually static condition. Its stonelike appearance masks a number of cellular activities that make it a living tissue. Proof of this is given by the observation that the death of its cells, especially osteocytes, causes tissue to die, i.e., transforms it into a mineralized foreign body that the organism tries to eliminate as quickly as possible. A clear example of this event is the resorption of bone that follows aseptic osteonecrosis in patients treated with corticosteroids.[6]

Although normal cell function is a prerequisite for the survival of any type of bone, the degree of cellular activity and, therefore, the reaction to fixation devices differ between bone types. This difference chiefly depends on divergences between types of bone structure, implying varying degrees of metabolic activity.[7,8] This appears to be mainly regulated by the topographic relationship of bone cells with blood vessels, many of which are present in spongy bone, but relatively few in compact bone.

Spongy bone (Figure 14.1), also called trabecular or cancellous bone, is found in the body of short bones (vertebrae), diploe of the skull, maxillofacial bones, the inner portion of some long and flat bones (osseous ribs, iliac bones, scapulae), and the metaphyseal spongiosa of long bones (femur, tibia, humerus, etc.). It is contained and surrounded by a thin layer of compact bone, which forms the cortical bone. Spongy bone consists of rod- or leaflike osseous trabeculae (Figure 14.1A) which are connected in a three-dimensional framework. The architectural arrangement of this frame is not casual. The trabeculae in a skeletal segment, in fact, are mostly oriented with their major axis parallel to the main direction of the mechanical forces that are physiologically supported by that segment. This typical arrangement can be found in the vertebral bodies, femoral neck, calcaneus, etc.[9] The connections between adjacent trabeculae (also referred to as bone connectivity), together with bone volume, are the factors mainly responsible for bone strength, as shown by the observation that even a slight and partial demolition of the trabecular frame may be followed by fractures.[10,11] The trabeculae delimit spaces that contain sinusoidal blood vessels and, closely related to them, the hemopoietic cells of the bone marrow, including stem cells, which may be osteoblast precursors.[12] The width of these spaces varies with the skeletal segment, and increases with age (see below and Figure 14.1B). Their content changes, too, because with aging the red bone marrow (i.e., the hemopoietically active marrow) is partly or totally transformed into yellow bone marrow (i.e., hemopoietic cells are substituted by adipose cells).

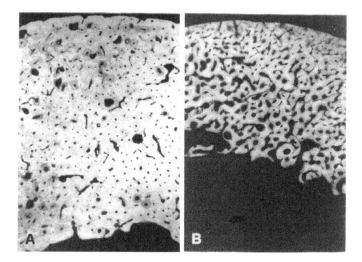

FIGURE 14.2 Microradiographs of cross sections of the middle part of the femoral diaphysis of (A) a young (30-year-old) and (B) an elderly (80-year-old) man. The compact bone mainly consists of osteons in (A) whereas it shows a spongy appearance and the resorption of the inner third of the compacta in (B). Ground sections, original magnification ×7.

Compact bone (Figure 14.2) mainly consists of mineralized matrix whose collagen fibrils may have a disordered arrangement (woven bone) or be gathered in lamellae (lamellar bone).[13] Woven bone is found in the skeleton of the fetus, and in cases of pathologic or reparative bone formation. Fetal bone may partly consist of lamellar bone, but this type of bone is characteristic of the adult skeleton, especially of the diaphysis of the long bones, where it forms an inner and an outer circumferential system and an intermediate, wide osteonic zone (Figure 14.2A).[14] All these parts change with age: compact bone may become osteopenic or osteoporotic, and the inner circumferential system may be completely resorbed (see below and Figure 14.2B). Hemopoietic cells are not found in compact bone, and most of the blood vessels run in canals of osteons. The structure of spongy and compact bone has been reviewed several times.[13-15]

The considerable diversity in structure and composition between spongy and compact bone clearly accounts for their different degrees of metabolic activity, which are much greater in the former than in the latter. More surprisingly, differences have also been reported between parts of the skeleton that have a similar structure and composition and might be expected to have comparable metabolic activities. This applies, for example, to periosteal zones in uremic rats, which have an appositional rate lower than that of the endosteal zones,[16] and to axial metaphyseal trabeculae, whose degree of bone resorption exceeds that of the peripheral trabeculae in normal dogs,[7] ovariectomized rats,[17-19] and immobilized skeletal segments.[20] These findings suggest that there may be two types of bone, one of which has essentially mechanical functions, whereas the other mainly reacts to metabolic demands.

III. THE REACTIVE, OR REPARATIVE, PROCESSES OF BONE

When the bone tissue is altered for any reason whatever, a reaction is set off that aims to remove the disturbing cause and repair any tissue damage already done. Similar to what occurs in any other tissue of the organism, the reaction process eventually becomes reparative, and its rapidity and completeness chiefly depend on the severity of the initial pathologic changes, and the degree of cellular activity of the tissue. Because of the structural differences reported above, especially in terms of vascularity, the reactivity of the spongy bone to pathologic stimulation, although it varies a little with the skeletal zone, is always more rapid and intense than that of the compact bone. The

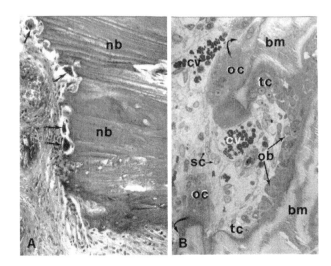

FIGURE 14.3 (A) Wall of the cavity left by the withdrawal of a mobilized osteosynthesis: osteoclasts (arrows) are in contact with fragments of necrotic bone (nb); inflammatory, granulomatous tissue is present on left. (Hematoxylin-eosin, original magnification ×220. (B) A BMU established on the surface of an osseous trabecula: a wide resorption lacuna has been produced by two osteoclasts (oc), which seem to be moving in the direction of the arrows, leaving behind them a few transitional cells (tc); most of the lacunar wall is covered by osteoblasts (ob). Calcified bone matrix (bm), capillary vessels (cv) and stromal cells (sc) are also visible. (Azure II–Methylene blue, original magnification ×350.)

cellular mechanism involved, however, is practically the same in all skeletal segments and is independent of bone type and structure.

The two cell types essentially responsible for the bone reaction, and eventually involved in bone repair, are osteoclasts, whose function is to remove the calcified matrix, bone fragments, or dead bone (Figure 14.3A), and osteoblasts, whose function is to synthesize new matrix. These cell types also govern so-called bone remodeling, i.e., the bone demolition–reconstruction process within bone, which is always active in the normal skeleton. Bone remodeling is a physiologic process comprising a series of coordinated cellular activities, which normally ensure a well-balanced sequence of bone resorption and formation. During the process, microscopic portions of bone matrix are resorbed by osteoclasts, and are then reconstructed by osteoblasts; the outcome is the complete reconstitution of the bone segment. This apparently useless process is governed by two principal mechanisms: the mechanical forces the tissue resists, and the regulation of serum calcium concentrations.

Mechanical forces have important effects on the way bone cells function. It has been proposed by Frost[21-25] that bone tissue is influenced by mechanical stresses according to a mechanism he called a "mechanostat." According to this concept, a stress induces a bone strain (that is, a deformation, which is actually a microstrain, measured in μm/m); this in its turn stimulates the metabolic activity of bone cells. If the strain is lower than the physiologic threshold, osteogenic activity is forestalled and bone volume falls; if, on the other hand, it is above the physiologic threshold, osteogenic activity is stimulated and bone volume rises. The stimulus induced by the microstrain might be transduced to the osteoblasts and/or the osteoclasts through the three-dimensional network formed by the cytoplasmic processes of the osteocytes, [26-28] with the triggering factor probably the synthesis of osteopontin.[29]

The second mechanism promoting bone remodeling is connected with the regulation of the serum calcium concentration.[30] It is known that, as far as possible, the value of calcemia is kept constant by the organism through three interrelated processes: intestinal calcium absorption, renal excretion of calcium ions, and bone resorption. This last process occurs whenever the serum calcium concentration tends to fall: the parathyroid glands are stimulated and produce parathyroid hormone; this itself stimulates the formation and activation of osteoclasts. These resorb the bone matrix, so releasing calcium ions from the mineral substance and raising serum calcium concentration.

If the osteoclastic resorption of the bone matrix were the only process triggered by hypocalcemia, bone volume would rapidly fall, causing severe osteopenia. In reality, the resorption of the calcified matrix is followed by its reconstitution by the osteoblast, whose activity leads to the complete repair of the resorption cavity left by the osteoclast. This balance between bone resorption and bone formation occurs in the so-called basic multicellular units (BMUs), i.e., transient complexes of cells that form in focal microscopic zones of the endosteal surfaces, and develop through different, almost contemporaneous phases, during which microscopic portions of calcified matrix are sequentially resorbed and rebuilt.[31-34] These phases include the activation phase, during which osteoclasts are recruited and collected on the endosteal surface; the resorption phase, during which they resorb a fraction, or quantum, of bone matrix, with the formation of a resorption lacuna; the reversion phase, during which they move away from the resorption lacuna, giving way to what appear to be transitional or post-osteoclastic cells; and the formation phase, during which osteoblasts synthesize new bone matrix until the lacuna has been completely rebuilt (Figure 14.3B).

The cellular activities that occur in the BMU, and the coupling between osteoclastic and osteoblastic functions, are regulated by a number of circulating substances (parathyroid hormone, $1,25(OH)_2D_3$, estrogens, calcitonin, etc.) and local growth factors (transforming growth factor-β, or TGF-β, superfamily, and, especially, the bone morphogenetic protein, or BMP).[35] All these substances and factors play a role in ensuring the delicate equilibrium that maintains the integrity of the skeleton during bone remodeling.

Obviously, any dysfunction in BMU regulation may have local or even general effects on the state of the skeleton and on the reactive, or reparative, processes of bone. The application of an internal fixation may cause osseous changes not only because of direct damage to the bone structure, but also because the normal process of bone remodeling is disturbed. As reported below, this may be mainly due to an upsetting of the balance between mechanical forces and to consequent shifts in the mechanostat control.

IV. FACTORS CONTROLLING THE REACTION OF BONE TO FIXATION DEVICES

Because the reaction to damage done to bone basically depends on the activity of osteoclasts and osteoblasts, it is controlled by the same systemic and local factors that regulate the function of the BMU. In any case, interactions between these factors, which have a high degree of complexity even in normal bone, may be further complicated by additional local or general factors when the reaction occurs in pathologic conditions. One typical example is the reaction of bone to internal fixation, because in this case the activity of the osseous cells may be modified both by the preexisting pathologic changes that make osteosynthesis necessary and by the new ones arising from osteosynthesis itself.

Systemic and local factors, and those connected with the bone state and the presence of implanted material, will steer the evolution of the osteosynthesis either toward a satisfactory degree of osseointegration or toward a greater or smaller degree of instability. The term *osseointegration* refers to a condition, recognizable under the light microscope, of perfect adhesion between the implanted device and bone without the interposition of fibrous tissue or other organic substance (Figure 14.4A and B).[36] In this case, the trabeculae formed around the implanted material are all alive, continuity is usually established with the preexisting trabeculae or the compact bone, and the osteosynthesis is fixed and stable. Perfect osseointegration is, however, difficult to attain, and

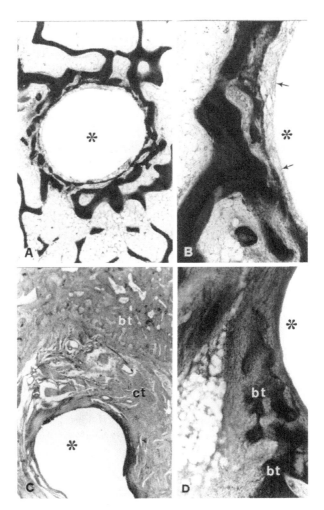

FIGURE 14.4 Relationship between osteosynthesis and bone; the implanted device has been removed to allow the histologic sections to be cut, and an empty space (asterisk) is visible in its place. (A) High degree of osseointegration: osseous trabeculae closely surround the implant; they are connected with the trabeculae of the neighboring spongy bone. (B) Detail of (A) showing the normal structure of the trabeculae and the very small amount of organic material (arrows) present between them and the implant. (C) Very low degree of osseointegration: the implant is surrounded by fibrous connective tissue (ct); there are few bone trabeculae (bt) and they are placed at a distance from the osteosynthesis. (D) Detail of (C) showing fibrous connective tissue containing small, irregular, randomly scattered bone trabeculae (bt). Hematoxylin-eosin; A and C, original magnification ×30; B and D, original magnification ×80.

the implanted material may be to some extent in contact with fibrous tissue instead of bone (Figure 14.4C and D). In this case, there are few osseous trabeculae, they are not connected with one another or with the preexisting bone, and the osteosynthesis remains unstable. The main factors capable of affecting the evolution of the osteosynthesis in one direction or another are the skeletal changes occurring prior to osteosynthesis, the bone alterations induced by surgery, the nature of the materials used for osteosynthesis, the characteristics of their surface and the formation of wear debris, the use of coated materials, and the mechanical forces applied to the osteosynthesis. These factors are active at the bone–implant interface, where processes promoting or inhibiting osteogenesis, or inducing the development of inflammation, can deeply affect osseointegration. Obviously, this also depends on the local and general condition of the bone tissue.

A. Bone Changes Prior to Osteosynthesis

The internal fixation of a skeletal segment is obviously carried out as a therapy for prior alterations in bone, whether traumatic, inflammatory, neoplastic, or of another type. The severity of these alterations may vary widely, so they may modify the reaction of bone to varying degrees, often slowing or even preventing healing. The multiplicity of bone fragments in a comminuted fracture, the soft tissue lesions that may occur in a compound fracture, the presence of neoplastic tissue or inflammatory exudate, or the onset of a metabolic bone disease, such as osteoporosis, are a few examples of conditions that can interfere with cellular activity and greatly influence the reaction of bone. They should never be disregarded in devising a plan for the internal fixation of bone.

B. Bone Changes Due to Surgery

The internal fixation of bone necessarily requires an invasive, bloody surgical operation that may itself induce fresh bone damage. Although the additional damage is usually mild and transitory, it should not be neglected, because it may prevent the primary fixation of the implant. On the other hand, it is difficult to eliminate, depending as it does on the difficulty of the operation and the ability of the surgeon, the type of osteosynthesis, the normal or pathologic condition of the skeleton, and other variables. In this connection, one need only recall that the simple application of a screw (or of any other fixation device), whether preceded or not by the preparation of an appropriate cavity by drilling, inevitably causes hemorrhage and necrosis in the bone matrix. Necrosis may also be produced by excessive heat production, or by the pressure that is needed to insert the fixation device (press-fit osteosynthesis) into the bone matrix. If excessive, the pressure may produce burst fractures or microfractures, especially if the cavity that has been prepared is too narrow, or if the bone is osteoporotic (see below). The dead tissue is subsequently removed by osteoclasts, and the resorption process, even if usually limited to a thin layer of the matrix close to the surface of the screw, may enlarge the osseous cavity and temporarily destabilize the fixation device.[37] A reparative osteoblastic process can then consolidate the screw, although the definitive consolidation may be prevented or slowed by the presence of bone particles at the interface.[38] To improve the primary fixation, Ogiso et al.[39] suggest first preparing the cavity and then waiting 2 weeks to apply the osteosynthesis after the necrotic bone and its particles have been removed.

The primary fixation of the osteosynthesis may be delayed or prevented by the intrusion of germs in the surgical area, either because they have an external origin or because the fixation device crosses an area of osteomyelitis. Similarly, the transportation and spread of neoplastic cells can occur if the osteosynthesis passes through a primary or secondary tumor.

An internal fixation through the medullary canal may induce the removal of the bone marrow and/or its necrosis. Theoretically, this should impair the reparative processes, because the stromal cells of the bone marrow are precursors of the cells of the osteoblastic lineage[40,41] and their removal might induce a defective formation of osteoblasts. This potential damage, however, appears to be balanced by the activity of osteoblastic cells that derive from the mesenchymal stem cells present on the endosteal surfaces.[42]

C. Materials for Osteosynthesis

Several of the reactions by bone to osteosynthesis depend on the nature, composition, and structure of the material used for internal fixation. Although such reactions have the primary aim of eliminating the foreign material inserted into bone, they inevitably induce secondary changes in the bone matrix. These develop slowly and, as a result, are especially prominent when a material has been left in bone for a long time. They are therefore more severe in the case of permanent osteoprostheses than of transitory osteosyntheses. The latter may, however, last long enough to produce dangerous effects, which sometimes develop very rapidly, so leading to the premature removal of the implant. For these reasons, there have been a large number of studies on the properties of implant and prosthetic materials.[43] They have led to the discovery of the so-called bioinert materials (oxide ceramics, carbon materials, some oxidized metals), that is, materials (often called biomaterials) that do not interfere with the reparative processes of bone or elicit adverse reactions. Bioactive materials (bioceramics and bioglasses) have also been described, i.e., biomaterials that should promote the formation of direct bonds with the bone matrix. On the basis of their characteristics, plenty of biomaterials have been tested in bone and soft tissues, so that as early as 1980 Hench[44] was able to list about 40 different types of them. It is outside the scope of this chapter to evaluate these materials in detail, or analyze each as to its stiffness or elasticity, resistance to stress, and persistence in the skeleton, although these properties may strongly affect the evolution of the internal fixation.

The most important feature for a biomaterial is its biological compatibility, i.e., its suitability for acceptance by the host tissue without eliciting particularly unfavorable biological reactions.[43-46] In the case of bone, a "biocompatible" material is one that is quickly surrounded by new bone, so that close contact between the surface of the material and that of bone is set up and persists. The process leads to a stabilization of the osteosynthesis, which thus becomes osseointegrated in the skeleton.

Unfortunately, fully biocompatible materials do not exist, and only a very few induce no more than a mild reaction in bone. Moreover, in the case of osteosynthesis they must be sufficiently strong to resist mechanical stresses, so that their number is further reduced and hardly goes beyond metallic materials. Organic, biodegradable polymers and composites (polyethylene, polylactic acid, polyglycolic acid, polydioxanone, etc.) have been proposed[46-48] and are currently being tested,[49-52] on the assumption that their slow biological degradation might avoid their surgical removal after healing. Although these substances are not completely inert[53,54] and their degradation is not yet under control,[50] their use in clinical practice will undoubtedly increase in the near future.[55]

The metals most commonly used in orthopaedics are titanium, stainless steel, cobalt, chromium, and their alloys.[56-59] They all display high mechanical strength and resistance to corrosion, are nontoxic to the host tissue, and are relatively inert with respect to osseous cells and associated structures. None of them, however, can completely replace bone, because none possesses complete biocompatibility. Moreover, their high stiffness limits the shifting of mechanical forces to the surrounding bone, which may tend to become underloaded and, therefore, osteoporotic.

D. Wear Debris

The presence of wear debris at the bone–implant interface is very frequent and depends mainly on the nature of the material used. Such debris is produced both by inorganic, nondegradable materials, and by organic, biodegradable materials. Moreover, quantities of wear debris are affected by local conditions, above all micromovements. These may not only abnormally compress focal zones of the bone surface, so inducing osteocyte death and necrosis, but can also loosen free particles by superficially abrading the material. Amounts of wear debris vary with the duration of the implant in bone. As a result, it is especially frequent in total hip or knee replacement,[60] but can also be found, sometimes very soon after surgery, in nonpermanent implants such as those used in osteosynthesis. Extraneous particles, on the other hand, may be unintentionally inserted into the interface by the surgeon.

Wear debris can have different shapes and sizes, can be birefringent under the polarizing microscope, and can have a heterogeneous composition, sometimes consisting of metalloproteic complexes that may give rise to "metallosis" in the surrounding tissues and even migrate to lymph nodes and other extraskeletal tissues. They are foreign bodies, and as such give rise to an aseptic, foreign-body inflammation.

E. Coated Materials

The surface of the implanted materials has been modified in various ways in an attempt to increase the degree of primary fixation, avoiding as far as possible the formation of wear debris at the interface, and improving and speeding the osseointegration process. Two main procedures have been tried: the use of materials with a porous surface, or a recourse to materials whose surface is coated with special substances.[61-63] As already discussed, the first procedure should increase bone–implant stabilization by improving vascular proliferation into, and bone formation within the pores; the second should improve the bone–implant contact by filling any gaps that may be present at the interface,[64] so reducing micromovements. It may also promote osteogenesis if the coated substance has osteogenic activity. Primary fixation can also be facilitated by using cements, especially in the case of prosthesis implantation. The cements may damage the bone surface, either because of heat development during their polymerization or by eliciting a foreign body, giant-cell reaction with the formation of a synovia-like membrane.[65,66]

The devices used for internal fixation may be coated with either osteoconductive or osteoinductive materials, or a combination of the two. Osteoconduction is promoted by spongy materials (for example, porous hydroxyapatite) whose pores may be permeated by capillary vessels and, together with these, by cells of the osteoblastic lineage.[67] Osteoinduction is due to substances that stimulate the modulation of mesenchymal cells into cells of the osteoblast lineage.[68] This effect may be produced by demineralized bone matrix,[69] or by growth factors, chiefly those of the TGF-β superfamily[70,71] and, specifically, BMP.[72,73] If adsorbed on osteoconductive materials, from which it may be gradually released after implantation, BMP can give them osteoinductive properties.[74-79] This procedure has been tested with other materials such as TGF-β and IGF to stimulate bone formation,[71,72] bisphosphonates to reduce bone resorption,[80] and antibiotics to treat osteomyelitis.[81]

The research done on this topic has, above all, been concerned with definitively implanted prostheses for which the problem of secondary fixation is much more important than for transitory osteosyntheses. In this connection, several coating materials, especially hydroxyapatite,[82] have been tested.[83] In several trials, no advantages have been observed with the use of hydroxyapatite-coated prostheses,[84,85] whereas in many others improved degrees of stabilization and osseointegration have been obtained.[62,83,86-88] Studies on hydroxyapatite-coated osteosyntheses have provided similarly favorable results, independent of the smoothness or roughness of the surface of the coated material.[89-93] In the author's personal experience, implants of porous hydroxyapatite mixed with fibrin glue have invariably ensured a very satisfactory degree of bone formation and regeneration (Figure 14.5B).[68,94]

F. Mechanical Forces

If successful, the internal fixation of a skeletal segment should hardly alter the distribution of forces normally applied to it. For a variety of reasons, this ideal result is only rarely achieved: slight anatomic and structural variations, in fact, frequently occur in reconstructing the integrity of bone; the bone–metal contact is unlikely to be uniform or complete, and gaps may be formed at the interface, so that the contact zones are overloaded, whereas those without contact are unloaded; the stiffness of the material itself, which is usually much greater than that of bone, easily induces segmental overloads or underloads, or stress-shielding, in the implanted segment.

In line with the mechanostat principle already mentioned, the unloading of skeletal segments leads to the uncoupling of osteoclast and osteoblast activity, with the prevalence of bone resorption and the development of localized osteoporosis. This process is often prominent in the case of hip prostheses, because the stiff intramedullary nail easily causes underloading of the upper portion of the femoral diaphyseal bone, which turns osteopenic. On the other hand, while some bone segments are underloaded, others are necessarily overloaded. The excessive pressure on circumscribed zones

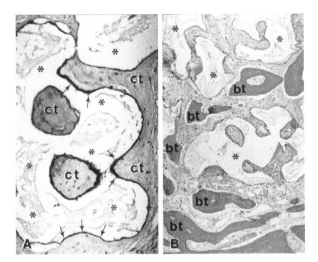

FIGURE 14.5 Implants of granular, porous hydroxyapatite mixed with fibrin glue; the specimens have been decalcified and the solubilized hydroxyapatite has left empty spaces (asterisks) which mirror its form. (A) Thirty days after implantation: organic material adsorbed on the hydroxyapatite surface appears as a deeply stained, thin border (arrows). The hydroxyapatite pores are filled by dense connective tissue (ct). (B) At 4 months after implantation, bone trabeculae (bt) have developed in the hydroxyapatite pores. (Azure II–methylene blue; original magnifications: A ×220, B ×60.)

of the skeleton, such as that often produced by compression plates, induces nutritional disturbance,[95] and increases the pressure of the interstitial fluid which itself causes osteocyte death and bone necrosis.[96-98] These events cause aseptic bone inflammation, which stimulates osteoclast activation and bone resorption, causing irregular enlargement of the interface, and allowing micromovements. If the excessive pressure persists, the inflammation becomes chronic and gives rise to the development of a granulation tissue at the interface (see below).

V. THE INTERFACE

The interaction between implanted materials and bone mainly occurs at their interface. As discussed above, the introduction of an internal fixation device, especially with the press-fit method, itself causes mechanical damage in bone that can, however, be quickly repaired. So the possibility of attaining a satisfactory primary fixation followed by a high degree of osseointegration is, initially, mainly dependent on the state of bone,[37] whereas it is later largely determined by the characteristics of the biomaterial, especially of its surface.[99] In this connection, Schwartz and Boyan[100] state that, at least *in vitro*, the mesenchymal cells are conditioned by the chemical composition of the material and by three main interrelated surface properties: surface energy, surface roughness (or porosity), and surface topography. Porosity promotes the ingrowth in the pores of capillaries, together with cells of osteoblastic lineage, enhancing the bonding of the metal with the bone tissue,[101] but it may also stimulate osteoblast proliferation and differentiation.[102] Moreover, the characteristics of the material surface may regulate the adsorption of organic molecules from the surrounding fluids[103-105] and may give rise to the formation of a surface coating to which the cells respond.[106] In this regard, the immunohistochemical demonstration that osteopontin is adsorbed on the implant surface[107-110] seems a special focus of interest. This protein, in fact, is not only potentially capable of allowing bone cells to adhere, but may also promote or constitute a bond between apposing substrates.[107] The metal surface may actually regulate cell adhesion by determining the type of integrins produced by the osteoblast.[111-113]

A. Evolution of the Interface

Once the bone changes directly caused by surgery have been repaired, the adsorption processes mentioned above lead to the formation at the interface of a thin layer of amorphous material, resembling a cementing line and containing osteopontin,[107-109,114] osteocalcin,[109] bone sialoprotein,[108] and proteoglycans.[115] *In vitro* studies show that there are no collagen fibrils in this early phase, which is characterized by the appearance of nanocrystalline calcium phosphate. The collagen fibrils are formed and mineralized at a later stage;[108] this leads eventually to the formation of osseous trabeculae around the implant. This sequence is confirmed by what occurs when porous hydroxyapatite is implanted to permit bone reconstruction (Figure 14.5): in this case, too, the first mark of osteogenesis is the appearance on the hydroxyapatite surface of a thin glycoproteic layer[94,116] containing glycoconjugates, osteopontin, osteocalcin, α2HS-glycoprotein, and albumin.[117]

The adsorption of organic material on the metal surface certainly favors the evolution of osteosynthesis, primarily because of the already noted adhesive properties of some of the components. The positive role of the metal surface may, however, be outweighed by negative effects arising from the presence of the metal itself. The dissolution and corrosion of its surface can, in fact, free soluble components that may damage cells or inhibit their development and function, so preventing the process of osseointegration. Other factors, especially abnormal mechanical forces applied to the osteosynthesis, micromovements, and the formation of wear debris, may have an inhibitory activity, or elicit an inflammatory reaction comprising the formation of a granulation tissue at the interface.

B. Development of Inflammation at the Bone–Implant Interface

Bone damage prior to osteosynthesis and produced at surgery both induce a usually mild aseptic inflammatory reaction that subsides as the hemorrhage, necrosis, and any other pathologic elements are absorbed and repaired. Conversely, a chronic, aseptic, granulomatous inflammation may develop at the interface if the osteosynthesis is left in the bone for a long time. Although the development of inflammation is multifactorial, it is mainly due to two factors: the abnormal distribution of mechanical forces, especially those dependent on micromovements, and the presence of wear debris.

As noted above, focal areas of bone may be overloaded, while others may be underloaded. Overloading may cause osteocyte death and bone necrosis, whereas underloading gives rise to alteration of the mechanostat control. In both cases, osteoclast activity is stimulated and erosion of the osseous interface may ensue; moreover, hemorrhages and focal necroses may stimulate macrophagic activation and inflammation (see Figure 14.3A). These effects may be enhanced by the presence of wear debris, especially that measuring less than 0.3 μm in thickness, which not only activates the macrophagic cells, but also modulates the release of cytokines, which are strong mediators of osteoclastogenesis[118-120] (especially, tumor necrosis factor-α[121]). The role of extraneous particles in inducing bone resorption may be less incisive than that of micromovements.[122] These not only may induce abrasion and compression of the bone surface, but may also inhibit the ossification process.[123]

The inflammatory tissue that develops at the bone–implant interface has been considered to be a synovia like membrane.[65] Obviously, it is the result of a chronic inflammatory reaction and its resemblance to a synovia is only apparent (Figure 14.6A). It is histologically characterized by the presence of lymphoid and macrophagic cells, giant cells, areas of necrosis, extravasated red cells, fragments of necrotic bone, dilated capillary vessels, and varying numbers of collagen fibrils (Figure 14.6A, C, and D). Foreign particles, either free or phagocytosed by macrophagic cells, become irregularly distributed through this tissue (Figure 14.6B). The macrophagic cells often appear as giant, polynucleated cells (Figure 14.6B and D), which show phagocytosis and give a positive reaction for tartrate-resistant acid phosphatase (TRAP), which is typical of osteoclasts[124]

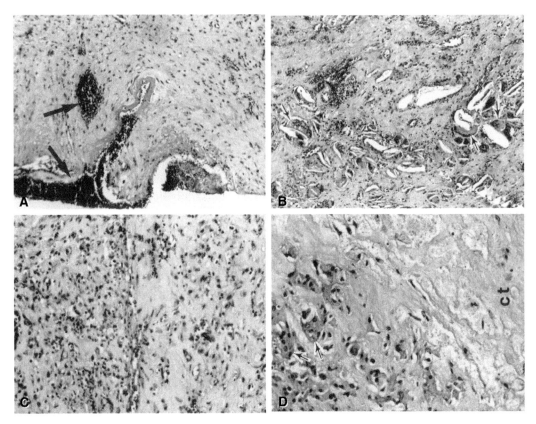

FIGURE 14.6 Various histologic aspects of the granulation tissue that may develop at the interface between osteosynthesis and bone. (A) The synovial-like granulation tissue is mainly fibrillar and there are relatively few inflammatory cells; its flat surface (left) shows that it was compressed against the implant. Extravasated red cells (arrows) appear within the tissue and at its surface. (B) A number of foreign bodies (appearing as empty clefts) are present in the granulation tissue; some of them are in contact with polynucleated giant cells (arrows). (C) Mononucleated, partly macrophagic and partly lymphoid cells represent the most frequent pattern of the granulation tissue. (D) Dense collagenous tissue (ct) often develops in the granulation tissue; note the presence of giant cells (arrows). (Hematoxylin-eosin; original magnifications: A and B ×110; C and D ×220.)

but is also expressed by activated macrophages.[125] Osteoclasts are present at the bone surface, in which varying numbers of resorption lacunae can be found. Metalloproteinases and their inhibitors can be detected in the granulomatous tissue.[126]

The development of inflammatory tissue at the interface is highly dangerous, not only because the macrophagic cells produce osteoclast-stimulating factors, thereby promoting the erosion of the osseous bed, but also because this tissue lies between the bone and the implant, and stops them coming into direct contact. This situation permits and favors micromovements, which themselves aggravate the bone damage and degree of inflammation, triggering a vicious circle that ends with the complete freeing of the implant. The development of interfascial granulomatous tissue is almost inevitable in the view of some authors.[127]

VI. REACTION OF OSTEOPOROTIC BONE

Osteoporosis can be defined as a disease characterized by normal bone matrix, bone mass lower than that which is normal on the basis of age, sex and race, and microarchitectural deterioration of the various skeletal segments (see Figures 14.1B and 2B), that is, a complex of skeletal changes that increases the probability of fractures. Independent of its etiology, the basic mechanism leading to osteoporosis implies abnormalities of bone remodeling in the BMUs, and consists in the uncoupling of bone resorption from bone formation, with the prevalence of the former over the latter.[34] This uncoupling may depend on transient but excessive osteoclastic bone resorption (rapid bone loss), like that found soon after menopause in women and after ovariectomy in rats, mice, and dogs,[19,128-131] and/or on reduced osteoblast activity (slow bone loss), with incomplete refilling of the resorption lacunae.[10]

The osteoporotic reduction of volume occurs both in compact and spongy bone. In compact bone, there is a progressive resorption of the inner lamellar system, with enlargement of the marrow canal, low numbers of osteons, and unusually high numbers of unrepaired resorption lacunae, which give the bone a spongy appearance (see Figure 14.2B). In spongy bone, where osteoporosis is usually more evident than in compact bone, there is a reduction in the numbers of and connections between trabeculae, with an evident upsetting of the whole microarchitecture (see Figure 14.1B). Because bone stiffness and strength depend not only on the mass and quality of the calcified matrix, but above all on its architecture,[132] osteoporotic bone offers little resistance to stress, and fractures are frequent.

The implantation of an osteosynthesis in osteoporotic bone is a demanding task, and may be unsuccessful. In spongy bone, this is probably mainly because the low number of trabeculae reduces contact between the bone and the fixation device,[133] which is therefore deprived of its necessary anchorage. As a result, the degree of primary fixation is poor, and micromovements of the fixation devices are frequent. Regarding compact bone, its thinness and spongy transformation both increase its fragility; this makes the failure of primary fixation more likely, and also raises the probability of fractures, especially burst fractures. Hydroxyapatite-coated and/or cemented fixation devices have been proposed to improve primary fixation in osteoporotic bone.[134,135] Cannulated screws with side ports that can be injected with cement might greatly improve fixation in osteoporotic bone.[136] Hydroxyapatite coating may also be helpful in improving the degree of ossification and secondary fixation, because the hydroxyapatite affinity index (the length of bone directly apposed to the implant surface/the total length of the bone–implant interface ×100) is the same in the tibiae of normal and osteoporotic rats, whereas that of titanium is lower in osteoporotic rats.[137,138]

The reaction of osteoporotic bone to internal fixation hardly differs from that which occurs in normal bone, including the development of a synovia-like membrane. The loss of balance between bone resorption and bone formation that is typical of the osteoporotic condition usually has no negative consequences on implant osseointegration. In his review of noncemented implants, Albrektsson[2] compares the reaction of bone around an implant to what happens in a fracture during callus formation. It is known that fracture repair and bone formation around implants are moderately impaired and delayed in osteoporosis,[139,140] especially at a late stage.[141] In fact, the removal torque of tibial implants in rabbits made osteoporotic by the administration of prednisolone is lower than in controls.[142] This impairment, however, does not prevent the formation of a callus, or the development of bone around an osteosynthesis,[139] if this is stable. The problem with patients with osteoporosis is to obtain a correct and durable primary fixation of an osteosynthesis, rather than to achieve a good secondary fixation. A long-standing implant may, however, increase the local degree of osteoporosis, especially in the case of compression plates.[95]

The primary fixation and later evolution of an osteosynthesis may be damaged by the concomitance of defective calcification of the osteoporotic bone (osteoporomalacia), or of Paget's disease. The frequency of both these pathologic conditions increases with aging, and the role of the former in senile skeletal pathology has probably been underestimated. Vignon et al.[143] reported osteoporomalacia in 35% and pure osteomalacia in 9% of 203 iliac bone samples from subjects over the age of 65; Hordon and Peacock[144] found osteomalacia in 27% of patients over 90, and Ballanti and

Bonucci[145] found osteoporomalacia in 23.5% and osteomalacia in 1.7% of 119 iliac crest biopsies from patients with the clinical diagnosis of osteoporosis.

VII. CONCLUSIONS

The main aim of internal fixation is that of restoring the anatomic pattern and the physiologic function of discontinuous bone segments, and of obtaining their definitive stabilization. These goals can be achieved if a balance is attained between two processes that may occur at the bone–implant interface: the tissue reparative processes that lead to bone reconstruction and osseointegration on the one hand, and the tissue reaction that tends to eliminate the foreign materials used in osteosynthesis on the other. A balance between these processes, or the prevalence of one of them, depends on a number of systemic and local factors, the most important of which are the severity of the skeletal damage that demands internal fixation and the severity of the damage usually produced by surgery; the distribution of loads, and their type and direction, both in the fixation devices themselves and in the restored skeletal segment; the degree of primary fixation, and the possible occurrence of micromovements; the type and arrangement of the materials used for internal fixation, and the shedding of particles from their surface; the severity of the granulomatous reaction developed at the interface; and the quality and amount of bone. In particular, the micromovements and the abnormal compressive loads may lead on the one hand to osteocyte death and to a focal necrosis of bone, which stimulates osteoclastic resorption, and, on the other, to osteoblast inhibition, which prevents any repair of the dead parts. Moreover, a breakdown of the mechanostat control may occur in the unloaded areas of the matrix, with consequent osteoclast–osteoblast uncoupling. These changes combine to increase the osteoclastic resorption of the inner surface of the osseous bed, which may gradually be enlarged. As a result, the stability of the osteosynthesis falls and the amplitude of the micromovements rises; this leads to further bone damage and the activation of a closed circle that ends in the total failure of the internal fixation. Besides, or alongside, this process, the presence of foreign particles at the interface may stimulate the formation of macrophagic cells, which phagocytose the particles and in so doing produce cytokines and other factors. These maintain the inflammatory process and lead to osteoclast stimulation, which further enlarges the interface and promotes mobilization. The process gives rise to a mechanically ineffectual synovia-like membrane, histologically characterized by the presence of mononucleated lymphoid cells, giant and polynucleated macrophagic cells, microscopic hemorrhages, small areas of necrosis, and varying amounts of collagen fibers.

The inflammatory process described above develops slowly and insidiously, and has a highly negative impact on the stabilization and osseointegration of the prostheses. It is less important in the case of internal bone fixations, which are transitory and often have too short a duration to permit full development of a chronic inflammatory reaction. Any evidence of this reaction, however, makes the early removal of the fixation devices a recognized necessity.

The quality of bone may have a great impact on the evolution of internal bone fixation. It has long been known that the mechanical resistance of osteoporotic bone is lower than that of normal bone. For this reason, burst fractures are possible during press-fit implantations, and microfractures or fractures easily develop when the osteosynthesis is loaded. Primary fixation is often unsatisfactory, especially in spongy bone, due to the low numbers of osseous trabeculae. The reaction that may occur at the interface because of micromovements and/or the presence of foreign particles is like that which may occur in normal bone, because reparative osteogenesis and foreign body inflammation are slightly influenced by osteoporosis. Defective calcification of the matrix (osteoporomalacia) can further hinder the primary fixation of the osteosynthesis; this facilitates micromovements and promotes the development of inflammatory reactions at the interface.

ACKNOWLEDGMENTS

The preparation of this chapter and the personal research mentioned have been supported by grants from the Italian Ministry of University and Scientific and Technological Research (MURST), the University of Rome la Sapienza, and the Italian National Research Council (CNR). The author is grateful to Paola Ballanti, Silvia Berni, Carlo della Rocca, Giuliana Silvestrini, and Lucio Virgilii for their technical and scientific support.

REFERENCES

1. Perren, S.M., "Physical and biological aspects of fracture healing with special reference to internal fixation," *Clin. Orthop.*, 138, 175, 1979.
2. Albrektsson, T., "The reactions of bone to non-cemented implants," in *Bone: Fracture Repair and Regeneration*, Hall, B.K., Ed., CRC Press, Boca Raton, FL, 1992, 153.
3. Plenk, H., Jr., "Prosthesis-bone interface," *J. Biomed. Mater. Res.*, 43, 350, 1998.
4. Perry, C.R., "Bone repair techniques, bone graft, and bone graft substitutes," *Clin. Orthop.*, 360, 71, 1999.
5. Al-Saffar, N. and Revell, P.A., "Pathology of the bone–implant interfaces," *J. Long-Term Eff. Med. Implants*, 9, 319, 1999.
6. Conrad, M.E. and Carpenter, J.T., "Bone marrow necrosis," *Am. J. Hematol.*, 7, 181, 1979.
7. Lozupone, E., "A quantitative analysis of bone tissue formation in different regions of the spongiosa in the dog skeleton," *Anat. Anz.*, 145, 425, 1979.
8. Gorski, J.P., "Is all bone the same? Distinctive distributions and properties of non-collagenous matrix proteins in lamellar vs. woven bone imply the existence of different underlying osteogenic mechanisms," *Crit. Rev. Oral Biol. Med.*, 9, 201, 1998.
9. Koch, J.C., "The laws of bone architecture," *Am. J. Anat.*, 21, 177, 1917.
10. Parfitt, A.M., "Age-related structural changes in trabecular and cortical bone: cellular mechanisms and biomechanical consequences," *Calcif. Tissue Int.*, 36, S123, 1984.
11. Goldstein, S.A., Goulet, R., and McCubbrey, D., "Measurement and significance of three-dimensional architecture to the mechanical integrity of trabecular bone," *Calcif. Tissue Int.*, 53, S127, 1993.
12. Tenenbaum, H.C., "Cellular origins and theories of differentiation of bone-forming cells," in *Bone: The Osteoblast and Osteocyte*, Hall, B.K., Ed., Telford Press, Caldwell, NJ, 1990, 41.
13. Marotti, G., "The structure of bone tissues and the cellular control of their deposition," *It. J. Anat. Embryol.*, 101, 25, 1996.
14. Bonucci, E., "Basic composition and structure of bone," in *Mechanical Testing of Bone and the Bone–Implant Interface*, An, Y.H. and Draughn, R.A., Eds., CRC Press, Boca Raton, FL, 2000, 3.
15. Hancox, N.M., *Biology of Bone*, Cambridge University Press, Cambridge, 1972.
16. Chan, Y.L., Alfrey, A.C., Posen, S., et al. "Effect of aluminum on normal and uremic rats: tissue distribution, vitamin D metabolites, and quantitative bone histology," *Calcif. Tissue Int.*, 35, 344, 1983.
17. Miller, S.C., Bowman, B.M., Miller, M.A., and Bagi, C.M., "Calcium absorption and osseous organ-, tissue-, and envelope-specific changes following ovariectomy in rats," *Bone*, 12, 439, 1991.
18. Yoshida, S., Yamamuro, T., Okumura, H., and Takahashi, H., "Microstructural changes of osteopenic trabeculae in the rat," *Bone*, 12, 185, 1991.
19. Ballanti, P., Martelli, A., Mereto, E., and Bonucci, E., "Ovariectomized rats as experimental model of postmenopausal osteoporosis: critical considerations," *It. J. Miner. Electrol. Metab.*, 7, 243, 1993.
20. Shen, V., Liang, X.G., Birchman, R., et al., "Short term immobilization-induced cancellous bone loss is limited to regions undergoing high turnover and/or modeling in mature rats," *Bone*, 21, 71, 1997.
21. Frost, H.M., "Bone 'mass' and the 'mechanostat': a proposal," *Anat. Rec.*, 219, 1, 1987.
22. Frost, H.M., "Perspectives: a proposed general model of the 'mechanostat' (suggestions from a new skeletal-biologic paradigm)," *Anat. Rec.*, 244, 139, 1996.
23. Frost, H.M., Ferretti, J.L., and Jee, W.S.S., "Perspectives: some role of mechanical usage, muscle strength, and the mechanostat in skeletal physiology, disease, and research," *Calcif. Tissue Int.*, 62, 1, 1998.

24. Frost, H.M., "Changing concepts in skeletal physiology: Wolff's law, the mechanostat, and the 'Utah paradigm,'" *Am. J. Hum. Biol.*, 10, 599, 1998.

25. Frost, H.M., "From Wolff's law to the mechanostat: a new 'face' of physiology," *J. Orthop. Sci.*, 3, 282, 1998.

26. Marotti, G., Canè, V., Palazzini, S., and Palumbo, C., "Structure-function relationships in the osteocyte," *It. J. Miner. Electrol. Metab.*, 4, 93, 1990.

27. Burger, E.H. and Klein-Nulend, J., "Mechanotransduction in bone — role of the lacuno-canalicular network," *FASEB J.*, 13, S101, 1999.

28. Mikuni-Takagaki, Y., "Mechanical responses and signal transduction pathways in stretched osteocytes," *J. Bone Miner. Metab.*, 17, 57, 1999.

29. Terai, K., Takano-Yamamoto, T., Ohba, Y., et al., "Role of osteopontin in bone remodeling caused by mechanical stress," *J. Bone Miner. Res.*, 14, 839, 1999.

30. Raisz, L.G. and Rodan, G.A., "Cellular basis for bone turnover," in *Metabolic Bone Disease and Clinically Related Disorders*, 2nd ed., Avioli, L.V. and Krane, S.M., Eds., W. B. Saunders, Philadelphia, 1990, 1.

31. Parfitt, A.M., "Quantum concept of bone remodeling and turnover: implications for the pathogenesis of osteoporosis," *Calcif. Tissue Int.*, 28, 1, 1979.

32. Bonucci, E., "The basic multicellular unit of bone," *It. J. Miner. Electrol. Metab.*, 4, 115, 1990.

33. Baron, R., Vignery, A., and Horowitz, M., "Lymphocytes, macrophages and the regulation of bone remodeling," in *Bone and Mineral Research,* Annual 2, Peck, W.A., Ed., Elsevier, Amsterdam, 1984, 175.

34. Burr, D.B. and Martin, R.B., "Errors in bone remodeling: toward a unified theory of metabolic bone disease," *Am. J. Anat.*, 186, 186, 1989.

35. Huffer, W.E., "Morphology and biochemistry of bone remodeling: possible control by vitamin D, parathyroid hormone, and other substances," *Lab. Invest.*, 59, 418, 1988.

36. Carlsson, L., Rostlund, T., Albrektsson, B., et al., "Osseointegration of titanium implants," *Acta Orthop. Scand.*, 57, 285, 1986.

37. Dhert, W.J.A., Thomsen, P., Blomgren, A.K., et al., "Integration of press-fit implants in cortical bone: a study of interface kinetics," *J. Biomed. Mater. Res.*, 41, 574, 1998.

38. Ishizaka, M., Tanizawa, T., Sofue, M., et al., "Bone particles disturb new bone formation on the interface of the titanium implant after reaming of the marrow cavity," *Bone*, 19, 589, 1996.

39. Ogiso, M., Yamashita, Y., Tabata, T., et al., "The delay method: a new surgical technique for enhancing the bone-binding capability of HAP implants to bone surrounding implant cavity preparations," *J. Biomed. Mater. Res.*, 28, 805, 1994.

40. Owen, M., "The origin of bone cells in the postnatal organism," *Arthritis Rheumat.*, 23, 1073, 1980.

41. Rickard, D.J., Kassem, M., Hefferan, T.E., et al., "Isolation and characterization of osteoblast precursor cell from human bone marrow," *J. Bone Miner. Res.*, 11, 312, 1996.

42. Bruder, S.P., Fink, D.J., and Caplan, A.I., "Mesenchymal stem cells in bone development, bone repair, and skeletal regeneration therapy," *J. Cell. Biochem.*, 56, 283, 1994.

43. Plenk, H., Jr. and Zitter, H., "Material considerations," in *Endosseous Implants: Scientific and Clinical Aspects*, Watzek, G., Ed., Quintessence Books, Berlin, 1996, 63.

44. Hench, L.L., "Biomaterials," *Science*, 208, 826, 1980.

45. Hench, L.L. and Wilson, J., "Surface-active biomaterials," *Science*, 226, 630, 1984.

46. Raiha, J.E., "Biodegradable implants as intramedullary nails. A survey of recent studies and an introduction to their use," *Clin. Mater.*, 10, 35, 1992.

47. Hollinger, J.O., Brekke, J., Gruskin, E., and Lee, D., "Role of bone substitutes," *Clin. Orthop.*, 324, 55, 1996.

48. Simon, J.A., Ricci, J.L., and Di Cesare, P.E., "Bioresorbable fracture fixation in orthopaedics: a comprehensive review. Part I. Basic science and preclinical studies," *Am. J. Orthop.*, 26, 665, 1997.

49. Daniels, A.U., Chang, M.K., and Andriano, K.P., "Mechanical properties of biodegradable polymers and composites proposed for internal fixation of bone," *J. Appl. Biomater.*, 1, 57, 1990.

50. van der Elst, M., Klein, C.P., de Blieck-Hogervorst, J.M., et al., "Bone tissue response to biodegradable polymers used for intramedullary fracture fixation: a long-term *in vivo* study in sheep femora," *Biomaterials*, 20, 121, 1999.

51. Furukawa, T., Matsusue, Y., Yasunaga, T., et al., "Biodegradation behavior of ultra-high-strength hydroxyapatite/poly (L-lactide) composite rods for internal fixation of bone fractures," *Biomaterials*, 21, 889, 2000.

52. Lewandrowski, K.U., Gresser, J.D., Wise, D.L., and Trantol, D.J., "Bioresorbable bone graft substitutes of different osteoconductivities: a histologic evaluation of osteointegration of poly(propylene glycol-co-fumaric acid)-based cement implants in rats," *Biomaterials*, 21, 757, 2000.

53. Goodman, S., Aspenberg, P., Song, Y., et al., "Polyethylene and titanium alloy particles reduce bone formation. Dose-dependence in bone harvest chamber experiments in rabbits," *Acta Orthop. Scand.*, 67, 599, 1996.

54. Nawrocki, B., Polette, M., Burlet, H., et al., "Expression of gelatinase A and its activator MT1-MMP in the inflammatory periprosthetic response to polyethylene," *J. Bone Miner. Res.*, 14, 288, 1999.

55. Woolf, S.K., An, Y.H., and Friedman, R.J., "Review of methods for evaluating orthopaedic bioabsorbable devices *in vivo*," *MUSC Orthop. J.*, 3, 27, 2000.

56. Albrektsson, T. and Hansson, H.A., "An ultrastructural characterization of the interface between bone and sputtered titanium or stainless steel surfaces," *Biomaterials*, 7, 201, 1986.

57. Johansson, C.B., Lausmaa, J., Ask, M., et al., "Ultrastructural differences of the interface zone betwen bone and Ti6A14V or commercially pure titanium," *J. Biomed. Eng.*, 1, 3, 1989.

58. Linder, L., "Osseointegration of metallic implants. I. Light microscopy in the rabbit," *Acta Orthop. Scand.*, 60, 129, 1989.

59. Linder, L., Obrant, K., and Boivin, G., "Osseointegration of metallic implants. II. Transmission electron microscopy in the rabbit," *Acta Orthop. Scand.*, 60, 135, 1989.

60. Schmalzried, T.P. and Callaghan, J.J., "Wear in total hip and knee replacements," *J. Bone Joint Surg.*, 81-A, 115, 1999.

61. Dorr, L.D., Wan, Z., Song, M., and Ranawat, A., "Bilateral total hip arthroplasty comparing hydroxyapatite coating to porous-coated fixation," *J. Arthroplasty*, 13, 729, 1998.

62. Simmons, C.A., Valiquette, N., and Pilliar, R.M., "Osseointegration of sintered porous-surfaced and plasma spray-coated implants: an animal model study of early postimplantation healing response and mechanical stability," *J. Biomed. Mater. Res.*, 47, 127, 1999.

63. Svehla, M., Morberg, P., Zicat, B., et al., "Morphometric and mechanical evaluation of titanium implant integration: comparison of five surface structures," *J. Biomed. Mater. Res.*, 51, 15, 2000.

64. Soballe, K., Hansen, E.S., Brockstedt-Rasmussen, H., et al., "Gap healing enhanced by hydroxyapatite coating in dogs," *Clin. Orthop.*, 272, 300, 1991.

65. Goldring, S.R., Schiller, A.L., Roelke, M., et al., "The synovial-like membrane at the bone-cement interface in loose total hip replacements and its proposed role in bone lysis," *J. Bone Joint Surg.*, 65A, 575, 1983.

66. Willert, H.G., and Puls, P., "Die Reaktion des Knochens auf Knochenzement bei der Allo-Arthroplastik der Hüfte," *Arch. Orthop. Unfall-Chir.*, 72, 33, 1972.

67. Cornell, C.N. and Lane, J.M., "Current understanding of osteoconduction in bone regeneration," *Clin. Orthop.*, 355, 267S, 1998.

68. Marini, E., Valdinucci, F., and Bonucci, E., "Bone reconstruction and/or augmentation with hydroxyapatite-fibrin glue: personal experience and review of the literature," *It. J. Miner. Electrol. Metab.*, 13, 5, 1999.

69. Riley, E.H., Lane, J.M., Urist, M.R., et al., "Bone morphogenetic protein-2. Biology and applications," *Clin. Orthop.*, 324, 39, 1996.

70. Lind, M., Overgaard, S., Soballe, K., et al., "Transforming growth factor-β1 enhances bone healing to unloaded tricalcium phosphate coated implants an experimental study in dogs," *J. Orthop. Res.*, 14, 343, 1996.

71. Linkhart, T.A., Mohan, S., and Baylink, D.J., "Growth factors for bone growth and repair: IGF, TGF-β and BMP," *Bone*, 19, 1S, 1996.

72. Aspenberg, P., Jeppsson, C., Wang, J.S., and Boström, M., "Transforming growth factor beta and bone morphogenetic protein 2 for bone ingrowth: a comparison using bone chambers in rats," *Bone*, 19, 499, 1996.

73. Heckman, J.D., Ehler, W., Brooks, B.P., et al., "Bone morphogenetic protein but not transforming growth factor-beta enhances bone formation in canine diaphyseal nonunions implanted with a biodegradable composite polymer," *J. Bone Joint Surg.*, 81A, 1717, 1999.

74. Arnaud, E., Morieux, C., Wybier, M., and De Vernejoul, M.C., "Potentiation of transforming growth factor (TGF-β1) by natural coral and fibrin in a rabbit cranioplasty model," *Calcif. Tissue Int.*, 54, 493, 1994.

75. Damien, C.J., Parsons, J.R., Prewett, A.B., et al., "Effect of demineralized bone matrix on bone growth within a porous HA material: a histologic and histometric study," *J. Biomater. Appl.*, 9, 275, 1995.

76. Gao, T.J., Lindholm, T.S., Kommonen, B., et al., "The use of a coral composite implant containing bone morphogenetic protein to repair a segmental tibial defect in sheep," *Int. Orthop.*, 21, 194, 1997.

77. Koempel, J.A., Patt, B.S., O'Grady, K., et al., "The effect of recombinant human bone morphogenetic protein-2 on the integration of porous hydroxyapatite implants with bone," *J. Biomed. Mater. Res.*, 41, 359, 1998.

78. Laffargue, Ph., Hildebrand, H.F., Rtaimate, M., et al., "Evaluation of human recombinant bone morphogenetic protein-2-loaded tricalcium phosphate implants in rabbits' bone defects," *Bone*, 25, 55S, 1999.

79. Yoshida, K., Bessho, K., Fujimura, K., et al., "Enhancement by recombinant human bone morphogenetic protein-2 of bone formation by means of porous hydroxyapatite in mandibular bone defects," *J. Dent. Res.*, 78, 1505, 1999.

80. Denissen, H., Montanari, C., Martinetti, R., et al., "Alveolar bone response to submerged bisphosphonate-complexed hydroxyapatite implants," *J. Periodontol.*, 71, 279, 2000.

81. Kawanabe, K., Okada, Y., Matsusue, Y., et al., "Treatment of osteomyelitis with antibiotic-soaked porous glass ceramic," *J. Bone Joint Surg.*, 80B, 527, 1998.

82. Ikeda, N., Kawanabe, K., and Nakamura, T., "Quantitative comparison of osteoconduction of porous, dense A-W glass-ceramic and hydroxyapatite granules (effects of granule and pore size)," *Biomaterials*, 20, 1087, 1999.

83. De Groot, K., Jansen, J.A., Wolke, J.G.C., et al., "Development in bioactive coatings," in *Hydroxyapatite Coating in Orthopaedic Surgery*, Geesink, R.G.T. and Manley, M.T., Eds., Raven Press, New York, 1993, 49.

84. McPherson, E.J., Dorr, L.D., Gruen, T.A., and Saberi, M.T., "Hydroxyapatite-coated proximal ingrowth femoral stems. A matched pair control study," *Clin. Orthop.*, 315, 223, 1995.

85. Yee, A.J., Kreder, H.K., Bookman, I., and Davey, J.R., "A randomized trial of hydroxyapatite coated prostheses in total hip arthroplasty," *Clin. Orthop.*, 366, 120, 1999.

86. Jaffe, W.L. and Scott, D.F., "Total hip arthroplasty with hydroxyapatite-coated prostheses," *J. Bone Joint Surg.*, 78A, 1918, 1996.

87. Lemons, J.E., "Ceramics: past, present, and future," *Bone*, 19, 121S, 1996.

88. Pazzaglia, U.E., Brossa, F., Zatti, G., et al., "The relevance of hydroxyapatite and spongious titanium coatings in fixation of cementless stems. An experimental comparative study in rat femur employing histologic and microangiographic techniques," *Arch. Orthop. Traumat. Surg.*, 117, 279, 1998.

89. Oonishi, H., Yamamoto, M., Ishimaru, H., et al., "The effect of hydroxyapatite coating on bone growth into porous titanium alloy implants," *J. Bone Joint Surg.*, 71B, 213, 1989.

90. Soballe, K., Hansen, E.S., Brockstedt-Rasmussen, H., et al., "Hydroxyapatite coating enhances fixation of porous coated implants. A comparison in dogs between press fit and noninterference fit," *Acta Orthop. Scand.*, 61, 299, 1990.

91. Tisdel, C.L., Goldberg, V.M., Parr, J.A., et al., "The influence of hydroxyapatite and tricalcium-phosphate coating on bone growth into titanium fiber-metal implants," *J. Bone Joint Surg.*, 76A, 159, 1994.

92. Moroni, A., Toksvig-Larsen, S., Maltarello, M.C., et al., "A comparison of hydroxyapatite-coated, titanium-coated, and uncoated tapered external-fixation pins. An *in vivo* study in sheep," *J. Bone Joint Surg.*, 80A, 547, 1998.

93. Lind, M., Overgaard, S., Bunger, C., and Soballe, K., "Improved bone anchorage of hydroxyapatite coated implants compared with tricalcium-phosphate coated implants in trabecular bone in dogs," *Biomaterials*, 20, 803, 1999.

94. Bonucci, E., Marini, E., Valdinucci, F., and Fortunato, G., "Osteogenic response to hydroxyapatite-fibrin implants in maxillofacial bone defects," *Eur. J. Oral Sci.*, 105, 557, 1997.

95. Hönig, J.F. and Merten, H.A., "Einfluss punktförmig gelagerter Osteosyntheseplatten in Vergleich zur Konventionellen Osteosyntheseplattenlagerung, auf das subimplantäre Lagerungsgewebe," *Vorläufige Mitt. Unfallchir.*, 95, 271, 1992.

96. Aspenberg, P. and van der Vis, H., "Fluid pressure may cause periprosthetic osteolysis. Particles are not the only thing," *Acta Orthop. Scand.*, 69, 1, 1998.

97. Aspenberg, P. and van der Vis, H., "Migration, particles, and fluid pressure. A discussion of causes of prosthetic loosening," *Clin. Orthop.*, 352, 75, 1998.

98. Skripitz, R. and Aspenberg, P., "Pressure-induced periprosthetic osteolysis: a rat model," *J. Orthop. Res.*, 18, 481, 2000.

99. Ducheyne, P. and Qiu, Q., "Bioactive ceramics: the effect of surface reactivity on bone formation and bone cell function," *Biomaterials*, 20, 2287, 1999.

100. Schwartz, Z. and Boyan, B.D., "Underlying mechanisms at the bone-biomaterial interface," *J. Cell. Biochem.*, 56, 340, 1994.

101. Welsh, R.P., Pilliar, R.M., and Macnab, I., "Surgical implants. The role of surface porosity in fixation to bone and acrylic," *J. Bone Joint Surg.*, 53A, 963, 1971.

102. Hatano, K., Inoue, H., Kojo, T., et al., "Effect of surface roughness on proliferation and alkaline phosphatase expression of rat calvarial cells cultured on polystyrene," *Bone*, 25, 439, 1999.

103. Wassell, D.T., Hall, R.C., and Embery, G., "Adsorption of bovine serum albumin onto hydroxyapatite," *Biomaterials*, 16, 697, 1995.

104. Wassell, D.T. and Embery, G., "Adsorption of bovine serum albumin on to titanium powder, " *Biomaterials*, 17, 859, 1996.

105. Browne, M., Gregson, P.J., and West, R.H., "Characterization of titanium alloy implant surfaces with improved dissolution resistance," *J. Mater. Sci. Mater. Med.*, 7, 323, 1996.

106. Boyan, B.D., Hummert, T.W., Dean, D.D., and Schwartz, Z., "Role of material surfaces in regulating bone and cartilage cell response," *Biomaterials*, 17, 137, 1996.

107. McKee, M.D. and Nanci, A., "Osteopontin at mineralized tissue interfaces in bone, teeth, and osseointegrated implants: ultrastructural distribution, and implications for mineralized tissue formation, turnover, and repair," *Microsc. Res. Technol.*, 33, 141, 1996.

108. Davies, J.E., "*In vitro* modeling of the bone/implant interface," *Anat. Rec.*, 245, 426, 1996.

109. Ayukawa, Y., Takeshita, F., Inoue, T., et al., "An immunoelectron microscopic localization of noncollagenous bone proteins (osteocalcin and osteopontin) at the bone–titanium interface of rat tibiae," *J. Biomed. Mater. Res.*, 41, 111, 1998.

110. Puleo, D.A. and Nanci, A., "Understanding and controlling the bone–implant interface," *Biomaterials*, 20, 2311, 1999.

111. Sinha, R.K. and Tuan, R.S., "Regulation of human osteoblast integrin expression by orthopaedic implant material," *Bone*, 18, 451, 1996.

112. Gronowicz, G. and McCarthy, M.B., "Response of human osteoblasts to implant materials: integrin-mediated adhesion," *J. Orthop. Res.*, 14, 878, 1996.

113. Anselme, K., "Osteoblast adhesion on biomaterials," *Biomaterials*, 21, 667, 2000.

114. Nanci, A., McCarthy, G.F., Zalzal, S., et al., "Tissue response to titanium implants in the rat tibia: ultrastructural, immunocytochemical and lectin-cytochemical characterization of the bone-titanium interface," *Cells Mater.*, 4, 1, 1994.

115. Klinger, M.M., Rahemtulla, F., Prince, C.W., et al., "Proteoglycans at the bone–implant interface," *Crit. Rev. Oral Biol. Med.*, 9, 449, 1998.

116. Marini, E., Valdinucci, F., Silvestrini, G., et al., "Morphological investigations on bone formation in hydroxyapatite-fibrin implants in human maxillary and mandibular bone," *Cells Mater.*, 4, 231, 1994.

117. Kawaguchi, H., McKee, M.D., Okamoto, H., and Nanci, A., "Immunocytochemical and lectin-gold characterization of the interface between alveolar bone and implanted hydroxyapatite in the rat," *Cells Mater.*, 3, 337, 1993.

118. Fadda, M., Espa, E., Marceddu, S., and De Santis, E., "I detriti metallici nei fallimenti delle artroprotesi d'anca non cementate. Studio morfologico e ultrastrutturale," *G. Ital. Ortop. Traumat.*, 22, 119, 1996.

119. Wang, J.Y., Wicklund, B.H., Gustilo, R.B., and Tsukayama, D.T., "Titanium, chromium and cobalt ions modulate the release of bone-associated cytokines by human monocytes/macrophages *in vitro*," *Biomaterials*, 17, 2233, 1996.

120. Shida, J., Trindade, M.C., Goodman, S.B., et al., "Induction of interleukin-6 release in human osteoblast-like cells exposed to titanium particles *in vitro*," *Calcif. Tissue Int.*, 67, 151, 2000.

121. Merkel, K.D., Erdmann, J.M., McHugh, F.P., et al., "Tumor necrosis factor-α mediates orthopaedic implant osteolysis," *Am. J. Pathol.*, 154, 203, 1999.

122. Aspenberg, P. and Herbertsson, P., "Periprosthetic bone resorption. Particles vs. movement," *J. Bone Joint Surg.*, 78B, 641, 1996.

123. Soballe, K., Brockstedt-Rasmussen, H., Hansen, E.S., and Bünger, C., "Hydroxyapatite coating modifies implant membrane formation. Controlled micromotion studied in dogs," *Acta Orthop. Scand.*, 63, 128, 1992.

124. Doty, S.B., "Histochemistry and enzymology of osteoclasts," in *Bone: The Osteoclast*, Hall, B.K., Ed., CRC Press, Boca Raton, FL, 1991, 61.

125. Bianco, P., Costantini, M., Dearden, L.C., and Bonucci, E., "Expression of tartrate-resistant acid phosphatase in bone marrow macrophages," *Basic Appl. Histochem.*, 31, 433, 1987.

126. Takagi, M., Santavirta, S., Ida, H., et al., "Matrix metalloproteinases and tissue inhibitors of metalloproteinases in loose artificial hip joints," *Clin. Prevent. Dent.*, 352, 35, 1998.

127. Lennox, D.W., Schofield, B.H., McDonald, D.F., and Riley, L.H., "A histologic comparison of aseptic loosening of cemented, press-fit and biologic ingrowth prostheses," *Clin. Orthop.*, 225, 171, 1987.

128. Faugere, M.C., Friedler, R.M., Fanti, P., and Malluche, H.H., "Bone changes occurring early after cessation of ovarian function in beagle dogs: a histomorphometric study employing sequential biopsies," *J. Bone Miner. Res.*, 5, 263, 1990.

129. Eriksen, E.F., Hodgson, S.F., Eastell, R., et al., "Cancellous bone remodeling in type I (postmenopausal) osteoporosis: quantitative assessment of rates of formation, resorption, and bone loss at tissue and cellular levels," *J. Bone Miner. Res.*, 5, 311, 1990.

130. Bonucci, E., Ballanti, P., Ramires, P.A., et al., "Prevention of ovariectomy osteopenia in rats after vaginal administration of Hyaff 11 microspheres containing salmon calcitonin," *Calcif. Tissue Int.*, 56, 274, 1995.

131. Most, W., van der Wee-Pals, L., Ederveen, A., et al., "Ovariectomy and orchidectomy induce a transient increase in the osteoclastogenic potential of bone marrow cells in the mouse," *Bone*, 20, 27, 1997.

132. Kleerekoper, M., Villanueva, A.R., Stanciu, J., et al., "The role of three-dimensional trabecular microstructure in the pathogenesis of vertebral compression fractures," *Calcif. Tissue Int.*, 37, 594, 1985.

133. Yamazaki, M., Shirota, T., Tokugawa, Y., et al., "Bone reactions to titanium screw implants in ovariectomized animals," *Oral Surg. Oral Med. Oral Pathol. Oral Radiol. Endod.*, 87, 411, 1999.

134. Dorr, L.D., Arnala, I., Faugere, M.C., and Malluche, H.H., "Five-year postoperative results of cemented femoral arthroplasty in patients with systemic bone disease," *Clin. Orthop.*, 259, 114, 1990.

135. Hara, T., Hayashi, K., Nakashima, K., et al., "The effect of hydroxyapatite coating on the bonding of bone to titanium implants in the femora of ovariectomised rats," *J. Bone Joint Surg.*, 81B, 705, 1999.

136. McKoy, B.E. and An, Y.H., "An injectable cementing screw for fixation in osteoporotic bone," *J. Biomed. Mater. Res.*, 53, 216, 2000.

137. Hayashi, K., Uenoyama, K., Mashima, T., and Sugioka, Y., "Remodeling of bone around hydroxyapatite and titanium in experimental osteoporosis," *Biomaterials*, 15, 11, 1994.

138. Fini, M., Nicoli Aldini, N., Gandolfi, M.G., et al., "Biomaterials for orthopaedic surgery in osteoporotic bone: a comparative study in osteopenic rats," *Int. J. Artif. Org.*, 20, 291, 1997.

139. Mori, H., Manabe, M., Kurachi, Y., and Nagumo, M., "Osseointegration of dental implants in rabbit bone with low mineral density," *J. Oral Maxillofac. Surg.*, 55, 351, 1997.

140. Walsh, W.R., Sherman, P., Howlett, C.R., et al., "Fracture healing in a rat osteopenia model," *Clin. Orthop.*, 342, 218, 1997.

141. Kubo, T., Shiga, T., Hashimoto, M., et al., "Osteoporosis influences the late period of fracture healing in a rat model prepared by ovariectomy and low calcium diet," *J. Steroid Biochem. Mol. Biol.*, 68, 197, 1999.

142. Fujimoto, T., Niimi, A., Sawai, T., and Ueda, M., "Effects of steroid-induced osteoporosis on osseointegration of titanium implants," *Int. J. Oral Maxillofac. Impl.*, 13, 183, 1998.

143. Vignon, G., Meunier, P., Pansu, D., et al., "Enquête clinique et anatomique sur l'étiopathogénie de l'ostéoporose sénile," *Rev. Rhumat.*, 37, 615, 1970.

144. Hordon, L.D. and Peacock, M., "Osteomalacia and osteoporosis in femoral neck fracture," *Bone Miner.*, 11, 247, 1990.

145. Ballanti, P. and Bonucci, E., "Histomorphometric aspects of bone in involutive osteoporosis," *G. Ital. Metab. Miner. Elettrol.*, 2, 203, 1988.

15 Management of Osteoporotic Fractures of Upper Extremities

Stephan W. Wachtl, Emanuel Gautier, and Roland P. Jakob

CONTENTS

I. INTRODUCTION

Osteoporosis is one of the major problems facing elderly people of both sexes, particularly women. The morbid event in osteoporosis is fracture. In the United States, approximately 1.5 million fractures are caused annually by osteoporosis. These include 700,000 vertebral fractures, 250,000 distal radius fractures, 250,000 hip fractures, and 300,000 fractures at other sites. Morbidity following these fractures is considerable. The annual cost of osteoporosis to the U.S. health-care system is at least $5 billion to $10 billion with similar incidence and cost in other developed countries. These already high costs will increase further with the continued aging of the population.[1]

Osteoporotic fractures of the upper extremities are of two main types: fractures of the proximal humerus and fractures of the distal radius. This chapter deals exclusively with these fractures. Other sites of the upper extremities can also fracture in older people, but their characteristics can also be found in younger patients. The treatment of the fractures of other sites is therefore the same as for young patients. Depending on the soft tissue conditions and accompanying injuries, the functional results of fracture sites other than the proximal humerus or the distal radius are often excellent or good and are generally comparable with those of younger patients.

Elderly patients with preexisting cardiovascular diseases or metabolic diseases such as diabetes mellitus have a predisposition to fall and could sustain a proximal humerus fracture. The risk for fracture rises due to a direct predisposition, in which osteoporosis plays the main role, accompanied by the painful arthritic joint of the upper and lower extremities and generalized muscle atrophy. These circumstances, a result of age, lead to a direct nonprotected effect of the trauma to the weakened bone.[2]

Fracture of the distal radius coupled with pathologic bone density is most often seen in elderly women. The typical patient is relatively healthy, still active in everyday activities, and has good neuromuscular functioning. The fracture incidence shows a close inverse relationship with incremental changes in bone density at the distal radial site. In a cohort of 460 women living in retirement centers, 31 distal radius fractures were reported during a 60-month period of observation.[3] In 28 of the 31 fractures, a bone density below the 325 mg/cm^2 risk value was reported. A 60-year-old woman with a life expectancy of 81 years had an estimated residual lifetime risk of radial or humeral fractures of 17 and 8%, respectively,[4] whereas the lifetime risk of fractures of the distal radius is 40% for white women and 13% for white men from 50 years of age onward.[1] The occurrence of a radial or humeral fracture is a predictive factor for the occurrence of a hip fracture. A 50-year-old woman with a radial or a humeral fracture has an estimated residual lifetime risk of sustaining a subsequent hip fracture of 17 and 16%, respectively, compared with 11% for the background population.[5]

Osteoporosis favors the occurrence of fractures but also causes a specific fracture pattern. Such osteoporotic fractures have certain characteristics and are sometimes difficult to range in the currently available fracture classification. The indirect trauma, which produces compression/distraction and shear forces, induces the direction of dislocation, the number of fragments involved or intra-articular fractures, a more or less severe and irreversible compression of cancellous bone, regardless of the geometry of the fracture. The severity of bone impaction depends on the energy absorbed during the trauma and the severity of osteoporosis. The reposition of the fracture will not restore the crushed porotic cancellous bone but will leave a bone cavity that will be surrounded by a comminuted thin cortical wall. The logical consequence would be to fill the hole with a bone graft or substitute. Nevertheless, because of the anatomic particularities of each region, the treatment has to be adapted to each individual case and problem.

II. PROXIMAL HUMERUS FRACTURE

Proximal humeral fractures represent 4 to 5% of all fractures seen in trauma and emergency departments, of which 15% need to be treated operatively.[6] Progression of the number of fractures of the proximal humerus will be dramatic in the next years. In Finland in 1970, 208 fractures and an incidence of 32 per 10^5 inhabitants were reported in the population over 60 years of age.[7] In 1998, the number rose to 1105 and the incidence to 110 per 10^5 inhabitants. During the same period, the mean age of patients increased from 72 to 77 years. Projections show that the number of fractures will greatly increase by the year 2030 to 3400 fractures and the incidence will rise to 200 per 10^5 inhabitants.

Optimal treatment of fractures of the proximal humerus still remains subject to controversy, especially in elderly patients, and precise, generally accepted guidelines for treatment are lacking.

A. Vascularization

The vascularization of the humeral head depends on the integrity of the arcuate artery and of the ascending branch of the anterior humeral circumflex artery.[8] Anastomosis between the anterior humeral circumflex artery with the dorsal artery or with the vessels of the rotator cuff has been described.[9] The branches of the anterior humeral circumflex artery can be disrupted at the time of injury, and also during surgery. Avascular necrosis has been reported to be as high as 34% in cases of extensive exposure and insertion of large metal devices.[10] Therefore, to avoid any damage to the humeral head, closed reduction, without opening the fracture area, and fixation by minimally invasive techniques have been recommended.[11]

B. Classification

Neer's classification[12] of humeral head fractures in one-, two-, three-, and four-part fractures is generally accepted. The one-part fracture represents a nondislocated fracture. The two-part fracture is one where the head is separated from the humerus at different levels between the surgical or anatomic neck, but can also include an avulsion of the lesser or the greater tuberosity. The three-part fracture is a fracture of the humeral head generally seen at the level of the surgical neck, accompanied by an avulsion of either the lesser or the greater tuberosity. The four-part fracture is a fracture of the head with avulsion of both tuberosities. This classification also has a prognostic value since the incidence of avascular humeral head necrosis is higher in the three- and four-part fractures.[13] The valgus impacted head fracture[14] is indeed a four-part fracture, as is the head-splitting fracture; it is considered as a separate entity. Other classifications have been proposed, but their reproducibility or intra- and interobserver reliability is poor.[15]

C. Conservative Treatment

Standard regimens with clear advice concerning the time of immobilization do not exist. In a prospective randomized study, Kristiansen et al.[16] did not find a statistically significant difference between a period of immobilization of 1 week vs. 3 weeks. On the other hand, Koval et al.[17] demonstrated that the percentage of good and excellent results was significantly greater and external rotation was significantly better for patients who had started supervised physical therapy sooner than 14 days after the injury, than for the patients who had started at 14 days or later. Therefore, the beginning of soft and gentle shoulder mobilization is recommended to start as soon as the pain disappears.

Conservative treatment is the treatment of choice for nondisplaced or minimally displaced proximal humerus fractures. Koval et al.[18] controlled 104 patients with a so-called one-part fracture treated conservatively with a follow-up of 41 months; 77% of the patients had a good or excellent result and functional recovery averaged 94%.

For three- and four-part fractures, conservative treatment is not indicated. Zyto et al.[19] found that 20 patients with a mean age of 75 years, who were treated conservatively for a three- or a four-part fracture, had a Constant score of 65 points. In a multicenter analysis with a follow-up of 4 years, Schai et al.[20] demonstrated that 19 patients with a three-part fracture reached a Constant score of 78 points, whereas 5 patients with a four-part fracture had a Constant score of 54 points.

D. Indications for Operative Treatment

The indications for nonoperative vs. operative treatments depend on the type of fracture and on the general condition of the patient. Neer's[12] criteria are very helpful. Generally, operative treatment should be performed if the fracture dislocation is more than 1 cm and/or if there is a tilt of the humeral head segment of more than 45°.

E. K-Wire Fixation

Stabilization of the proximal humerus fracture with K-wire after it has been reduced indirectly with a closed technique and controlled with a biplanar image intensifier is a mix of operative treatment and conservative treatment, as the fracture area remains untouched. This method was proposed by Böhler[21] in 1962. Reports seemed to be encouraging since Jaberg et al.[22] showed that 34 of a cohort of 44 patients treated with closed reduction and stabilized with percutaneously introduced K-wires had a good to an excellent result after a 3-year follow-up. The technique of percutaneous pinning is a very demanding procedure. K-wire migration remains a problem, especially in osteoporotic bone and/or when functional rehabilitation is started early.[23]

F. Screw Fixation

The use of a cannulated screw alone introduced percutaneously is a variation of the stabilization of the proximal humerus fracture with K-wire. Resh et al.[24] reported a series of 27 patients with a mean age of 54 years and a mean follow-up of 2 years. The 9 patients with three-part fractures had a mean Constant score of 85 points and the 18 patients with four-part fractures had a mean Constant score of 82 points. Two patients in the four-part group developed avascular head necrosis. The operation is technically very demanding. It remains questionable whether the screw can hold in osteoporotic bone and the danger that it may penetrate into the glenohumeral joint remains high. This procedure is therefore not recommended for elderly patients.

G. Plate Fixation

The use of a plate implies a surgical exposure of the fracture and dissection of the surrounding soft tissues. The standard approach is the deltopectoral approach reclining the vena cephalica with the deltoid muscle. The extensive dissection can lead to avascular head necrosis. Kristiansen and Christensen[25] noted four cases of avascular head necrosis in a group of 20 controlled patients with a mean follow-up of 4 years out of a cohort of 32 patients operated with insertion of an AO T-plate. In the group of 20 controlled patients, 11 patients had an unsatisfactory or a poor result. The high prevalence of bad results was also attributed to the fact that the AO T-plate used was too bulky. Paavolainen et al.[26] made the same observation; they noted postoperative restriction in the movements of the glenohumeral joint because the implant impinged under the acromion during abduction.

H. Tension-Band Fixation

Tension-band fixation can be considered a minimally invasive technique as it requires only a limited exposure of the proximal humerus. The principle of this technique uses the so-called healthy and strong tissues of the rotator cuff for fixation. Another advantage of this technique is that no hardware is placed close to the subacromial space, thus preventing impingement. Cornell et al.[27] reported that from a sample 13 patients with a mean age of 71 years and a follow-up of 20 months, 10 patients presented a good result according to the functional Hawkins scale. There was no avascular necrosis. They concluded that tension band wiring afforded sufficient fracture stability to allow early aggressive functional rehabilitation in older patients and that this technique has advantages in elderly patients with osteoporosis. Other authors do not share Cornell's optimism. Zyto et al.[19] reported a series of 19 three-part fractures and 1 four-part fracture in 20 patients with a mean age of 73 years. They were treated with semirigid fixation with tension band wiring and obtained a Constant score of only 60 points after a 50-month follow-up. Koval et al.[17] reported on a sample of 14 patients with 15 fractures treated with a tension band wiring technique, with a 33-month follow-up. Despite 80% good or excellent results, they found a rate of 26% of early loss of fixation, leading the authors to cease recommending this technique.

I. INTRAMEDULLARY FIXATION

In an attempt to optimize the biomechanical efficacy of implants, fixation of subcapital humeral fractures using intramedullary pinning seemed to provide sufficient stability without damaging the vascularity of the fracture fragments, while leaving the soft tissue layers surrounding the shoulder untouched.[28]

Prévot nails, made of a titanium alloy (Landos, Chaumont, France), are introduced in the medullary canal of the humerus through the radial epicondyle and advanced to the fracture level. Reduction is controlled and eventually definitively corrected using image control in two planes. The Prévot nails are finally pushed up in divergent directions to different segments of the humeral head. Postoperatively, the shoulder is immobilized for 6 weeks and fixed to the body in a Desault bandage. Wachtl et al.[29] reported on 61 patients with a proximal humeral fracture who were treated by closed reduction and fracture fixation with intramedullary Prévot (or Nancy) nails. The mean Constant score was 63, the mean Neer score 74, and the mean visual analogue scale 73. The 14 patients under 24 years of age reached a Constant score of 86, a Neer score of 99, and a visual analogue scale of 97, whereas 13 patients aged between 25 and 60 years presented a Constant score of 67, a Neer score of 75, and a visual analogue scale of 71. The 26 patients over 61 years had a Constant score of 48, a Neer score of 61, and a visual analogue scale of 61. One patient with total humeral head necrosis and six with partial humeral head necrosis as well as five pseudarthroses were noted (Figure 15.1). Proximal nail perforation of the humeral head due to fracture collapse was seen in 22 cases. Complications were more frequently observed in the elderly patients. End results were not related to the type of fracture. The low rate of humeral head necrosis is encouraging, particularly when considering that only one patient presented total head involvement. Because iatrogenic vascular damage seems to be a relevant factor for the development of humeral head necrosis just as the fracture itself, closed fracture reduction associated with intramedullary nailing is justified. However, the rate of nonunion and of complications is embarrassing. Age is an important prognostic factor, whereas the type of fracture had no or little influence on the final outcome. Other studies have so far failed to relate the results after operative treatment of proximal humeral fractures to the patient's age, probably because not all age categories were included in such studies. One problem with aging is the well-documented concomitant osteoporosis. In the proximal humerus, osteoporosis is an important factor as the bone mineral density of the base of the humeral head represents only about 65% of the density of the base of the femoral head.[30] The fact that the shoulder is a non-weight-bearing articulation may further enhance demineralization. Osteoporosis mainly weakens the cancellous bone, so bone impaction is a frequent sequel of a fracture. After reduction with de-impaction of the fragments, a bone defect will be present. With a posterior tilt of the humeral head, bone impaction is observed in the posterolateral region. The phenomenon is also particularly evident in the case of valgus impacted fractures where the defect is observed in the lateral side of the humeral head.[13] The bone defect is responsible for the remaining instability at the fracture level, after reduction and de-impaction (Figure 15.2). Fracture fixation alone is insufficient as secondary displacement may occur, especially in patients more than 61 years of age. The high rate of nail perforation through the humeral head is another sign of persistent fracture instability in elderly people. Secondary displacement and nail perforation does not occur in patients less than 24 years whose bone stock is optimal. Thus, bone defects should be filled with autologous cancellous bone in patients over 60 years of age. This type of management is actually not routinely applied for the proximal humerus because it is thought to necessitate an open reduction with extensive dissection. Therefore, percutaneous insertion of bone substitutes or bone cement into the bone defect, once closed reduction and fixation have been performed, should be evaluated separately.

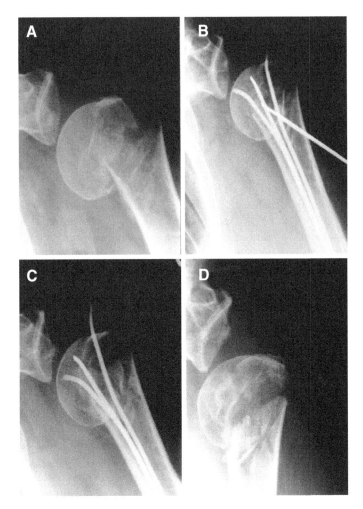

FIGURE 15.1 Proximal two-part humerus fracture with inferior subluxation of the humeral head (A). Treatment with three intramedullary Prévot nails and one Kirschner wire: immediate postoperative fracture dislocation and persistent humeral head subluxation. Migration of the Kirschner wire, which was removed 3 weeks after surgery. The Prévot nails perforated the humeral head (B). Humeral head perforation (C). Pseudoarthrosis after implant removal (D).

J.   New Trends and Implants

To avoid implant migration, new intramedullary implants have been designed. Corkscrew twisted nails can be introduced in the humerus, distal to the insertion of the deltoid, and brought up to the humeral head (Figures 15.3 and 15.4). The corkscrew twisted form of the nail allows fixation in the weakened cancellous bone. Thus, perforation should be less frequent and fracture reduction maintained until healing, despite the presence of the posterolateral bone defect. The question will be whether the defect will fill itself with bone or scar tissue, rendering it unstable and thus leading to implant breakage.

Plating is regaining popularity. Hessmann et al.[31] used a buttress plate after indirect fracture reduction. They evaluated retrospectively 98 patients with an average follow-up of 34 months. Results were good to excellent in 69% of the patients according to the Constant score and in 59% according to the Neer score. The avascular necrosis rate was 4%. The authors concluded that plate fixation may be adequate if an indirect reposition of the unstable and displaced two- to four-part

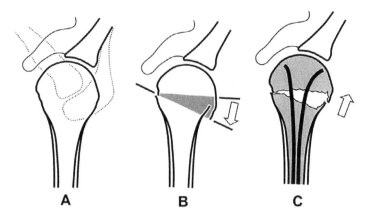

FIGURE 15.2 Proximal humerus fracture with dorsal tilt of the proximal fragment. Axial view of the proximal humerus (A). The humeral head is tilted dorsally so that impaction and comminution of the dorsal cortex are present (B). Reposition of the fracture induces a bone defect. This bone defect has to be filled; otherwise, fracture instability will persist (C).

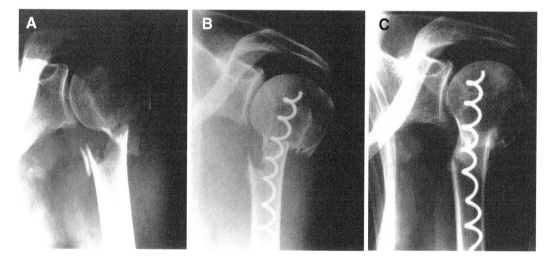

FIGURE 15.3 Proximal two-part humerus fracture (A). Treatment with an intramedullary corkscrew-shaped implant and immediate translation of the distal fragment because of the pull on the tendon of the pectoralis major (B). Consolidation was obtained at 4 months with clinically acceptable shoulder function (C).

fracture had been performed, enabling early function after treatment. The authors pointed out that poor rotational and angular stability could lead to a loss of reduction.

Palmer ct al.[32] treated nine patients with a mean age of 62 years with a customized interlocked blade plate. The plates are standard AO dynamic compression plates of a suitable length that are bent to an acute angle in an industrial vice and interlocked. At a mean follow-up of 7 months all fractures had healed, with one patient presenting a subacromial impingement as the only complication.

New plates with locked screws are now seen on the market. Following a deltopectoral approach, the lateral aspect of the humeral head is exposed. The fracture is exposed at the level of the greater and lesser tuberosity. Great care is taken not to disrupt the blood supply of the humeral head. The fracture is reduced, the humeral head is eventually elevated with an instrument, and the tuberosities

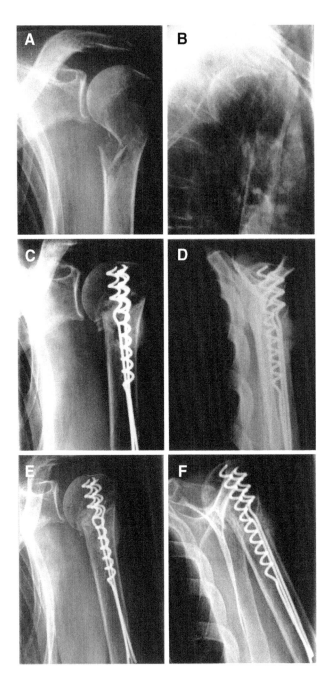

FIGURE 15.4 Proximal two-part humerus fracture. The displacement is less important on the anteroposterior view (A) than on the Neer view (B). Treatment with modified corkscrew-shaped implant. Persistent fracture gap at 3 months (C). Presence of callus on the posterior aspect of the humerus (D). Consolidation at 6 months (E, F).

are placed in position. The fracture is temporarily fixed with K-wires. The plate is then fixed on the lateral side of the proximal humerus (Figure 15.5).

The main problem in the treatment of osteoporotic proximal humerus fracture remains the bone defect that has to be solved with bone grafting. Promising reports are available: Vandenbussche et al.[33] reported on eight cases with four-part valgus-impacted proximal humeral fractures, which

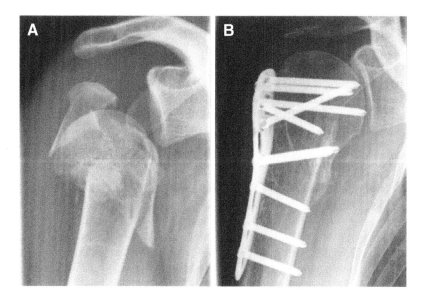

FIGURE 15.5 Proximal four-part humerus fracture anteroposterior view (A). The fracture was reduced through an open procedure and stabilized with a locked screw. At 3 months after operation bone consolidation occurs with good alignment. One screw is slightly too long (B), but no scratching is felt during shoulder mobilization.

were operated on with open reduction and stabilized with autologous bone only. By using a deltopectoral approach, the impacted segment of the humeral head was raised, the void was filled with autologous three-cortical iliac bone graft, and the tuberosities were relocated. The average Constant score was 62 after a 16-month follow-up. Magnetic resonance imaging (MRI) results showed only one asymptomatic partial avascular necrosis. Resch et al.[34] treated 22 patients with a valgus-impacted four-part fracture with a mean follow-up of 3 years. The bone defect was filled with cancellous bone graft and the fracture was stabilized with percutaneous pinning during a period of 5 weeks. The mean Constant score was 81 points and represented 84% of the score of the opposite shoulder. A Japanese group proposed to fill the void with bone cement. Matsuda et al.[35] reported on five cases of proximal humeral fractures with advanced osteoporosis treated with conventional plate and intramedullary bone cement. The outcome was similar to that of fractures seen in younger patients without osteoporosis.

K. PROSTHESIS

Prosthetic replacement of the humeral head for the treatment of three- or four-part fracture is highly controversial. The only consensus is that the results after primary prosthesis are better than with implantation 4 weeks after the injury. Dimakopoulos et al.[36] stated that patients with acute trauma who were operated on early had no difficulty in performing all tasks of the American Shoulder and Elbow Surgeons evaluation form[37] within 3 to 6 months postoperatively. In contrast, patients with an old trauma and a late reconstruction could accomplish these tasks only after 1 year of continuous exercise. Bosch et al.[38] studied 25 patients with a mean follow-up of 42 months from a series of 39 consecutive patients treated with hemiarthroplasty. The 11 patients who were operated on less than 4 weeks after injury obtained a Constant score of 65 points, whereas the patients who were operated on more than 4 weeks after the injury had a Constant score of 45 points.

Prostheses have the advantage that they allow early mobilization of the shoulder, do not require special care, and permit rapid discharge from the hospital. Pain disappears a few days after surgery. They represent a single operation, avoiding complications such as implant migration, pseudoarthrosis, or aseptic head necrosis. Activity level can be restored to the preinjury level. Skutek et al.[39] reported on 10 patients, of a cohort of 13 patients with an average follow-up of 50 months, who regained their physical activities without a change in their participation level. Function of the shoulder seemed not to be fully reestablished in cases of implantation of a shoulder prosthesis. Another series of 27 patients, average age 71 years (48 to 91), treated by humeral head replacement only obtained a Constant score of 51 in cases of a three-part fracture and 46 in cases of four-part fracture.[40] The question of long-term survival is still open and is still not answered. Despite these considerations, the solution of implanting a prosthesis should still be considered in older patients.

L. Comparison of Methods

Comparison of results with other studies is difficult. Prospective and randomized studies are rare. Nevertheless, it seems that the reported results on the management of proximal humeral fractures are often disappointing whatever method of treatment is chosen.[19] Ilchmann et al.[41] compared 16 patients treated without osteosynthesis with 18 patients treated with tension-band fixation. Most of the three-part fractures healed with good pain relief and good function in daily life but often with a loss of motion. For the patients with four-part fractures, pain, and loss of motion and function were reported. Conservative treatment seemed superior to tension-band fixation for three-part fractures. Four-part fractures healed with better function and range of motion after tension-band fixation.

M. Conclusion

The elderly patient who comes to the emergency room with a proximal humerus fracture usually suffers from osteoporosis, dysfunction of the rotator cuff, cardiopulmonary comorbidity, and a low insurance coverage. All these factors influence the prognosis, but this is the situation with which we must deal and the solution is not clearly evident. Operative management has not shown superiority over conservative management. Surgery should therefore be reserved for fractures with severe displacement. Neer's criteria give clear indication for surgery and should be taken into consideration. Moreover, dislocation or angulation that are more important than Neer's criteria can be accepted in the elderly patient. The problem of the bone void that results from the fracture reduction needs to be solved with bone grafting. Because harvesting of bone at the iliac crest raises the morbidity of the treatment of the proximal humeral fracture in elderly patients, the use of a bone substitute such as Endobon® (Merck, Darmstadt, Germany) or Tutoplast® (Tutogen, Erlangen, Germany) seems to be preferable.

III. DISTAL RADIUS FRACTURE

According to Baron et al.,[42] distal radius fractures represent 15% of the incidence of limb fractures in the population over 65 years. Women have higher rates than men of the same race and Caucasian people generally have higher rates than black people of the same gender.

A. Classification

Fractures of the distal radius are classified as extra-articular and intra-articular fractures. In cases of an extra-articular fracture (the so-called A-fracture in the AO comprehensive classification[43]), the distal fragment can be tilted or shifted to palmar or dorsal. Some intra-articular fractures involve only the palmar or dorsal margin of the distal end of the radius and represent the B-type in the AO classification. The C-type consists of intra-articular fractures, which can involve the radiocarpal joint or the distal radioulnar joint and which are combined with a metaphyseal fracture.

The typical osteoporotic fracture of the distal radius, the so-called Colles' fracture, consists of a metaphyseal fracture with a dorsal tilt of the distal fragment. This dorsal tilt implies a dorsal

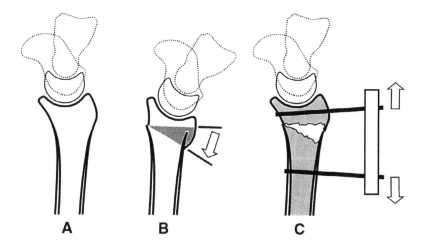

FIGURE 15.6 Distal radius fracture with dorsal tilt of the distal fragment. Lateral view of the anatomic form of the distal radius (A). Impaction and comminution of the dorsal cortex (B). Reposition of the fracture and stabilization with a nonbridging external fixator. The fracture reduction induced a bone defect that had to be filled; otherwise, fracture instability may have persisted (C).

zone of comminution of the thin and brittle corticalis and a zone of compression and impaction of the cancellous bone of the distal radius metaphysis. Flinkkila et al.[44] demonstrated that the relative size of the defect correlated with the severity of dorsal angulation of the fracture but not with the shortening of the radius. Association of such a metaphyseal fracture with an undisplaced intra-articular fracture is not uncommon. A dorsal translation of the distal fragment may be present.

The reposition of a typical osteoporotic distal radius fracture with manipulation of the distal fragment will lead to a bone cavity surrounded by a thin and brittle cortical bone (Figure 15.6). Secondary dislocation will be observed after plaster fixation, because no buttress can act against the compressive force crossing the wrist and the distal radius. The application of an external fixator will neutralize the forces crossing the wrist, so that no secondary displacement occurs as long as the external fixator stays *in situ*, but loss of reduction has been described after removal of the external fixator even at 3 months. Only the filling of the bone void with a sufficient amount of bone graft or bone substitute will prevent secondary dislocation.

In addition to the difficulty of maintaining reduction in osteoporotic fractures, others factors will also influence the end results such as Sudeck's algodystrophia or intracarpal ligament disorders.[45] Lindau et al.,[46] in a series of 92 distal radial fractures, demonstrated that instability at clinical examination of the distal radioulnar joint has been associated with a bad wrist score and doubled the visual analogue measure for pain. In another series of 51 patients with distal radial fractures, Lindau et al.[47] documented with arthroscopy that 43 of the patients presented a complete or partial tear of the triangular fibrocartilage complex. Of 11 patients with complete peripheral triangular fibrocartilage complex tears, 10 had distal radioulnar joint instability. Instability was not associated with any radiographic finding either at the time of fracture or at the follow-up examination. Initial fracture or nonunion of the styloid was not regarded as a poor prognostic factor.

B. CONSERVATIVE TREATMENT

Conservative treatment does not seem to be able to maintain reduction. Van der Linden and Ericson[51] analyzed 250 cases treated conservatively, immobilized according to five different techniques, thus creating five groups. The original dorsal angle was 26 to 28° and the dorsal angle at final follow-up was 15 to 18° for the five groups. The mean loss of dorsiflexion compared with uninjured side was 12 to 17° and the loss of palmar flexion was 15 to 17°. Villar et al.[52] studied 90 consecutive

Colles' fractures treated with immobilization for 5 weeks in either plaster or plaster combined with Viscopaste. Mean grip score of the injured wrist was 90% of the uninjured side. Of the patients, 27% reported pain that had persisted for 3 years after their injury.

The common belief that restoration of normal anatomy should absolutely be obtained to regain normal function has been placed in doubt by Young and Rayan[53] in a study of 25 sedentary low-demand patients older than 60 years. Mean age was 72 years and follow-up 34 months. The final radiographic scores revealed that 24% of patients had excellent results and 44% had good results. Five of eight patients with intra-articular fractures that healed with a residual articular incongruency of more than 2 mm had satisfactory functional outcome. The functional assessment showed that results were good or excellent in 88% of the patients. Radiographic outcome did not correlate with functional outcome. In all, 88% of the patients were able to regain their previous activities. Thus, nonoperative treatment of distal radius fractures seems to be adequate in patients with low functional demands.

C. INDICATIONS FOR SURGERY

Indications for surgical repair have been defined as follows: presence of a severe dorsal comminution; severe displacement such as a radial shortening more than 2 mm or a dorsal tilt more than 20°; intra-articular fracture; associated ulna fracture and/or distal radioulnar instability.[48]

The goal of treatment should be restoration of normal anatomy as normal radiographic appearance correlates with normal function.[49,50]

D. K-WIRE FIXATION

The stabilization of a distal radius fracture after closed reduction with percutaneous K-wires is a minimally invasive procedure and is particularly suited for elderly patients with multiple illnesses. Clancey[54] reported on 30 patients treated with percutaneus fixation with two K-wires. Only 2 patients had a minor loss of reduction. Mean volar angle was 4°. Results were excellent or satisfactory in all except 1 patient.

The stabilization of the distal radius fracture with K-wire can be performed according to Kapandji's method in which the K-wire is introduced dorsally into the fracture line, angulated palmar, and drilled in the proximal main fragment so that the K-wire is buttressing the distal fragment. Board et al.[55] reported that functional results were excellent or good in 19 patients in a cohort of 23 patients with a mean follow-up of 17 months treated according to the methods of Kapandji.

Lenoble et al.[56] compared 42 patients treated with trans-styloid K-wire fixation with 54 patients treated according to Kapandji. The radiologic reduction was better soon after Kapandji fixation, but some loss of reduction was observed. The clinical result at 2 years was similar in both groups.

The stabilization of the distal radius fracture with K-wire can be completed with bone graft. McBirnie et al.[57] treated 83 patients with open reduction, bone grafting, and fixation with a single K-wire. At a mean follow-up of 13 months, a recovery of 63% of mass grip strength was observed with an excellent return of specialized grip strength and range of motion. The advantage of this method is the ability to regain the volar tilt.

E. EXTERNAL FIXATION

External fixation is a minimally invasive procedure and can be used by itself or in combination with other implants. Threaded K-wires are inserted into the proximal radius and the second metacarpal. The reduction of the fracture is performed under image intensifier control. The bar joining the K-wires is mounted and definitive reduction is performed if needed. A tube-to-tube configuration of the external frame allows a completely free positioning of the wrist joint in all possible six degrees of freedom, better possibility of postponing manual reduction, and easy correction of axial, flexural, or rotational malalignment during surgery.[58]

Cooney et al.[59] reported a series of 65 patients with a mean age of 63 years followed for at least 2 years. Objective analysis revealed that 90% of the patients had a good or excellent result with an average of a wrist dorsiflexion of 58° and an average volar flexion of 50°. The mean grip strength was 20 kg compared with 30 kg for the uninjured side. Shortening was a median of 2 mm and dorsal tilt of the distal radial articulation was 3°. Subjective evaluation showed that 85% of the patients had a good result.

External fixation can be combined with cancellous bone grafting. Cannegieter and Juttmann[60] presented 32 fractures with a mean follow-up of 3 years treated by external fixation and cancellous grafting with minimal exposure. Results were excellent or good in 84% of the patients. All patients had satisfactory functional recovery. The average grip strength was 95% of normal.

Because of the risks inherent to bone autograft such as pain or development of hematoma at harvesting site, cancellous bone allograft seems to be a valuable alternative, despite the rise in cost that will accompany the generalized use of allograft. Herrera et al.[61] treated 17 patients with a mean age of 70 years with bone allograft and external fixation. The outcome at a mean follow-up of 23 months demonstrated three excellent, eight good, six fair, and no poor results.

Other bone substitutes such as coralline hydroxyapatite graft have been used in association with external fixation. Wolfe et al.[62] reported on 18 patients followed for 35 months out of a cohort of 21 patients. Wrist motion averaged 90% of the uninjured side and grip strength measured 75% of the uninjured side. Results in 17 of the 18 cases were rated as good or excellent. The volar tilt was 4°.

The nonbridging external fixator (Figure 15.7) presents the advantage that it does not cross the wrist, hence allowing early mobilization of the wrist. The two distal K-wires are inserted in the distal radial fragment instead of the second metacarpal. The reduction can be performed with the help of the K-wires, used as joysticks. Nevertheless, the anchorage of the K-wires in the distal fragment can be critical if osteoporosis is too severe, if the size of the distal fragment is too small, or if the distal fragment presents an intra-articular fracture not recognized on the preoperative radiographs. McQueen et al.[63] reported a series of 20 patients with an unstable redisplaced fracture of the distal radius with sufficient space in the distal fragment to allow use of a nonbridging technique. Volar tilt was maintained at a mean of 4° and radial shortening was a mean of 1 mm at final follow-up. Of the 20 patients, 19 regained normal carpal alignment. Grip strength returned to a mean of 74% of the normal side. Range of motion was restored to 80%. The rate of complication was 15%. In a randomized prospective study including 60 patients comparing the nonbridging technique with the bridging technique, McQueen[64] demonstrated that the functional result showed better grip strength and flexion in the nonbridging group in all stages of review.

F. PLATES

Plates are used in combination with open reduction. They allow stable fixation and early rehabilitation. They can be used alone or in combination with bone graft or even in combination with an external fixator if one judges that additional stability is needed.

Multiple implants have been proposed. Hove et al.[65] used open reduction and fracture fixation with an AO 3.5-mm T-plate in 31 patients and achieved excellent or good function in 26 patients at a mean follow-up of 4 years. Jakob et al.[66] reported a series of 74 fractures of the distal radius treated with two 2.0-mm titanium plates placed on the radial and ulnar faces of the dorsal distal radius angulated 50 to 70° apart. Anatomic results were excellent or good in 72 patients; 71 patients regained their previous activity levels (Figure 15.8).

Complications are not unusual when using plates. Hove et al.[65] reported six complications in the series presented just above. In a series of 34 patients treated by open reduction and osteosynthesis

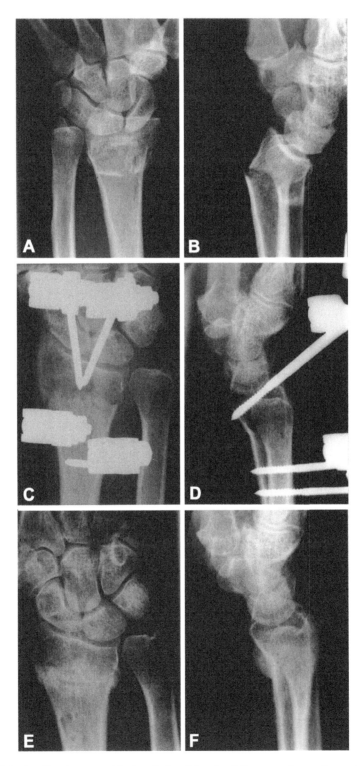

FIGURE 15.7 Distal radius fracture with dorsal tilt of the distal fragment. Impaction and comminution of the dorsal cortex (A, B). Treatment with a nonbridging external fixator (C, D). The radiographs taken after external fixator removal showed good axial alignment (E, F).

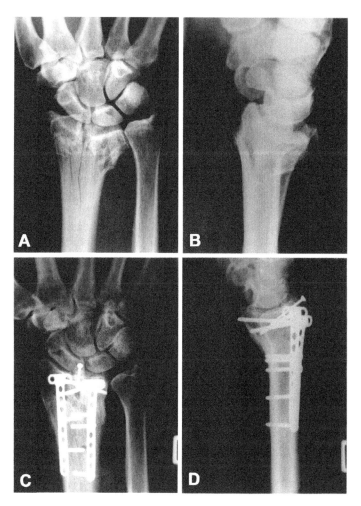

FIGURE 15.8 Distal intra-articular radius fracture with severe displacement (A, B). Treatment with two AO 2-mm T-shaped plates. The distal screw fixes a small-sized fragment of the dorsal lip of the radius. Good axial alignment and no osteoarthritis at the 1 year follow-up were found (C, D).

with plate and screws, Fitoussi et al.[67] showed a 26% complication rate despite an overall good or excellent result at final follow-up in 82% of the patients. A marked change in fracture alignment between the postoperative period and final follow-up was noted in 9% and presence of osteoarthritis was seen in 18% of the patients.

Other plates especially shaped for the distal radius have been proposed. The π-plate (Stratek, Oberdorf, Switzerland), shaped like the Greek letter π, is a device that matches the anatomy of the distal radius and allows a near half-circumferential dorsal buttress of comminuted intra-articular and extra-articular radial fractures. The juxta-articular band of the plate can be fixed with self-tapping screws or with locked buttress pins protecting the articular reconstruction.[68] Ring et al.[69] reported a prospective study of 22 complex fractures of the distal radius, which were treated with a π-plate and achieved, after a mean follow-up of 14 months, an average wrist motion of 76% and an average grip strength of 56% of the contralateral side. Irritations of the tendons in the second dorsal compartment were seen in 22% of the patients. Hahnloser et al.,[70] in a prospective randomized study, compared a group of 21 patients operated with the new π-plate with a group of 25 patients treated with two ¼ tube plates. Bone grafting was performed in both groups. Results were good to excellent in 56% of the patients in the π-plate group, whereas in the two ¼ tube plates 82% of the patients achieved excellent to good results. The complication rate in the π-plate group was 14%. No complications were observed in the second group. The authors conclude they can no longer recommend this plate.

G. New Trends

Norian SRS (Norian Corp., Cupertino, USA) is a percutaneously injectable, fast-setting, high-strength calcium phosphate. The material cures *in vivo* to form a carbonated apatite of low crystallinity and small grain size similar to the mineral phase of bone. It begins to harden 10 min after injection, at which time the paste is cured. It attains an initial compressive strength of 10 MPa within 10 min and a final compressive strength of 55 MPa as well as a final tensile strength of 2.1 MPa. The plasticity of Norian SRS during implantation offers the potential for filling irregular bony voids. Norian SRS is bioabsorbable as it appears to be recognized by osteoclasts as the inorganic phase of bone and osteoclastic cells have been observed tunneling through the bone cement.[71] Jupiter et al.[72] treated 20 patients with Norian SRS injected into the fracture area, followed by an immobilization with a cast for 6 weeks. Five patients were controlled at 1-year follow-up. The volar angle was 6.8°. Range of motion was between 85 and 100% of the contralateral wrist. Grip strength was 88% of the contralateral side. Kopylov et al.[73] observed six patients treated with Norian SRS followed by an external splint for 2 weeks. After 1 year, all patients had a satisfactory clinical outcome. The material maintained reduction except in one case in which the cement fragmented into small pieces. In a second study, Kopylov et al.[74] compared 20 patients treated with Norian SRS and immobilized by a cast for 2 weeks with 20 patients treated with an external fixator for 5 weeks. Patients treated with a cement injection had better grip strength, wrist extension, and forearm supination at 7 weeks. There were no differences at 3 months or later. Radiographs showed a progressive redislocation in both groups. None of the methods could completely stabilize the fracture. Long-term studies on resorption or integration of Norian SRS are yet not available; thus routine recommendations cannot be made at this time.

To act as a buttress, plates are placed on the dorsal side of the radius. A new concept proposes to put a T-shaped plate with angular locked pins to the volar aspect of the radius, through a volar approach. The pins are placed next to the distal radial articulation so that the pins support the distal radial fragment. Because the angular stabilized pins rest on the subchondral plate of the distal radial, the complex plate-pins provide a fixed-angle support to the fracture reconstruction. The morbidity of the approach is low and the wrist can be mobilized after operation. Depending on the size of the dorsal defect, the defect can be filled through a minidorsal approach or it can be filled using the palmar approach. The danger lies in the fact that the pins can be placed in the joint. The advantage is that the plate is not in contact with tendons, as the plate can be covered with the muscle belly of the muscle quadratus pronator.

We performed six osteosyntheses of the distal radius with a volar plate with locked pins and screws through a volar approach for extra-articular dorsal tilted distal radius in six patients (four women and two men) with a mean age of 46 years (range, 31 to 69). Preoperative dorsal tilt was 17° (range, 9 to 29), radial tilt was 14° (range, 0 to 30), and radial shortening was 3 mm (range, 0 to 7.5). Postoperative reconstruction resulted in a mean dorsal tilt of –6° (range, –10 to –2), a mean radial tilt of 24° (range, 19 to 28), and a radial shortening of 0 mm (range, –1 to 1). Mean range of motion after an average follow-up of 10 months (range, 6 to 12) showed a volar flexion of 45° (range, 30 to 60) and a dorsal extension of 42° (range, 20 to 70). Radial abduction was 15° (range, 10 to 20) and ulnar adduction 18° (range, 15 to 20). Functional recovery occurred in all patients. A single complication was noted, namely, the intra-articular placement of pins, which was corrected by a second operation. Final outcome was excellent (Figure 15.9).

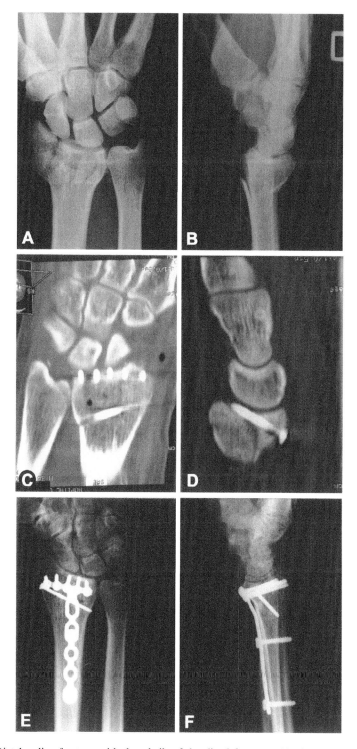

FIGURE 15.9 Distal radius fracture with dorsal tilt of the distal fragment (A, B). Treatment with a palmar plate with fixed angled locked screw. Postoperative computerized tomography scan showed that the locked screw is placed in the radiocarpal joint (C, D). The position of the screw was corrected. At 3 months after this second operation the fracture was healed. The reconstruction of the articulation is anatomic. The function of the wrist fully recovered (E, F).

H. COMPARISON OF METHODS

Following a comparison of the different methods used today, it remains difficult to determine generally accepted guidelines for the treatment of the distal radius fracture. One study seems to indicate that external fixation is the treatment of choice. Comparing conservative treatment, external fixation, and open reduction with internal fixation, in the treatment of 90 displaced intra-articular distal radial fracture, Kapoor et al.[75] demonstrated that functional results were good or excellent in 43% of the cast patients, in 80% of the external fixation group, and in 63% of the open reduction and internal fixation group. On the other hand, McQueen et al.,[76] comparing (1) remanipulation and casting, (2) open reduction and bone grafting, and (3) closed external fixation with and (4) without mobilization of the wrist at 3 weeks, could not determine a difference in functional results. Mean grip strength was 63% and mean recovery of range of motion was 91% when expressed as a percentage of the normal hand, without statistically significant differences among the four groups. Radiologic assessment showed improvement in angulation of the distal radius for the open reduction and bone grafting group which present a dorsal angulation of –3°, compared to a mean of dorsal tilt of 8° for the three other groups.

I. CONCLUSION

Restoration of the anatomy is an important factor for the recovery of the function of the wrist, but is not the only factor influencing functional results. Carpal alignment, defined as the longitudinal axis of the capitate with respect to the axis of the radius, also seems to be an important factor.

Maintaining reduction is the challenge in the treatment of the osteoporotic fracture of the distal radius, because the dorsal bone defect at the dorsal side of the radius induces instability of the fracture with inherent danger of redislocation. Filling this defect after fracture reduction will provide an inherent stability so the fracture can heal in anatomic position. The filling can be done with bone autograft or bone substitute, which is particularly promising as it avoids donor site morbidity.

REFERENCES

1. Riggs, B.L. and Melton, L.J., III, "The worldwide problem of osteoporosis: insights afforded by epidemiology," *Bone*, 17, 505S, 1995.
2. Kelsey, J.L., Browner, W.S., Seeley, D.G., et al., "Risk factors for fractures of the distal forearm and proximal humerus. The study of osteoporotic fractures research group," *Am. J. Epidemiol.*, 135, 477, 1992.
3. Lester, G.D., Anderson, J.J., Tylavsky, F.A., et al., "Update on the use of distal radial bone density measurements in prediction of hip and Colles' fracture risk," *J. Orthop. Res.*, 2, 220, 1990.
4. Lauritzen, J.B., Schwarz, P., Lund, B., et al., "Changing incidence and residual lifetime risk of common osteoporosis-related fractures," *Osteoporos. Int.*, 3, 127, 1993.
5. Lauritzen, J.B., Schwarz, P., McNair, P., et al., "Radial and humeral fractures as predictors of subsequent hit, radial or humeral fractures in women, and their seasonal variation," *Osteoporos. Int.*, 3, 133, 1993.
6. Horak, J. and Nilsson, B.E., "Epidemiology of fracture of the upper end of the humerus," *Clin. Orthop.*, 112, 250, 1975.
7. Kannus, P., Palvanen, M., Miemi, S., et al., "Osteoporotic fractures of the proximal humerus in elderly Finnish persons," *Acta Orthop. Scand.*, 71, 465, 2000.
8. Laing, P.G., "The arterial supply of the adult humerus," *J. Bone Joint Surg.*, 38A 1105, 1956.
9. Gerber, C., Schneeberger, A.G., and Vinh, T., "The arterial vascularization of the humeral head. An anatomic study," *J. Bone Joint Surg.*, 72A, 1486, 1990.
10. Sturzenegger, M., Fornaro, E., and Jakob, R.P., "Results of surgical treatment of multifragmented fractures of the humeral head," *Arch. Orthop. Trauma Surg.*, 100, 249, 1982.

11. Cuomo, F., Flatow, E.L., Maday, M.G., et al., "Open reduction and internal fixation of two- and three-part displaced surgical neck fractures of the proximal humerus," *J. Shoulder Elbow Surg.*, 1, 287, 1992.
12. Neer, C.S., "Displaced proximal humerus fractures. Part I: classification and evaluation," *J. Bone Joint Surg.*, 52A, 1077, 1970.
13. Esser, R.D., "Open reduction and internal fixation of three- and four-part fractures of the proximal humerus," *Clin. Orthop.*, 299, 244, 1994.
14. Jakob, R.P., Miniaci, A., Anson, P.S., et al., "Four-part valgus impacted fractures of the proximal humerus," *J. Bone Joint Surg.*, 73B, 295, 1991.
15. Siebenrock, K.A. and Gerber, C., "The reproducibility of classification of fractures of the proximal end of the humerus," *J. Bone Joint Surg.*, 75A, 1751, 1993.
16. Kristiansen, B., Angermann, P., and Larsen, T.K., "Functional results following fractures of the proximal humerus: a controlled clinical study comparing two periods of immobilization," *Arch. Orthop. Trauma Surg.*, 108, 339, 1989.
17. Koval, K.J., Sanders, R., Zuckerman, J.D., et al., "Modified-tension band wiring of displaced surgical neck fractures of the humerus," *J. Shoulder Elbow Surg.*, 2, 85, 1993.
18. Koval, K.J., Gallagher, M.A., Marsicano, J.G., et al., "Functional outcome after minimally displaced fractures of the proximal part of the humerus," *J. Bone Joint Surg.*, 79A, 203, 1997.
19. Zyto, K., Ahrengart, L., Sperber, A., and Törnkvist, H., "Treatment of displaced proximal humeral fractures in elderly patients," *J. Bone Joint Surg.*, 79B, 412, 1997.
20. Schai, P., Imhoff, A., and Preiss, S. "Comminuted humeral head fractures: a multicenter analysis," *J. Shoulder Elbow Surg.*, 4, 319, 1995.
21. Böhler, J., "Perkutane Osteosynthese mit dem Röntgenbildverstärker," *Wien. Klin. Wochenschr.*, 74, 485, 1962.
22. Jaberg, H., Warner, J.J.P., and Jakob, R.P., "Percutaneous stabilization of unstable fractures of the humerus," *J. Bone Joint Surg.*, 74A, 508, 1992.
23. Lyons, F.A. and Rockwood, C.A., "Migration of pins used in operations on the shoulder," *J. Bone Joint Surg.*, 72A, 1262, 1992.
24. Resch, H., Povacz, P., Fröhlich, R., and Wambacher, M., "Percutaneous fixation of three- and four-part fractures of the proximal humerus," *J. Bone Joint Surg.*, 79B, 295, 1997.
25. Kristiansen, B. and Christensen, S.W., "Plate fixation of proximal humeral fractures," *Acta Orthop. Scand.*, 57, 320, 1986.
26. Paavolainen, P., Björkenhein, J.M., Slätis, P., and Paukku, P., "Operative treatment of severe proximal humeral fractures," *Acta Orthop. Scand.*, 54, 374, 1983.
27. Cornell, C.N., Levine, D., and Pagnani, M.J., "Internal fixation of proximal humerus fractures using the screw-tension band technique," *J. Orthop. Trauma*, 8, 23, 1994.
28. Gautier, E., Slongo, T., and Jakob, R.P., "Die Behandlung der subkapitalen Humerusfraktur mit dem Prévot-Nagel," *Z. Unfallchir. Vers. Med.*, 85, 145, 1992.
29. Wachtl, S.W., Marti, C.B., Hoogewoud, H.M., et al., "Treatment of proximal humerus fracture using multiple intramedullary flexible nails," *Arch. Orthop. Trauma Surg.*, 120, 171, 2000.
30. Saitoh, S. and Nakatsuchi, Y., "Osteoporosis of the proximal humerus: comparison of bone-mineral density and mechanical strength with the proximal femur," *J. Shoulder Elbow Surg.*, 2, 78, 1993.
31. Hessmann, M., Baumgaertel, F., Gehling, H., et al., "Plate fixation of proximal humeral fractures with indirect reduction: surgical technique and results utilizing three shoulder scores," *Injury*, 30, 453, 1999.
32. Palmer, S.H., Handley, R., and Willett, K., "The use of interlocked 'customised' blade plates in the treatment of metaphyseal fractures in patients with poor bone stock," *Injury*, 31, 187, 2000.
33. Vandenbussche, E., Peraldi, P., Naouri, J.F., et al., "Four part valgus impacted fractures of the proximal humerus: graft reconstruction," *Rev. Chir. Orthop.*, 82, 658, 1996.
34. Resch, H., Beck, E., and Bayley, I., "Reconstruction of the valgus-impacted humeral head fracture," *J. Shoulder Elbow Surg.*, 4, 73, 1995.
35. Matsuda, M., Kiyoshige, Y., Takagi, M., and Hamasaki, M., "Intramedullary bone-cement fixation for proximal humeral fracture in elderly patients," *Acta Orthop. Scand.*, 70, 283, 1999.
36. Dimakopoulos, P., Potamitis, N., and Lambiris, E., "Hemiarthroplasty in the treatment of comminuted intra-articular fractures of the proximal humerus," *Clin. Orthop.*, 341, 7, 1997.
37. Rockwood, C.A. and Matsen, F.A., *The Shoulder*, W. B. Saunders, Philadelphia, 1990, 161.

38. Bosch, U., Skutek, M., Fremerey, R.W., and Tscherne, H., "Outcome after primary and secondary hemiarthroplasty in elderly patients with fractures of the proximal humerus," *J. Shoulder Elbow Surg.*, 7, 479, 1998.

39. Skutek, M., Fremerey, R.W., and Bosch, U., "Level of physical activity in elderly patients after hemiarthroplasty for three- and four-part fractures of the proximal humerus," *Arch. Orthop. Trauma Surg.*, 117, 252, 1998.

40. Zyto, K., Wallace, W.A., Frostick, S.P., and Preston, B.J., "Outcome after hemiarthroplasty for three and four part fractures of the proximal humerus," *J. Shoulder Elbow Surg.*, 7, 85, 1998.

41. Ilchmann, T., Ochsner, P.E., Wingstrand, H., and Jonsson, K., "Nonoperative treatment vs. tension-band osteosynthesis in three- and four-part proximal humeral fractures. A retrospective study of 34 fractures from two different trauma centers," *Int. Orthop.*, 22, 316, 1998.

42. Baron, J.A., Karagas, M., Barrett, J., et al., "Basic epidemiology of fractures of the upper and lower limb among Americans over 65 years of age," *Epidemiology*, 7, 612, 1996.

43. Müller, M.E., Allgöwer, M., Schneider, R., and Willenegger, H., *Manual of Internal Fixation*, Springer, Berlin, 1991.

44. Flinkkila, T., Nikkola-Sihto, A., Raatikainen, T., et al., "Role of metaphyseal cancellous bone defect size in secondary displacement in Colles' fracture," *Arch. Orthop. Trauma Surg.*, 119, 319, 1999.

45. Wachtl, S.W. and Sennwald, G.R., "Arthroscopie du poignet: apport diagnostique et thérapeutique," *Int. Orthop.*, 19, 339, 1995.

46. Lindau, T., Hagberg, L., Adlercreutz, C., et al., "Distal radioulnar instability is an independent worsening factor in distal radial fractures," *Clin. Orthop.*, 376, 229, 2000.

47. Lindau, T., Adlercreutz, C., and Aspenberg, P., "Peripheral tears of the triangular fibrocartilage complex cause distal radioulnar joint instability after distal radial fractures," *J. Hand Surg.*, 25, 464, 2000.

48. Jupiter, J.B., "Fractures of the distal end of the radius," *J. Bone Joint Surg.*, 73A, 461, 1991.

49. Howard, P.W., Stewart, H.D., Hind, R.E., and Burke, F.D., "External fixation or plaster for severely displaced comminuted Colles' fractures? A prospective study of anatomic and functional results," *J. Bone Joint Surg.*, 71B, 68, 1989.

50. Sennwald, G.R., *L'entité Radius-Carpe*, Springer, Berlin, 1987, 115.

51. Van der Linden, W. and Ericson, R., "Colles' fracture. How should its displacement be measured and how should it be immobilized?" *J. Bone Joint Surg.*, 63A, 1285, 1981.

52. Villar, R.N., Marsh, D., Rushton, N., and Greatorex, R.A., "Three years after Colles' fracture. A prospective review," *J. Bone Joint Surg.*, 69B, 635, 1987.

53. Young, B.T. and Rayan, G.M., "Outcome following nonoperative treatment of displaced distal radius fractures in low-demand patients older than 60 years," *J. Hand Surg.*, 25, 19, 2000.

54. Clancey, G.J., "Percutaneous Kirschner-wire fixation of Colles' fractures. A prospective study of thirty cases," *J. Bone Joint Surg.*, 66A, 1008, 1987.

55. Board, T., Kocialkowski, A., and Andrew, G., "Does Kapandji wiring help in older patients? A retrospective comparative review of displaced intra-articular distal radial fractures in patients over 55 years," *Injury*, 30, 663, 1999.

56. Lenoble, E., Dumontier, C., Goutallier, D., and Apoil, A., "Fracture of the distal radius. A prospective comparison between trans-styloid and Kapandji fixations," *J. Bone Joint Surg.*, 77B, 562, 1995.

57. McBirnie, J., Court-Brown, S.M., and McQueen, M.M., "Early open reduction and bone grafting for unstable fractures of the distal radius," *J. Bone Joint Surg.*, 77B, 571, 1995.

58. Gautier, E. and Stutz, P., "Combination of the small external fixator and standard tubular system," *Injury*, 25, S 35, 1994.

59. Cooney, W.P., Linscheid, R.L., and Dobyns, J.H., "External pin fixation for unstable Colles' fractures," *J. Bone Joint Surg.*, 61A, 840, 1979.

60. Cannegieter, D.M. and Juttmann, J.W., "Cancellous grafting and external fixation for unstable Colles' fractures," *J. Bone Joint Surg.*, 79B, 428, 1997.

61. Herrera, M., Chapman, C.B., Roh, M., et al., "Treatment of unstable distal radius fractures with cancellous allograft and external fixation," *J. Hand Surg.*, 24, 1269, 1999.

62. Wolfe, S.W., Pike, L., Slade, J.F., III, and Katz, L.D., "Augmentation of distal radius fracture fixation with coralline hydroxyapatite bone graft substitute," *J. Hand Surg.*, 24, 816, 1999.

63. McQueen, M.M., Simpsson, D., and Court-Brown, C.M., "Use of the Hoffman 2 compact external fixator in the treatment of redisplaced unstable distal radial fractures," *J. Orthop. Trauma*, 13, 501, 1999.
64. McQueen, M.M., "Redisplaced unstable fractures of the distal radius. A randomised, prospective study of bridging vs. non-bridging external fixation," *J. Bone Joint Surg.*, 80B, 665, 1998.
65. Hove, L.M., Nilsen, P.T., Furnes, O., et al., "Open reduction and internal fixation of displaced intra-articular fractures of the distal radius. 31 patients followed for 3–7 years," *Acta Orthop. Scand.*, 68, 59, 1997.
66. Jakob, M., Rikli, D.A., and Regazzoni, P., "Fractures of the distal radius treated by internal fixation and early function. A prospective study of 73 consecutive patients," *J. Bone Joint Surg.*, 82B, 340, 2000.
67. Fitoussi, F., Ip, W.T., and Chow, S.P., "Treatment of displaced intra-articular fractures of the distal end of the radius with plates," *J. Bone Joint Surg.*, 79A, 1303, 1997.
68. Ring, D. and Jupiter, J.B., "A new plate for internal fixation of the distal radius," *AO/ASIF Dialogue*, 9, 1996.
69. Ring, D., Jupiter, J.B., Brennwald, J., et al., "Prospective multicenter trial of a plate for dorsal fixation of distal radius fractures," *J. Hand Surg.*, 22A, 777, 1997.
70. Hahnloser, D., Platz, A., Amgwerd, M., and Trentz, O., "Internal fixation of distal radius fractures with dorsal dislocation: π-plate or two 1/4 tube plates? A prospective randomized study," *J. Trauma*, 47, 760, 1999.
71. Constantz, B.R., Ison, I.C., Fulmer, M.T., et al., "Skeletal repair *in situ* formation of the mineral phase of bone," *Science*, 267, 1796, 1995.
72. Jupiter, J.B., Winters, S., Sigman, S., et al., "Repair of five distal radius fractures with an investigational cancellous bone cement: a preliminary report," *J. Orthop. Trauma*, 11, 110, 1997.
73. Kopylov, P., Jonsson, K., Thorngren, K.G., and Aspenberg, P., "Injectable calcium phosphate in the treatment of distal radial fractures," *J. Hand Surg.*, 21B, 768, 1996.
74. Kopylov, P., Runnqvist, K., Jonsson, K., and Aspenberg, P., "Norian SRS vs. external fixation in redisplaced distal radial fractures. A randomised study in 40 patients," *Acta Orthop. Scand.*, 70, 1, 1999.
75. Kapoor, H., Agarwal, A., and Dhaon, B.K., "Displaced intra-articular fractures of distal radius: a comparative evaluation of results following closed reduction, external fixation and open reduction with internal fixation," *Injury*, 31, 75, 2000.
76. McQueen, M.M., Hajducka, C., and Court-Brown, C.M., "Redisplaced unstable fractures of the distal radius. A prospective randomised comparison of four methods of treatment," *J. Bone Joint Surg.*, 78B, 404, 1996.

16 Management of Osteoporotic Fractures of Lower Extremities

Dariusz Palczewski

CONTENTS

I. INTRODUCTION

Simultaneous growth and aging of the global population has resulted in an increased incidence of osteoporotic fractures and has considerably raised the related health-care expenses.[1] At the beginning of the 1980s, the noted incidence of osteoporotic fractures in the United States was 250,000 fractures per year. The national health-care system expenses were established at $10 billion, while the number of inhabitants was 250 million. The prognoses then predicted that the annual number of fractures would reach 650,000 by the year 2050.[2] In the National Osteoporosis Foundation report from 1995, a cost of $13.8 billion was cited, of which $8.6 billion (63%) was due to fractures of the proximal femur alone.[3] In 1990, it was predicted that the cost of treatment of proximal femoral fractures would be as high as $240 billion in 2040.[4] These data suggest the size of economic, therapeutic, and social problems created by these fractures and highlight the prominence of fractures of the hip. The role of osteoporosis in proximal tibial fractures and ankle fractures is not as marked as in fractures of the hip.

This chapter presents the current standards of treatment of osteoporotic fractures with the main focus placed on femoral neck fractures and intertrochanteric fractures. A broad account of the historical development of treatment methods is given and recent innovations creating new therapeutic possibilities for the future are presented. In the discussion of treatment methods, widely accepted standards are presented as well as contradictory opinions, as controversy has always been the motor of progress in medicine.

II. FRACTURES OF THE PROXIMAL FEMUR

A. INTRODUCTION

Femoral neck fractures present the largest and most common threat for patients' health and life. At the beginning of the 19th century, Sir Astley Cooper commented on how difficult it was to find examples of fracture in the proximal region of the thigh.[5] During the last few decades, there has been a significant increase in the number of hip fractures in urbanized societies. The aging of the population is the most important factor behind this increase; the number of fractures increases exponentially when analyzed using this parameter.[6] The risk is doubled every 5 years after the age of 65.[7] The most important etiologic factor in this increase is senile osteoporosis, secondary to hormonal dysfunction and other physiologic deficiencies in the elderly population.[8-12] Other factors include malnutrition, neuromuscular conditions,[13-15] and reduced physical activity of aged subjects, which is particularly common in cities.[16,17] Statistical data reflect the magnitude of the problem. In Spain, the incidence of hip fractures is 27 per 100,000 inhabitants per year,[18] whereas in the United States it is three times higher,[19] and in Sweden twice as high.[20] In Poland, the incidence is 35 fractures per 100,000 inhabitants per year.[21] In the United States, hip fracture incidence is approximately 250,000 per year, producing annual health-care expenditures of $8.7 billion. The actual number of fractures in the United States doubled between 1960 and 1980, and is predicted to triple relative to current rates by the year 2050.[22] Hip fracture patients occupy 20% of all orthopaedic beds and have an average length of stay of 30 days.[23]

B. ANATOMY

The proximal femoral epiphysis generally is closed by the age of 16 years, thus establishing the anatomy of the proximal part of the femur in an adult.[24] The neck shaft angle is approximately $130 \pm 7°$ and the femoral neck is normally anteverted with respect to the femoral shaft. This anteversion has been measured as $10 \pm 7°$ in normal specimens; neither of these parameters varies substantially between the sexes. The diameter of the femoral head varies according to the size of the individual and ranges from 40 to 60 mm. The thickness of the articular cartilage covering the femoral head averages from 4 mm at the superior portion to 3 mm at the periphery.[25] A synovial membrane covers the entire femoral neck anteriorly but only the proximal half posteriorly. The length and shape of the femoral neck show considerable variation in normal specimens. According to Harty[26] and Griffin,[27] the calcar femorale (a dense vertical plate of bone that originates from the posteromedial portion of the femoral shaft, radiates superiorly toward the greater trochanter, and fuses with the posterior cortex of the femoral neck) plays a central role in the development of fracture patterns of the proximal part of the femur. Trueta and Harrison[28] studied the vascular anatomy of the proximal aspect of the femur using injection techniques and found that most of the femoral head is supplied by the lateral epiphyseal artery (two thirds to four fifths). The inferior metaphyseal vessel supplies the more distal metaphyseal bone anteriorly and inferiorly. The third major blood supply to the femoral head is the artery of the ligamentum teres, which generally anostomoses with the system of the lateral epiphyseal artery.[29,30] Many authors have noted that the important vessels that supply the major part of femoral head — the lateral epiphyseal artery system — are contained within the retinacular reflection on the femoral neck (the retinaculum of Weitbrecht).[30,31]

C. EPIDEMIOLOGY

Fractures of the hip have occurred with increasing frequency as longevity has increased,[32] and in an older population there is inevitably a higher proportion of patients who have a chronic illness. Increased age, dementia, a malignant tumor, and cardiopulmonary disease have all been associated with an increased risk of fracture of the femoral neck, a poorer outcome, and a higher mortality rate.[33,34] Fractures of the hip occur more commonly in Caucasian individuals than in black individuals, but when a fracture of the hip occurs in a black patient it is more likely to be a subcapital or a femoral neck fracture. The risk of a second fracture of the hip is twice the risk of a first fracture because of the increased likelihood of falling.[35] Long-term physical activity has been shown to reduce the risk of hip fracture,[36] and the use of supplemental vitamin D_3 and calcium has been

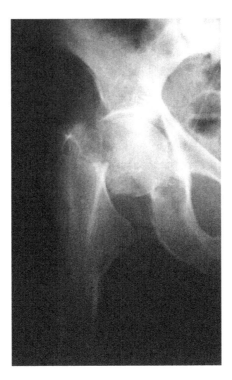

FIGURE 16.1 Femoral neck fracture. Anteroposterior view.

shown to reduce the risk of hip fracture in elderly women.[37] Fractures of the proximal femur are divided into femoral neck fractures and intertrochanteric fractures.

III. FEMORAL NECK FRACTURES

A. BIOMECHANICS OF THE FRACTURE

The type of trauma that is associated with most femoral neck fractures (more than 90%) is a fall from a standing position.[38] Such a fall may not cause a fracture in a femoral neck (Figure 16.1) of normal density, and the issue has been raised as to whether the fracture precedes the fall or the fall causes the fracture. Sloan and Holloway[39] found that 13 of 54 (24%) patients had increased pain in the groin before the lower limb gave way. Freeman et al.[40] found numerous fatigue fractures in control specimens, with the highest concentration in the subcapital region. Although fatigue fractures of the femoral neck occur and may displace, most authors have believed that the trauma of the fall produces the fracture in most patients.[33] Because the number of fatigue fractures of trabeculae in the femoral neck increases as bone density decreases, most fractures that occur before a fall or without a fall do so in the presence of severe osteoporosis.[40] Less common are fractures of the femoral neck resulting from high-energy traumata, which are capable of damaging a femoral neck of normal density; those are not included in this chapter.

B. HISTORY

Ambrose Paré, the famous French surgeon, recognized the existence of hip fractures over 400 years ago.[41] In 1783, Pott described the technique of exerting traction in flexion on the fractured limb to reduce the severe shortening that usually resulted. This technique was later refined by Dupuytren and by Malgaigne.[42] Usually, however, the overall results were poor. In the early 19th century, Sir Astley Cooper expressed the sense of pessimism that prevailed about the eventual outcome of hip fractures.[5] He appears to have been the first to attempt to delineate clearly between fractures of the femoral neck, or intracapsular fractures, and other fractures and dislocations of the hip. He believed that nonunion of intracapsular fractures was related to the loss of blood supply to the proximal fragment. In 1867, Philips introduced a technique for longitudinal and lateral traction to be used in the treatment of femoral neck fractures to eliminate shortening and deformity of the limb.[43] In 1902, Whitman[44] introduced a combination of abduction, internal rotation, and traction under the then-new general anesthesia. This was followed by a 3-month period of immobilization in a spica cast. The first significant improvement in results occurred in those who survived this treatment. The earliest attempt at internal fixation of a fractured femoral head by driving a metallic nail through the trochanter was apparently by Langenbeck[45] in 1850. Similar procedures were reported by Konig[46] and Trendelenburg[47] in 1878, but the results were poor. The internal fixation techniques were abandoned until nailing by open reduction was reported by Smith-Petersen and Cave[48] in 1931. This was improved in 1932 with the introduction of "blind nailing" fixation under roentgenographic control by Westcott[49] in the United States. The technique of closed reduction and fixation was improved over the years with the introduction of various fixation devices, fracture tables for reduction and control of the fragments, image intensifiers for shorter surgical time, improved anesthesia technique, and antibiotics for sepsis control. As a result, internal fixation proved to be an improvement over closed reduction and traction.[50-52] The incidence of nonunion, failure of fixation, and avascular necrosis after these procedures prompted the development of prostheses to replace the femoral head. The prostheses introduced by Moore[53] and Thompson[54] were first used by surgeons for salvage after failure of internal fixation, but with increased experience surgeons used them for primary treatment of these fractures. The single-unit prosthesis introduced by Moore and Thompson came in variable head sizes with the stem size varying proportionally with the head size. Their early experiences were published in 1954[54] and 1957.[53] In the following years various complications were described. Early complications included perioperative death,[55,56] fractures of the greater trochanter or shaft of the femur,[55-57] dislocation,[55,56,58] and infection.[55,56] Late complications inclined cartilage wear and protrusion[59-61] and component loosening.[61-63] Another step forward was made with the introduction of the total hip arthroplasty. The first hip endoprosthesis was designed by Adam Gruca in 1949,[64] who was followed by McKee and Farrar in 1957,[65] and by Charnley in 1958.[66] Negative features of these early prostheses included low mechanical endurance of materials and low stability of anchoring in bone. Only with the introduction of "bone glue," or cement, were the results of treatment significantly improved.[67] However, the negative features of cement, such as the large amount of heat emitted in the process of binding, and polymer degradation, which may result in implant loosening, stimulated the development of noncemented prostheses. These implants were positioned in bone mechanically. Later versions were coated with porous material so that union between bone tissue and prosthesis may occur. In 1974, Bateman[68] introduced the bipolar prosthesis, a self-articulating prosthesis designed as a femoral head replacement. The majority of motion theoretically occurs between a small, 22-mm inner stainless steel sphere and a polyethylene socket, which in turn fits into a metallic acetabular sphere. Since the introduction of the Bateman prosthesis, additional versions of the original have been developed.

C. PATHOPHYSIOLOGY VS. TREATMENT OBJECTIVES

A fracture of the femoral neck has a devastating effect on the blood supply to the femoral head.[69,70] The severity of the damage to the major blood supply (the lateral epiphyseal artery system) depends on the extent of displacement of the bones. The studies by Sevitt[71] and Catto[72] confirmed histologically that femoral neck fracture damages the vascular supply leading to loss of osteocytes and irreversible cellular changes after 12 h. Increased intercapsular pressure, which has been documented by numerous authors in studies of patients who had a fracture of femoral neck,[73-75] also has an adverse effect on blood flow to the femoral head and may produce cellular death.[76] Although the adverse effect of a fracture of the femoral neck on the blood flow to the femoral head has been documented with certainty, some elements of the situation remain under a surgeon's control. Optimal reduction of the femoral neck has been shown to be associated with a lower rate of avascular necrosis of the femoral head.[77,78] This may be true because all the vessels of the lateral epiphyseal artery system may not be torn and the reduction may unkink a vessel. Claffey[79] showed that a displaced fracture of the femoral neck may occur without disruption of this critical vascular supply. Extension and internal rotation of the hip elevate the intracapsular pressure substantially because of the effect on the volume of the capsule. This position should therefore be avoided before an operation, and the position of flexion and external rotation should be encouraged.[74,80] Furthermore, stabilization of the fracture by internal fixation creates an optimum mechanical environment for revascularization to proceed.[70] While further vascular damage to the femoral head is unlikely with standard techniques of fixation, Brodetti[81] demonstrated that the posterosuperior quadrant of the femoral head should be avoided.

D. CLASSIFICATIONS

The two most common classifications of intracapsular fractures are those of Garden[82,83] and Pauwels.[84] Pauwels' classification, published in 1935, was the first to focus on the biomechanics of femoral neck fractures and, on this basis, was used as a therapeutic guideline. Although it is still mentioned in articles and monographs dealing with femoral neck fractures, its significance has declined and in clinical practice it has been replaced by Garden's classification. This seems to be due to several factors:

1. Accurate evaluation of the inclination of the fracture line, especially in dislocated fractures, is rather difficult. Such statements were mentioned by Linton[85] as early as 1949.
2. The current techniques of internal fixation and modern implants, such as a sliding hip screw, allow stable internal fixation in younger patients, even in fractures of Type III.
3. Garden's classification also appears to be more reliable in terms of evaluating the risk of avascular necrosis.

Despite this, Pauwels' classification still has its significance in the planning of reconstruction surgeries (valgus intertrochanteric osteotomy) in postfracture malunions of the femoral neck. Garden's classification describes subcapital intracapsular fractures and is based on the degree of displacement evident on an anteroposterior radiograph of the hip. Garden's grades (I to IV) correspond to the likelihood of osteonecrosis and collapse of the femoral head, with grade IV representing the worst prognosis; thus, they are useful as a tool for outcome audit. Rotational malalignment is not considered with the current classifications systems.

E. TREATMENT

Surgical treatment should be regarded as the method of choice in treatment of femoral neck fractures due to osteoporosis. This opinion is based on the fact that in the typical patient with femoral neck fracture, who is elderly and has coexisting morbidities, lengthy immobilization in bed required by conservative treatment may lead to serious complications: pressure sores, cardiopulmonary complications, secondary displacement of reduced or undisplaced fractures, and nonunion. Furthermore, current surgical options (internal fixation, hemiarthoplasty, total hip arthoplasty) allow for the choice of the most suitable treatment and create a chance for the patient's return to previous living activities. In our institution, the rules of treatment of femoral neck fractures are as follows: (1) treatment method matching demands of each individual patient; (2) early, intensive rehabilitation; (3) minimalization of bed rest length and of hospital stay duration; and (4) antithrombotic prophylaxis in all patients.[86]

1. Conservative Treatment

Nonoperative treatment is restricted to two cases only: (1) patient's medical condition precludes surgery and (2) patient refuses operative treatment. Two approaches are possible. Patients with undisplaced fractures, capable of walking without weight bearing on an injured limb, are made ambulatory after the acute period and then the amount of weight bearing on an affected limb is gradually increased. If the patient's condition does not allow for ambulation, general rehabilitation is introduced and the patient is prepared for "chair" lifestyle.

2. Operative Treatment

Treatment of fractures of the femoral neck should be conducted by an experienced surgeon, as a number of factors must be considered for deciding the correct method of treatment: patient's age, type of femoral neck fracture, bone quality (degree of osteoporosis), existing comorbidities, and patient's overall vitality and functional demands.

Swiontkowski[87] presented the treatment algorithm for the femoral neck fractures. Patients who are younger than 65 years old and do not have a chronic illness should be managed with immediate reduction and internal fixation of the femoral head fracture with multiple pins or screws. Patients who are older than 75 years should be managed with prosthetic replacement. Patients who are 65 to 75 years old may be treated with internal fixation, total hip arthroplasty, or bipolar replacement, the choice depending on their general medical condition, functional demands, and bone quality. One should always remember that the method of treatment chosen should meet with patients' demands and expectations. This author thinks that in patients older than 50 years of age with high functional demands, who are still working, the use of uncemented prosthesis should be considered for treatment of Garden grade III to IV fractures. Similarly, in patients between 60 and 70 years of age with functional demands as above, one may consider using either a cemented or uncemented prosthesis instead of internal fixation, because of the high risk of nonunion and avascular necrosis of the femoral head that is associated with the latter method in this age group. Indications for bipolar replacement in younger patients should also be carefully analyzed, as this method has been in use for a relatively short time and divergent opinions are expressed in the literature.

Medically stable patients with planned internal fixation should be reduced and internally fixed with compression within 8 hours after the injury,[88] as many authors have shown that reduction of a displaced fracture of the femoral neck improves blood flow to the femoral head.[69,70,77,79] In older patients, stability of secondary conditions (cardiac, renal, or pulmonary) must take precedence over treatment of a femoral neck fracture, so that mortality can be decreased.[89] However, in the medically stable elderly patient, the chance of postoperative morbidity (confusion, pressure sores, or pulmonary complications) is decreased substantially if surgery is performed in the first 24 hours after the fracture. It may be said that femoral neck fractures present a true orthopaedic emergency.

a. Internal Fixation

To perform closed reduction of a displaced femoral neck fracture the surgeon should flex the hip to 45° while it is in slight abduction, extend the hip while gently increasing traction, and then internally rotate it to 30 to 45° in full extension. This technique has been described, with minor differences, by many authors, including Smith-Petersen,[90] Cotton,[91] and Leadbetter.[92] If the reduction is achieved, it should be fixed with two or three Kirschner wires. However, if the reduction is not successful, one should refrain from repeating the attempts with greater force, as this could damage the blood supply to the femoral head.[93] Instead, open reduction should be performed. According to Watson-Jones,[94] the technique of open reduction begins with a straight lateral incision, which is extended proximally in the interval between the tensor fascie latae and the gluteus medius muscles. The hip capsule is opened anteriorly and the fracture site is exposed. The fragments are reduced under visual control and held with a Kirschner wire. Afterward the stabilization with

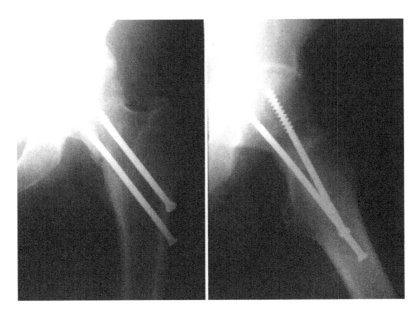

FIGURE 16.2 Femoral neck fracture after treatment with two cancellous screws. Anteroposterior view.

internal fixation may be performed under fluoroscopic guidance. At present, two types of screws, mainly cannulated (this allows for using previously inserted Kirschner wires as guide wires), are in use: cancellous screws (Figure 16.2) (such as AO) and large screws (such as Garden). Those implants are designed to produce compression across the fracture site. Implants that do not possess this characteristic (triflange nails) should not be used in the treatment of femoral neck fractures, as with the disturbance of fragments blood flow to the femoral head is further impaired.[95] Usually, two to three cancellous screws or one large screw may be used. The use of more than three implants does not seem to provide an increased mechanical advantage.[31,96,97] This author prefers cancellous screws, because of certain advantages of this method of fixation: (1) small incision if closed reduction has been performed; (2) good control of rotational movements of the proximal fragment; (3) small loss of cancellous bone due to insertion of implants; and (4) short operative time.

Large hip-compression screws, such as those recommended for intertrochanteric fractures of the hip, should not be used routinely. They provide the same mechanical duration as two or three cancellous screws,[98] but their use in the treatment of femoral neck fractures has some disadvantages: (1) considerable loss of bone from the center of the femoral neck, (2) the risk of damaging the blood supply to the femoral head if implants are placed suboptimally in the posterior and superior aspects of the femoral head,[81] and (3) lower rotational stability.

Avascular necrosis of the femoral head is the most common complication after the internal fixation of the femoral neck. The risk of avascular necrosis generally corresponds to the degree of displacement of the fracture of the femoral neck on the initial radiographs.[71] Another complication is the failure of fixation, with the lack of stable reduction as the critical factor. This complication is related to the failure of weak, osteoporotic bone around the implants, and often results from the inappropriate selection of the patient for the procedure. Technical problems, such as the use of implants that are too short, that have threads that cross the fracture line, or that are widely divergent and prevent settling of the fracture, can lead to a failure of fixation. Traumatic osteoarthrosis can also result from a failure of fixation as an implant may penetrate the joint.[99,100] Nonunion is still another complication. In a younger patient in whom adequate bone remains in the femoral head, refixation with a cancellous graft or muscle-pedicle graft may be indicated.[101] A valgus osteotomy is the procedure of choice when a patient has a shortened limb. For older patients hip arthroplasty

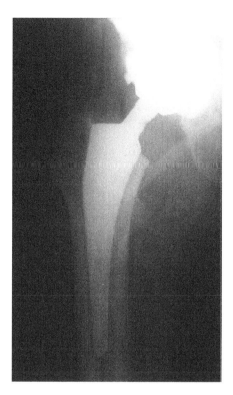

FIGURE 16.3 Uncemented total hip arthroplasty. Anteroposterior view.

has provided good functional results.[102] Boyd and Salvatore[103] and Sikorsky and Barrington[60] suggested that internal fixation should not be used in elderly patients because of high morbidity, significant mortality, and serious problems with achieving satisfactory functional results. Moreover, they described a high incidence of technical failures (60%); one third of patients in these series required repeated surgical procedures. Numerous authors share this point of view.[104-106]

b. Prosthetic Replacement

Total hip arthroplasty (Figures 16.3 and 16.4) is generally reserved for the treatment of patients with degenerative changes and for the treatment of femoral neck fractures in patients about 50 to 60 years of age with high functional demands, with good (for uncemented prostheses) or medium (for cemented prostheses) bone quality, and in good overall health. In the United States, England, and Poland, the use of hemiarthroplasty is considered the optimal treatment for femoral neck fractures in elderly patients with severe osteoporosis. Two types of unipolar prostheses are currently in use: noncemented Moore-type prostheses (Figure 16.5) and cemented Thompson-type prostheses (Figure 16.6). Painful loosening and acetabular erosion often occur after the use of these implants.

Variants of anterior or posterior approach may be used for the insertion of prosthetic replacement. Kenzora et al.[107] found no differences in medical complication rates, postoperative confusion, or length or cost of hospitalization between patients who had an anterior or posterior approach for hemiarthroplasty. Patients who had a posterior approach had a somewhat higher rate of surgical complications. When analyzed specifically for the type of surgical complications, six (2.2%) cases of prosthetic hip dislocation were identified; all occurred in patients who had posterior approach. There were no differences between the two groups of patients concerning mortality or any of the functional measures recorded. However, studies also exist that suggest that there is a higher mortality rate after a posterior approach.[108]

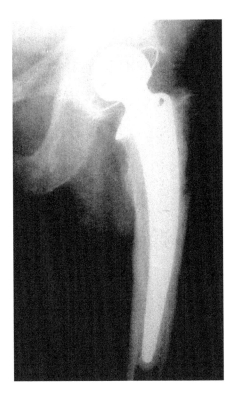

FIGURE 16.4 Cemented total hip arthroplasty. Anteroposterior view.

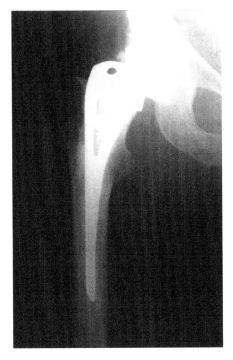

FIGURE 16.5 Uncemented hip hemiarthroplasty. Anteroposterior view.

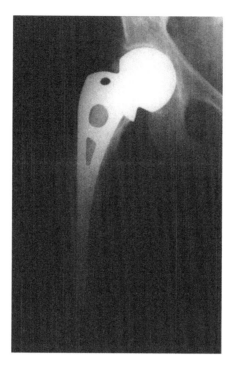

FIGURE 16.6 Cemented hip hemiarthroplasty. Anteroposterior view.

c. New Devices: Bipolar Replacement

Bipolar replacement (Figure 16.7) was expected to bring substantial improvement in the treatment of femoral neck fractures. However, a review of current literature comparing the results with bipolar and with unipolar prostheses shows that considerable controversy is associated with the subject.

Calder et al.[109] reported better functional scores in patients between 65 and 79 years of age with bipolar rather than unipolar prostheses. Lestrange[110] reviewed 469 patients with bipolar replacements for displaced neck fractures and compared them with patients having unipolar replacements. He found that the bipolar prosthesis offered advantages over one-piece designs in terms of fit, decreased acetabular erosion, and improved function. LaBelle et al.[111] in a long-term follow-up of bipolar vs. unipolar protheses concluded that there was less pain and decreased acetabular protrusion in the bipolar group. Likewise, Merlo et al.[112] attested to the superiority of bipolar components when compared with conventional hemiarthoplasties. The average patient age in their group was 69 years. Wathne et al.[113] prospectively reviewed 140 geriatric patients with femoral neck fractures: 92 received cemented bipolar replacements; 48 received cemented unipolar replacements. Wathne et al. found no difference in the rates of complications, length of hospital stay, and subsequent functional activity of the patients. Similarly, Drinker and Murray[114] retrospectively evaluated 101 bipolar and 160 Thompson unipolar prostheses. They found no significant advantage in the bipolar group. Calder et al.[115] conducted a prospective randomized study of people in their 80s with displaced neck fractures treated with unipolar and bipolar prostheses and concluded that there was no justification for the use of a bipolar component in patients older than 80 years of age.

Numerous studies focused on the motion in the intraprosthetic joint. West and Mann[116] found shared motion at the intraprosthetic and extraprosthetic articulations. Drinker and Murray[114] described inner bearing motion as long as 4 years after surgery. Opinions to the contrary were expressed by other authors. Verberne[117] reported that intraprosthetic motion was absent 3 months after surgery. Tsukamoto et al.[118] suggested that motion during walking occurred mainly at the

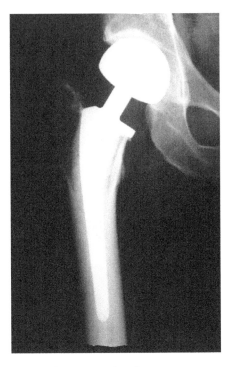

FIGURE 16.7 Bipolar hip replacement. Anteroposterior view.

outer bearing. Brueton et al.[119] showed that the size of the inner head was an important determination in allowing inner bearing motion. Small heads (22 mm) allowed bipolar motion, whereas large heads (32 mm) hindered inner bearing motion. Chen et al.,[120] looking at non-weight-bearing radiographic movement, found outer bearing motion in 70% of patients evaluated. Tsukamoto et al.[118] conducted cadaver motion studies of bipolar implants. They found that in stems loaded with less than 10 kg, motion occurred at both bearings. If the load was greater than 20 kg, then the outer bearing was the primary site of articulation.

Because of the faults of unipolar prostheses, the brief experience with bipolar replacements, and the controversies presented above, many authors now recommend total hip arthroplasty in patients with a displaced femoral neck fracture.[121-123]

IV. INTERTROCHANTERIC FRACTURES

A. INTRODUCTION

Intertrochanteric fractures (Figure 16.8) occur mainly in elderly patients, more frequently in women than in men. Of patients who sustain this type of injury, 80% are between 70 and 90 years of age. These fractures are located on the metaphyseal–epiphyseal border or in the area between metaphysis and the femoral shaft. For this reason they are also described as extracapsular fractures of the proximal femur.[124,125] In this area age-related structural changes (senile osteoporosis) are often present. As a consequence, low-energy trauma may produce fractures in elderly patients. At the same time, this region is well supplied with blood and surrounded by numerous muscles. The conditions for fracture healing are good and nonunion is a rare complication. The main challenge presented by these fractures lies in achieving a stable reduction of transversally oriented fragments and maintaining it until healing is completed.

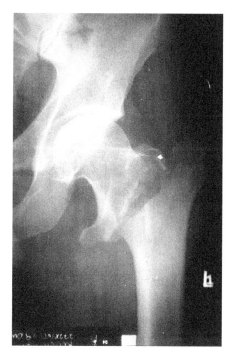

FIGURE 16.8 Intertrochanteric fracture of the proximal femur. Anteroposterior view.

B. CLASSIFICATIONS

1. Boyd and Griffin Classification[126]

Type 1: Fractures that extend along the intertrochanteric line from the greater trochanter to the lesser trochanter.

Type 2: Comminuted fractures, the main fracture being along the intertrochanteric line but with multiple fractures in the cortex.

Type 3: Fractures that are basically subtrochanteric with at least one fracture passing across the proximal end of the shaft just distal to the lesser trochanter. Varying degrees of comminution are associated.

Type 4: Fractures of the trochanteric region and the proximal shaft, with fracture in at least two planes.

2. Evans Classification[127]

Evans divided intertrochanteric fractures into stable and unstable groups. The unstable fractures are further divided into those in which stability could be restored by anatomic or near anatomic reduction and those in which anatomic reduction would not create stability. In type I fracture, the fracture line extends upward and outward from the lesser trochanter. In type II, the reversed obliquity fracture, the major fracture line extends outward and downward from the lesser trochanter. This tends to be unstable. The most important element in classification of intertrochanteric fractures is whether the fracture is stable or unstable, as this directly determines the choice of method of treatment.

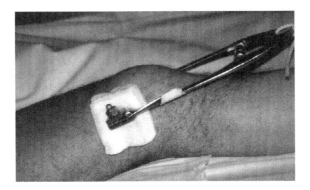

FIGURE 16.9 Conservative treatment of intertrochanteric fracture with the use of skeletal supracondylar traction.

C. Treatment

The patient's age, overall medical condition, fracture pattern (stable or unstable), and consent to operative treatment are the factors determining the choice of a method of treatment.

1. Conservative Treatment

Patients in good overall health with stable undisplaced intertrochanteric fractures should be addressed with casting and encouraged to walk with the aid of crutches, gradually increasing weight bearing on the injured limb. If the patient is not capable of such effort, functional treatment may be employed. The patient is treated in traction for 3 to 4 weeks, then active exercises of the knee and hip joints are introduced. Noncompliant patients disqualified from surgery may be treated with supracondylar skeletal traction (Figure 16.9) maintained for a period of 6 to 8 weeks. Such patients require regular radiographic study so that correction of reduction may be performed in case of fragment displacement. They also demand intensive medical and nursing care. All methods of conservative treatment are associated with a high rate of general complications and high mortality ranging from 8.7 to 31%.[128] Malunion is also common. For these reasons, most authors recommend primary operative treatment for intertrochanteric fractures.

2. Operative Treatment

Surgical stabilization of the intertrochanteric fracture is one of the most commonly performed orthopaedic procedures. Internal fixation of intertrochanteric fractures, popularized by Jewett,[129] gained rapid acceptance because it allowed early mobilization of patients while reducing deformity secondary to malunion. However, because this implant does not have a sliding mechanism, impaction at the fracture site resulted in failure by intra-articular penetration of the Jewett nail through the femoral head.[130,131] The results of treatment with this method were good only in stable, two-part intertrochanteric fractures. Later, similar, not very satisfactory results were achieved with the use of Smith-Petersen's nail plate, McLaughlin nail plate, or with different variants of the angular plate. Numerous complications were described including secondary fracture displacement, delayed healing, nonunion, and "fatigue" implant failure. A sliding nail plate modification of the Jewett nail was introduced to avoid these complications,[132] and was replaced by the sliding screw plate (dynamic hip screw, DHS). The sliding screw plate construct has been the standard in treating patients with intertrochanteric fractures during the past two decades.[33,133,134] At the same time, research on intramedullary fixation of intertrochanteric fractures has been carried out. In the late 1960s, Küntscher[135] presented the technique of condylocephalic approach using a single elastic nail inserted through the medial condyle of the femur. Ender[136] designed the method of fixation of

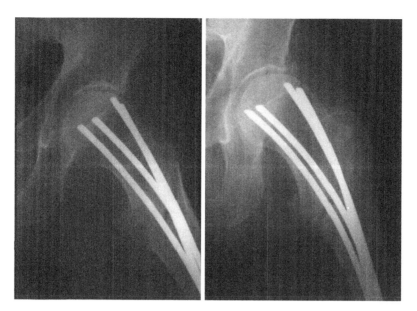

FIGURE 16.10 Intertrochanteric fracture after fixation with Ender rods. Anteroposterior view.

intertrochanteric fractures with the use of 4.5-mm elastic nails inserted into the femoral head through the medial aspect of the distal femoral epiphysis. The method became very popular, particularly in the 1970s and 1980s. This method is still used and new designs of implants for intramedullary fixation are being introduced.

a. Ender Rod Fixation

In this procedure, after reduction under image intensification is performed, fixation is achieved by inserting three to five Ender's rods (Figure 16.10) into the medullary canal through the medial condyle and advancing them to the femoral head.

The advantages of the method include the following:

1. Minimal invasiveness
2. The possibility of rapid mobilization and weight bearing
3. Lower mortality as compared with other methods (3 to 14.8%)
4. Low rate of infection: 0 to 3.8% for superficial infections and 0 to 0.7% for deep infections
5. Low incidence of delayed healing (0 to 2%)
6. Extremely rare implant failure
7. Elasticity of fixation enabling spontaneous fracture compression[137-145]

The reported disadvantages are as follows:

1. Comparatively low rotational stability in 30% of cases resulting in external rotation deformity
2. Nail migration occurring proximally (0.3 to 7.7%) or, more often, distally (1.7 to 16.6%)
3. The risk of supracondylar femur fracture at the moment of wire insertion (0 to 1%) or postoperatively (2 to 12%)
4. Knee pain and decreased range of motion[137-145]

Many authors proposed different solutions to eliminate the disadvantages of the method. Chapman et al.[142] recommended cutting the tips of the rods off flush at the insertion portals to

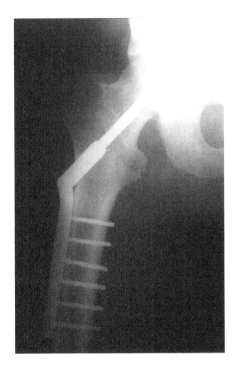

FIGURE 16.11 Intertrochanteric fracture after fixation with dynamic hip screw. Anteroposterior view.

prevent backing out. Butterfield et al.[141] left the distal tips of the rods within the intermedullary canal. Farcy and Grelsamer[146] described an Ender rod insert that locks into the distal eyelet of the rods and is secured to the femur with an anchoring screw. Olerud et al.[147] achieved a decrease in the rate of external rotation deformity with the use of Ender rods with a 25° anteversion bend. However, these methods did not bring substantial improvement of results and new, method-specific complications occurred. For this reason, present indications for Ender rod fixation are limited to the treatment of elderly, medically compromised patients with severe osteoporosis.

b.   DHS Fixation

In this procedure, a lateral incision is used to expose the fracture site and open reduction is performed. Then, one screw is inserted through the femoral neck into the femoral head under image intensification. Finally, this screw is fixed with a metal plate placed on the femoral shaft (Figure 16.11).

The advantages of the method are as follows:

1. Anatomic reduction (allows controlled fracture collapse)
2. Good fracture compression[148]
3. Very high success rate (over 95%)

The disadvantages are the following:

1. Large incision increasing potential for infection
2. Relatively high surgical blood loss
3. Postoperative full weight bearing not possible
4. 25% incidence of mechanical complications, most frequently cut-out of the femoral head screw through osteoporotic bone[7,149-151]

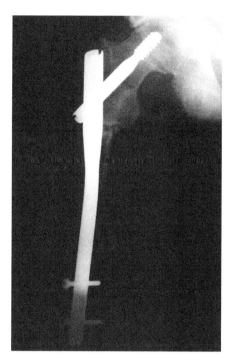

FIGURE 16.12 Gamma nail fixation of subtrochanteric fracture. Anteroposterior view.

Considering the extension of surgical incision and the amount of inserted hardware with a large screw coming through the center of the femoral neck, this author prefers using this method in younger patients with better bone quality

c.   New Devices — Gamma Nail Fixation

In 1987, Grosse and Taglag[152] designed the Gamma nail (Figure 16.12). This device combines the advantages of the sliding lag screw, which allows controlled fracture collapse, with the advantages of intramedullary fixation.

The procedure starts with closed reduction under image intensification. Then, a 2- to 4-cm incision is made proximal to the greater trochanter and taken to the level of fascia. The fascia is penetrated with a Küntscher awl, which is then positioned on the medial tip of the greater trochanter and advanced within the canal to the level of the lesser trochanter. A beaded guide rod is advanced into the medullary canal, and a handheld reamer, 0.5 mm larger than the anticipated nail diameter, is used to sound the canal. An intramedullary nail is then introduced by hand. Next, a guide pin is advanced from the lateral cortex of the femur to the subchondral bone of the femoral head and is positioned along the calcar into the center of the femoral head. The correct length of the pin should be confirmed intraoperatively using the calibrated reamer before screw placement. Traction then is released and a flywheel mechanism is used to compress the fracture. The achieved compression is blocked with a screw.

The advantages of the method are as follows:

1. Rapid percutaneous placement (insertion)
2. Reduced surgical blood loss
3. Low incidence of wound complications
4. Decreased potential for screw cutout (migration)[157]
5. Early return to full weight bearing[153-156]

The disadvantages of the method are as follows:

1. The risk of intra- or postoperative femoral shaft fracture[153-155]
2. The risk of screw cut-out through osteoporotic femoral head, reported in 1 to 25% of cases[153-155,148]

Multiple factors, involving implant design and operative technique, have been reported with these complications.[158,159] The most common errors in operative technique include mismatch in implant size and canal diameter, inadequate reaming of the medullary canal, and forceful nail insertion (difficulty with distal locking screw insertion). Decreases in implant curvature, length, and diameter (recommended diameters are 11 and 12 mm),[160] overreaming of the femoral canal, insertion of the implant only by hand, and meticulous placement of distal interlocking screws without creating additional stress risers have significantly decreased the occurrence of femoral shaft fracture.[157,161,162]

Improvements in implant design and operative technique have increased the popularity of this method, which is now recommended in most intertrochanteric fractures.

V. TIBIAL PLATEAU FRACTURES

A. INTRODUCTION

Tibial plateau fractures are usually caused by indirect injuries such as a fall from height, rapid adduction and abduction of the tibia, and motor vehicle injuries. Less frequently they result from direct trauma like an impact on medial or lateral aspect of the knee joint occurring at a moment when the foot is fixed. In younger patients, macroenergetic injury is needed, whereas in older individuals with osteoporosis much lower force is required to produce a fracture. Fracture of the lateral condyle (Figure 16.13) is the most frequent, bicondylar fractures (Figure 16.14) are less frequent, and isolated fractures of the medial condyle are the least frequent. Proximal tibial fractures are often accompanied by injuries of nerves, vessels, and soft tissues. In a study of 190 proximal tibial articular fractures, Tscherne and Lobenhoffer[163] found a 67% rate of meniscal injury, a 96% rate of cruciate injuries, an 85% rate of medial collateral ligament injuries, and a high rate of peroneal nerve injury. Complex fractures involving both the femoral and tibial articular surfaces had a 25% incidence of vascular injury and 25% incidence of compartment syndrome.[163]

B. CLASSIFICATIONS

1. Schatzker Classification[164]

Type I: Pure cleavage. A typical wedge-shaped uncomminuted fragment is split off and displaced laterally and downward.
Type II: Cleavage combined with depression. A lateral wedge is split off, but in addition the articular surface is depressed down into the metaphysis.
Type III: Pure central depression.
Type IV: Fractures of medial condyle.
Type V: Bicondylar fractures. Both tibial plateaus are split off. The distinguishing feature is that the metaphysis and diaphysis retain continuity.
Type VI: Plateau fractures with dissociation of metaphysis and diaphysis.

2. Fracture–Dislocation Classification (Hohl and Moore)[165]

Type I: Coronal split fracture
Type II: Entire condyle fracture

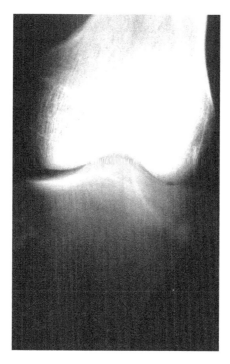

FIGURE 16.13 Fracture of the lateral tibial condyle with the large depression of the articular surface. Anteroposterior view.

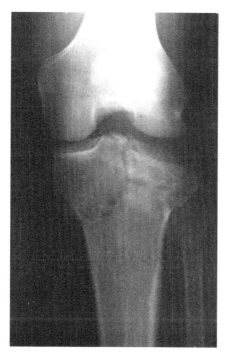

FIGURE 16.14 Bicondylar fracture of the proximal tibia with the distinct depression of the lateral condyle. Anteroposterior view.

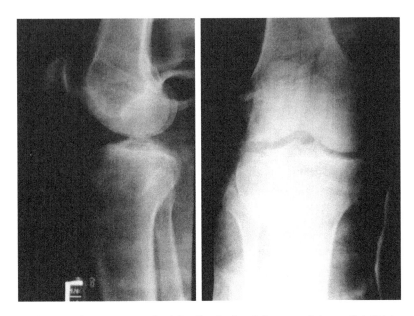

FIGURE 16.15 Conservative treatment of minimally displaced fracture of the medial tibial condyle. Cast immobilization. Anteroposterior view.

Type III: Rim avulsion fracture
Type IV: Rim compression fracture
Type V: Four part fracture

C. TREATMENT

When determining the choice of treatment approach, the degree of depression of the articular surfaces and associated injury of soft tissues are decisive factors.

1. Conservative Treatment

Nonoperative treatment includes casting, traction, and functional treatment. In our institution,[86] patients with an isolated fracture of one condyle and an articular step-off not larger than 5 mm qualified for treatment with a cast positioned in slight valgus or varus depending on which condyle was fractured (Figure 16.15). The cast was maintained for 6 to 8 weeks.

That 5 mm is the maximum step-off allowing for conservative treatment was suggested by Blokker et al.[166] and Hohl,[167] whereas Waddell et al.[168] suggested 10 mm. Most authors agree that the acceptable range of intra-articular step-off is in the range of 2 to 10 mm.[169-171] Some authors consider that the major indication for open reduction is more than 5° of clinical valgus or varus instability.[172,173]

Traction and functional treatment were used in patients with multifragment proximal tibial fracture in whom an articular depression was smaller than 5 mm.[86] Supracondylar skeletal traction was applied for a period of 6 weeks. At 2 weeks passive exercises were introduced and were followed by active exercises at 4 weeks. After traction was removed, walking with crutches was encouraged and the patient was instructed to increase frequency of weight bearing on the injured limb. One patient from the group of 23 had the 1-cm depression of articular surface of the lateral condyle diagnosed after 4 weeks of treatment. In this patient, reconstructive surgery was performed at 5 weeks after injury. Like other authors,[174] we achieved a high rate of good functional results.

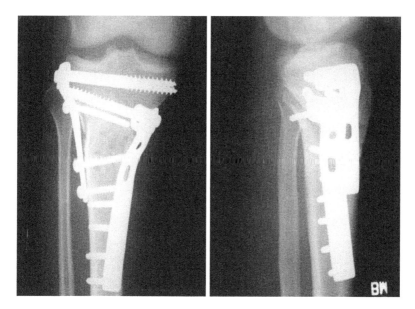

FIGURE 16.16 Bicondylar fracture of the proximal tibia after treatment with plates and screws. Anteroposterior and lateral radiographs.

2. Operative Treatment

Complex fractures of the proximal tibia are difficult to treat. Fracture reduction is hard both to obtain and maintain, and the rates of wound breakdown and infection are high, particularly with approaches that expose both medial and lateral plateaus.[175-177] These complications are probably due to a compromise in the local blood supply, which is exacerbated by an extensive surgical dissection. Another complication is aseptic nonunion, which is particularly common in high-energy injuries, such as Schatzker V and VI fractures.[176] These complex fractures are commonly bone-grafted as soon as delays in healing become apparent.[171]

a. Metal Fixators

Currently used methods of operative treatment may be summarized as follows:

1. Extensile exposure with arthrotomy and reconstruction of the joint surface with plate and screw fixation, with or without bone grafting.[178,179]

   In these procedures extensive surgical incision was used for the reconstruction of the joint surface. The depressed articular surface was elevated together with a small layer of cancellous bone and the reposition was held with plates and screws (Figures 16.16 and 16.17). The achieved stability was good and allowed for early motion. However, this method does not create good biomechanical conditions for the healing of cancellous bone and the insertion of the considerable amount of metallic elements increases potential for complications, e.g., compartment syndrome. This method is often complicated with wound dehiscence and infection. Moore et al.[180] reported a 23% incidence of infection in bicondylar tibial plateau fractures treated with internal fixation. Those complications are particularly frequent in complex fractures when double plating is used. In Young and Barrack's[177] study, seven of eight fractures treated with double plating were complicated by infection. To decrease the incidence of complications, Benirschke et al.[181] used smaller incisions made on the basis of the location of bone pathology. Tscherne and Lobenhoffer[163] recommended temporarily immobilizing the knee with an external fixator

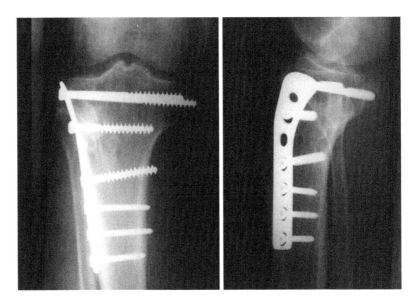

FIGURE 16.17 Fracture of the lateral tibial condyle after treatment with plate and screws. Anteroposterior view.

in patients with severe soft tissue injury and performing internal fixation when the swelling has subsided.

An angular stabilization system for plates (LISS) has been designed for the proximal tibia. Angular stability in plates is a significant development for the treatment of complex tibial plateau fractures.[182,183] The implant allows for the stabilization of both medial and lateral columns using a single plate through a unilateral approach. This implant is inserted through a lateral approach and is sufficient for most fractures that are amenable to minimally invasive plating. However, the potential disadvantages of a laterally inserted implant include (1) the requisite elevation of muscle from the bone, which further devitalizes the fracture; (2) the potential risk for injury to the superficial peroneal nerve; (3) the potentially increased risk of developing compartment syndrome; and (4) the difficulty in placement of a long implant into the limited space of the distal tibiofibular joint to stabilize a distal fracture. For these reasons, Krettek et al.[184] developed a medial approach for minimally invasive plating of complex plateau fractures.

2. Arthroscopy or limited arthrotomy and percutaneous screw fixation or external fixation with pin or wire fixators.[185,186]

Minimization of surgical incision and of the amount of inserted implants was aimed at decreasing the rate of complications. However, in the author's opinion, these methods very often are not sufficient for adequate management of the depression of the articular surface and often after the elevation of fragments there remains an inferior bone void, which results in decreased mechanical endurance and delayed bone healing.

3. Open reconstruction with bone grafting and external fixation.

Morandi and Pearse[187] and Watson[188] advocated the use of Illizarov external fixation for treatment of complex tibial fractures. In Morandi and Pearse's series, 26% of patients required elevation and bone grafting. The advantage of this method lies in stability and elasticity of fixation that allows for walking with weight bearing. Disadvantages of this method include pin site infection, skin injury with Kirschner wires, pain, and low tolerance of this device by patients.

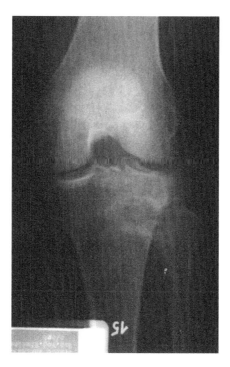

FIGURE 16.18 Fracture of the lateral tibial condyle after treatment with frozen cancellous bone graft. Anteroposterior view. For preoperative radiograph see Figure 16.13.

b.   Management of Proximal Tibial Fractures without Metal Fixators

Since 1995, a method of our own design has been used in our institution for the treatment of proximal tibial fractures.[86]

The anterolateral approach was used for the treatment of fractures of the lateral condyle, and the anteromedial approach was used for fractures of the medial condyle. The incision reached about 1 cm above the joint line and 4 to 5 cm below the biggest depression of the articular surface. In intraoperative evaluation, the fractures were characterized as the depression and cleavage-depression types. The biggest depression was usually located in the posteromedial part of the condyle. Osteotomy was performed 2 cm below the level of the biggest step-off. Next, the detached fragment was repositioned and the articular surface was reconstructed under visual control. The bone defect that resulted inferiorly was tightly filled with appropriately adjusted bone graft from frozen femoral heads.

In the case of cleavage-depression fractures of the lateral condyle, exposure of the fracture site revealed that the lateral part of the condyle was separated, while the depression was mainly located in the medial and posterior parts. The lateral part was moved aside and the reconstruction of the articular surface was performed in the same way as previously described. Then the lateral fragment was fixed with a cancellous screw. The wound was closed in layers over a drain, and casting in valgus or varus position ended the procedure. The results of treatment are shown in Figures 16.18 and 16.19.

In roentgenographic study after 4 weeks, healing cancellous bone union was visible, while there was no union of cortical bone. The cast was maintained for 6 to 8 weeks. After removal of the cast, rehabilitation began. Positive features of the method are as follows:

1. Reposition of the articular cartilage with the base of cancellous bone creates favorable conditions for rapid primary union between the displaced fragment and its surroundings, increasing the chances for the survival of the articular cartilage.

3. Short oblique fracture of the fibula above the level of the joint
4. Rupture of posterior tibiofibular ligament or avulsion fracture of the posterolateral tibia

e. *Pronation-Dorsiflexion (PD)*

1. Fracture of the medial malleolus
2. Fracture of the anterior margin of the tibia
3. Supramalleolar fracture of the fibula
4. Transverse fracture of the posterior tibial surface

2. Danis–Weber (AO) Classification[192]

This classification is based on the location and appearance of the fibular fracture.

Type A: Fracture is caused by internal rotation and adduction that produce a transverse fracture of the lateral malleolus at or below the plafond, with or without an oblique fracture of the medial malleolus.

Type B: Fracture is caused by external rotation that results in an oblique fracture of the lateral malleolus, beginning on the anteromedial surface and extending proximally to the posterolateral aspect.

Type C-1: Fracture is caused by abduction injury producing an oblique fracture of the fibula proximal to the disrupted tibiofibular ligaments.

Type C-2: Fracture is caused by abduction-external rotation injuries that result in a more proximal fracture of the fibula and more extensive disruption of the interosseus membrane. Type C injuries may involve a medial malleolar fracture or a deltoid ligament rupture. Fracture of the posterior malleolus may accompany any of the three types.

At present, the Lauge-Hansen system is the most widely used classification, both in the literature and in planning of operative treatment. However, Nielsen et al.[193] cautioned against using the Lauge-Hansen classification alone to determine treatment, noting that of 118 ankle fractures, only 43% were classified identically by four observers.

C. Treatment

The goals of treatment are the same for all ankle injuries: anatomic positioning of the talus in the mortise, a joint line that is parallel to the ground, and a smooth articular surface. Unless these requisites are achieved by treatment, post-traumatic arthritis is likely to occur.[194] Even slight talar shift may cause sufficient joint incongruity to result in degenerative changes. Ramsey and Hamilton[194] have shown that a lateral shift of the talus of just 1 mm can lead to abnormal wear on the tibiotalar joint.

1. Conservative Treatment

In our institution, cast immobilization (Figure 16.21) was used in undisplaced and displaced ankle fractures that were amenable to closed reduction. Knowledge of the mechanism of injury is necessary to carry out manipulative reduction; as with any method employed, the principle is the same: reversal of the injuring forces. For example, fractures produced by external rotation and abduction are reduced by internal rotation and adduction of the foot. Interposition of periosteum at the fracture site or impingement of the lateral malleolus on the proximal fibular fragment may prevent reduction.[195] Opinions on the treatment of fractures of the lateral malleolus are divided. Although fractures of the lateral malleolus without significant medial injury are common, the indications for open reduction of these fractures are still controversial. Yablon et al.[195] demonstrated

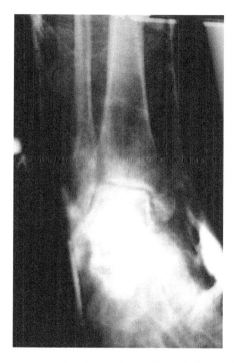

FIGURE 16.21 Bimalleolar fracture after closed reduction and immobolization in a cast. Anteroposterior view.

that displacement of the talus accompanies displacement of the lateral malleolus in bimalleolar ankle fractures and emphasized the importance of anatomic reduction of the lateral malleolus in these injuries. A recent biomechanical study by Brown et al.[196] showed that isolated fractures of the lateral malleolus do not disturb joint kinematics or cause talar displacement with axial loading. A long-term clinical follow-up study by Bauer et al.[197] of closed treatment of supination-external rotation stage II fractures reported good functional results in 94 to 98%, even with 3 mm of fibular displacement. Yde and Kristensen[198] found the results of operative treatment no better than those of closed treatment in supination-external rotation stage II injuries, even though only 1 in 35 patients (3%) who had closed treatment had anatomic reduction, compared with 28 of 34 (82%) with operative treatment. If swelling precludes definitive treatment of external rotation-abduction injuries by either open or closed methods, the foot may be suspended in stockinette as recommended by Quigley.[199] After application of stockinette from toe to groin, the limb is suspended at the knee and foot by means of weights. Thus balanced, the foot will assume a position of internal rotation and adduction, which often accomplishes the reduction by the time the swelling subsides.

2. Operative Treatment

Primary operative treatment for ankle fractures has been recommended with increasing frequency in recent years, in spite of tenuous data to support this position and infection rates as high as 18%.[200,201] Open reduction and internal fixation may be possible within the first 12 hours after injury but may not be possible again for 2 to 3 weeks because of excessive swelling. Breederveld et al.[202] found equally good functional results with immediate and delayed open reduction and internal fixation; however, hospitalization was briefer and pain was diminished with immediate surgery. A similar opinion was expressed by Eventov et al.[200] If surgery is planned, it should be done promptly, because operative delay, especially after repeated manipulations, has been correlated with less satisfactory end results. In retrospective study of closed Danis–Weber type B bimalleolar fracture or bimalleolar-equivalent ankle fractures treated with open reduction and internal fixation,

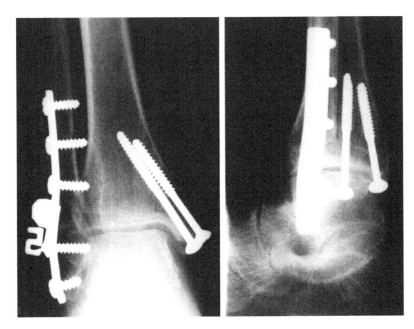

FIGURE 16.22 Bimalleolar fracture. Treatment with plate and screws fixation was used for the lateral malleolus and two screws were used for the medial malleolus. Anteroposterior and lateral radiographs.

Konvath et al.[203] found no significant differences in complications, adequacy of reduction, range of motion, or operative time in 105 fractures treated within 5 days of injury compared with 97 fractures treated more than 5 days after injury.

a. Medial Malleolar Fractures

Displaced fractures of the medial malleolus require operative treatment because resulting instability causes the talus to shift into varus. The fracture site is exposed using anteromedial approach or posteromedial incision. A single screw, directed perpendicular to the fracture line, is sufficient for most medial malleolar fractures. If a fragment is large, two screws are inserted and in case of fragment comminution combination of a Kirschner wire and tension band wiring may be used (Figure 16.22).

b. Lateral Malleolar Fractures

Isolated fractures of the lateral malleolus comprise up to 40% of all ankle fractures.[204] The fracture site is exposed using lateral incision. After open reduction, fixation is typically performed with plate osteosynthesis using a one third tubular plate, which is placed on the lateral aspect of the fibula. The plate should allow for three bicortical screws proximally and at least two screws distally that cross the malleolus to engage in the medial cortex, but not to penetrate it. Because the lateral border of the fibula is subcutaneous, these plates are often palpable. As such, they may cause irritation,[205] and require removal to allow for freedom of shoe wear.[206] Jacobson et al.[205] reported that 66% of patients with lateral plates had complaints related to the implant that led to removal. Of these patients, 75% had relief after plate removal. Intramedullary fixation and antiglide plating have been advocated to decrease the amount of laterally placed hardware.[207,208]

One method of lateral malleolus fixation is lag-screw-only fixation of the lateral malleolus. This method, however, is suitable mainly for patients younger than 50 years of age with good bone quality and simple noncomminuted oblique fractures of the lateral malleolus that are long enough to accept two lag screws placed at least 1 cm from each other. The advantages of the method include smaller incision and decreased patient complaints, as compared with patients treated by fixation with standard plates.

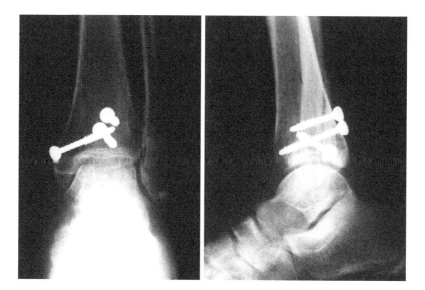

FIGURE 16.23 Bimalleolar fracture: fracture of the medial malleolus is accompanied by fracture of the posterior tibial surface. Treatment with screw fixation. Anteroposterior view.

Antiglide plate fixation is another method. There are several advantages of placing the plate as an antiglide plate on the posterolateral surface of the fibula for treatment of oblique fractures (Lauge-Hansen supination-external rotation type injury). Any method chosen for fixation of these fractures must resist proximal migration and rotation of the distal fragment, and a posterolaterally applied antiglide plate is much more effective at resisting these forces than standard lateral plating.[208] Furthermore, lag screws may be placed through the plate adding even greater stability to the construct. Perhaps the most obvious advantage of posterolateral plating of fibula, however, is the avoidance of problems with painful implant providence and the potential need for hardware removal.[209]

c. Posterior Malleolar Fractures

McDaniel and Wilson[210] recommended surgical reduction and fixation of posterior malleolar fractures (Figure 16.23) if more than 25% of the joint surface is involved. In their report, those patients treated surgically for large displaced fractures of the posterior malleolus had better clinical and radiographic results than those receiving nonsurgical treatment. Fixation for posterior malleolar fractures may be applied from either the anterior or posterolateral approach. Several problems are connected with the anterior approach. This method of treatment requires indirect reduction of the fracture, so it may be difficult to achieve or distinguish truly anatomic restoration of the joint surface. A quality lateral radiograph must be carefully scrutinized to assess joint reduction. "Shingling" or overlap of the posterior tibial cortex at the level of the superior fracture spike is a useful sign indicating imperfect joint reduction. Moreover, lag screws directed from anterior to posterior may not provide rigid fixation of a fracture that may encounter significant shear stresses. Bone in this area is mostly cancellous with a thin cortical rim and the posterior malleolar fragment quickly narrows as the fracture line moves away from the ankle joint. Thus, lag screws may gain only few millimeters of screw purchase and partially threaded lag screws may, if used, need to be excessively long to ensure that threads are not crossing the fracture line. In contrast, the posterior approach allows for direct reduction of the posterior malleolar fracture using bony landmarks to assess the quality of reduction. Lag screws may be easily placed at the plafond level with abundant bone available for screw purchase. What is more, adding a short, flattened tubular plate posteriorly over the superior fracture spike gives the construct tremendous resistance to shearing forces across the fracture.[209]

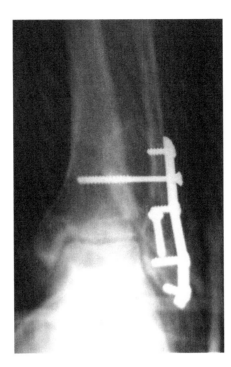

FIGURE 16.24 Fracture of the lateral malleolus with accompanying syndesmotic injury. Plate and screws fixation. Syndesmotic screw is inserted in a standard position 2 cm above articular surface, parallel to the joint line. Anteroposterior view.

d. Syndesmotic Injury

Injuries of the tibiofibular syndesmosis are typically fixed with a 3.5 mm cancellous screw that is inserted through a small incision over the lateral aspect of the fibula. A screw is placed through both cortices of the fibula and either one or two cortices of the tibia, parallel to the joint line, 2 cm above the articular surface. If a plate is used for fixation of an ankle fracture with accompanying syndesmotic injury, a screw should be inserted through a window 2 cm above the articular surface of the tibia (Figure 16.24). In the case of high fractures with disruption of the syndesmosis, a screw should be inserted above the syndesmosis, parallel to the articular surface (Figure 16.25).[179]

In a recent biomechanical study, Peter et al.[211] found that the stability achieved by two oblique, trans-syndesmotic, 1.5-mm Kirschner wires was equivalent to fixation with a 3.5-mm tricortical neutralization screw. Xenos et al.[212] found that fixation with two screws is more secure than fixation with one screw and that suture repair had the least mechanical strength. Van der Griend et al.[213] suggested using two syndesmotic screws in large or noncompliant patients.

Karges[214] claims that the unstable ankle fracture is one of the most underrated articular injuries sustained in the lower extermity. Open reduction and internal fixation provide a superior, more predictable long-term outcome than nonoperative management of the unstable ankle fracture. The operative technique employed is determined by the fracture pattern, soft tissue compromise, bone quality, and surgeon preference. The displaced trans-syndesmotic ankle fracture-dislocation with an associated posterior malleolar fracture involving more than 35% of the plafond with deltoid ligament injury represents an unstable ankle injury warranting immediate closed reduction and splinting. Early reconstruction is recommended, although operative timing can be delayed if soft tissue compromise precludes immediate surgery. A long-term follow-up study by Bauer et al.[197] also demonstrated superior results after operative treatment of supination-external rotation stage IV fractures. Tile[215] and the AO group recommend open reduction and internal fixation of both malleoli for almost all bimalleolar fractures.

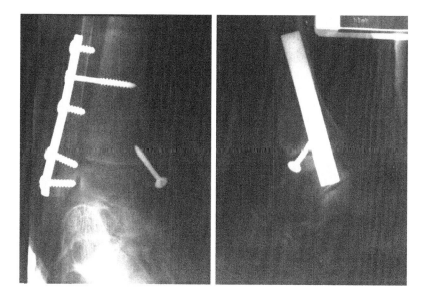

FIGURE 16.25 Bimalleolar fracture (low transversal fracture of the lateral malleolus and accompanying syndesmotic injury). Screw is inserted above syndesmosis, parallel to the joint line. Severe osteoporosis. Anteroposterior view.

e.   New Trends and Devices

Recently, a shift from a conservative approach to more aggressive, operative treatment may be observed. Ankle movement can be improved by early mobilization and partial weight bearing, which provides better cartilage nutrition and recovery.[216-218] Rigid internal fixation is essential for early joint movement and postoperative mobilization.[216,217,219,220]

Introduction of bioabsorbable implants for internal fixation is also a recent trend. Böstman[221] and Frokjaer and Möller[222] used polyglycolide rods and screws for fixation of ankle fractures and achieved high rates of union. However, 5 to 10% developed late drainage thought to be related to the breakdown of the polyglycolide. In a study of 155 patients with medial malleolar fractures addressed with 4-mm polylactide screws, Bucholz et al.[223] found no difference in functional results as compared with stainless steel implants.

VII. PERIOPERATIVE CARE

In an elderly patient waiting for surgical treatment of an osteoporotic fracture, multiple comorbidities are often present, including diabetes, hypertension, and cardiac and pulmonary disorders. Therefore, consultation with an internal medicine specialist should always precede operative treatment. As soon as the patient's medical condition is stabilized, antibiotic prophylaxis is introduced (usually second-generation cephalosporins).

Operative treatment of osteoporotic fractures should provide stable, anatomic reduction, so that early postoperative limb motion and mobilization may be possible. In choosing the operative approach, several factors should be considered. The incision should allow for fixation to be performed in a short time and with small surgical blood loss. Moreover, it should not be too extensive, because the increased potential for infection is associated with large surgical dissections.

Postsurgical patients and patients immobilized with a cast are routinely administered standard antithrombotic prophylaxis (Clexane, Fraxiparine) until return to full ambulation and until a cast is removed, respectively. Research in our institution showed that, in about 30% of patients treated with a cast, vein thrombosis, often asymptomatic, was present. The increased risk of thrombosis associated with such morbidities as diabetes, diseases of the cardiovascular system, or varices of lower extremities requires a double dose of anticoagulants.

Changes in bone density in older people do not seem to be as much related to the process of aging itself as to the decrease in overall physical activity.[224-226] As bone density and mass of accompanying muscles are correlated, it is believed that exercise, by improving the latter parameter, may positively influence the former.[226-229] Therefore, rehabilitation, particularly when accompanying surgery, is of great importance. Rapid mobilization, together with well-balanced diet, provides protection against general and local complications and inhibits the progress of psychomotor insufficiency.[230]

In our institution patients are subjected to pre- and postoperative rehabilitation, which comprises (1) respiratory exercises, (2) contralateral exercises of the uninjured limb, (3) isometric tensing of the muscles of lower extremities, and (4) exercises of upper extremities.

Patients who do not require immobilization in a cast after surgical treatment begin exercises of the operated joint on the second or third day postoperatively. All patients are mobilized as soon as possible and are taught to walk in a walker or with the aid of crutches. Such treatment improves patients' fitness, reduces the risk of pulmonary and neurologic complications, and decreases the length of hospital stay.

REFERENCES

1. Norris, R.J., "Medical costs of osteoporosis," *Bone,* 13, 11, 1992.
2. Cummings, S.R., Rubin, S.M., and Black, D., "The future of hip fractures in the United States: numbers, costs, and potential effects of postmenopausal estrogen," *Clin. Orthop.*, 252, 163, 1990.
3. Rat, N.F., Chan, J.K., Thamer, M., and Melton, L.J., "Medical expenditures for the treatment of osteoporotic fractures in the United States 1995: report from the National Osteoporosis Foundation," *J. Bone Miner. Res.,* 12, 24, 1997.
4. Cummings, S.R., Rubin, S.M., and Black, D., "The future of hip fractures in the United States: numbers, costs, and potential effects of postmenopausal estrogen," *Clin. Orthop.,* 252, 163, 1990.
5. Cooper, A., *Fractures and Dislocations of the Joints,* Longman, Hurst, Rees, Orme, and Brown, London, 1822.
6. White, B.L., Fisher, W.D., and Laurin, A., "Rate of mortality for elder patients after fracture of the hip in the 1980s," *J. Bone Joint Surg.,* 69A, 1335, 1987.
7. Jensen, J.S., Tondevold, E., and Mossing, N., "Unstable trochanteric fractures treated with the sliding screw-plate system. A biomechanical study of unstable trochanteric fractures," *Acta Orthop. Scand.,* 49, 392, 1978.
8. Buchanan, J.R., Nyers, C., Greer, R.B., et al., "Assessment of the risk of vertebral fracture in menopausal women," *J. Bone Joint Surg.,* 69A, 212, 1987.
9. Kristensen, K.D. and Hansen, T., "Closed treatment of ankle fractures: stage II supination-eversion fractures followed for 20 years," *Acta Orthop. Scand.,* 56, 107, 1985.
10. Ferris, B.B., Doods, R.A., Klenerman, L., et al., "Major components of bone in subcapital and trochanteric fractures. A comparative study," *J. Bone Joint Surg.,* 69B, 234, 1987.
11. Lindsay, R., "Prevention of osteoporosis," *Clin. Orthop.,* 222, 44, 1987.
12. Makin, M., "Osteoporosis and proximal femoral fractures in the female elderly of Jerusalem," *Clin. Orthop.,* 218, 19, 1987.
13. Cooper, C., Baker, D.J.P., Morris, J., and Briggs, R.S.J., "Osteoporosis, falls and age in fracture of the proximal femur," *Br. Med. J.,* 295, 13, 1987.
14. Cummings, S.R., "Are patients with hip fractures more osteoporotic? Review of the evidence," *Am. J. Med.,* 78, 487, 1985.
15. Melton, L.J., Whaner, H.V., Richelson, L.S., et al., "Osteoporosis and the risk of the hip fracture," *Am. J. Epidemiol.,* 124, 254, 1986.
16. Falch, J.A., Ilebekk, A., and Slungaard, U., "Epidemiology of the hip fractures in Norway," *Acta Orthop. Scand.,* 56, 218, 1985.

17. Sernbo, I., Johnell, O., and Anderson, T., "Differences in the incidence of the hip fracture. Comparison of an urban and a rural population in Southern Sweden," *Acta Orthop. Scand.*, 59, 382, 1988.

18. Diez Perez, A., Puig Mamesa, J., and Martinez Izquierdo, M.T., "Approximacion a los costos de la fractura osteoporotica de femur en Espana," *Med. Clin. (Barcelona)*, 92, 721, 1989.

19. Lewinnek, G.E., Kelsez, J., White, A.A., and Kreiger, N.J., "The significance and a comparative analysis of the epidemiology of the hip fractures," *Clin. Orthop.*, 152, 35, 1980.

20. Zatteberg, C., Elmerson, S., and Anderson, G.B.J., "Epidemiology of the hip fractures in Goteborg, Sweden, 1940–1983," *Clin. Orthop.*, 191, 43, 1984.

21. Lebiedowski, M., Ipnarska, A., and Muszynska, M., "Zlamania szyjki kosci udowej w krajowej populacji lat 1986–1987 w swietle danych o hospitalizacji," Medycyna 2000, PRO PHARMA Sp. 2.0.0., Warsaw, 1996.

22. Protzman, R.R. and Burkhalter, W.E., "Femoral-neck fractures in young adults," *J. Bone Joint Surg.*, 58A, 689, 1976.

23. Stromqvist, B. and Nilsson, L.T., "The femoral neck fracture treatment controversy," *Semin. Orthop.*, 3, 156, 1989.

24. Garden, R.S., "The structure and function of the proximal end of the femur," *J. Bone Joint Surg.*, 43B, 576, 1961.

25. Hoaglund, F.T. and Low, W.D., "Anatomy of the femoral neck and head, with comparative data from Caucasians and Hong Kong Chinese," *Clin. Orthop.*, 152, 10, 1980.

26. Harty, M., "The calcar femorale and the femoral neck," *J. Bone Joint Surg.*, 39A, 625, 1957.

27. Griffin, J.B., "The calcar femorale redefined," *Clin. Orthop.*, 164, 211, 1982.

28. Trueta, J. and Harrison, M.H.M., "The normal vascular anatomy of the femoral head in adult man," *J. Bone Joint Surg.*, 35B, 442, 1953.

29. Chandler, S.B. and Kreuscher, P.H., "A study of the blood supply of the ligamentum teres and its relation to the circulation of the head of the femur," *J. Bone Joint Surg.*, 14A, 843, 1932.

30. Crock, H.V., "An atlas of the arterial supply of the head and neck of the femur in man," *Clin. Orthop.*, 152, 17, 1980.

31. Holmes, C.A., Edwards, W.T., and Myers, E.R., "Biomechanics of pin and screw fixation of femoral neck fractures," *J. Orthop. Trauma*, 7, 242, 1993.

32. Rowe, S.M., Yoon, T.R., and Ryang, D.H., "An epidemiologic study of hip fracture in Honam, Korea," *Int. Orthop.*, 17, 139, 1993.

33. Jarnlo, G.B. and Thorngren, K.G., "Background factors to hip fractures," *Clin. Orthop.*, 287, 41, 1993.

34. Wood, D.J., Ions, G.K., Quinby, J.M., et al., "Factors which influence mortality after subcapital hip fracture," *J. Bone Joint Surg.*, 74B, 199, 1992.

35. Schroder, H.M., Petersen, K.K., and Erlandsen, M., "Occurrence and incidence of the second hip fracture," *Clin. Orthop.*, 289, 166, 1993.

36. Michel, B.A., Bloch, D.A., and Fries, J.F., "Physical activity and fractures over the age of fifty years," *Int. Orthop.*, 16, 87, 1992.

37. Chapuy, M.C., Arlot, M.E., Duboeuf, F., et al., "Vitamin D3 and calcium to prevent hip fractures in the elderly women," *N. Engl. J. Med.*, 327, 1637, 1992.

38. Christodoulou, N.A. and Dretakis, E.K., "Significance of muscular disturbances in the localization of fractures of the proximal femur," *Clin. Orthop.*, 187, 215, 1984.

39. Sloan, J. and Holloway, G., "Fractured neck of the femur: the cause of the fall?" *Injury*, 13, 230, 1981.

40. Freeman, M.A.R., Todd, R.C., and Pirie, C.J., "The role of fatigue in the pathogenesis of senile femoral neck fractures," *J. Bone Joint Surg.*, 56B, 698, 1974.

41. Paré, A., *The Work of That Famous Chirurgion, Ambroise Paré*, translated from the Latin and compared with the French by Tho. Johnson, Book XV, T. Cotes and R. Young, London, 1634.

42. Malgaigne, J.F., *Treatise on Fractures*, translated by Packard, J.H., J.B. Lippincott, Philadelphia, 1859.

43. Phillips, G.W., "Fracture of the neck of the femur: treatment by means of extension with weights, applied in the direction of the axis of limb, and also laterally in axis of neck: recovery without shortening or other deformity," *Am. J. Med. Sci.*, 58, 398, 1869.

44. Whitman, R., "A new method of treatment for fractures of the neck of the femur, together with remarks on coxa vara," *Ann. Surg.*, 36, 746, 1902.

45. Langenbeck, B., Vorstellung eines Falles von veraltaten Querbuga der Patella, durch Analgung von Silberdrahten geheilt, *Verth. Dtsch. Ges. Chir. Kong. VII*, 1, 92, 1878.

46. Konig, J., Vorstellung eines Falles von veraltaten Querbuga dur Patella, durch Analgung von Silber-drahten geheilt, *Verth. Dtsch. Ges. Chir. Kong. VII*, 1, 93, 1878.

47. Trendelenburg, F., Vorstellung eines Falles von veraltaten Querbuga der Patella, durch Analgung von Silberdrahten geheilt, *Verth. Dtsch. Ges. Chir. Kong. VII*, 1, 89, 1878.

48. Smith-Petersen, M.N. and Cave, W.S., "Hip arthroplasty with the metallic prosthesis," *J. Bone Joint Surg.*, 44A, 6, 1962.

49. Westcott, H.H., "Preliminary report of method of internal fixation of transcervical fractures of the neck of the femur in the aged," *Va. Med.*, 59, 197, 1932.

50. Cram, R.H., "The unstable intertrochanteric fracture," *Surg. Gynecol. Obstet.*, 101, 15, 1955.

51. Ecker, M.L., Joyce, J.J., and Kohl, E.J., "The treatment of trochanteric hip fractures using a compres-sion screw," *J. Bone Joint Surg.*, 57A, 1, 1975.

52. Harrington, K.D. and Johnston, J.O., "The management of comminuted unstable intertrochanteric fractures," *J. Bone Joint Surg.*, 55A, 7, 1973.

53. Moore, A.T., "The self-locking metal hip prosthesis," *J. Bone Joint Surg.*, 39A, 811, 1957.

54. Thompson, F.R., "Two and a half years' experience with a Vitallium intramedullary hip prosthesis," *J. Bone Joint Surg.*, 36A, 489, 1954.

55. Hinchey, J.J. and Day, P.L., "Primary prosthetic replacement in fresh femoral neck fractures," *J. Bone Joint Surg.*, 46A, 223, 1964.

56. Hunter, G.A., "A comparison of the use of internal fixation and prosthetic replacement for fresh fractures of the neck of the femur," *Br. J. Surg.*, 56, 229, 1969.

57. Stinchfield, F.E., Cooperman, B., and Shea, C.E., "Replacement of the femoral head by Judet or Austin-Moore prosthesis," *J. Bone Joint Surg.*, 39A, 1043, 1957.

58. D'Arcy, L. and Devas, M., "Treatment of fractures of the femoral neck by replacement with the Thompson prosthesis," *J. Bone Joint Surg.*, 58B, 279, 1976.

59. Meyer, S., "Prosthetic replacement in hip fractures and comparison between the Moore and Chris-tiansen endoprostheses," *Clin. Orthop.*, 160, 57, 1981.

60. Sikorsky, J.M. and Barrington, R., "Internal fixation vs. hemiarthroplasty for the displaced subcapital fracture of the femur: a prospective randomised study," *J. Bone Joint Surg.*, 63B, 4, 1981.

61. Whittaker, R.P., Abeshaus, M.M., Scoll, H.W., et al., "Fifteen years' experience with metallic endoprosthetic replacement of the femoral head for femoral neck fractures," *J. Trauma*, 12, 799, 1972.

62. Coventry, M.B., "An evaluation of the femoral head prosthesis after ten years of experience," *Surg. Gynecol. Obstet.*, 109, 243, 1959.

63. Gingras, M.B., Clarke, J., and Evans, C.M., "Prosthetic replacement in femoral neck fractures," *Clin. Orthop.*, 152, 147, 1980.

64. Garlicki, M. and Kreczko, R., *Arthrosis Deformas Coxae*, Wydawnictwo Lekarskie PZWL, Warszawa, 1974.

65. McKee, G. and Farrar, W., "Replacement of osteoarthritic hips by the McKee-Farrar prosthesis," *J. Bone Joint Surg.*, 48B, 236, 1966.

66. Charnley, J., "The bonding of prosthesis to bone by cement," *J. Bone Joint Surg.*, 45B, 518, 1964.

67. Charnley, J., "A biomechanical analysis of the use of cement to anchor the femoral head prosthesis," *J. Bone Joint Surg.*, 47B, 354, 1965.

68. Bateman, J.E., "Single-assembly total hip prosthesis: preliminary report," *Orthop. Dig.*, 2, 15, 1974.

69. Stromqvist, B., "Femoral head vitality after intracapsular hip fracture. 490 cases studied by intravital tetracycline labeling and TC-MDP radionuclide imaging," *Acta Orthop. Scand. Suppl.*, 200, 5, 1983.

70. Swiontkowski, M.F., Tepic, S., Rahn, B.A., and Perren, S., "The effect of femoral neck fracture on femoral head blood flow," in *Bone Circulation and Bone Necrosis*, Fourth International Symposium on Bone Circulation, Springer, New York, 1990, 105.

71. Sevitt, S., "Avascular necrosis and revascularisation of the femoral head after intracapsular fractures. A combined arteriographic and histologic necropsy study," *J. Bone Joint Surg.*, 46B, 270, 1964.

72. Catto, M., "A histologic study of avascular necrosis of the femoral head after transcervical fracture," *J. Bone Joint Surg.*, 47B, 749, 1965.

73. Crawfurd, E.J.P., Emery, R.J.H., Hansell, D.M., et al., "Capsular distension and intracapsular pressure in subcapital fractures of the femur," *J. Bone Joint Surg.*, 70B, 195, 1988.

74. Jacobsson, B., Dalen, N., Jonsson, B., and Ackerholm, P., "Intra-articular pressure during operation of cervical hip fractures," *Acta Orthop. Scand.*, 59, 16, 1988.

75. Wingstrand, H., Stromqvist, B., Egund, N., et al., "Hemiarthrosis in undisplaced cervical fractures. Tamponade may cause reversible femoral head ischemia," *Acta Orthop. Scand.,* 57, 305, 1986.
76. Swiontkowski, M.F., Tepic, S., Perren, S.M., et al., "Laser Doppler flowmetry for bone blood flow measurement: correlation with microsphere estimates and evaluation of the effect of intracapsular pressure on femoral head blood flow," *J. Orthop. Res.,* 4, 362, 1986.
77. Garden, R.S., "Malreduction and avascular necrosis in subcapital fractures of the femur," *J. Bone Joint Surg.,* 53B, 183, 1971.
78. Smyth, E.H. and Shah, V.M., "The significance of good reduction and fixation in displaced subcapital fractures of the femur," *Injury,* 5, 197, 1974.
79. Claffey, T.J., "Avascular necrosis of the femoral head. An anatomic study," *J. Bone Joint Surg.,* 42B, 802, 1060.
80. Stromqvist, B., Nilsson, L.T., Egund, N., et al., "Intracapsular pressures in undisplaced fractures of the femoral neck," *J. Bone Joint Surg.,* 70B, 192, 1988.
81. Brodetti, A., "The blood supply of the femoral neck and head in relation to the damaging effects of nails and screws," *J. Bone Joint Surg.,* 42B, 794, 1960.
82. Garden, R.S., "Reduction and fixation of subcapital fractures of the femur," *Orthop. Clin. North Am.,* 5, 683, 1974.
83. Garden, R.S., "Stability and union in subcapital fractures of the femur," *J. Bone Joint Surg.,* 46B, 630, 1964.
84. Pauwels, F., *Der Schenkelhalsbruch. Ein mechanisches Problem,* Beilageheft Z. Orthop. Chir., Enke, Stüttgart, 1935, 63.
85. Linton, P., "Types of displacement in fractures of the femoral neck and observation on impaction of fractures," *J. Bone Joint Surg.,* 31B, 184, 1949.
86. Palczewski, D., Kordala, K., and Waniewski, M., "Wyniki leczenia zlaman klykci kosci piszczelowych w materiale Oddzialu Ortopedyczno Urazowego w Siedlcach," *Chir. Narzadow Ruchu Ortop. Pol.,* 57, 3, 1997.
87. Swiontkowski, M.F., "Intercapsular fractures of the hip," *J. Bone Joint Surg.,* 76A, 131, 1994.
88. Swiontkowski, M.F., Winquist, R.A., and Hansen, S.T., Jr., "Fractures of the femoral neck in patients between the ages of twelve and forty-nine years," *J. Bone Joint Surg.,* 66A, 837, 1984.
89. Mullen, J.O. and Mullen, N.L., "Hip fracture mortality. A prospective, multifactorial study to predict and minimize death risk," *Clin. Orthop.,* 280, 214, 1992.
90. Smith-Petersen, M.N., "Treatment of fractures of the neck of the femur by internal fixation," *Surg. Gynecol. Obstet.,* 64, 287, 1937.
91. Cotton, F.J., "Artificial impaction in hip fractures," *Surg. Gynecol. Obstet.,* 45, 307, 1927.
92. Leadbetter, G.W., "Closed reduction of fractures of the neck of the femur," *J. Bone Joint Surg.,* 20A, 108, 1938.
93. Jaadet, R., "Traitement des fractures du col du femur par greffe pediculee," *Acta Orthop. Scand.,* 23, 421, 1952.
94. Watson-Jones, R., "Fractures of the neck of the femur," *Br. J. Surg.,* 23, 787, 1936.
95. Stromqvist, B., Hansson, L., Palmer, J., et al., "Scintimetric evaluation of nailed femoral neck fractures with special reference to type of osteosynthesis," *Acta Orthop. Scand.,* 54, 340, 1989.
96. Smith, M.D., Cody, D.D., Goldstein, S.A., et al., "Proximal femoral bone density and its correlation to fracture load and hip screw penetration load," *Clin. Orthop.,* 283, 244, 1992.
97. Springer, E.R., Lachiewicz, P.F., and Gilbert, J.A., "Internal fixation of femoral neck fractures. A comparative biomechanical study of Knowles pins and 6.5-mm cancellous screws," *Clin. Orthop.,* 267, 85, 1991.
98. Ort, P.J. and LaMont, J., "Treatment of femoral neck fractures with a sliding compression screw and two Knowles pins," *Clin. Orthop.,* 190, 158, 1984.
99. Chapman, M.W., Stehr, J.H., Eberle, C.F., et al., "Treatment of intracapsular hip fractures by the Deyerle method. A comparative review of one hundred and nineteen cases," *J. Bone Joint Surg.,* 57A, 735, 1975.
100. Swiontkowski, M.F. and Hansen, R.T., Jr., "The Deyerle device for fixation of femoral neck fractures. A review of one hundred twenty-five consecutive cases," *Clin. Orthop.,* 206, 248, 1986.
101. Meyers, M.H., Hanvey, J.P., Jr., and Moore, T.M., "Delayed treatment of subcapital and transcervical fractures of the neck of the femur with internal fixation and a muscle pedicle bone graft," *Orthop. Clin. North Am. Suppl.,* 5(4), 743, 1974.

102. Marti, R.K., Schuller, H.M., and Raaymakers, E.L.F.B., "Intertrochanteric osteotomy for nonunion of the femoral neck," *J. Bone Joint Surg.*, 71B, 782, 1989.

103. Boyd, H.B. and Salvatore, J.E., "Acute fracture of the femoral neck: internal fixation or prosthesis?" *J. Bone Joint Surg.*, 46A, 5, 1964.

104. Johnson, L.L., Lottes, J.O., and Arnot, J.P., "The utilization of the Holt nail for proximal femoral fractures: a study of one hundred and forty-six patients," *J. Bone Joint Surg.*, 50A, 1, 1968.

105. Lindholm, R.V., Puranen, J., and Kinnunen, P., "The Moore vitallium femoral-head prosthesis in fractures of the femoral neck," *Acta Orthop. Scand.*, 47, 70, 1976.

106. Wrighton, J.D. and Woodyard, J.E., "Prosthetic replacement for subcapital fractures of the femur: a comparative study," *Injury*, 2, 4, 1971.

107. Kenzora, J.E., Magaziner, J., Hudson, J., et al., "Outcome after hemiarthroplasty for neck fractures in the elderly," *Clin. Orthop.*, 348, 51, 1998.

108. Lu-Yao, G.L., Keller, R.B., Littenberg, B., and Wennberg, J.E., "Outcomes after displaced fractures of the femoral neck. A meta-analysis of one hundred and six published reports," *J. Bone Joint Surg.*, 76A, 15, 1994.

109. Calder, S.J., Craig, J.S.J., Hinves, B.L., and Heatley, F.W., "Effect of femoral component head size on movement of the two-component hemiarthroplasty," *Injury*, 24, 231, 1993.

110. Lestrange, N.R., "Bipolar arthroplasty for 496 hip fractures," *Clin. Orthop.*, 251, 7, 1990.

111. LaBelle, L.W., Colwill, J.C., and Swanson, A.B., "Bateman bipolar hip arthroplasty for femoral neck fractures. A five- to ten-year follow-up study," *Clin. Orthop.*, 251, 20, 1990.

112. Merlo, L., Augereau, B., and Apoil, A., "Bipolar prosthesis in femoral neck fractures," *Rev. Chir. Orthop. Reparatrice Appar. Mot.*, 78, 536, 1992.

113. Wathne, R.A., Koval, K.J., Aharonoff, G.B., and Zuckerman, J.D., "Modular unipolar vs. bipolar prosthesis: a prospective evaluation of functional outcome after femoral neck fracture," *J. Orthop. Trauma*, 9, 298, 1995.

114. Drinker, M. and Murray, W.R., "The universal proximal femoral endoprosthesis. A short term comparison with conventional hemiarthroplasty," *J. Bone Joint Surg.*, 61A, 1167, 1979.

115. Calder, S.J., Anderson, G.H., Jagger, C., et al., "Unipolar or bipolar prosthesis for displaced intracapsular hip fractures in octogenarians. A randomized prospective study," *J. Bone Joint Surg.*, 78B, 391, 1996.

116. West, W.F. and Mann, R.A., "Evaluation of the Bateman self-articulating femoral prosthesis," *Orthop. Trans.*, 3, 17, 1979.

117. Verberne, V.H.M., "A femoral head with a built-in joint," *J. Bone Joint Surg.*, 65B, 544, 1983.

118. Tsukamoto, Y., Mabuchi, K., Futami, T., and Kubotera, D., "Motion of the bipolar hip prosthesis components," *Acta Orthop. Scand.*, 63, 648, 1992.

119. Brueton, N., Craig, J.S.S., Hinves, B.L., and Heatley, F.W., "Effect of femoral component head size on movement of the two-component hemiarthroplasty," *Injury*, 24, 231, 1993.

120. Chen, S.C., Badrinath, K., Pell, L.H., and Mitchell, K., "The movements of the components of the Hastings bipolar prosthesis. A radiographic study in 65 patients," *J. Bone Joint Surg.*, 71B, 186, 1989.

121. Gebhard, J.S., Amstutz, H.C., Zinar, D.M., and Dorey, F.J., "A comparison of total hip arthroplasty and hemiarthroplasty for treatment of acute fracture of the femoral neck," *Clin. Orthop.*, 282, 123, 1992.

122. Sim, F.H. and Sigmond, E.R., "Acute fractures of the femoral neck managed by total hip replacement," *Orthopaedics*, 9, 35, 1986.

123. Taine, W.H. and Armour, P.C., "Primary total hip replacement for displaced subcapital fractures of the femur," *J. Bone Joint Surg.*, 67B, 214, 1985.

124. Tylman, D. and Dziak, A., *Traumatologia Narzadu Ruchu*, PZWL, Warszawa, 1985.

125. Zwierzchowski, H. and Olejniczak, A., "Wczesne wyniki leczenia zlaman blizszego konca kosci udowej na zrownowazonym wyciagu szkieletowym u osob w wieku starszym," *Chir. Narzadow Ruchu Ortop. Pol.*, 33, 145. 1968.

126. Boyd, H.B. and Griffin, L.L., "Classification and treatment of trochanteric fractures," *Arch. Surg.*, 58, 853, 1949.

127. Evans, E.M., "The treatment of trochanteric fractures of the femur," *J. Bone Joint Surg.*, 31B, 190, 1949.

128. Tkaczyk, T. and Sokolowski, J., "Leczenie zachowawcze zlaman okolicy kretarzowej kosci udowej," *Kwart. Ortop.*, 2, 56, 1994.

129. Jewett, E.L., "One-piece angle nail plate for trochanteric fractures," *J. Bone Joint Surg.*, 23A, 803, 1941.

130. Bannister, G.C. and Gibson, A.G.F., "Jewett nail plate or AO dynamic hip screw for trochanteric fractures? A randomised prospective controlled trial," *J. Bone Joint Surg.*, 65B, 218, 1983.

131. Dimon, J.H., "The unstable intertrochanteric fracture," *Clin. Orthop.*, 92, 1000, 1973.

132. Pugh, W.L., "A self-adjusting nail-plate for fractures about the hip joint," *J. Bone Joint Surg.*, 37A, 1085, 1955.

133. Flores, L.A., Harrington, I.J., and Heller, M., "The stability of intertrochanteric fractures treated with a sliding screw-plate," *J. Bone Joint Surg.*, 72B, 37, 1990.

134. Rao, J.P., Banzon, M.T., Weiss, A.B., and Rayhack, J., "Treatment of unstable intertrochanteric fractures with anatomic reduction and compression hip screw fixation," *Clin. Orthop.*, 175, 65, 1983.

135. Küntscher, G., "A new method of treatment of pertrochanteric fractures," *Proc. R. Soc. Med.*, 63, 1120, 1970.

136. Ender, H.G., "Treatment of peritrochanteric fractures and subtrochanteric fractures of the femur with Ender pins," in *The Hip: Proceedings of the Sixth Open Scientific Meeting of the Hip Society*, Mosby, St. Louis, 1978, 43.

137. Ayers, D.S., Pellergrini, V.D., and Evarts, C.M., "Prevention of heterotopic ossification in high risk patients by radiation therapy," *Clin. Orthop.*, 263, 87, 1991.

138. Bremen-Kuhne, R., Stock, D., and Franke, C., "Indometacin-Kurzzeittherapie vs. Einzetige Low-Dose-Radiation zur Prophylaxe periartikularer Ossifikation (PAO) nach Huft-TEP," *Z. Orthop.*, 135, 422, 1997.

139. Bruckl, R. and Frey, M., "Prophylaxe paraartikularer Ossifikationen durch Strahlentherapie nach zementloser Huft-TEP-Implantation," *Z. Orthop.*, 135, 430, 1997.

140. Kreczko, R., Szulc, W., Serafin, J., et al., "Ocena wynikow totalnej alloplastyki biodra sposobem Parhofera," Pamietniki XVII Zjazdu Naukowego PTO I Tr., 118, Warszawa, 1988.

141. Butterfield, S., Qussou, S.S., and Reschaurer, R., "Ender intramedullary nailing of pertrochanteric fractures," *Orthopaedics*, 2, 507, 1979.

142. Chapman, M., Bowman, W., Soongradi, J., et al., "The use of Ender's pins in extracapsular fractures of the hip," *J. Bone Joint Surg.*, 63A, 14, 1981.

143. Levy, R.N., Seigel, M., Sedlin, E., and Siffen, R., "Complications of Ender-pin fixation in basicervical, intertrochanteric, and subtrochanteric fractures of the hip," *J. Bone Joint Surg.*, 65A, 66, 1983.

144. Pankovich, A. and Tirabaishy, I., "Ender nailing of intertrochanteric and subtrochanteric fractures of the femur," *J. Bone Joint Surg.*, 62A, 63S, 1980.

145. Russin, L.A. and Sanni, A., "Treatment of intertrochanteric and subtrochanteric fractures with Ender's intramedullary rods," *Clin. Orthop.*, 148, 203, 1980.

146. Farcy, J. and Grelsamer, R.P., "Stabilizing insert for Ender nail," *Orthop. Rev.*, 13, 11, 1984.

147. Olerud, S., Stark, A., and Gillstrom, P., "Malrotation following Ender nailing," *Clin. Orthop.*, 147, 139, 1980.

148. Rantanen, J. and Aro, H.T., "Intramedullary fixation of high subtrochanteric femoral fractures. A study comparing two implant designs, the gamma nail and the intramedullary hip screw," *J. Orthop. Trauma*, 12, 249, 1998.

149. Doherty, J.H.J. and Lyden, J.P., "Intertrochanteric fractures of the hip treated with the hip compression screw: analysis of problems," *Clin. Orthop.*, 141, 184, 1979.

150. Manoli, A., "Malassembly of the sliding screw-plate device," *J. Trauma*, 26, 916, 1986.

151. Simpson, A.H., Varty, K., and Dodd, C.A., "Sliding hip screws: modes of failure," *Injury*, 20, 227, 1989.

152. Grosse, A. and Taglag, G., "The history of gamma nails," presented at *International Symposium on Recent Advances in Locking Nails*, Hong Kong, 1992, 63.

153. Bridle, S.H., Patel, A.D., Brichter, M., and Calvert, P.T., "Fixation of intertrochanteric fractures of the femur. A randomised prospective comparison of the gamma nail and the dynamic hip screw," *J. Bone Joint Surg.*, 73B, 330, 1991.

154. Leung, K.S., So, W.S., Shen, W.Y., and Hui, P.W., "Gamma nails and dynamic hip screws for pertrochanteric fractures. A randomised prospective study in elderly patients," *J. Bone Joint Surg.*, 74B, 345, 1992.

155. Lindsey, R.W., Teal, P., Probe, R.A., et al., "Early experience with the gamma nail interlocking nail for peritrochanteric fractures of the proximal femur," *J. Trauma*, 31, 1649, 1991.

156. Loch, D.A., Kyle, R.F., Bechtold, J.E., et al., "Forces required to initiate sliding in second-generation intramedullary nails," *J. Bone Joint Surg.,* 80A, 1626, 1998.

157. Leung, K.S., Chen, C.M., So, W.S., et al., "Multicenter trial of modified gamma nail in East Asia," *Clin. Orthop.,* 323, 146, 1996.

158. Mahaisavariya, B. and Laupattarkasem, W., "Cracking of the femoral shaft by the gamma nail," *Injury,* 23, 493, 1992.

159. Radford, P.J., Needoff, M., and Webb, J.K., "A prospective randomised comparison of the dynamic hip screw and the gamma locking nail," *J. Bone Joint Surg.,* 75B, 789, 1993.

160. Alvares, J.R., Gonzales, R.C., Aranda, R.L., et al., "Indications for use of the long gamma nail," *Clin. Orthop.,* 350, 62, 1998.

161. Boriani, S., De Lure, F., Campanacci, L., et al., "A technical report reviewing the use of the 11 mm gamma nail: interoperative femur fracture incidence," *Orthopaedics,* 19, 597, 1996.

162. Lyddon, D.W.J., "The prevention of complications with the gamma locking nail," *Am. J. Orthop.,* 25, 357, 1996

163. Tscherne, H. and Lobenhoffer, P., "Tibial plateau fractures: management and expected results," *Clin. Orthop.,* 292, 87, 1993.

164. Schatzker, J., McBroom, R., and Bruce, D., "The tibial plateau fracture. The Toronto experience 1968–1975," *Clin. Orthop.,* 138, 94, 1979.

165. Hohl, M., "Treatment methods in the tibial condylar fractures," *South. Med. J.,* 68, 985, 1975.

166. Blokker, C.P., Rorabeck, C.H., and Bourne, R.B., "Tibial plateau fractures. An analysis of the results of treatment in 60 patients," *Clin. Orthop.,* 182, 193, 1984.

167. Hohl, M., "Tibial condylar fractures," *J. Bone Joint Surg.,* 49A, 1455, 1967.

168. Waddell, J.P., Johnston, D.W., and Neidre, A., "Fractures of the tibial plateau: a review of ninety-five patients and comparison of treatment methods," *J. Trauma,* 21, 376, 1981.

169. Brown, T.D., Anderson, D.D., Nepola, J.V., et al., "Contact stress aberrations following imprecise reduction of simple tibial plateau fractures," *J. Orthop. Res.,* 6, 851, 1988.

170. Lachiewicz, P.F. and Funcik, T., "Factors influencing the results of open reduction and internal fixation of tibial plateau fractures," *Clin. Orthop.,* 259, 210, 1990.

171. Watson, J.T. and Schatzker, J., "Tibial plateau fractures," in *Skeletal Trauma,* Browner, B.D., Trafton, P.G., Jupiter, J.B., and Levine, A.M., Eds., W. B. Saunders, Philadelphia, 1998.

172. Honkonen, S.E., "Indications for surgical treatment of tibial condyle fractures," *Clin. Orthop.,* 302, 199, 1994.

173. Lansinger, O., Bergman, B., Korner, L., et al., "Tibial condylar fractures. A twenty-year follow-up," *J. Bone Joint Surg.,* 68A, 13, 1986.

174. Duvelius, P.J. and Connolly, J.F., "Closed reduction of tibial plateau fractures: a comparison of functional and roentgenographic end results," *Clin. Orthop.,* 230, 116, 1988.

175. Stokel, E.A. and Sadesivan, K.K., "Tibial plateau fractures standardized evaluation of operative results," *Orthopaedics,* 14, 263, 1991.

176. Weiner, L.S., Kelley, M., Yang, E., et al., "The use of combination internal fixation and hybrid external fixation in severe proximal tibia fractures," *J. Orthop. Trauma,* 9, 244, 1995.

177. Young, M.J. and Barrack, R.L., "Complications of internal fixation of tibial plateau fractures," *Orthop. Rev.,* 23, 149, 1994.

178. Garlicki, M. and Kreczko, R., "Wyniki leczenia srodstawowych zlaman blizszej nasady kosci piszczelowej," *Chir. Narzadow Ruchu Ortop. Pol.,* 34, 489, 1969.

179. Ramatowski, W., "Osteosynteza stabilna w leczeniu zlaman blizszej nasady piszczeli," *Chir. Narzadow Ruchu Ortop. Pol.,* 52, 247, 1977.

180. Moore, T.M., Patzakis, M.J., and Harvey, J.P., "Tibial plateau fractures: definition, demographics, treatment rationale, and long-term results of closed traction management or operative reduction," *J. Orthop. Trauma,* 1, 97, 1987.

181. Benirschke, S.K., Agnew, S., Mayo, K.A., et al., "Immediate internal fixation of open, complex tibial plateau fractures: treatment by a standard protocol," *J. Orthop. Trauma,* 6, 78, 1992.

182. Frankhauser, C., Frenk, A., and Marti, A.A., "Comparative biomechanical evaluation of three systems for the internal fixation of distal fractures of the femur," *Trans. Orthop. Res. Soc.,* 24, 498, 1999.

183. Schandelmaire, P., Krettek, C., Miclau, T., et al., "Stabilization of distal femoral fractures using the LISS," *Tech. Orthop.,* 14, 230, 1999.

184. Krettek, C., Gerich, T., and Miclau, T., "A minimally invasive medial approach for proximal tibial fractures," *Injury,* 32, SA4, 2001.

185. Chapman, M.W., *Operative Orthopaedics,* Vol. 1–3, J.B. Lippincott, Philadelphia, 1988.

186. Kus, W.M. and Gorecki, A., "Wykorzystanie artroskopu do leczenia zlaman blizszej nasady kosci piszczelowej z obnizeniem powierzchni stawowej," *Chir. Narzadow Ruchu Ortop. Pol.,* 52, 296, 1987.

187. Morandi, M. and Pearse, M.F., "Management of complex tibial plateau fractures with the Illizarow external fixator," *Tech. Orthop.,* 11, 125, 1996.

188. Watson, J.T., "High-energy fractures of the tibial plateau," *Orthop. Clin. North Am.,* 25, 723, 1994.

189. Lindsjo, U., "Operative treatment of ankle fractures," *Acta Orthop. Scand. Suppl.,* 52, 1, 1981.

190. Daly, P.J., Fitzgerald, R.H., Melton, L.J., and Ilstruo, D.M., "Epidemiology of ankle fractures in Rochester, Minnesota," *Acta Orthop. Scand.,* 50, 539, 1987.

191. Lauge-Hansen, N., "Fractures of the ankle. II. Combined experimental-surgical and experimental-roentgenologic investigations," *Arch. Surg.,* 60, 957, 1950.

192. Müller, M.E., Allgöwer, M., and Willenegger, H., *Manual of Internal Fixation,* Springer-Verlag, New York, 1970.

193. Nielsen, J.O., Dons-Jensen, H., and Sorensen, H.T., "Lauge-Hansen classification of malleolar fractures: an assessment of the reproducibility in 118 cases," *Acta Orthop. Scand.,* 61, 385, 1990.

194. Ramsey, P.L. and Hamilton, W., "Changes in tibiotalar area of contact caused by lateral talar shift," *J. Bone Joint Surg.,* 58A, 356, 1976.

195. Yablon, I.G., Heller, F.G., and Shouse, L., "The key role of the lateral malleous in displaced fractures of the ankle," *J. Bone Joint Surg.,* 57A, 169, 1997.

196. Brown, T.D., Hurlbut, P.T., Hale, J.E., et al., "Effects of imposed hindfoot constraint on contact mechanics of displaced lateral malleolar fractures," *Trans. Orthop. Res. Soc.,* 40, 257, 1994.

197. Bauer, M., Jonsson, K., and Nilsson, B., "Thirty-year follow-up of ankle fractures," *Acta Orthop. Scand.,* 56, 103, 1985.

198. Yde, J. and Kristensen, K.D., "Ankle fractures: supination-eversion fractures of stage II-primary and late results of operative treatment," *Acta Orthop. Scand.,* 51, 695, 1980.

199. Quigley, T.B., "Management of ankle injuries sustained in sports," *J. Am. Med. Assoc.,* 169, 1431, 1959.

200. Eventov, L., Salama, R., Goodwin, D.R.A., and Weissman, S.L., "An evaluation of surgical and conservative treatment of fractures of the ankle in 200 patients," *J. Trauma,* 18, 271, 1978.

201. Mast, J.W. and Teipner, W.A., "Reproducible approach to the internal fixation of adult ankle fractures: rationale, technique, and early results," *Orthop. Clin. North Am.,* 11, 661, 1980.

202. Breederveld, R.S., van Straaten, J., Patka, P., and van Mourik, J.C., "Immediate or delayed operative treatment of fractures of the ankle," *Injury,* 19, 436, 1988.

203. Konvath, G., Karges, D., Watson, J.T., et al., "Early vs. delayed treatment of severe ankle fractures: a comparison of results," *J. Orthop. Trauma,* 9, 377, 1995.

204. Ryd, L. and Bengtsson, S., "Isolated fracture of the lateral malleolus requires no treatment: 49 prospective cases of supination-eversion type II ankle fractures," *Acta Orthop. Scand.,* 63, 443, 1992.

205. Jacobsen, S., Honnens de Lichtenberg, M., Jensen, C., et al., "Removal of internal fixation — the effect on patients' complaints: a study of 66 cases of removal of internal fixation after malleolar fractures," *Foot Ankle Int.,* 15, 170, 1994.

206. Tornetta, P., III, "Ankle injuries," in *Principles of Orthopaedic Practice,* Dee, R., Ed., McGraw-Hill, New York, 1997, 531.

207. Bankston, A., Anderson, L., and Nimityongskul, P., "Intramedullary screw fixation of lateral malleolus fractures," *Foot Ankle Int.,* 15, 599, 1994.

208. Schaffer, J.J. and Manoli, A., "The antiglide plate for distal fibular fixation: a biomechanical comparison with fixation with a lateral plate," *J. Bone Joint Surg.,* 69A, 596, 1987.

209. Tornetta, P., "Ankle fracture," *J. Orthop. Trauma,* 4, 304, 2001.

210. McDaniel, W.J. and Wilson, F.C., "Trimalleolar fractures of the ankle: an end result study," *Clin. Orthop.,* 122, 37, 1977.

211. Peter, R.E., Harrington, R.M., Henley, M.B., and Tencer, A.F., "Biomechanical effects of internal fixation of the distal tibiofibular syndesmotic joint: comparison of two fixation techniques," *J. Orthop. Trauma,* 8, 215, 1994.

212. Xenos, J.S., Hopkinson, W.J., Mulligan, M.E., et al., "The tibiofibular syndesmosis," *J. Bone Joint Surg.,* 77A, 847, 1995.

213. Van der Griend, R., Michelson, J.D., and Bone, L.B., "Fractures of the ankle and the distal part of the tibia," *J. Bone Joint Surg.*, 78A, 1772, 1996.

214. Karges, D.E., "Open reduction with lateral plate and anterior-posterior lag screws for posterior malleolar fracture," *J. Orthop. Trauma*, 4, 305, 2001.

215. Tile, O.N., "Fractures of the ankle," in *The Rationale of Operative Fracture Care*, Schatzker, J. and Tile, O.N., Eds., Springer-Verlag, New York, 1987.

216. Kellam, J.F. and Waddel, J.P., "Fractures of the distal tibia metaphysis with intra-articular extension: the distal tibial explosion fracture," *J. Trauma*, 19, 593, 1979.

217. Mast, J., "A test of surgical judgment," in *Major Fractures of the Pilon, the Talus, and the Calcaneus*, Tscherne, H. and Schatzker, J., Eds., Springer-Verlag, Berlin, 1993, 7.

218. Saleh, M., Shanahan, G., and Fern, E.D., "Intra-articular fractures of the distal tibia: surgical management by limited internal and articulated distraction," *Injury*, 24, 37, 1993.

219. Heim, U. and Naser, M., "Die operative Behandlung der Pilon Tibial-Fraktur: Technik der Osteosynthese und Resultate bei 128 Patienten," *Acta Orthop. Unfallchir.*, 86, 341, 1976.

220. Ruedi, T. and Allgower, M., "Spatresultate nach operativer Behandlung der Gelenkbruche am distalen Tibiaende," *Unfallheikunde*, 81, 319, 1978.

221. Böstman, O.M., "Intense granulomatous inflammatory lesions associated with absorbable internal fixation devices," *Clin. Orthop.*, 278, 193, 1992.

222. Frokjaer, J. and Möller, B.N., "Biodegradable fixation of ankle fractures: complications in a prospective study of 25 cases," *Acta Orthop. Scand.*, 63, 434, 1992.

223. Bucholz, R.W., Henry, S., and Henley, M.B., "Fixation with bioabsorbable screws for the treatment of fractures of the ankle," *J. Bone Joint Surg.*, 76A, 325, 1994.

224. Cheng, S., Souminen, H., and Roitenen, T., "Bone mineral density and physical activity in 50- to 60-year-old women," *Bone Miner.*, 12, 123, 1991.

225. Eisman, J.A., "OsteoPPPorosis — prevention, prevention and prevention," *Aust. N. Z. J. Med.*, 21, 205, 1991.

226. Mazess, R. and Barden, H., "Bone density in premenopausal women: effects of age, dietary intake, physical activity, smoking and birth-control pills," *Am. J. Clin. Nutr.*, 53, 132, 1991.

227. Eisman, J.A., Sambrook, P.N., and Kelly, P.J., "Exercise and its interaction with genetic influences in the determination of bone mineral density," *Am. J. Med.*, 91, 186, 1991.

228. Gutin, B. and Kasper, M.J., "Can vigorous exercise play a role in osteoporosis prevention?" *Osteoporos. Int.*, 2, 55, 1992.

229. Michel, B., Bloch, D., and Fries, J., "Weight-bearing exercise, overexercise and lumbar bone density over age 50 years," *Arch. Intern. Med.*, 7, 91, 1989.

230. Goralczyk, B., Mikula, W., and Jozwiak-Kaczocha, B., "Rehabilitacja pourazowa pacjentow w podeszlym wieku," *Nowa Med.*, 9, 30, 1996.

17 The Use of Bone Cement in the Treatment of Osteoporotic Fractures

Jeffrey M. Walker and Subrata Saha

CONTENTS

I. INTRODUCTION

Fractures that develop in osteoporotic bone are often difficult to treat because of the lack of structural integrity that exists in these bones. As the disease progresses, the bone density decreases and the trabecular network begins to thin and gradually disappear. Without the support of the trabecular bone, fractures become much more likely and are most common in the vertebrae, ribs, proximal femur, humeri, and distal radius. However, comminuted fractures of the trochanter and compression fractures of the vertebrae present some of the most serious problems. Surgeons have investigated the use of bone cement as a tool in the treatment of osteoporotic fractures for several decades and have reported good results from using polymethylmethacrylate (PMMA) as an augmentation method in treating these fractures.[1-5]

A. BENEFITS OF USING PMMA

Müller[6] was one of the first to propose the use of bone cement as an adjunct to internal fixation with bone screws in the treatment of neoplastic pathologic fractures as well as fractures with evidence of osteoporosis. Bone screws rely on the quality of bone to provide adequate fixation; yet when trabecular bone is compromised, as with osteoporosis, loosening of the screws is common. If the screws become loose, adequate fixation may not be possible and nonunions and malunions may occur. Injecting bone cement into the trabecular bone provides much better fixation for the plates and screws and allows for early mobilization that may be beneficial to the normal healing process. Early mobilization also eliminates many of the potential problems with prolonged bed rest. Injecting cement to enhance the fixation increases the interfacial surface area of the implant and reduces the shear stresses at the bone–implant interface.[7] Although the recommendation has not always been followed, Cameron et al. have indicated that the screws should be inserted into the holes before the cement has cured to ensure maximum strength of the fixation.[8]

B. ADVERSE EFFECTS OF USING PMMA

Despite the improvement in fixation strength and subsequent healing, the use of PMMA in treating fractures has never been widespread due to the potential complications that may arise, which include necrosis and bone resorption as well as other concerns. A large amount of heat is generated during the exothermic polymerization of the cement and this could pose significant dangers including thermal necrosis of the surrounding tissue. Necrosis of bone tissue is reported to occur for exposure to temperatures in excess of 50°C for longer than 1 min, and an Arrhenius relationship is also thought to exist, whereby the extent of thermal damage is associated with the duration of exposure to elevated temperatures.[9] Studies have shown that temperatures at the surface of polymerizing PMMA reach as high as 90°C.[10]

A fibrous membrane often forms around the bone–cement interface as well, which may lead to increased motion of the implant with accumulation of wear particles and loosening of the implant with the subsequent loss of mechanical function. And because PMMA is inert and not biodegradable, an inflammatory response can possibly occur. Macrophages are believed to become activated in response to wear particles with the release of a number of pro-inflammatory cytokines (IL-1β, IL-6, and TNF-α), inflammatory mediators (e.g., prostaglandin E_2), and proteolytic enzymes (e.g., collagenase) that may play a role in bone resorption activity.[11-14] Another disadvantage of using PMMA is that cement may leak from the intended location and escape into the fracture site as well as the joint causing additional problems. Therefore, the adjunctive use of PMMA in fracture fixation has recently been advocated only for elderly patients with a short life expectancy.[7]

C. CALCIUM PHOSPHATE CEMENT

The recent development of *in situ* setting calcium phosphate bone cements has renewed the interest in the adjunctive use of cement for improving the stability of internal fixation of osteoporotic fractures. Several calcium phosphate derivatives are mixed dry and when an aqueous solution is added, a paste is created that remains formable and injectable for about 5 min.[15] These calcium phosphate cements are biocompatible and resorb with time, being replaced by host bone. They undergo a remodeling phase similar to that of normal bone and also have a similar mineral content. The paste begins to harden in about 10 min as it begins to crystallize into dahllite, which is similar to the mineral phase of bone.[15] The cement hardens within minutes and reaches maximum strength in about 12 hours.[15,16] There have also been reports of calcium phosphate bone cements that cure and reach maximum strength even faster. Stryker Leibinger Bone Source® Hydroxyapatite Cement (HAC) (manufactured by Orthofix/Osteogenics, Richardson, TX) is reported to reach a compressive strength in excess of 50 MPa in only 4 hours.[17,18]

A number of biomechanical studies have been conducted demonstrating the improvement in the fixation strength with the adjunctive use of calcium phosphate cements.[7,18-22] Calcium phosphate cement has also been shown to provide similar anchoring to that of PMMA.[7] The compressive strength of approximately 55 MPa (SRS®, Norian Corporation, Cupertino, CA)[15,16] greatly exceeds that of cancellous bone, which has been reported to be on the order of 1.9 MPa.[23] Important to note, however, is that the tensile and shear strengths are less than or equal to those of cancellous bone with maximum values of about 3 to 5 MPa for the SRS cement.[16] Constantz et al.[15] have reported the tensile strength of SRS calcium phosphate cement to be about 2.1 MPa, while the ultimate tensile strength of cancellous bone has been reported to be about 2.42 MPa.[23] Great care must therefore be taken to ensure that the implant devices chosen do not place undesirable loading onto the bone cement. Probably the most important characteristic is that the calcium phosphate cements undergo an endothermic reaction and cure at normal body temperature and pH, eliminating much of the concern regarding the use of acrylic bone cement.

Histocompatibility studies have been performed in animals, demonstrating the biocompatibility of calcium phosphate cements and the associated osteoblast-osteoclast coupled bone remodelling.[21] Small particles of cement have been noticed during the remodeling with associated cellular response.[24,25] However, this response did not persist, and no fibrosis or unexpected resorption of bone was seen. Some authors, however, have questioned the possible effect the particulate debris may have on osteoblast function,[26] which could inhibit the expected remodeling. Early clinical results have shown promise for the use of calcium phosphate bone cements in treating fractures of the proximal femur and distal radius.[15,16,20,27-29]

II. FRACTURES OF THE PROXIMAL FEMUR

Fractures of the proximal femur are among the most feared complications of osteoporosis and can make the disease a life-threatening disorder.[30] The mortality rates for fractures of the proximal femur range from 12% to more than 30% at 1 year.[31-34] Intertrochanteric fractures are generally associated with a slightly higher mortality rate than the intracapsular, femoral neck fractures.[32] Conventional treatment for fractures of the proximal femur had customarily been traction and long-term immobilization. However, elderly patients are not able to sustain long periods of bed rest very well, and the mortality rate for traction has been reported to be between 33 and 64%.[1] Because of the very high rates of nonunion and malunion associated with the use of traction, treatment using internal fixation has become much more prevalent in recent years. Yet, despite improvements in devices and techniques, failure rates are still too high. In a recent meta-analysis of 52 studies of femoral neck fracture treated with internal fixation, Lu-Yao et al.[33] found reports of nonunions in 33% of the cases, late collapse in 16%, and avascular necrosis in 16%. Sliding hip screw devices generally work well for intertrochanteric fractures, but excessive impaction of the fracture site can present problems. Bendo et al.[35] have reported poor functional outcome in 93% of the fractures treated with the sliding hip screw that were associated with moderate to severe fracture collapse. If the cases of older individuals with osteoporosis were considered alone, the rates of complication likely would be even higher.

A. FEMORAL NECK FRACTURES

Conventional treatment for femoral neck fractures by many surgeons now involves the use of either two or three cannulated screws.[16,20] Stankewich et al.[19] investigated the improvement in fixation strength using SRS calcium phosphate bone cement to treat femoral neck fractures. Fractures were created in the midcervical neck region of 16 pairs of proximal cadaveric femora (10 female and 6 male). The mean age of the retrieved femurs was 70.9 years (range 49 to 88), and prior to testing, the bone mineral density was measured using dual-energy X-ray absorptiometry (DEXA; mean t-score, –2.0; range 0 to –3.6). (See Table 17.1 for a description of the t-score rating system.) The fractures were anatomically reduced and three 7.0×32 mm cancellous bone screws were inserted in an inverted triangular configuration. On the contralateral femurs, calcium phosphate cement was used to augment the screw fixation. Both augmented and unaugmented test specimens were then kept at 37°C for 24 hours to allow curing at normal body temperature.

TABLE 17.1
Densitometry Measurements: *t*-scores

Bone density measurements are made for an individual generally using
DEXA and then compared with standardized bone density values for young
adults of peak bone mass to establish the degree of bone loss.

An Alternative Rating System for Bone Density[a]

1.0–1.5 SD below	Borderline osteopenia
1.6–2.0 SD below	Mild osteopenia
2.1–2.5 SD below	Moderate osteopenia
>2.5 SD below	Severe osteopenia

[a] This modification of the classification by the World Health Organization
allows for the inclusion of factors other than just osteoporosis that cause a
reduction in bone density.

Source: Adapted from Seeger, L.L., *Spine,* 22(Suppl. 24), 49S, 1997.

The femurs were then mounted with the long axis of the femoral shaft oriented at 12° of adduction to represent anatomic position and were tested on a materials testing machine (828 Bionix®, MTS Systems, Minneapolis, MN). After pretreating the femurs for ten cycles at a reduced load, they were loaded for 1000 cycles at 0.5 Hz with a peak compressive force of 611.6 N. This loading represents approximately one body-weight for an elderly woman.

Following the cyclical loading, a quasi-static compressive load was applied until the fixation failed. Results showed that cement injected into the screw holes and the fracture site provided a significant increase in the initial stiffness and the strength of fixation (average improvement of 169.6%). All but one of the augmented femurs failed at a higher load. The bone cement never filled the inferior cortex to provide a buttress in the one that failed at a lower load. Also significant to note is that all six specimens with severe osteoporosis (*t*-scores >3.0) failed with a significantly higher load. Some of the augmented femurs were less stiff after 1000 cycles yet still required a larger load to failure. Inferior migration of the femoral head was reduced in the group augmented with calcium phosphate cement (average of 0.12 vs. 0.27 mm) and less varus rotation was also noted.

In early clinical trials of using calcium phosphate cement to augment femoral neck fractures, results from initial pilot studies have shown excellent results with minimal complications.[16,20] Goodman et al.[20] reported 52 patients (44 female, 8 male) with displaced femoral neck fractures who were treated with cannulated cancellous bone screws in two medical centers.[20] In Sweden, two Uppsala cannulated screws (Olmed AB, Uppsala, Sweden) were used and, in Belgium, three 7-mm cannulated screws (Synthes, Paoli, PA) were used. The average age of the patients in the study was 79 (range 62 to 93). Channels were drilled over guide wire pins, SRS calcium phosphate cement was injected, and the screws were inserted. Additional cement was packed into the posteromedial femoral neck after inserting the screws. The cement was allowed to harden for 10 min while the lower extremity was kept stationary.

The average follow-up was 6 months and 43 of the 52 patients healed without problems. Revisions with total hip arthroplasty were required in 9 patients because of nonunion or loss of fixation. However, 8 of these 9 cases were from the initial period of the trial when the technique was still evolving. All 8 of these showed poor filling of the cement into the screw tract and the fracture void. Any time a material, even one that is biocompatible, is placed into voids in the bones, there is a risk for vascular damage.[20] Necrosis of the femoral head was seen in 1 patient with subsequent nonunion. In 43 of the 52 patients, the cement filled the fracture area fully and was well centered. Seven cases showed leaking of the cement into the surrounding soft tissue and two cases had leaking into the intracapsular area of the joint, but no discomfort or any other complications were

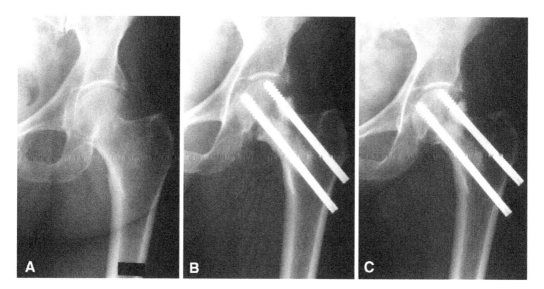

FIGURE 17.1 Fixation of a femoral neck fracture with internal fixation supplemented by biodegradable bone cement. (A) Preoperative radiograph of a displaced femoral neck fracture. (B) Postoperative radiograph showing excellent reduction and fixation of the fracture with two Uppsala screws supplemented with Norian SRS bone cement. C. One year later, the fracture has healed with minor impaction. (From Goodman, S.B. and Larsson, S., in *Internal Fixation in Osteoporotic Bone,* An, Y.H., Ed., Thieme Medical, New York, 2002. With permission.)

reported. All of the cement that escaped had resorbed after a period of time. Figure 17.1 shows an example of fixation of a femoral neck fracture with internal fixation supplemented with biodegradable cement.

B. INTERTROCHANTERIC FRACTURES

Nonunions are generally rare for intertrochanteric fractures. Getting the femur heal in the proper anatomic position, though, can be difficult. Closed reduction and internal fixation using sliding hip screw plates has become the current standard of treatment for these fractures.[7] However, compression hip screws with an intramedullary nail are also becoming more popular. Despite some of the complications that have been reported with devices such as the Gamma nail® (Howmedica, Rutherford, NJ) and the stigma that has been attached to these intramedullary devices, very good to excellent results have been reported by some.[34,37] Unstable fractures of the trochanter may still prove difficult to stabilize with internal fixation, even in the absence of osteoporosis. One of the primary causes for implant failure with hip screws and nails is screw cutout through the femoral head, and considerable limb shortening may also occur as a result of excessive impaction. Screw loosening with the compression plate devices does not occur very often and does not appear to be a major factor.[34]

Biomechanical studies have recently been conducted to determine the potential success of the adjunctive use of calcium phosphate cement with compression hip screw plates for the treatment of unstable fractures of the trochanter. In a study by Elder et al.,[22] a three-part intertrochanteric fracture with a displaced posteromedial fragment was created in ten pairs of cadaver femora and then stabilized with a sliding hip screw. All cadaver femurs were from women older than 65 years (mean 78.5; range 68 to 94) and were moderately osteopenic (*t*-scores at least 2 standard deviation below that of young, gender-matched population) as determined from DEXA. Contralateral femurs were augmented with SRS bone cement. The cement was injected around the screw threads and the shank of the lag screw and was packed into the posteromedial defect as well. A load simulating approximate body weight was used and the specimens were tested for 1000 cycles, then loaded to failure. The fracture loads for the augmented group were only slightly higher, but significantly less sliding was seen in the devices that were aided with cement. Strain gauges were also used to evaluate the conditions further and more load sharing was seen in the medial side of the femur in those with SRS cement. The load in the plate of the augmented group was 55% of the control on average, indicating that much more of the load was transferred to the femur. Therefore, this study indicates that calcium phosphate cement may be beneficial for patients with osteoporotic, intertrochanteric fractures, providing more suitable conditions for healing.

In a recent pilot study, 39 patients had been treated with a dynamic hip screw (32 female, 7 male).[20] The mean age of the patients was 81 (range 57 to 94) and they were all ambulatory before the injury. The severity of the fracture was classified according to the Hennepin system (also known as the Kyle–Gustilo classification[32,38]) and the bone quality was evaluated according to the Singh index.[39] Of the fractures, 30% were unstable (Hennepin Type III or IV) and 34% showed severe signs of osteoporosis (Singh Grade I or II) while a moderate degree of osteoporosis was seen in 46% of the cases (Singh Grade III). The surgical technique involved a routine closed reduction followed by injection of SRS bone cement into the intertrochanteric region and the posteromedial defect. Initially, cement was also injected into the tract of the lag screw, but inserting the screw was difficult and this was stopped early in the study. New needles were also developed during the study to improve the infiltration of the cement and were used after the first 16 patients. Periodic follow-up was conducted to evaluate the sliding of the lag screw in the barrel of the implant, any changes in screw position, and eventual fracture union. The improvement in technique and surgical instruments resulted in reduced sliding of the lag screw from an average of 15.6 mm (range 1.5 to 29.3 mm) to 11.9 mm (range 5.2 to 18.6 mm). All fractures showed union by 6 months. Two minor complications were reported, both in cases treated early in the study. In one, a small amount of bone cement escaped into the joint, but no discomfort or problems were reported and the cement decreased in size after 6 months. In another of the early patients, the lag screw could not be fully inserted and projected laterally. Union was still achieved, though, and no pain was reported. Figure 17.2 shows an example of fixation of an intertrochanteric fracture with internal fixation supplemented with biodegradable cement.

Theoretically, the intramedullary device offers a mechanical advantage over the sliding hip screws with plates in that the lever arm is reduced and there should be a decrease in the potential for screw cutout.[37] In a randomized study of 100 elderly patients (all older than 60 years of age) treated with either a compression hip screw and plate or an intramedullary hip screw, Hardy et al.[34] found similar results for the two groups. Few of the lag screws were noted to be placed in a poor position and subsequently there was no screw cutout in either of the groups. Increased compression of the lag screw with more limb shortening was reported with the use of the compression hip screw plate devices. Slightly better mobility was noted in the intramedullary group, and this was attributed possibly to less limb shortening. Cortical hypertrophy in the diaphyseal region of the femur at the level of the distal nail was reported in 14 of 35 patients treated with the intramedullary device after 1 year and significant pain was noted in many of these patients. The use of the distal locking nails could be partially responsible for these problems.

A number of improvements in the intramedullary device and the surgical techniques have since been developed and significantly better results have been reported.[37] In a study by Bellabarba et al.,[37] 90 of 100 patients (age 16 to 100, average 71) were treated using a Gamma nail and were evaluated at least 6 months postoperatively; 98% healed at an average of 13 weeks (range 7 to 20 weeks). Of these cases, 75 involved intertrochanteric fractures and the remaining were either basicervical or subtrochanteric fractures. No distal interlocking screws were used in any of the patients. There were some complications in a few of the cases requiring revision surgery in 4%, but this is the same value reported for dynamic hip screws.

Despite a shorter lever arm providing better device mechanics, cutout has been reported in 1 to 25% of cases treated with the Gamma nail, and this has been attributed primarily to the improper

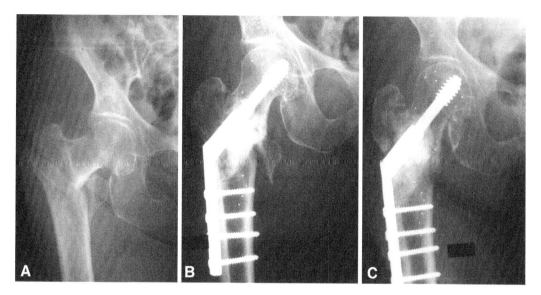

FIGURE 17.2 Fixation of an intertrochanteric fracture with internal fixation supplemented by biodegradable cement. (A) Preoperative radiograph of a displaced intertrochanteric femur fracture. Note the large, displaced lesser trochanteric fragment. (B) Postoperative radiograph showing that an excellent reduction and fixation have been achieved. Note the large bolus of Norian SRS bone cement that has filled the posteromedial calcar defect. The lesser trochanteric fragment has not been reduced. Numerous tantalum balls are present for radiostereometric analysis. (C) One year later, the fracture has healed in excellent position. The bone and SRS have remodeled extensively. (From Goodman, S.B. and Larsson, S., in *Internal Fixation in Osteoporotic Bone, An*, Y.H., Ed., Thieme Medical, New York, 2002. With permission.)

position of the lag screw in the femoral head.[37] Bellabarba et al. found only one case of late screw cutout, yet this was for a screw that appeared to be positioned properly. The authors attributed the reduced rate of screw cutout to the better biomechanical principles of the intramedullary device and overall correct positioning of the screw in the femoral head. Regardless of the device used, failure still does occur, especially in older patients with osteoporosis. Therefore, there is considerable opportunity for bone cements to improve the surgical outcomes in many cases.

III. FRACTURES OF THE UPPER EXTREMITIES

A. DISTAL RADIUS FRACTURES

Fractures of the distal radius are another common injury and can prove considerably difficult to treat, especially when dealing with osteoporotic bone. Fractures of the distal radius are typically referred to as Colles' fractures. Falling onto an outstretched hand is common with elderly people and fractures often occur as a result of the compressive forces through the carpals with splitting of the bone in the sagittal and coronal direction.[40] Colles' fractures have been estimated as ⅙ of all emergency room fractures with two predominant age groups accounting for most: children from 6 to 10 years old, and elderly people (in their 60s).[41] The goal of treatment is to restore and maintain the anatomy and to attain an early return to function, but most of the current methods of treatment result in failure. Simple fractures with little or no displacement or comminution can generally be treated with success by reducing the fracture and stabilizing it in a cast.[28,40] However, comminuted fractures often become redisplaced within weeks when only casting[42] or external fixation[43] is used to immobilize the fractured area. Methods of treating unstable fractures have included percutaneous pinning, a combination of pins and plaster casting, and external fixation, but all these treatment methods have resulted in a high degree of complication and failure.[21,41] Open reduction and internal fixation have become popular, but have also been associated with a number of problems, including loss of fixation. Kirschner wires and adjuvant use of external fixation have been suggested as an effective method for treating intra-articular fractures of the distal radius,[40,44] but complications may still occur.[21,44] The additional use of bone grafts may also be necessary with complex intra-articular fractures.[40] PMMA alone has been used with success as a tool in treating these types of fractures,[43,45] but the dangers of using PMMA are widely recognized. Yetkinler et al.[21] compared the use of calcium phosphate cement (SRS) to Kirschner wires in treating three-part intra-articular fractures created in ten pairs of human cadaveric radii, and found that significantly less settling and more consistent stability was achieved with SRS cement fixation than with the Kirschner wires.

In a limited clinical study, Jupiter et al.[28] found that calcium phosphate bone cement (SRS) could be delivered percutaneously and support unstable, displaced, extra-articular fractures of the distal radius. Five patients, all women (age 49 to 57, average 52.6), had distal radii fractures that were treated with SRS cement, placed in a cast for 6 weeks following reduction and fixation, and then followed for 12 months with periodic examination (one patient withdrew from the study voluntarily after 6 months). The fractures in two of these cases, including the patient who withdrew from the study, were discovered to have intra-articular fracture extensions after reduction and treatment with cement, yet were still included in the study. The results showed little shortening in radial length (<1 mm at 12 months), radial angle within the normal range, good wrist motion (averaging 89 to 100% of the contralateral wrist at 12 months), improved grip strength in all of the cases (mean of 88% at 12 months), minimal motion-related pain, and good clinical progress overall in all five of the patients. There was limited extrusion of the cement, none into the articular area, and the cement showed resorption over time as expected. There was one case, in the patient who withdrew and who also had intra-articular involvement, that showed a progressive loss of volar angle due to the failure of the bone cement to penetrate the site of injury completely. However, the other patient with intra-articular involvement showed much better results. Although the number of patients was small, this study demonstrated the relative effectiveness of calcium phosphate cement in treating unstable fractures of the distal radius. Since only two of these patients had intra-articular fractures, it is unclear how effective these techniques are in treating injuries affecting the articulating joint.

A large randomized study of distal radius fractures was conducted by Sanchez-Sotelo et al.[29] comparing operative treatment using SRS cement and casting for 2 weeks (55 patients, average age 65.18) to conservative treatment with casting for 6 weeks (55 patients, average age 66.87). Inclusion in the study required all of the patients to be older than the age 50 and the fractures to be of either type A3 (comminuted, extra-articular fracture; 73 patients total) or type C2 (simple, intra-articular with metaphyseal comminution; 37 patients total) based on the AO system.[41,46,47] The patients were followed for 1 year and the group treated with SRS had an earlier return to function with significantly better range of motion and grip strength as well as less pain (Figure 17.3). Some progressive settling was reported in both groups, but was greater in the control group receiving conservative treatment. Malunion was more common in the control group (41.8%), yet was still somewhat high (18.2%) in the SRS group. With this significant degree of malunion reported, additional fixation such as Kirschner wires may be necessary to adequately stabilize the fracture in certain cases. Cement extravasation into the soft tissue was noted in 69.1% of the SRS cases and 30 of the 34 cases that escaped into the dorsal soft tissue were associated with occasional discomfort. The cement did resorb over time, but was still present in 18 (32.73%) of the cases at 1 year. Mechanical loading does appear to be a factor in the remodeling of calcium phosphate cements, and a longer period of time may be necessary before the cement is replaced with bone in non-weight-bearing bones such as the wrist.[24,29] However, no cases of infection were reported and the cement escape does not appear to affect the successful return to function, as some degree of pain was the only reported complication. One patient, with an intra-articular extension of the fracture, had cement escape into the radio-carpal joint and required surgical removal of the cement to treat the pain. In studies involving the femur, no clinical effects were reported for the cases that

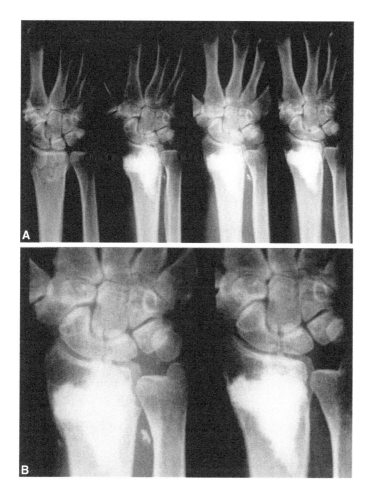

FIGURE 17.3 Radiographs of an extra-articular unstable fracture treated by Norian SRS and immobilization in a cast for 2 weeks. Note the stability provided by SRS in this case with no changes in radiologic position from 6 weeks to 1 year. (A) Anteroposterior views of the fracture shown prior to treatment and at 6 weeks, 6 months, and 1 year. (B) Close-up view of the anteroposterior radiographs shown at 6 weeks and 1 year. (From Sanchez-Sotelo, J. et al., *J. Bone Joint Surg.*, 82B, 856, 2000. With permission.)

had cement extravasation into the joint space.[20] In the study by Sanchez-Sotelo et al., less cement was noted to have escaped as the surgical techniques improved during the course of the study. However, because the degree of complications related to cement presence in the joint cavity varies, it is critical to avoid cement escape into the articulating region. Overall, wrist and hand function was restored earlier in the patients treated with SRS cement than those treated with casting alone.

Calcium phosphate cement has been used with success in treating complex fractures of the distal radius. Figure 17.4 shows fixation of an intra-articular, closed fracture of the distal radius with severe comminution treated using internal fixation supplemented with biodegradable bone cement (HAC Bone Source, Stryker Leibinger, Plantage, MI). There was no evidence of osteoporosis, but the patient was a 51-year-old smoker with non-insulin-dependent diabetes and gout. Therefore, successful healing was already in question. The fracture was sustained after a 20-ft fall from a roof and the patient was subsequently enrolled in a clinical trial for the hydroxyapatite cement 30 days following the initial injury. The external fixator and Kirschner wires were scheduled for removal after 3 months of immobilization and were only left in for a longer period of time (6 months) because the patient did not return for the scheduled visit. At the 12-month postoperative

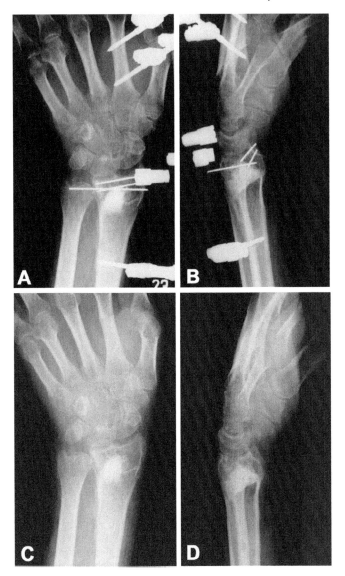

FIGURE 17.4 Fixation of an intra-articular closed fracture of the distal radius with severe comminution using internal fixation supplemented with biodegradable cement. (A,B) Anteroposterior and lateral radiographs at 6 months postoperative showing a bolus of Stryker Leibinger Bone Source Hydroxyapatite Cement with external fixator and Kirschner wires still in place. (C,D) Anteroposterior and lateral radiographs at 6 months postoperative following removal of the fixation devices. (Courtesy of Stryker Leibinger, Plantage, MI and Orthofix International, Richardson, TX.)

visit, the patient did complain of some numbness and weakness in the right hand, but showed good healing and return to function.

To date, however, calcium phosphate cement has only been approved by the U.S. Food and Drug Administration (FDA) for treatment of simple, low-impact fractures of the distal radius where early mobilization is indicated. Following reduction and treatment with the cement, the patients wear a cast for 2 weeks and then a removable splint for 2 to 4 weeks. This treatment allows an earlier return to function and is thought to produce better end results, probably because of the shorter period of immobilization.[29] As more research is done on the use of calcium phosphate cement, expanded use can eventually be expected and these cements should be useful in treating more complex fractures of the distal radius.

SRS calcium phosphate cement was approved by the FDA for limited use in treating fractures of the distal radius on December 23, 1998, but is the only calcium phosphate cement that has received approval at the time this chapter was written. The clinical indications for the cement are use as an adjunct for fracture stabilization in the treatment of low-impact, unstable, metaphyseal distal radius fractures, in cases where early mobilization (cast for 2 weeks, then removable splint for 2 to 4 weeks) is indicated. Use of SRS alone in highly comminuted fractures is not indicated. SRS cement should not be used (1) in the presence of active or suspected infection, (2) in diaphyseal fractures, and (3) as a substitute for external fixation.

B. Proximal Humerus Fractures

The treatment of severe proximal humeral fractures generally requires internal fixation; yet results have been relatively disappointing, especially with older patients where osteoporosis is likely. Two-part fractures based on the classification scheme of Neer[48] seem to heal adequately for the most part with conservative treatment.[48,49] Results, however, have varied considerably for conservative treatment of more complex fractures, with success rates ranging from only 39% up to 80%.[50,51] Paavolainen et al.[49] reported excellent to satisfactory results in 74.2% of 41 patients treated for severe proximal humeri fractures by open reduction and internal fixation, but a large number of these were younger patients who were less likely to have a reduction in bone mass. In 32 cases of proximal humeral fractures treated with internal fixation, Kristiansen and Christiansen[52] reported unsatisfactory or poor results in 11 of 20 that were available for postoperative evaluation (2- to 7-year follow-up). More than half of the patients available for follow-up were women and the average age was 63.6 (range 44 to 82). The functional assessment was based on the 100 point rating system of Neer, where pain, function, range of motion, and anatomy are considered.[48] Their observations suggested that successful treatment was unlikely and there was a high risk for complications.

In more recent studies published for only a small group of patients, the adjunctive use of bone cement has led to much better results. In a study by Trotter and Dobozi,[53] five patients (55 to 66, average age 65) were treated for humeral nonunions using open reduction and internal fixation with compression plating augmented with methylmethacrylate. The average follow-up was 24 months (8 to 38 months) and all five nonunions healed at an average of 5 months. Matsuda et al.[5] compared five patients (75 to 84, mean age 81) with advanced osteoporosis and proximal humeral fractures treated using conventional plate and screw fixation with intramedullary bone cement augmentation to five younger patients (54 to 68) with no radiographic indications of osteoporosis. The younger group of patients was treated with plate and screw fixation without the use of cement. Similar functional results were reported at both 3-month and 1-year follow-up with bone healing in all the patients. Although no complications were reported in these two studies from the use of methylmethacrylate, it is apparent that much less risk is present with the use of calcium phosphate cements and similar results can be expected based on studies for the treatment of injuries to other bones.

Another alternative to bone cement has been investigated on a limited basis in treating osteoporotic humeral fractures, and early studies have indicated results as good as with the use of the cement. The Schuli nut® (Synthes U.S.A., Paoli, PA) has three sharp projections on one side to engage the cortical bone and, when used with a plate, can possibly provide enhanced fixation in osteoporotic bone.[54] Biomechanical studies using cadaveric humeri have been conducted comparing the Schuli locking nut to a dynamic compression plate with standard screws as well as standard screws augmented with PMMA. DEXA showed that the bone was moderately osteoporotic and the screw holes were overdrilled to simulate osteoporotic purchase. The specimens were tested nondestructively in four-point bending, offset axial compression, and torsion. Results demonstrated that the Schuli nut could provide stability equivalent to cement-augmented screws and could be maintained after cyclic loading. The standard screws alone were significantly loosened after cyclic loading and gross motion was evident at the screw–plate and the screw–bone interfaces. Further studies are obviously necessary to fully evaluate the efficacy of this hardware, but the Schuli nut or similar implants may provide an additional alternative to cement-augmented internal fixation of osteoporotic fractures in the humerus as well as other locations.

IV. VERTEBRAL COMPRESSION FRACTURES

Although vertebral compression fractures are common in patients with osteoporosis, surgical intervention is rarely indicated.[55,56] Despite a high degree of pain and discomfort, internal fixation does not necessarily improve the healing. Unstable fractures, however, often resulting from trauma, also occur with patients who are affected by osteoporosis, and these do require surgery, typically stabilization and spinal fusion. Newer devices are being developed for use in spinal fusion such as interbody fusion cages, but most of the devices involve rods or plates and rely on the use of screws to anchor the implant to the bone. If the mechanical integrity of the bone has been compromised, as with osteoporosis, achieving a strong bone–screw interface is difficult and device failure due to screw pullout is possible. Often, there are not many alternatives and the chance of a solid fusion is questionable, with short-term fixation the best-case scenario.

One of the most common systems for spinal fusion has been the transpedicular implants, which use rods that span multiple levels of the spine. These rods are then anchored with screws inserted into the pedicles. Axial pullout tests with monotonically increasing loads have been used most often to assess the fixation strength of pedicle screws. However, it may also be useful to test fixation strength by analyzing other modes of failure such as fatigue. Studies have been performed to determine the relationship between the pullout force and the degree of osteoporosis for pedicle screw devices.

Soshi et al.[57] conducted tests on cadaveric lumbar spine and found that the mean pullout force was greater than 1000 N for normal bone, but was 300 N or lower when osteoporosis had reached Grade II or Grade III in severity according to the Jikei grading scale. These tests were for 7.0 × 35 mm Steffee VSP® (Variable Screw Placement, DePuy AcroMed, Raynham, MA) system screws. The Jikei method is based on simple lateral lumbar vertebral roentgenograms and the spine is classified into five grades of osteoporosis (normal, initial onset of osteoporosis, and Grades I to III) based on the density of the trabecular bone apparent on the radiograph. The degree of osteoporosis might be more accurately characterized when the bone mineral density (BMD) is used as the critical parameter, and Soshi also compared the pullout force to the BMD. This group and others have described a correlation between the Jikei scale and BMD *in vivo*.[57] Earlier reports, however, have indicated that a loss in bone density might not be detectable on radiographs until bone loss of 30% or more has occurred.[31,58] Moreover, some recent results have shown no correlation between the bone density from DEXA and radiographic evaluations such as the Singh system and the Jikei method.[36] Therefore, what may be classified as normal bone from the Jikei method could actually have a loss of bone mass that may not be detected from the roentgenogram. Soshi indicates that screw loosening is not as likely when the pullout force is greater than 500 N, and values of 300 N or lower were described as a danger.

By injecting bone cement into the pedicles, the cement can fill into the trabecular region of the pedicular bone and provide a more suitable anchor for the screws. If the cement is able to interdigitate with what remains of the trabecular bone, stronger fixation can be achieved. Soshi et al.[57] used a disposable syringe, injected 2 to 3 ml of bone cement into the pedicles, and then inserted the screws into the vertebrae through the pedicles. They found that the pullout force was doubled for cases of Grade I or Grade II osteoporosis and the mean pullout force was in excess of 500 N. Note, however, that for Grade III, which is the most severe stage of osteoporosis, the mean pullout force was 300 N or less, indicating that this type of implant may not provide proper fixation for severe osteoporosis. Other types of implants or treatment should probably be used if possible because any device that relies solely on screw fixation as its primary anchor may fail in a short period of time.

It should also be noted that just obtaining proper fixation of the implant might not be sufficient to generate bony fusion because the surrounding bone is still osteoporotic. Fusion requires that some type of graft be placed into the defect to provide stability and allow for remodeling of bone with eventual fusion throughout the indicated area. Even though proper fixation may be possible by using cement to anchor the screws, fusion may be unlikely because the ability of the surrounding bone to produce new bone has been inhibited by the osteoporosis. If this is the case, the device may eventually fail in fatigue, because no implant can withstand the repeated high loading that may be present unless some of the load is eventually transmitted through the bone in that area.

Cement augmentation has also been suggested for anterior instrumentation in spinal fusion procedures where secure fixation is questionable,[59,60] but cases of improving the fixation of spinal instrumentation by using bone cement appear to be limited. No reports that document the clinical use of bone cement for augmentation of instrumentation in spinal fusion of patients with osteoporosis were found in the literature. Methylmethacrylate has been used in treating traumatic fractures and dislocations of the spine,[61,62] as well as malignant tumors.[62-68] However, complications have been relatively common,[62-64,66] especially with traumatic lesions, often inhibiting the neurologic recovery or leading to progressive neural deficits.[69] Most authors seem to agree that PMMA should not be used as the initial method of treating traumatic lesions, where conventional means of grafting and fusion have results that are much more successful and predictable.[63,69] Methylmethacrylate has achieved the most merit as a vertebral replacement for metastatic disease and primary tumors of the spine.[64,66,68] The use of PMMA provides immediate stability postoperatively, usually eliminating the need for cumbersome external braces, and offers the potential for dramatically improved quality of life. The sole use of bone grafts, or in combination with the PMMA, has been strongly recommended whenever possible if survival is expected to be longer than 6 months.[65,67,69,70] Concerns over the possible negative effects radiation and chemotherapy have on the incorporation of the graft have led many to suggest not using bone grafts or to perform the rehabilitative treatment either before the surgery or about 6 weeks postoperatively.[64,65,70] This has not been universally accepted, and some authors have reported successful long-term stability with bone grafts even with postoperative radiotherapy.[67] Nonetheless, the use of PMMA does have benefits for patients with terminal conditions and appears to be relatively safe and effective as long as rigid metal fixation is used to stabilize the spine sufficiently.

Although bone cement has been used in the spine as well as other areas when optimal fixation cannot be achieved, concern still exists regarding the use of a material that undergoes a highly exothermic reaction in the vertebrae. Therefore, PMMA has generally been used only with patients having a relatively short life expectancy. A large amount of heat is produced during the polymerization of the cement, and this could pose significant dangers, especially when used in close proximity to the neural elements of the spine. Reports have indicated that temperatures above 42 to 47°C are sufficient to kill a number of different cells, including embryonal, blood, cartilage, and carcinoma cells.[71] Even so, in a study using rabbits, Wang et al.[10] have reported minimal temperature elevation in the subdural tissues when methylmethacrylate has been applied directly to the lamina and also directly over the exposed dura. And additional *in vivo* studies in dogs over longer periods of time have shown no evidence of damage to the neural elements.[72] The constant flow of cerebrospinal fluid is thought to dissipate the heat from the reaction, and the connective tissues and the presence of blood and/or fluids between the cement and dura may also be a factor. The potential damage to the surrounding neurologic and vascular structures is therefore unclear, but extreme caution is obviously warranted. The more recently developed biocompatible cements may prove more useful and safer in treating fractures of the spine.

Calcium phosphate cements have been studied on a limited basis for use in treating burst fractures of the spine and may be capable of providing the additional anchorage necessary to use instrumentation with osteoporotic bone. Mermelstein et al.[18] studied the ability of calcium phosphate cement to reduce the bending moments on pedicle screw constructs and improve the stability of short segment pedicle screw instrumentation (SSPI). In this study, they compared the stiffness of the Cotrel-Dubousset® (Medtronic Sofamor Danek, Memphis, TN) instrumentation on six thoracolumbar (T10–L3) cadaveric spines with experimentally created L1 burst fractures with and without cement augmentation (HAC Bone Source, Stryker Leibinger, Plantage, MI). There was a 40% increase in the mean initial stiffness of the construct in flexion and extension when bone cement was used. Generally, there was also a slight increase in the stiffness for lateral bending and torsion, but the results were not statistically significant. Significant reduction in screw bending moments was also reported in flexion (59% decrease) and extension (38% decrease) and there was a definite trend for the bending moments to be decreased in lateral bending. Results from this study indicate the potential benefit calcium phosphate cements can provide in improving the stability of spinal instrumentation when bone stock is compromised.

As an additional tool, McKoy and An[73] performed *in vitro* biomechanical testing on cadaveric lumbar vertebrae to evaluate a new screw design. Side ports were created along the shaft of a cannulated screw to allow cement to exit the holes, and this screw was shown to enhance the purchasing power in bone. A larger cement mantle is created around the screw shaft allowing greater interdigitation with the trabecular bone than is possible with simply injecting cement into a hole prior to inserting the screw. Axial pullout tests demonstrated that the cannulated screw injected with PMMA had a 278% greater holding power than a solid screw augmented with PMMA. Radial spokes of cement could be seen emanating from the shaft of the screw and providing more secure fixation. This type of design could prove useful in cement augmentation of spinal instrumentation as well as other fractures throughout the body.

A. VERTEBROPLASTY

Percutaneous transpedicular vertebroplasty has evolved more recently as a tool in restoring the strength and stiffness of the vertebral body following compression fractures and compression fractures resulting from osteoporosis and tumors.[55,74] This procedure involves injecting PMMA cement into the cancellous interior of the vertebral body to provide strength and support. Osteoporotic bones are at risk of refracture, and therefore it is beneficial not only to restore the vertebral body height, but also to increase the strength to normal levels. Reports have indicated that this treatment results in good relief of pain with minimal complications.[75-78] Only two studies of percutaneous vertebroplasty have been reported in the United States to date.[76,78]

In 1997, Jensen et al.[76] reported short-term results for 29 patients (19 women, 10 men) and found 90% to have initial reduction in pain and improved mobility. Minor complications were reported in several of the patients. Nondisplaced rib fractures occurred in 2 patients being treated for thoracic fractures. In 2 other patients a small amount of PMMA escaped into the inferior vena cava and embolization to the lungs was presumed to have occurred; yet, no respiratory changes were seen. Fractures apparently developed in the end plates in 9 patients with cement leaking into the disc space, but no clinical effects were detected. One patient developed an additional fracture and computerized tomography (CT) scans showed PMMA presence in the internal venous plexus at L4 that caused the thecal sac to flatten. However, no radicular findings were noted on the neurologic examination. Three of the patients in the study had no significant relief of pain. Overall, no worsening of the pain was reported in any of the patients and all of the complications were relatively minor.

In a study by Barr et al.,[78] 38 patients were treated for a total of 70 osteoporotic fractured vertebrae; 9 other patients were treated for either neoplasms (*n* = 8) or a hemangioma (*n* = 1). The entire study comprised 24 females and 23 males (age 33 to 88, mean 69.4). From one up to six vertebrae were treated; yet results seemed to indicate that much more success is realized when only one fracture level is treated. For the patients with osteoporosis, the follow-up ranged from 2 to 42 months (mean 18) with lasting pain relief in 94% of the cases. There were five cases of recurrent pain, three of which presented with markedly different pain than preoperatively, suggesting possible effects from the vertebroplasty. Minor complications occurred in only 6.4% of the patients, which is in line with the results reported by others, yet none of these complications was a result of cement extravasation. Another important consideration is the additional stress the augmented vertebrae place on the surrounding vertebrae. Strengthening individual vertebra by injecting cement causes more mechanical stress to be placed on the inferior vertebrae than before the augmentation, which in rare cases can cause subsequent fracture, especially when marked kyphosis is also present.[78] Prophylactic treatment of the surrounding vertebrae as a preventive measure may be indicated.

In an open prospective study in France, 20 vertebrae in 16 patients (9 female, 7 male) with a mean age of 66 (range 47 to 79) were treated by percutaneous vertebroplasty.[77] DEXA was used to evaluate the bone mineral density and average t-scores of -2.3 were reported for the lumbar spine. Inclusion in the study required painful vertebral fractures that had been unsuccessfully treated with conservative treatment after 3 months. The efficacy of the treatment was evaluated with periodic follow-up over the course of 6 months and was based on two different pain scoring systems, the visual analog scale (VAS) and a verbal scale (VS, McGill Melzack scoring system), as well as quality of life assessment (Nottingham Health Profile Scores). Patients were monitored closely for harmful side effects due to PMMA by periodic interpretation of CT scans and were then evaluated radiographically at 180 days to assess any new vertebral fractures or worsening of previous fractures.

Three thresholds were defined to determine the extent of improvement and were based on pain scores at day 3 (level 1 = 50% improvement, level 2 = 33% improvement, and level 3 = 25% improvement). Of the patients, 88% showed 25% improvement, 75% showed 33% improvement, and 44% improved more than half. A mean decrease of 53% was reported for VAS scores at day 3. The treatment appeared to be stable over time without any increases in the VAS scores. Nor were there any incident vertebral fractures or worsening of prevailing fractures at day 180. However, studies with a longer follow-up[75,78] have demonstrated a risk of new vertebral fractures, although these were still reported only in a select few cases. The average follow-up by Grados et al.[75] was 48 months and by Barr et al.[78] was 18 months, compared with only 6 months in the French study,[77] indicating possible risks over a longer period of time.

No clinically relevant side effects were reported in the study, but there were several instances of cement extravasation into surrounding areas. Some cement leakage occurred in 13 of the 20 vertebrae, including the paravertebral soft tissue, the peridural space, the adjacent discs, and the lumbar venous plexus. However, no epidural or foraminal leakage was seen, which can lead to spinal cord or nerve root compression. Vertebroplasty has been used in treating tumoral lesions and the prevalence of leakage into the epidurus and foramen appears to occur with much more prevalence with these cases.[79] This could very well be due to the cortical destruction that occurs with tumors, making cement leakage and needle breakthrough much more likely.[77-79] For the most part, cement leakage has generally been limited, with no clinical significance, but a few reported cases of vertebroplasty treatment of metastatic or myeloma lesions have required additional surgical intervention for decompression of affected nerve roots.[79] The thermal effects are still a major issue regarding the use of PMMA and could pose significant neurologic dangers as well as other problems. Therefore, additional studies with a longer follow-up are necessary to document fully the dangers of PMMA fully, and the use of newer, biocompatible bone cements may be necessary before the benefits of vertebroplasty can be fully realized. *In vitro* studies have been performed on several biocompatible cements to determine the potential for use in vertebroplasty; Table 17.2 summarizes some of these materials.

Orthocomp© (Orthovita, Malvern, PA) is a new bioactive composite material that is biocompatible and has potential applications for vertebroplasty as well as other augmentation procedures including screw fixation and cortical bone repair.[80,81] The material is composed of a matrix of highly cross-linked dimethacrylate resins reinforced with biocompatible glasses.[80] CORTOSS© (Orthovita, Malvern, PA) is exactly identical in chemical composition and material properties and is indicated for screw and vertebral augmentation including vertebroplasty.[81] The cement is not resorbable, but does have a hydrophilic surface that allows direct chemical bonding between bone and cement. This cement has a lower setting exotherm (58 to 62 $\pm$ 5°C)[81] than that of PMMA and biomechanical testing has demonstrated much greater material properties as well.[80,82,83-85] Only minimal static creep

TABLE 17.2
Biocompatible Bone Cements for Potential Use in Vertebroplasty

Orthocomp[a]
(Orthovita, Malvern, PA)[80-82]

Bioactive, glass-ceramic-reinforced composite material

Matrix of bis-phenol glycidyl dimethacrylate (BisGMA), bis-phenol ethoxy dimethacrylate (BisEMA), and triethyleneglycol dimethacrylate (TEGDMA)

Biocompatible and exhibits a lower setting exotherm than PMMA cements

Is not resorbable, but does have a hydrophilic surface that allows bone to bond chemically to the cement

Stronger material properties than PMMA;[83-85] reported compressive strength of 210 MPa and tensile strength of 56.7 MPa (*Note:* Is also stronger in compression as compared with the reported properties of cortical bone and has about 40% of the tensile strength reported for cortical bone)[86,87]

Only *in vitro* study so no conclusion can be made regarding the palliative effects and the ability of this cement to reduce or limit pain

Skeletal Repair System[b]
(SRS, Norian, Cupertino, CA)[15,88]

Cures *in situ* under normal physiologic body conditions and crystallizes into dahllite, which is similar to the mineral phase of bone

Biocompatible and undergoes a remodeling phase similar to normal bone, being resorbed by osteoclasts over time and replaced by new bone tissue

For potential use in vertebroplasty, the liquid-to-solid ratio of the apatite was increased considerably to achieve the desired flow characteristics appropriate for percutaneous injection reducing the material properties somewhat

Ultimate compressive strength for a number of curing conditions used averaged from 11.6 to 17.7 MPa, which is less than the 55 MPa compressive strength of the cement used for other osteoporotic augmentation,[15,16,20] but still is significantly greater than the reported strength of cancellous bone in the human spine (Failure Stress, 1.55 to 4.6 MPa)[70,89,90]

Demonstrated significantly greater energy absorption for vertebral bodies that were injected with the Norian cement than the controls that were not injected with anything indicating potential for use in augmenting osteoporotic compression fractures of the spine

[a] CORTOSS (Orthovita, Malvern, PA) has the same chemical composition and mechanical properties as Orthocomp and has been discussed more often in the recent literature in screw and vertebral augmentation including vertebroplasty; because of its superior compressive and tensile properties it is also indicated as a synthetic cortical bone void filler. (Neither material has been approved for use in the United States at the time this manuscript was written.)

[b] Schildhauer et al.[88] actually tested a calcium phosphate cement that is a precursor to the more recently developed SRS cement.

resulted over a period of 24 hours, and because of the extensively cross-linked components of the polymer matrix and the high molecular weight of the resins as well, the material should offer improved durability over PMMA.[82] Orthocomp and CORTOSS are naturally more radiopaque than PMMA, even after the addition of 20% barium sulfate, offering considerably better imaging both radiographically and flouroscopically.[80] This should help in reducing the cement extravasation during vertebroplasty,[81] which is one of the greatest problems with this procedure. Thermal analysis and biomechanical studies of Orthocomp have demonstrated improvements over the use of PMMA in vertebroplasty.[9,80]

In vitro studies performed on osteoporotic cadaveric vertebra have shown that Orthocomp reaches lower peak temperatures than PMMA and for much more transient periods of time.[9] Thermocouples were placed interior to the anterior cortex, at the geometric center of the vertebral body, and between the periosteum of the posterior cortex and the posterior longitudinal ligament to evaluate the temperatures caused during vertebroplasty. As mentioned earlier, temperatures above 50°C for longer than 1 min are reported to cause thermal necrosis of bone tissue and the duration of exposure to elevated temperatures may also be important.[9] At the center of the vertebral bodies,

Orthocomp produced lower peak temperatures (51.2 ± 6.2°C) and temperatures above 50°C lasted for a shorter duration (1.3 ± 1.4 min) than what occurred with Simplex P® (Howmedica, Rutherford, NJ; 61.8 ± 12.7°C; 3.6 ± 2.1 min). Conditions at the posterior aspect of the vertebral body reveal potential danger to the spinal cord and nerve roots. The group treated with Simplex P experienced temperatures above 50°C for significantly longer periods of time (1.2 ± 1.6 min vs. 0.2 ± 0.6 min), but the peak temperatures were not significantly different (50.3 ± 9.8°C vs. 45.2 ± 4.9°C). Because these were *in vitro* studies, the ability of the blood and the cerebrospinal fluid to dissipate heat would likely reduce these temperatures. This would seem to indicate that the neural elements are not at great risk, even with the use of PMMA.[9,81] As previously stated, this was supported by findings from Wang et al.[10,72] for PMMA studies in rabbits and dogs.

Mechanical testing involved creating compression fractures in osteoporotic lumbar spines (mean *t*-score of –5.0, range –3.4 to –6.4) and then augmenting them with either Orthocomp or PMMA (Simplex P).[80] Results from compression testing after augmentation showed that the strength of the specimens in each group was significantly greater than the original values. However, the specimens augmented with Orthocomp were much stronger than those augmented with PMMA and the stiffness was restored to initial values with Orthocomp, but not with PMMA. Pain is a complex phenomenon and the cause for the palliative effects from vertebroplasty is not well understood. Therefore, this *in vitro* testing gives no indication of the ability to reduce and limit the degree of pain, but does demonstrate the improvement in strength and stiffness that is possible. This cement may therefore offer a potential alternative to PMMA and its numerous drawbacks for use in vertebroplasty as well as other augmentation procedures including enhanced screw fixation.

The Norian SRS cement may also be more appealing for use in vertebroplasty procedures due to its properties. As this cement is biocompatible and undergoes a non-exothermic reaction as it cures and is replaced with host bone, it offers a number of advantages over the use of PMMA. Schildhauer et al.[88] performed *in vitro* biomechanical testing using cement similar to the Norian SRS (the cement they tested is actually a precursor to the SRS cement, which was developed shortly after testing was complete) to determine the potential for use in vertebroplasty.[88] Cadaver thoracic vertebrae were infiltrated with the biocompatible cement and then compressed in a hydraulic mechanical testing machine until they were collapsed 25, 50, and 70%. The infiltrated specimens showed significantly greater energy absorption than control specimens, indicating the advantages the cement offers. The liquid-to-solid ratio was increased to attain the appropriate flow characteristics and this reduced the material properties somewhat. The ultimate compressive strength ranged from 11.6 to 17.7 MPa for a number of curing conditions, which is less than the compressive strength of the Norian SRS cement used for other osteoporotic augmentation, which is reported to be about 55 MPa.[15,16,20] However, the ultimate compressive strength was still significantly greater than the reported compressive strength of cancellous bone in the human spine (Failure Stress, 1.55 to 4.66 MPa).[70,89,90] Once again, no inferences can be made regarding the ability to reduce and limit pain and morbidity following vertebroplasty with this cement as only *in vitro* testing was performed, but because of more beneficial properties, this cement may be a more suitable alternative to the use of PMMA.

B. KYPHOPLASTY

Kyphoplasty is an even more recently developed technique that seems to enhance the efficacy of the vertebroplasty procedure. Vertebroplasty has been effective at restoring the strength and stiffness of the vertebrae following compression fractures, but it may also be important to restore the normal height and anatomy. Belkoff et al.[91] performed *ex vivo* biomechanical testing on osteoporotic cadaveric vertebral bodies with induced compression fractures to compare kyphoplasty with vertebroplasty. Kyphoplasty involves inserting a balloonlike device ("inflatable bone tamp") into the crushed vertebra, inflating the tamp to restore the anatomy of the vertebral body, and then filling the void with bone cement to restore the strength and stiffness of the vertebra, reducing the likelihood of a recurring fracture. Inflating the tamp compresses the cancellous bone, creating a void within the vertebral body, and in effect reducing the fracture. The cavity within the vertebral body allows the cement to be introduced under less pressure than with percutaneous vertebroplasty and, therefore, may potentially limit the likelihood of cement extravasation.[91,92] In fact, five of the eight vertebrae treated with vertebroplasty were associated with cement extravasation whereas no leakage occurred in the kyphoplasty group. They found that both the kyphoplasty and vertebroplasty groups were significantly stronger after simulated treatment. However, only the kyphoplasty group was restored to the initial stiffness values. More importantly, they found that 97% of the vertebral body height was restored in the kyphoplasty group while only 30% of the height was restored in the vertebral bodies given only vertebroplasty.

The initial clinical experience with the kyphoplasty procedure has shown it to be effective at reducing the bodily pain and improving the physical function and role as well as restoring the vertebral height.[92,93] However, based on a comparison of preoperative and postoperative radiograhs, only 38% of the vertebral body height was restored,[93] significantly less than that reported from the *in vitro* studies.[91] Nonetheless, kyphoplasty appears to be an additional technique of use in treating osteoporotic compression fractures of the vertebrae.

V. CONCLUSION

Osteoporotic fractures occur quite frequently, especially in the proximal femur and the vertebrae, as well as the distal radius and humerus. Treating these injuries can prove very difficult because loss of bone stock prevents secure attachment of fracture fixation devices. Conventional treatment used traction in treating femoral fractures with long periods of immobilization and prolonged hospital stays. Vertebral compression fractures have also been customarily treated by conservative means. However, osteoporosis generally occurs in elderly individuals and long periods of bed rest and immobilization often produce various complications in these patients. Conservative treatment that has been customarily used in treating osteoporotic fractures of the distal radius and humerus has often proved ineffective as well. Therefore, the use of bone cement to improve the fixation of the implants in treating osteoporotic fractures may provide enormous benefits.

The adjunctive use of bone cement in osteoporotic fractures allows for early mobilization, which eliminates many of the problems with prolonged bed rest and conservative treatment, and significantly aids in the recovery. Excellent results have been reported for fracture fixation of osteoporotic bones in the proximal femur as well as the supracondylar region, when PMMA was used to augment the implants.[1-4] However, concerns over the use of PMMA have generally limited its use to elderly patients with a short life expectancy. The recent advent of biocompatible cements has renewed interest in the use of bone cement for treating osteoporotic fractures and other fractures where fixation strength of the implant is in question. The newer calcium phosphate cements form a paste-on mixture that remains injectable for about 5 min, hardens in 10 min, undergoes a remodeling phase similar to normal bone, and reaches maximum strength in 12 h or less.

Vertebroplasty was developed in France in the 1980s to treat vertebral compression fractures, whereby PMMA is injected into the vertebral bodies to restore strength and stability.[74] Early results have shown that this procedure provides excellent relief of pain with minimal complications even though the use of PMMA may pose some danger.[76-78] Because of the ill effects possible, PMMA has not gained widespread acceptance. With the development of non-exothermic cements such as those composed of calcium phosphate derivatives, vertebroplasty may become even more effective and common in treating compression fractures of the vertebrae. Other biocompatible cements with lower setting exotherms than PMMA and greater mechanical properties have proved effective as well.[80,81] Kyphoplasty is a recently developed technique that may enhance the benefits of vertebroplasty. This procedure involves inserting an inflatable bone tamp into the crushed vertebra to restore the anatomy prior to infiltrating the vertebral body with cement. Early *in vitro* biomechanical testing and clinical results have shown that not only can strength and stiffness be restored, but the height of the crushed vertebra can also be restored, which is not possible with vertebroplasty.

Extensive research is being performed on the use of biocompatible cements, and early clinical results for use in treating fractures of the proximal femur and distal radius have been promising.[15,16,20,28,29] Overall, results are encouraging, with bone cement dramatically improving the opportunity for recovery. Thus far, the Norian SRS calcium phosphate cement has been approved by the FDA for limited use in treating fractures of the distal radius. As more is learned from the use of these alternative cements, their role should expand and their use in treating osteoporotic fractures of all kinds is likely to increase.

ACKNOWLEDGMENTS

The authors gratefully acknowledge Drs. Stuart Goodman, Sune Larsson, Joaquin Sanchez-Sotelo, and Ms. Kathy McDermott and Orthofix International for providing the clinical radiographs used in this chapter.

REFERENCES

1. Harrington, K.D., "The use of methylmethacrylate as an adjunct in the internal fixation of unstable comminuted intertrochanteric fractures in osteoporotic patients," *J. Bone Joint Surg.*, 57A, 744, 1975.
2. Benum, P., "The use of bone cement as an adjunct to internal fixation of supracondylar fractures of osteoporotic femurs," *Acta Orthop. Scand.*, 48, 52, 1977.
3. Muhr, G., Tscherne, H., and Thomas, R., "Comminuted trochanteric femoral fractures in geriatric patients: the results of 231 cases treated with internal fixation and acrylic cement," *Clin. Orthop.*, 138, 41, 1979.
4. Zehntner, M.K. and Ganz, R., "Internal fixation of supracondylar fractures after condylar total knee arthroplasty," *Clin. Orthop.*, 293, 219, 1993.
5. Matsuda, M., Kiyoshige, Y., Takagi, M., and Hamasaki, M., "Intramedullary bone-cement fixation for proximal humeral fracture in elderly patients: a report of 5 cases," *Acta Orthop. Scand.*, 70, 283, 1999.
6. Müller, M.E., "Die Verwendung von Kunstharzen in der Knockenchirurgie," *Arch. Orthop. Unfall-Chir.*, 54, 513, 1962.
7. Moore, D.C., Frankenburg, E.P., Goulet, J.A., and Goldstein, S.A., "Hip screw augmentation with an *in situ*-setting calcium phosphate cement: an *in vitro* biomechanical analysis," *J. Orthop. Trauma*, 11, 577, 1997.
8. Cameron, H.U., Jacob, R., MacNab, I., and Pilliar, R.M., "Use of polymethylmethacrylate to enhance screw fixation in bone," *J. Bone Joint Surg.*, 57A, 655, 1975.
9. Deramond, H., Wright, N.T., and Belkoff, S.M., "Temperature elevation caused by bone cement polymerization during vertebroplasty," *Bone*, 25, 17S, 1999.
10. Wang, G.J., Reger, S.J., McLaughlin, R.E., et al., "The safety of cement fixation in the cervical spine: studies of a rabbit model," *Clin. Orthop.*, 139, 276, 1979.
11. Goldring, S.R., Schiller, A.L., Roelke, M., et al., "The synovial-like membrane at the bone-cement interface in loose total hip replacements and its proposed role in bone lysis," *J. Bone Joint Surg.*, 65A, 575, 1983.
12. Jasty, M.J., Floyd, W.E., III, Schiller, A.L., et al., "Localized osteolysis in stable, non-septic total hip replacement," *J. Bone Joint Surg.*, 68A, 912, 1986.
13. Whitehill, R., Drucker, S., McCoig, J.A., et al., "Induction and characterization of an interface tissue by implantation of methylmethacrylate cement into the posterior part of the cervical spine of the dog," *J. Bone Joint Surg.*, 70A, 51, 1988.
14. Ingham, E., Green, T.R., Stone, M.H., et al., "Production of TNF-α and bone resorbing activity by macrophages in response to different types of bone cement particles," *Biomaterials*, 21, 1005, 2000.
15. Constantz, B.R., Ison, I.C., Fulmer, M.T., et al., "Skeletal repair by *in situ* formation of the mineral phase of bone," *Science*, 267, 1796, 1995.
16. Larsson, S., Mattsson, P., and Bauer, T.W., "Resorbable bone cement for augmentation of internally fixed hip fractures," *Ann. Chir. Gynaecol.*, 88, 205, 1999.

17. Osteogenics, Inc., Premarket Notification to the FDA, "Bone Source™ Hydroxyapatite (HAC) for cranial defects," July 1995.

18. Mermelstein, L.E., McLain, R.F., and Yerby, S.A., "Reinforcement of thoracolumbar burst fractures with calcium phosphate cement: a biomechanical study," *Spine*, 23, 664, 1998.

19. Stankewich, C.J., Swiontkowski, M.F., Tencer, A.F., et al., "Augmentation of femoral neck fracture fixation with an injectable calcium-phosphate bone mineral cement," *J. Orthop. Res.*, 14, 786, 1996.

20. Goodman, S.B., Bauer, T.W., Carter, D., et al., "Norian SRS cement augmentation in hip fracture treatment," *Clin. Orthop.*, 348, 42, 1998.

21. Yetkinler, D.N., Ladd, A.L., Poser, R.D., et al., "Biomechanical evaluation of fixation of intra-articular fractures of the distal part of the radius in cadavera: Kirschner wires compared with calcium-phosphate bone cement," *J. Bone Joint Surg.*, 81A, 391, 1999.

22. Elder, S., Frankenburg, E., Goulet, J., et al., "Biomechanical evaluation of calcium phosphate cement-augmented fixation of unstable intertrochanteric fractures," *J. Orthop. Trauma*, 14, 386, 2000.

23. Rohl, L., Larsen, E., Linde, F., et al., "Tensile and compressive properties of cancellous bone," *J. Biomech.*, 24, 1143, 1991.

24. Frankenburg, E.P., Goldstein, S.A., Bauer, T.W., et al., "Biomechanical and histologic evaluation of a calcium phosphate cement," *J. Bone Joint Surg.*, 80A, 1112, 1998.

25. Yuan, H., Li, Y., de Bruijn, J.D., et al., "Tissue responses of calcium phosphate cement: a study in dogs," *Biomaterials*, 21, 1283, 2000.

26. Pioletti, D.P., Takei, H., Lin, T., et al., "The effects of calcium phosphate cement particles on osteoblast functions," *Biomaterials*, 21, 1103, 2000.

27. Kopylov, P., Jonsson, K., Thorngren, K.G., and Aspenberg, P., "Injectable calcium phosphate in the treatment of distal radial fractures," *J. Hand Surg.*, 21B, 768, 1996.

28. Jupiter, J.B., Winters, S., Sigman, S., et al., "Repair of five distal radius fractures with an investigational cancellous bone cement: a preliminary report," *J. Orthop. Trauma*, 11, 110, 1997.

29. Sanchez-Sotelo, J., Munuera, L., and Madero, R., "Treatment of fractures of the distal radius with a remodelable bone cement: a prospective, randomised study using Norian SRS," *J. Bone Joint Surg.*, 82B, 856, 2000.

30. Glaser, D.L. and Kaplan, F.S., "Osteoporosis: definition and clinical presentation," *Spine*, 22(Suppl. 24), 12S, 1997.

31. Davies, R. and Saha, S., "Osteoporosis," *Am. Fam. Physician*, 32, 107, 1985.

32. Kyle, R.F., "Intertrochanteric fractures," in *The Hip and Its Disorders*, Steinberg, M.E., Ed., W. B. Saunders, Philadelphia, 1991, chap. 16

33. Lu-Yao, G.L., Keller, R.B., Littenberg, B., and Wennberg, J.E., "Outcomes after displaced fractures of the femoral neck," *J. Bone Joint Surg.*, 76A, 15, 1994.

34. Hardy, D.C.R., Descamps, P.Y., Krallis, P., et al., "Use of an intramedullary hip-screw compared with a compression hip-screw with a plate for intertrochanteric femoral fractures," *J. Bone Joint Surg.*, 88A, 618, 1998.

35. Bendo, J.A., Wiener, L.S., Strauss, E., and Yang, E., "Collapse of intertrochanteric hip fractures fixed with sliding screws," *Orthop. Rev.*, 23, S30, 1994.

36. Seeger, L.L., "Bone density determination," *Spine*, 22(Suppl. 24), 49S, 1997.

37. Bellabarba, C., Herscovici, D., Jr., and Ricci, W.M., "Percutaneous treatment of peritrochanteric fractures using the Gamma nail," *Clin. Orthop.*, 275, 30, 2000.

38. Kyle, R.F., Gustilo, R.B., and Premer, R.F., "Analysis of six-hundred and twenty-two intertrochanteric hip fractures," *J. Bone Joint Surg.*, 61A, 216, 1979.

39. Singh, M., Nagrath, A.R., and Maini, P.S., "Changes in trabecular pattern of the upper end of the femur as an index of osteoporosis," *J. Bone Joint Surg.*, 52A, 457, 1970.

40. Jupiter, J.B., "Complex articular fractures of the distal radius: classification and management," *J. Am. Acad. Orthop. Surg.*, 5, 119, 1997.

41. Jupiter, J.B., "Current concepts review: fractures of the distal end of the radius," *J. Bone Joint Surg.*, 73A, 461, 1991.

42. McQueen, M.M., MacLaren, A., and Chalmers, J., "The value of remanipulating Colles' fractures," *J. Bone Joint Surg.*, 68B, 232, 1986.

43. Kofoed, H., "Comminuted displaced Colles' fractures: treatment with intramedullary methylmethacrylate stabilisation," *Acta Orthop. Scand.*, 54, 307, 1983.

44. Mehta, J.A., Bain, G.I., and Heptinstall, R.J., "Anatomic reduction of intra-articular fractures of the distal radius: an arthroscopically-assisted approach," *J. Bone Joint Surg.*, 82B, 79, 2000.

45. Schmalholz, A., "Bone cement for redislocated Colles' fracture: a prospective comparison with closed treatment," *Acta Orthop. Scand.*, 60, 212, 1989.

46. Jupiter, J.B. and Lipton, H., "The operative treatment of intra-articular fractures of the distal radius," *Clin. Orthop.*, 292, 48, 1993.

47. "The comprehensive classification of fractures of long bones," in *Manual of Internal Fixation: Techniques Recommended by the AO-ASIF Group*, 3rd ed., corrected 3rd printing, Müller, M.E. et al., Eds., Springer-Verlag, New York, 1995, appendix A.

48. Neer, C.S., II, "Displaced proximal humeral fractures: classification and evaluation," *J. Bone Joint Surg.*, 52A, 1077, 1970.

49. Paavolainen, P., Björkenheim, J.M., Slätis, P., and Paukku, P., "Operative treatment of severe proximal humeral fractures," *Acta Orthop. Scand.*, 54, 374, 1983.

50. Einarsson, F., "Fractures of the upper end of the humerus: discussion based on the follow-up of 302 cases," *Acta Orthop. Scand. Suppl.*, 32, 1, 1958.

51. Svend-Hansen, H., "Displaced proximal humeral fractures: a review of 49 patients," *Acta Orthop. Scand.*, 45, 359, 1974.

52. Kristiansen, B. and Christiansen, S.W., "Plate fixation of proximal humeral fractures," *Acta Orthop. Scand.*, 57, 320, 1986.

53. Trotter, D.H. and Dobozi, W., "Nonunion of the humerus: rigid fixation, bone grafting, and adjunctive bone cement," *Clin. Orthop.*, 204, 162, 1986.

54. Jazrawi, L.M., Bai, B., Simon, J.A., et al., "A biomechanical comparison of Schuhli nuts or cement augmented screws for plating of humeral fractures," *Clin. Orthop.*, 377, 235, 2000.

55. Bostrom, M.P. G. and Lane, J.M., "Future directions: augmentation of osteoporotic vertebral bodies," *Spine*, 22(Suppl. 24), 38S, 1997.

56. Hu, S.S., "Internal fixation in the osteoporotic spine," *Spine*, 22(Suppl. 24), 43S, 1997.

57. Soshi, S., Shiba, R., Kondo, H., and Murota, K., "An experimental study on transpedicular screw fixation in relation to osteoporosis of the lumbar spine," *Spine*, 16, 1335, 1991.

58. Harrington, K.D., "Current concepts review: metastatic disease of the spine," *J. Bone Joint Surg.*, 68A, 1110, 1986.

59. Ghanayem, A.J. and Zdeblick, T.A., "Anterior instrumentation in the management of thoracolumbar burst fractures," *Clin. Orthop.*, 335, 89, 1997.

60. Karaikovic, E.E., Kaneda, K., Akbarnia, B.A., and Gaines, R.W., Jr., "Kaneda instrumentation for spinal fractures," in *The Textbook of Spinal Surgery*, 2nd ed., Bridwell, K.H. and DeWald, R.L., Eds., Lippincott-Raven, Philadelphia, 1997, 1918.

61. Duff, T.A., "Methyl methacrylate in spinal stabilization," in *Techniques in Spinal Fusion and Stabilization*, Hitchon, P.W., Traynelis, V.C., and Rengachary, S.S., Eds., Thieme Medical, New York, 1995, chap. 14.

62. Clark, C.R., Keggi, K.J., and Panjabi, M.M., "Methlymethacrylate stabilization of the cervical spine," *J. Bone Joint Surg.*, 66A, 40, 1984.

63. Dunn, E.J., "The role of methyl methacrylate in the stabilization and replacement of tumors of the cervical spine: a project of the Cervical Spine Research Society," *Spine*, 2, 15, 1977.

64. Harrington, K.D., "The use of methylmethacrylate for vertebral-body replacement and anterior stabilization of pathologic fracture-dislocations of the spine due to metastatic malignant disease," *J. Bone Joint Surg.*, 63A, 36, 1981.

65. Fidler, M.W., "Pathologic fractures of the cervical spine," *J. Bone Joint Surg.*, 67B, 352, 1985.

66. Siegal, T., Tiqva, P., and Siegal, T., "Vertebral body resection for epidural compression by malignant tumors," *J. Bone Joint Surg.*, 67A, 375, 1985.

67. Caspar, W., Pitzen, T., Papavero, L., et al., "Anterior cervical plating for the treatment of neoplasms in the cervical vertebrae," *J. Neurosurg.*, 90, 27S, 1999.

68. Miller, D.J., Lang, F.F., Walsh, G.L., et al., "Coaxial double-lumen methylmethacrylate reconstruction in the anterior cervical and upper thoracic spine after tumor resection," *J. Neurosurg.*, 92, S181, 2000.

69. McAfee, P.C., Bohlman, H.H., Ducker, T., and Eismont, F.J., "Failure of stabilization of the spine with methylmethacrylate," *J. Bone Joint Surg.*, 68A, 1145, 1986.

70. Panjabi, M.M. and White, A.A., "Physical properties and functional biomechanics of the spine," in *Clinical Biomechanics of the Spine*, 2nd ed., Panjabi, M.M. and White, A.A., Eds., J.B. Lippincott, Philadelphia, 1990, 35.

71. Leeson, M.C. and Lippitt, S.B., "Thermal aspects of the use of polymethylmethacrylate in large metaphyseal defects in bone," *Clin. Orthop.*, 295, 239, 1993.

72. Wang, G.J., Wilson, C.S., Hubbard, S.L., et al., "Safety of anterior cement fixation in the cervical spine: *in vivo* study of dog spine," *South. Med. J.*, 77, 178, 1984.

73. McKoy, B.E. and An, Y.H., "An injectable cementing screw for fixation in osteoporotic bone," *J. Biomed. Mater. Res.*, 53, 216, 2000.

74. Galibert, P., Deramond, H., Rosat, P., and Le Gars, D., "Note préliminaire sur le traitement des angiomes vertébraux par vertébroplastie acrylique percutanée [Preliminary note on the treatment of vertebral angioma by percutaneous acrylic vertebroplasty]," *Neurochirurgie*, 33, 166, 1987.

75. Grados, F., Hardy, N., Cayrolle, G., et al., "Percutaneous vertebroplasty for the treatment of osteoporotic vertebral fractures," *Rev. Rhum. [Engl. Ed.]*, 64, 38, 1997.

76. Jensen, M.E., Evans, A.J., Mathis, J.M., et al., "Percutaneous polymethylmethacrylate vertebroplasty in the treatment of osteoporotic vertebral body compression fractures: technical aspects," *Am. J. Neuroradiol.*, 18, 1897, 1997.

77. Cortet, B., Cotton, A., Boutry, N., et al., "Percutaneous vertebroplasty in the treatment of osteoporotic vertebral compression fractures: an open prospective study," *J. Rheum.*, 26, 2222, 1999.

78. Barr, J.D., Barr, M.S., Lemley, T.J., and McCann, R.M., "Percutaneous vertebroplasty for pain relief and spinal stabilization," *Spine*, 25, 923, 2000.

79. Cotten, A., Dewatre, F., Cortet, B., et al., "Percutaneous vertebroplasty for osteolytic metastases and myeloma: effects of percentage of lesion filling and the leakage of methyl methacrylate at clinical follow-up," *Radiology*, 200, 525, 1996.

80. Belkoff, S.M., Mathis, J.M., Erbe, E.M., and Fenton, D.C., "Biomechanical evaluation of a new bone cement for use in vertebroplasty," *Spine*, 25, 1061, 2000.

81. Erbe, E.M., Personal communication, February 14, 2001.

82. Erbe, E.M., Pomrink, G.J., and Murphy, J.P., "A comparison of the mechanical properties of a new synthetic cortical bone void filler (Cortoss™/Orthovita) with those of polymethyl methacrylate," presented at the 2nd Annual Meeting of the Spine Society of Europe, Antwerp, Belgium, October 10–14, 2000, *Eur. Spine J. [Abstr.]*, 9, 288, 2000.

83. Taitsman, J.P. and Saha, S., "Tensile strength of wire-reinforced bone cement and twisted stainless-steel wire," *J. Bone Joint Surg.*, 59A, 419, 1977.

84. Saha, S. and Pal, S., "Improvement of mechanical properties of acrylic bone cement by fiber reinforcement," *J. Biomech.*, 17, 467, 1984.

85. Saha, S. and Pal, S., "Mechanical properties of bone cement: a review," *J. Biomed. Mater. Res.*, 18, 435, 1984.

86. Lindahl, O. and Lindgren, G.H., "Cortical bone in man. II: Variation in tensile strength with age and sex," *Acta Orthop. Scand.*, 38, 141, 1967.

87. Lindahl, O. and Lindgren, G.H., "Cortical bone in man. III: Variation of compressive strength with age and sex," *Acta Orthop. Scand.*, 38, 129, 1968.

88. Schildhauer, T.A., Bennett, A.P., Wright, T.M., et al., "Intravertebral body reconstruction with an injectable *in situ*-setting carbonated apatite: biomechanical evaluation of a minimally invasive technique," *J. Orthop. Res.*, 17, 67, 1999.

89. Lindahl, O., "Mechanical properties of dried defatted spongy bone," *Acta Orthop. Scand.*, 47, 11, 1976.

90. Hansson, T.H., Keller, T.S., and Panjabi, M.M., "A study of the compressive properties of lumbar vertebral trabeculae: effects of tissue characteristics," *Spine*, 11, 56, 1986.

91. Belkoff, S.M., Mathis, J.M., Fenton, D.C., et al., "An *ex vivo* biomechanical evaluation of an inflatable bone tamp used in the treatment of compression fractures," *Spine*, 26, 151, 2001.

92. Lieberman, I.H., Dudeney, S., Phillips, F.M., and Bell, G.R., "Initial clinical outcome with kyphoplasty for osteoporotic vertebral compression fractures," in *Proceedings from the 15th Annual Meeting of the North American Spine Society*, New Orleans, October 25–28, 2000.

93. Lieberman, I., Dudeney, S., and Philips, F., "Inflatable bone tamp kyphoplasty in the treatment of osteoporotic compression fractures," presented at the 2nd Annual Meeting of the Spine Society of Europe, Antwerp, Belgium, October 10–14, 2000, *Eur. Spine J. [Abstr.]*, 9, 287, 2000.

Part IV

Surgical Management of Osteoporotic Spine

18 Challenges of Internal Fixation in Osteoporotic Spine

Gary L. Lowery, Leon J. Grobler, and Samir S. Kulkarni

CONTENTS

I. INTRODUCTION

With an increase in the geriatric age population as a result of rising life expectancy, today's spine surgeon must consider osteoporosis an important factor in the orthopaedic management of elderly patients. The number of surgical procedures performed on the spine in elderly patients is also increasing due to improving surgical and medical technology and advances in minimally invasive techniques. Patients in the older age group have more active lifestyles than in previous generations and refuse to accept disability and deformity as a part of the aging process.[1] In addition there exists a relatively younger subgroup of patients with spine problems and secondary osteoporosis due to factors like hypercortisolism, hyperthyroidism, hyperparathyroidism, alcohol abuse, and immobilization, and this group needs special consideration in management of the spinal pathology. Approximately 30% of postmenopausal white women in the United States have osteoporosis, and 16% have osteoporosis of the lumbar spine in particular.[1]

Spinal osteoporosis and compression fractures can lead to significant disability and have a negative impact on the patient's quality of life.[2-4] The lifetime risk of a vertebral fracture from age 50 onward is 16% in white women and only 5% in white men. The incidence of vertebral fractures in postmenopausal women has been quoted to be as high as 25%, and vertebral fractures are second only to hip fractures as a cause of morbidity and mortality in elderly patients.[1] The presence of multiple osteoporotic vertebral fractures has been reported by a recent study to increase the mortality risk in elderly women by 1.3 to 2.6 times. Physical and occupational therapy, psychosocial support, bed rest, pain management, bracing, and back school programs suffice to treat most vertebral fractures.[2] However, increasing pain, spinal stenosis, neurologic deficit, or severe postural deformity could necessitate surgical correction. Multiple osteoporotic fractures could lead to severe kyphotic or scoliotic deformities resulting in postural problems and cardiopulmonary compromise needing surgical intervention. The reduced bone density and mechanical strength of the bones in these patients has been shown by various studies[5-7] to result in poor purchase for the screws leading to increase in screw pullout, screw displacement, and eventually failure of instrumentation. In addition, patients undergoing surgery for vertebral collapse due to metastatic tumors also pose the problem of reconstructive surgery in bone with poor mechanical qualities in which obtaining adequate purchase for instrumentation for stabilization becomes a challenge.

Awareness of the possible complications, judicious selection of patients, and use of appropriate instrumentation at the correct levels are of paramount importance to help ensure that spinal surgery will be a safe and effective means of restoration of function in this difficult group of patients.

II. COMMON METHODS OF SPINAL INSTRUMENTATION

A large variety of instrumentation is available for stabilization of the cervical and thoracolumbar spine and it is the responsibility of the surgeon to choose judiciously the appropriate instrumentation for the patient.

Upper cervical spine stabilization can be obtained via the posterior approach by a posterior fusion and wiring (i.e., Gallies') method with or without transarticular screw fixation or with the use of plates and screws (occipitocervical junction). The anterior approach is also used for fixation of odontoid fractures using anterior screws.

In the lower cervical spine, posterior instrumentation may include interspinous, facet, or interlaminar wiring, articular pillar and pedicle screws with posterior plates, and also hybrid rod plate constructs spanning the cervicothoracic junction. Anterior plating of the cervical spine has also been shown to be a safe and reliable method of cervical decompression and stabilization, especially in multilevel pathology.

Posterior hook and rod fixation has been the most popular method for stabilization of the thoracic spine and correction of deformities. Anterior reconstruction methods with grafts supplemented with fixation systems (plates or rods) have been employed but stand-alone anterior reconstructions have a higher failure mode in osteoporotic bone.

In the lumbar spine, pedicle screw fixation has proved to be an effective way of stabilization of anterior interbody fusions and corpectomy reconstructions. Recent advances in technology have enabled more and more accurate placement of pedicle screws using flouroscopic or computer guidance and have promoted the use of minimally invasive percutaneous techniques for posterior stabilization of the spine.

Anterior stabilization of the spine with anterior implants has proved to be useful for management of fractures, tumors, and spinal deformities, but also carries the risk of fixation failure without concomitant posterior instrumentation.

III. CHOOSING FIXATION METHODS

The choice of instrumentation in the patient with osteoporosis must take into consideration the increased fragility of the bones leading to problems of inadequate purchase for the screws as well as the increased likelihood of screw pullout by pedicle stripping or fracture of pedicles. Laminar hooks may fail by cutting through the laminae, leading to pullout. Adjacent-level fractures can lead to increased deformity secondary to excessive forces on the stiffer instrumented segment. The possibility of subsidence of the anterior strut grafts (corpectomy reconstruction) adds to the diffi-culty in treating these patients.

Because the chances of failure at the points of fixation are higher in patients with poor bone quality, the number of points of fixation must be increased to distribute the forces more evenly. As previously stated, utilization of supplementary fixation such as laminar hooks, wires, or transverse bars may help in improving the performance of the pedicle screws. The possibility of hardware pullout during the procedure while manipulating the instrumentation for deformity correction is also a problem that can be addressed by obtaining fixation in vertebrae at least two levels above and below the actual kyphotic deformity to be corrected. In patients with severe osteoporosis where the possibility of failure is high, we may have to accept a lower degree of correction to avoid the problem of complete failure.

IV. COMMON CONDITIONS

The quality of life in elderly patients is significantly affected by the presence of osteoporosis. It not only causes deformities, pain, and neurologic problems in patients with fractures, but also produces a significant negative impact on the quality of life measurements.

A prospective study of vertebral fractures and mortality in 9575 women aged 65 years or older over a period of 8.3 years demonstrated the incidence of vertebral fractures to be 20%.[8] Compared with women who did not have a vertebral fracture, women with one or more fractures had a 1.23-fold greater age-adjusted mortality rate. Mortality rose with greater numbers of vertebral fractures, from 19 per 1000 woman-years in women with no fractures to 44 per 1000 woman-years in those with five or more fractures. In particular, vertebral fractures were related to the risk of subsequent cancer and pulmonary compromise. Severe kyphosis was 2.6 times more frequently related to pulmonary deaths.

A. OSTEOPOROTIC PAIN

Backache in elderly patients is often attributed to osteoporotic changes. Ettinger et al.[9] investigated the contribution of vertebral deformities to chronic back pain and disability among 2992 Caucasian women aged 65 to 70 years by measuring radiographic vertebral dimensions of T5 to L4 and calculating ratios of heights: anterior/posterior, mid/posterior, and posterior/posterior of either adjacent vertebra. Only 39.4% of the study population had no vertebral deformity and 10.2% had a deformity greater than or equal to 4 standard deviations (SD). Vertebral deformities less than 4 SD below the mean were not associated with increased back pain, disability, or loss of height. In contrast, women whose deformity was greater than or equal to 4 SD had a 1.9 times higher risk of moderate to severe back pain and a 2.6 times higher risk of disability involving the back. They were also 2.5 times more likely to have lost greater than or equal to 4 cm in height. All three types of vertebral deformity (wedge, end plate, and crush) were equally associated with these outcomes. This large cross-sectional study suggests that vertebral deformities led to substantial pain, disability, or loss of height only if vertebral height ratios fell 4 SD below the normal mean. Nevitt et al.[10] studied 7223 Caucasian women aged 65 years and older for prevalent and incident radiographic vertebral fractures, the frequency and severity of back pain, disability in performing six activities involving the back, and days of bed rest and days of limited activity due to back pain over a period of 3.7 years. Women with or without a fracture at baseline who had an incident fracture during this period showed a greater incidence of back pain, back disability, and functional limitation irrespective of whether the fracture was discovered because of clinical symptoms or was discovered at regular yearly screening.

A study of the pain and disability experienced by 85 consecutive postmenopausal Caucasian women (average age 64 years, range 50 to 82) with spinal osteoporosis revealed persistent back pain in 54 (63%) in the lumbar spine and 53 (62%) in the thoracic spine.[11] Sleep was disturbed in 60%, difficulty obtaining suitable clothes was found in 42%, and difficulties with functional activities in 47%, although these were severe in only 10%. Although osteoporosis is thought to represent one of the main causes of back pain in perimenopausal women, other causes of back pain have to be ruled out. Kann et al.[12] have reported that, in perimenopausal women (45 to 60 years old), 20% had disc degeneration and 19% had other degenerative disorders (osteoarthritis) of the spine without coincident scoliosis. Scoliosis due to different leg length was detected in 15%, idiopathic scoliosis in 13%, and spondylolisthesis occurred in 7% (even more frequently than osteoporosis with vertebral deformities, 6%). Also significant is the fact that newly occurring fractures are more significantly associated with pain and disability than existing fractures. In a longitudinal analysis by Ross et al.[13] of pain and disability associated with new vertebral fractures, new fractures were three times more likely to be associated with back pain. The association with prevalent fractures was weaker and not significant.

B. Compression Fractures

Fractures of the spine result from a discrepancy between the applied load on the vertebral bone and the structural strength of the bone. In an osteoporotic spine, even loads generated by activities of daily living such as bending and lifting or by low-energy trauma such as a minor fall can result in compressive failure and a resultant fracture. Low-energy compression fractures caused by minor injuries like a trivial fall are characteristic of the osteoporotic spine and the presence of multiple such fractures can lead to spinal deformity. The fractures may be asymptomatic in many cases but sometimes can lead to progressive deformity, spinal stenosis, and neurologic deficit necessitating surgical correction. Burst fractures of the vertebra can also occur with propulsion of fragments into the spinal canal causing myelopathy and requiring surgery.

Many osteoporotic compression fractures can be treated via vertebroplasty for pain relief. Kyphoplasty has been utilized for acute compression fractures either to aid in reducing deformity or to prevent further deformity in addition to alleviating pain. These two techniques will be covered in other chapters.

Over the past several years, we have advanced a minimally invasive posterior approach to osteoporotic burst fractures. A limited anterior exposure is performed for decompression and anterior column reconstruction. A percutaneous approach is then utilized posteriorly to insert pedicle screws and the rods are placed subcutaneously above the fascia (suprafascial).[14] This allows the musculature and fascial envelope to remain intact and there is no surgical compromise to the facet capsules and posterior supportive structures. The patients' muscles aid in biomechanical support posteriorly and the recovery is faster with less morbidity (see case examples 1 and 2 at the end of the chapter).

Spine bone mineral density (BMD) as determined by dual-energy X-ray absorptiometry (DEXA) correlates strongly with the compressive failure load and therefore should be a convenient and specific indicator of the compressive strength of the vertebrae *in vivo*. Earlier grading systems based on the disappearance of the normal trabecular pattern usually seen in the femoral neck (Singh index) and X-ray absorptiometry have given way to more accurate methods such as photon absorptiometry, DEXA, and quantitative computerized tomography (QCT).

DEXA scans have a precision range of 1 to 2% and can be used as an accurate and precise method to monitor changes in bone density in patients undergoing treatments. Measurement of BMD by QCT uses most standard CT scanners with software packages that allow them to determine bone density in the hip or spine. This technique provides for true three-dimensional imaging and reports BMD as a true volume density measurement. The advantage of QCT is its ability to isolate the area of interest from surrounding tissues. QCT can localize an area in a vertebral body of only trabecular bone leaving out the elements most affected by degenerative change and sclerosis. The

QCT radiation dose is about ten times that of DEXA and QCT tests may be more expensive than DEXA. Lower-cost portable devices that determine BMD at peripheral sites, such as the radius, the phalanges, or the calcaneus, are also being utilized, but the problem with peripheral testing is that only one site is tested and low bone density in the hip or spine may be missed. In the early postmenopausal years, bone density in the spine decreases first because the turnover in this highly trabecular bone is higher than in other skeletal sites. Bone density at various skeletal sites begins to coincide at about age 70. Caution must be used in interpreting spine scans in elderly patients because of degenerative changes falsely elevating the BMD values. There are a number of studies that have attempted to quantify the actual BMD at which vertebral fractures are most likely to occur. Norimatsu et al.[15] studied BMD of the spine and proximal femur with dual photon absorptiometry, using gadolinium-153. They found that the peak bone mass of the spine (L2–L4) was 1.20 g/cm^2 in women, which was lower than that of men by 4.7. Fracture threshold evaluated at the 90th percentile for BMD of L2–L4 in patients with vertebral crush fractures was 0.97 g/cm^2 at the spine. Using the DEXA technique, Jahng and Lee[16] compared BMD in 283 postmenopausal and senile women. BMD of the vertebral body in the osteoporotic fracture group was compared with that in the osteoporotic group to investigate the correlation among BMD, age distribution, and fracture type, and to estimate fracture threshold in the osteoporotic fracture group. BMD decreased rapidly (10%) from 50 and 60 years of age and decreased slowly after 60 years of age. Osteoporotic spine fractures were found in 98 cases (35%) and there was significant difference in BMD between the osteoporotic group and osteoporotic fracture group. There was no spine fracture when BMD was above 1.00 g/cm^2 and the fracture threshold was 0.85 g/cm^2 at the 90th percentile. BMD in multiple spine fracture and old fracture groups was lower than in the single and fresh fracture groups and this was statistically significant.

Ryan et al.[17] reported the fracture threshold as 0.81 g/cm^2 at the lumbar spine and that 5% of normal women aged 40 to 49 years, 20% aged 50 to 59 years, and 45% aged 60 to 69 years had a BMD below this threshold.

Radiologic identification of vertebral fractures is difficult and different methods using vertebral height measurements for fracture identification have therefore been developed. The methods of Hedlund and Gallagher,[18] Melton,[1] and Davies et al.[19] are based on the ratio of heights within one vertebra or of the height ratios of adjacent vertebrae. All three methods rely on counting the number of vertebral fractures. The fourth method, that of Sauer et al.,[20] relates anterior, middle, and posterior heights of the vertebrae between T5 and L5 to the respective heights of T4. The relative vertebral heights of patients with osteoporosis are compared to the respective relative heights (anterior, middle, and posterior) of normal subjects from T5 to L5. This allows the identification of fractured vertebrae, as well as a quantification of the extent of deformation due to these fractures (spine deformity index, SDI). Vertebral fractures as identified by SDI were not detected by the other three methods in 12 to 29% of the cases, even if vertebral height reduction was more than 6 mm.[20]

C. Spinal Deformity

Compressive osteoporotic vertebral fractures commonly occur in the anterior part of the body and lead to thoracic kyphosis. However, lateral wedge fractures can also occur, causing or exacerbating preexisting lateral deformities.[21] In either case, multiple fractures can lead to severe spinal deformity causing stenosis of the spinal canal or neural foramina resulting in neurologic deficit. Loss of height and cardiopulmonary compromise can also result from severe kyphosis.

Kyphotic deformity of the spine is associated with low BMD levels. Ettinger et al.[22] found in a study of 610 women aged 65 to 91 years that the 10% of women with the most severe kyphosis had 7 to 17% lower BMD ($p < 0.001$) and had lost an additional 2.4 cm in height. Ryan et al.[11] found that the severity of thoracic back pain is significantly related to degree of kyphosis, numbers of collapsed vertebrae, and the severity of collapse.[11]

D. Tumors

Surgical management of metastatic tumors of the spine from breast, prostate, lungs, or other primaries also poses a problem for operating on elderly patients with poor-quality bone tissue for stabilization of the spine after tumor resection and reconstruction.

In patients with bone involvement in the absence of structural deformity, adjuvant therapy usually is appropriate. In cases of bone collapse, with or without neurologic compromise, surgical consideration should be given to patients with appropriate life expectancy.

To date, the treatment of spinal tumors is only palliative, and surgery must be considered for cases with unremitting neck pain, major vertebral destruction with loss or impending loss of cervical spine stability, and neurologic deficits due to local tumor compression.

V. VERTEBROPLASTY

Percutaneous injection of polymethylmethacrylate (PMMA) is often proposed for prophylactic stabilization of osteoporotic vertebral bodies at risk for fracture or for augmentation of vertebral bodies that have already fractured. The procedure has been shown to provide significant pain relief in a high percentage of patients with osteoporotic fractures and also provides spinal stabilization in patients with malignancies and osteoporosis. Vertebral body augmentation can also be used as an adjunct to fixation of internal hardware such as pedicle screws in osteoporotic spines.[23] A number of products are now available or are in clinical trials including injectable PMMA or mineral bone cement, glass-ceramic-reinforced composites, and injectable non-exothermic, biocompatible carbonated apatite cancellous bone cements. Osteoconductive granular coral particles have also been used in a human cadaveric study and in a sheep model by Cunin et al.[24] They found increased osteogenesis in cavities filled with coral as compared to control group in the sheep.[24]

Barr et al.[25] conducted a retrospective review of 47 consecutive patients in whom percutaneous intraosseous methylmethacrylate cement injection (percutaneous vertebroplasty) was used to treat osteoporotic vertebral compression fractures and spinal column neoplasms. Percutaneous vertebroplasty provided significant pain relief in a high percentage of patients with osteoporotic fractures. The procedure provided spinal stabilization in patients with malignancies but did not produce consistent pain relief.

PMMA has the disadvantage of undergoing an exothermic reaction during setting that can damage nearby neural structures. Also, the chances of exudation and dislodgment and the difficulty of carrying out revision surgeries in PMMA-injected patients have led to the search for alternatives. Schildhauer et al.[26] explored the use of a carbonated apatite cement by infiltration of the cement into thoracic vertebral bodies using a combined suction–injection technique. The energy-absorption capabilities of the reinforced vertebral bodies were then measured during axial compressive tests and compared with those of nonreinforced vertebrae. Energy absorption was significantly higher ($p < 0.05$) between 25 and 70% collapse of the vertebral body in the specimens that received the apatite injection as compared with the controls. The osteoconductive nature of the cement and its ability to be remodeled by bone, together with its compressive strength, which is higher than that of cancellous bone, could provide better clinical results than those of current treatments with acrylic cement.

VI. MANAGEMENT AND COMPLICATIONS

A. Preoperative Evaluation

Adequate preoperative evaluation of the patient with osteoporosis or with suspected osteoporosis is essential before planning surgical intervention.

BMD of the spine has been shown by various studies to be a significant factor in the success or failure of spinal instrumentation, especially of pedicle screws.[5] BMD evaluation is necessary to confirm a diagnosis of osteoporosis in patients with existing fractures, to predict chances of fracturing in the future, and also to determine the rate of bone loss and/or to monitor the effects of treatment when conducted at intervals of a year or more. BMD is reported as the amount of bony tissue in a unit volume (g/cm^2). The t-score is the number of SD above or below the young adult mean, which is the peak bone density at about age 20 of a reference population of the same sex and ethnicity. The z-score is the number of standard deviations of the patient's bone density above or below the values expected for the patient's age. By comparing the patient to the expected BMD for his or her own age, the z-score can help classify the type of osteoporosis. A z-score lower than −1.5 is reason to suspect secondary osteoporosis due to thyroid or parathyroid abnormalities, malabsorption, alcoholism, smoking, and the use of certain medications, especially corticosteroids. If secondary causes are suspected, the patient should usually undergo further workup including laboratory testing to discover if there is an underlying reason for the osteoporosis that requires correction.

The therapeutic strategies for treating osteoporosis are designed to maximize peak bone mass through proper nutrition, appropriate intake of calcium and vitamin D, maintenance of physiologic menstrual cycles in premenopausal women, and a program of weight-bearing and strengthening exercises. Measurement of serum albumin and prealbumin may also be helpful in some cases with appropriate dietary supplementation if required. For conditions involving high bone turnover (osteoporosis in which osteoclastic resorption is increased) efficacious treatment options include hormone replacement therapy, calcitonin, and bisphosphonates. Osteoporosis with low bone turnover results from deficient osteoblastic bone formation and responds to the experimental drug programs of fluoride, parathyroid hormone, and parathyroid hormone–related peptide analogals.[27] Determination of bone density defines the patient's current condition. Measurement of the level of N-telopeptides (collagen breakdown products) predicts the patient's future regarding osteoporotic fractures, and the presence of risk factors for hip fracture establish the therapeutic window for treatment. Biomarkers such as bone-specific alkaline phosphatases and osteocalcin levels can be used in conjunction with DEXA scans to help quantify the degree of osteoporosis.[28]

B. Spinal Instrumentation and Associated Problems

Odontoid fracture is the most frequent lesion in cervical spine in elderly individuals due to increased fragility of the trabecular structure of the dens and increasing stiffness of the cervical spine with age.[29] Gallies' posterior fusion with or without transarticular screws or occipitocervical plate fixation with screws, rods with wires, or anterior screw fixation are commonly used for management of these fractures. However, in patients with osteoporosis, the anterior approach may be difficult owing to the higher possibility of comminution at the fracture site and limited ability to extend the neck. In a retrospective analysis of 29 patients with odontoid fractures treated by conservative halopelvic immobilization (10 patients), posterior C1–C2 fusion (7 patients) and with anterior Bohler screw fixation (8 patients), Andersson et al.[30] found an unacceptably high rate of complications including failed fusion in 75%, as well as loosening of screws, redisplacement, and systemic complications with anterior screw fixation. The anterior approach had to be abandoned in 2 patients due to difficulty in exposure.

In contrast, Berlemann and Schwarzenback[31] investigated the outcome of direct anterior screw fixation of type 2 dens fractures in 19 patients over 65 years of age and reported satisfactory results with the anterior procedure with a high rate of fusion (16/19) and recommended the technique for elderly patients.

Occipitocervical fixation with plates or screws is also used for the treatment of nontraumatic upper cervical instabilities. However, these devices are not indicated in the treatment of patients with severe osteoporosis or in instances of significant thinning of the occipital bone. Paquis et al.[32] have described the use of cervical interlaminar hooks and occipital claws with hooks or screws with significant improvement of neck pain and improvement or stabilization of neurologic symptoms.

Stable fractures of the upper cervical spine may be treated conservatively with halopelvic external stabilization but it is important to recognize type II dens fractures, where instability may cause immediate or delayed problems such as pain and myelopathy, and these patients should be considered surgical candidates. In fact, surgical treatment of these patients decreases the hospital stay and immobilization, thus decreasing the morbidity and mortality associated with odontoid fractures. Nonunion of odontoid fractures, however, does not essentially mean a bad result and a stable fibrous union might also be an acceptable end point.[21]

Zink[33] studied the effect of BMD on the insertion torque for screws used in anterior lower cervical plating as well as the axial force generated at the plate screw junction at the end of screw tightening (F_{ax}). A strong correlation was found between the two measurements and the BMD. It was felt that increasing the screw length and obtaining bicortical engagement significantly increases the torque and the F_{ax}. He also concluded that a stable fixation of 3.5 mm screws cannot be achieved if the BMD remains below 150 mg/ml as measured by the QCT method. In such cases he has recommended the use of external immobilization for additional stabilization.

One of the problems faced in the osteoporotic thoracic spine is the pullout of hooks and wires during surgical deformity correction and during postoperative management. To prevent this from occurring, we need to obtain purchase at additional sites or accept a lesser degree of deformity correction. Anterior spinal release may improve flexibility and decreases the need for excessive force.[21]

Segmental fixation with multiple point fixation may prove to be a useful technique by distributing the forces over a larger number of pressure points and reducing the chances of failure. Postoperative pullout or displacement of hardware can also occur due to the stresses and strains imposed on the instrumentation by the loading caused by activities of daily life. The osteoporotic spine is less able to withstand these forces and this may be evidenced as a sudden giving way with pain, neurologic problems, or hardware prominence. Symptomatic failure may need surgical revision that may be achieved by extension of the number of instrumented segments or by using larger-size screws. Asymptomatic failure may be seen as either hardware displacement or a radiolucent halo around the screws on radiographs and may not need any surgical intervention.

Sublaminar wiring has been suggested to be a safe and well-tested method of thoracic spine stabilization providing multiple fixation points; however, it does not provide axial control and hence proximal hooks have been advised to prevent junctional kyphosis at the proximal end of the construct.[21]

Coe et al.[5] studied the mechanisms of failure of different thoracic implants such as spinous process wire/button implants, laminar hooks, and two different types of pedicle screws in spines of elderly patients under cyclic loading. The most common mode of failure of the spinous process wiring was by cutting through the bone posteriorly. Failure through lamina or pedicle occurred in only 5% of the segments. Laminar hooks failed mainly by cutting through the posterior lamina but up to 30% of the failures occurred through the pedicle or the pedicle body junction. The most common mode of failure for the pedicle screw was direct pullout. However, in 6.8% there was ipsilateral pedicle or pedicle body junction failure with cracking or complete failure of the contralateral pedicle. The laminar hooks were the most resistant to failure and the difference between load to failure for the hooks vs. the other implants was statistically significant.

Correlation of the BMD to the load to failure revealed a linear relationship. The load to failure decreased linearly with decrease in BMD and there was no threshold level below which failure occurred precipitously. Hence, they could not define a minimum BMD that could predict a secure fixation.

In another study conducted by Butler et al.[34] comparing the strength of different sublaminar wiring constructs, 83% of the failures occurred through the pedicles and not at the actual site of the anchor itself. They also reported that the T2 pedicle was stronger than T3–T6 pedicles. The stiffness of the claw implants was greater than sublaminar wiring. However, the subpars wiring showed equivalent strength to the claws, probably because the point of contact was the thicker subpars bone as compared with the thin laminar edge in the sublaminar wires. They have also suggested that subpars wiring might provide more transverse plane angulation force. However, lateralization of the wires into the subpars position raises the concerns of foraminal encroachment and nerve root irritation. Sublaminar wires tended to pull through more easily with decreasing BMD, but the performance of laminar hooks as well as pedicle hooks did not suffer with osteoporosis. This study therefore recommends the use of pedicle hooks, laminar hooks, or subpars wires in patients with significant osteoporosis as well as the inclusion of T2 vertebral level in the fixation as it is the strongest anchor point.

Anterior vertebral screw fixation for the thoracolumbar spine has been used for management of spinal fractures, tumors, and deformities. The pullout of anterior instrumentation also has been shown to have a direct correlation with the BMD.

Lim et al.[35] correlated the BMD of vertebral bodies as measured by DEXA with the pullout strength of bicortical Kaneda screws inserted in the transverse direction along the midline of the vertebral body. Screw insertional torque was also measured and was found to have a linear correlation with the BMD. This suggests that the osteoporotic spine has a higher chance of instrumentation failure, and augmentation with PMMA or carbonated apatite cement could improve the performance.

Pullout strength of the screws was also directly related to bone density and increased linearly. By using the grading by Soshi et al.[7] patients with Grade I osteoporosis (0.6 to 0.8 g/cm^2) had significantly greater mean pullout strength and insertional torque measurements as compared with Grade II (0.4 to 0.6 g/cm^2) and Grade III (0.3 to 0.4 g/cm^2).

Minimal-access surgery in managing osteoporotic vertebral fractures with neurologic deficits has been reported by Huang et al.[36] Using formal anterior spinal surgery might significantly violate the patient's respiratory mechanism and increase operative morbidity or mortality that can be avoided by a minimally invasive approach as it can obviate the necessity of dividing the diaphragm to facilitate exposure. However, the stability of the vertebral screw purchase in the osteoporotic spine is still a matter of concern.

In the lumbar spine, pedicle screws have gained wide acceptance as a safe and effective means of stabilization. Flexion/extension movements of the spine *in vivo* produce a pullout load along the direction of the screw as well as tilting or cutout load, especially in constrained devices. This can result in screw loosening and displacement with loss of correction for patients having instrumentation at more than one level.[37] Many studies have reported a direct correlation between the pullout loads and the BMD of the vertebrae. A study of transpedicular screw fixation in osteoporotic lumbar spines by Soshi et al.[7] showed that screws in patients with Grade I osteoporosis had a significantly higher pullout strength than screws placed in the pedicles of patients with severe osteoporosis of Grades II and III. Augmentation with cement resulted in increasing the pullout strength in the Grade I and II patients by almost double, but had no significant effect in Grade III patients. Increasing the screw size resulted in greater pullout forces but the combination of cement and increased screw size had a positive effect only in patients with Grade I or Grade II osteoporosis while it had no effect in osteoporosis of Grade III severity. They concluded that transpedicular fixation technique cannot be used for patients with BMD less than 0.3 to 0.4 g/cm^2.

Yamagata et al.[38] have shown that a 100 mg/cm^2 decrease in BMD as measured by DEXA technique caused a 10 kP decrease in the pullout force. Okuyama et al.,[39] using the QCT method for BMD measurement, have reported a decreased rate of pullout force of about 60 N when the BMD decreased by 10 mg/ml. They also reported that the cutout of the screw through the vertebral end plate on cyclic flexion/extension loading was directly related to the BMD and that there is a possibility of cutout in an osteoporotic vertebrae (BMD of 130 ± 53.2 mg/ml) at even physiologic flexion loads of 7.5 Nm. They also found that the torque required for screw insertion was directly proportional to the BMD and could be a useful predictor of the mechanical stability of the screws.

Halvorson et al.[6] have also reported that the BMD was a strong influence on screw pullout strength. Average pullout force in osteoporotic spines (BMD = 0.818 mg/ml) was only 206 ± 159 N as compared to 1540 ± 61 N in normal spines (BMD = 1.17 mg/ml). In normal spines, the technique of screw insertion did not have a significant effect. However, in osteoporotic spines, untapped pedicles or pedicles tapped with a smaller diameter than the screw showed statistically significant higher pullout strength. Supplementation of the pedicle screw fixation with laminar hooks improved the fixation strength of moderately osteoporotic spines to almost the level of normal spine. In normal bone it was possible to salvage a stripped screw hole by packing with corticocancellous graft, but similar packing did not augment the pullout strength of osteoporotic pedicles.

Various solutions have been suggested for the problem of pedicle screw pullout such as increasing the size of pedicle screws, supplementary laminar hooks, or transverse connections and augmentation with bone cement or other strengthening materials.

The use of larger screws brings with it the risk of pedicle fracture. Incidence of pedicle fracture has been described to be 0.4 to 2.3%. Sjostrom et al.[40] have shown that 85% of the pedicles expanded when the screw diameter exceeded 65% of the outer diameter of the pedicle while Misenhimer et al.[41] found that pedicle fracture or cutout occurred when the screw diameter was greater than 80% of the outer diameter of the pedicle as measured by CT scan. Hirano et al.[42] studied the risk of pedicle fracture in normal as well as osteoporotic pedicles. They found that the BMD as well as the percentage of cortical bone was significantly lower in the osteoporotic group and found that the highest risk of fracture was seen in pedicles with BMD of 0.7 gm/cm^2 when screws diameter was >70% of the pedicle diameter. The lateral pedicle wall was more often fractured than the medial wall that is two to three times thicker than the lateral wall. They suggest that medial wall fracture may represent malposition rather than screw–pedicle size discrepancy. George et al.[43] have shown that the pullout strength of fractured pedicles is 11% less than that of screws in intact pedicles. Correction of this problem again may be addressed by repair with bone graft or bone cements such as PMMA or the recently available biocompatible cements like carbonated apatite or calcium phosphate bone cement.

Use of methylmethacrylate to increase the pullout strength has been described by Kleeman et al.[44] Zindrick et al.[45] have reported that bone cement augments the strength of fixation by up to 226%. This increase in strength, however, is seen only when the cement is injected under pressure.[45] The risk of extravasation of the heated cement causing injury to neural structures and difficulty in removing it during revision surgery should be kept in mind. An injectable, biocompatible, non-exothermic carbonated apatite cancellous bone cement has been suggested as an alternative. Lotz et al.[46] have described its use to augment pedicle screw fixation by testing pullout strength and cyclic transverse loading force in lumbar pedicle screws. They found that the pullout strength of the augmented pedicles was 68% greater than the control group's and the biomechanical response to cyclic loading was improved by 30 to 63%.

Hilibrand et al.[47] compared the pullout strength of pedicle screws alone with pedicle screws supplemented with supralaminar hooks for intact and compromised pedicles stripped by pulling out previously placed pedicle screws. They found no significant difference between the two constructs in case of intact bone, but found that in stripped bone the pedicle screw alone restored only 19% of the intact pedicle pullout strength as compared to 89% restoration by the pediculolaminar construct. A study by Hasegawa et al.[48] also confirmed the fact that augmentation of pedicle screw fixation with hooks increased the stiffness of the construct under cyclic loading by about 49%. McAfee et al.[49] have suggested that transverse linking of pedicle screws at the same level with a metallic device also increases the axial pullout strength of the screws.

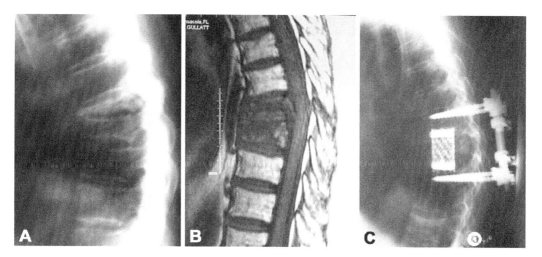

FIGURE 18.1 (A) Lateral radiograph showing severe osteoporosis with compression fractures at T7 and T8 level. (B) MRI and CT scans revealed severe cord compression at T7–T8. (C) Transthoracic corpectomy T8–T9 and reconstruction using titanium surgical mesh plus iliac crest bone graft plus rib plus coralline hydroxyapatite along with posterior suprafascial stabilization using moss-miami polyaxial screws and cross-links.

VII. SUMMARY

Osteoporosis is a growing problem in surgical treatment of spinal disorders due to an increase in the geriatric population. Problems like compression fractures, spinal deformity, postural problems, spinal stenosis, and neurologic compromise caused by osteoporosis need to be treated following certain principles.

Adequate preoperative evaluation of the patient, differentiation between primary and secondary osteoporosis, management of secondary causes, and adequate nutritional, medical, and rehabilitational measures are necessary along with a judicious choice of patients for surgical intervention.

In patients undergoing surgery, the instrumentation chosen should have multiple point fixation to distribute loads. Application of instrumentation that gains purchase at stronger bony points (e.g., laminar hooks, subpars wires) and the use of supplementary instrumentation (combined pediculolaminar hooks) also helps to reduce failure.

In cases of deformity correction, using instrumentation-spanning levels beyond the actual level of the deformity can help prevent failure. Anterior release and acceptance of lesser degrees of correction may also be necessary to avoid excessive forces on the purchase points. Use of larger-sized or longer screws, bicortical purchase, and use of transverse connections spanning pedicle screws have also been found to be beneficial. Cement augmentation of vertebral bodies or pedicles can decrease chances of pullout.

Supplementary external immobilization can be useful in patients with severe osteoporosis where high risk of failure is expected.

VIII. CASE EXAMPLES

CASE 1

A 68-year-old female complained of acute pain in her back when she tried to get up from sitting. Radiographic study showed severe osteoporosis with compression fracture at T7–T8 level (Figure 18.1A). She was admitted to the hospital and treated conservatively for a period of 6 weeks. Her symptoms worsened over the next few weeks and she had bilateral paresthesias from hip to

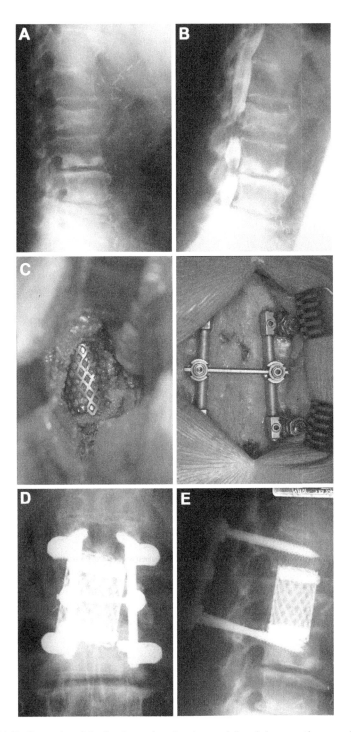

FIGURE 18.2 (A) Radiographs of the lumbar spine showing multilevel degenerative spondylosis with 50 to 60% loss of vertebral body height at the L2 vertebra. (B) Myelography showed retropulsion of a bony fragment at the level of the fracture and narrowing of the spinal canal. (C) Patient underwent corpectomy with reconstruction using titanium surgical mesh (left) and suprafascial stabilization of L1 to L3 using titanium USS fracture module (right). (D) Postoperative radiographs demonstrated some asymmetric collapse of the titanium cage into the end plate of L3. (E) Radiographs 7 months after surgery showed no motion on flexion extension with no further sinking of the cage into the end plate.

toes and was not able to bear weight on either leg. On examination she was quite tender within the thoracic spine. Radiographs showed a severe compression fracture at T7–T8. Magnetic resonance imaging (MRI) and CT scans revealed severe cord compression (Figure 18.1B). The patient underwent left-sided transthoracic decompression and corpectomy at T8–T9 with reconstruction using titanium surgical mesh plus left iliac crest bone graft plus rib plus coralline hydroxyapatite. Posterior suprafascial stabilization of T6 through T9 using moss-miami polyaxial screws and cross lengths was also performed (Figure 18.1C). Postoperatively the patient had significant reduction in the thoracic axial pain but continued to have some pain over the hardware. At 9 months after the surgery, the posterior hardware was removed. Anterior solid fusion was confirmed during hardware removal by stressing the pedicle screws under fluoroscopy.

CASE 2

A 68-year-old male had pain in the lumbar region after a fall on his back. Radiographs of the lumbar spine showed multilevel degenerative spondylosis with 50 to 60% loss of vertebral body height at the L2 vertebra (Figure 18.2A). Myelo-CT showed retropulsion of a bony fragment at the level of the fracture with associated narrowing of the spinal canal (Figure 18.2B). The patient underwent anterior lumbar corpectomy with reconstruction using titanium surgical mesh, local and autologous iliac crest bone graft and suprafascial stabilization of L1 to L3 using titanium USS fracture module (Figure 18.2C). Radiographs taken 2 weeks postoperatively demonstrated some asymmetric collapse of the titanium cage into the end plate of L3, more to the right side than to the left (Figure 18.2D). At latest follow-up, 7 months after surgery, the patient is ambulatory and functional status is better than before surgery, as is his pain status. Radiographs showed no motion on flexion extension and the anterior fusion appears solid with no further sinking of the cage into the end plate (Figure 18.2E).

REFERENCES

1. Melton, L.J., III, "Epidemiology of spinal osteoporosis," *Spine,* 22, 2S, 1997.
2. Lukert, B.P., "Vertebral compression fractures: how to manage pain, avoid disability," *Geriatrics,* 49, 22, 1994.
3. Lyles, K.W., Gold, D.T., Shipp, K.M., et al., "Association of osteoporotic vertebral compression fractures with impaired functional status," *Am. J. Med.,* 94, 595, 1993.
4. Myers, E.R. and Wilson, S.E., "Biomechanics of osteoporosis and vertebral fracture," *Spine,* 22, 25S, 1997.
5. Coe, J.D., Warden, K.E., Herzig, M.A., and McAfee, P.C., "Influence of bone mineral density on the fixation of thoracolumbar implants. A comparative study of transpedicular screws, laminar hooks, and spinous process wires," *Spine,* 15, 902, 1990.
6. Halvorson, T.L., Kelley, L.A., Thomas, K.A., et al., "Effects of bone mineral density on pedicle screw fixation," *Spine,* 19, 2415, 1994.
7. Soshi, S., Shiba, R., Kondo, H., and Murota, K., "An experimental study on transpedicular screw fixation in relation to osteoporosis of the lumbar spine," *Spine,* 16, 1335, 1991.
8. Kado, D.M., Browner, W.S., Palermo, L., et al., "Vertebral fractures and mortality in older women: a prospective study. Study of Osteoporotic Fractures Research Group," *Arch. Intern. Med.,* 159, 1215, 1999.
9. Ettinger, B., Black, D.M., Nevitt, M.C., et al., "Contribution of vertebral deformities to chronic back pain and disability. The Study of Osteoporotic Fractures Research Group," *J. Bone Miner. Res.,* 7, 449, 1992.
10. Nevitt, M.C., Ettinger, B., Black, D.M., et al., "The association of radiographically detected vertebral fractures with back pain and function: a prospective study," *Ann. Intern. Med.,* 128, 793, 1998.
11. Ryan, P.J., Blake, G., Herd, R., and Fogelman, I., "A clinical profile of back pain and disability in patients with spinal osteoporosis," *Bone,* 15, 27, 1994.

12. Kann, P., Schulz, G., Schehler, B., and Beyer, J., "[Backache and osteoporosis in perimenopausal women]," *Med. Klin.,* 88, 9, 1993.

13. Ross, P.D., Davis, J.W., Epstein, R.S., and Wasnich, R.D., "Pain and disability associated with new vertebral fractures and other spinal conditions," *J. Clin. Epidemiol.,* 47, 231, 1994.

14. Lowery, G.L. and Kulkarni, S.S., "Posterior percutaneous spine instrumentation," *Eur. Spine J.,* 9, S126, 2000.

15. Norimatsu, H., Mori, S., Uesato, T., et al., "Bone mineral density of the spine and proximal femur in normal and osteoporotic subjects in Japan," *Bone Miner.,* 5, 213, 1989.

16. Jahng, J.S. and Lee, W.I., "Measurement of bone mineral density in osteoporotic fractures of the spine using dual energy X-ray absorptiometry," *Orthopaedics,* 19, 951, 1996.

17. Ryan, P.J., Blake, G.M., and Fogelman, I., "Fracture thresholds in osteoporosis: implications for hormone replacement treatment," *Ann. Rheum. Dis.,* 51, 1065, 1992.

18. Hedlund, L.R. and Gallagher, J.C., "Vertebral morphometry in diagnosis of spinal fractures," *Bone Miner.,* 5, 59, 1988.

19. Davies, K.M., Stegman, M.R., Heaney, R.P., and Recker, R.R., "Prevalence and severity of vertebral fracture: the Saunders County Bone Quality Study," *Osteoporos. Int.,* 6, 160, 1996.

20. Sauer, P., Leidig, G., Minne, H.W., et al., "Spine deformity index (SDI) vs. other objective procedures of vertebral fracture identification in patients with osteoporosis: a comparative study," *J. Bone Miner. Res.,* 6, 227, 1991.

21. Hu, S.S., "Internal fixation in the osteoporotic spine," *Spine,* 22, 43S, 1997.

22. Ettinger, B., Black, D.M., Palermo, L., et al., "Kyphosis in older women and its relation to back pain, disability and osteopenia: the study of osteoporotic fractures," *Osteoporos. Int.,* 4, 55, 1994.

23. Bostrom, M.P. and Lane, J.M., "Future directions. Augmentation of osteoporotic vertebral bodies," *Spine,* 22, 38S, 1997.

24. Cunin, G., Boissonnet, H., Petite, H., et al., "Experimental vertebroplasty using osteoconductive granular material," *Spine,* 25, 1070, 2000.

25. Barr, J.D., Barr, M.S., Lemley, T.J., and McCann, R.M., "Percutaneous vertebroplasty for pain relief and spinal stabilization," *Spine,* 25, 923, 2000.

26. Schildhauer, T.A., Bennett, A.P., Wright, T.M., et al., "Intravertebral body reconstruction with an injectable *in situ*-setting carbonated apatite: biomechanical evaluation of a minimally invasive technique," *J. Orthop. Res.,* 17, 67, 1999.

27. Lane, J.M., "Osteoporosis. Medical prevention and treatment," *Spine,* 22, 32S, 1997.

28. Eyre, D.R., "Bone biomarkers as tools in osteoporosis management," *Spine,* 22, 17S, 1997.

29. Blauth, M., Lange, U.F., Knop, C., and Bastian, L., "[Spinal fractures in the elderly and their treatment]," *Orthopade,* 29, 302, 2000.

30. Andersson, S., Rodrigues, M., and Olerud, C., "Odontoid fractures: high complication rate associated with anterior screw fixation in the elderly," *Eur. Spine J.,* 9, 56, 2000.

31. Berlemann, U. and Schwarzenbach, O., "Dens fractures in the elderly. Results of anterior screw fixation in 19 elderly patients," *Acta Orthop. Scand.,* 68, 319, 1997.

32. Paquis, P., Breuil, V., Lonjon, M., et al., "Occipitocervical fixation using hooks and screws for upper cervical instability," *Neurosurgery,* 44, 324, 1999.

33. Zink, P.M., "Performance of ventral spondylodesis screws in cervical vertebrae of varying bone mineral density," *Spine,* 21, 45, 1996.

34. Butler, T.E., Jr., Asher, M.A., Jayaraman, G., et al., "The strength and stiffness of thoracic implant anchors in osteoporotic spines," *Spine,* 19, 1956, 1994.

35. Lim, T.H., An, H.S., Evanich, C., et al., "Strength of anterior vertebral screw fixation in relationship to bone mineral density," *J. Spinal Disord.,* 8, 121, 1995.

36. Huang, T.J., Hsu, R.W., and Chen, Y.J., "Minimal-access surgery in managing osteoporotic vertebral fractures with neurologic deficits: a preliminary report," *Changgeng. Yi. Xue. Za Zhi.,* 23, 542, 2000.

37. Kumano, K., Hirabayashi, S., Ogawa, Y., and Aota, Y., "Pedicle screws and bone mineral density," *Spine,* 19, 1157, 1994.

38. Yamagata, M., Kitahara, H., Minami, S., et al., "Mechanical stability of the pedicle screw fixation systems for the lumbar spine," *Spine,* 17, S51, 1992.

39. Okuyama, K., Sato, K., Abe, E., et al., "Stability of transpedicle screwing for the osteoporotic spine. An *in vitro* study of the mechanical stability," *Spine,* 18, 2240, 1993.

40. Sjostrom, L., Jacobsson, O., Karlstrom, G., et al., "CT analysis of pedicles and screw tracts after implant removal in thoracolumbar fractures," *J. Spinal Disord.*, 6, 225, 1993.

41. Misenhimer, G.R., Peek, R.D., Wiltse, L.L., et al., "Anatomic analysis of pedicle cortical and cancellous diameter as related to screw size," *Spine*, 14, 367, 1989.

42. Hirano, T., Hasegawa, K., Washio, T., et al., "Fracture risk during pedicle screw insertion in osteoporotic spine," *J. Spinal Disord.*, 11, 493, 1998.

43. George, D.C., Krag, M.H., Johnson, C.C., et al., "Hole preparation techniques for transpedicle screws. Effect on pull-out strength from human cadaveric vertebrae," *Spine*, 16, 181, 1991.

44. Kleeman, B.C., Takeuchi, T., Gerhart, T.N., and Hayes, W.C., "Holding power and reinforcement of cancellous screws in human bone," *Clin. Orthop.*, 284, 260, 1992.

45. Zindrick, M.R., Wiltse, L.L., Widell, E.H., et al., "A biomechanical study of intrapedicular screw fixation in the lumbosacral spine," *Clin. Orthop.*, 203, 99, 1986.

46. Lotz, J.C., Hu, S.S., Chiu, D.F., et al., "Carbonated apatite cement augmentation of pedicle screw fixation in the lumbar spine," *Spine*, 22, 2716, 1997.

47. Hilibrand, A.S., Moore, D.C., and Graziano, G.P., "The role of pediculolaminar fixation in compromised pedicle bone," *Spine*, 21, 445, 1996.

48. Hasegawa, K., Takahashi, H.E., Uchiyama, S., et al., "An experimental study of a combination method using a pedicle screw and laminar hook for the osteoporotic spine," *Spine*, 22, 958, 1997.

49. McAfee, P.C., Farey, I.D., Sutterlin, C.E., et al., "1989 Volvo Award in basic science. Device-related osteoporosis with spinal instrumentation," *Spine*, 14, 919, 1989.

19 Biomechanics of Interbody Fusion in Osteoporotic Spine

Lisa A. Ferrara and William E. McCormick

CONTENTS

I. INTRODUCTION

Osteoporosis is a condition of reduced bone mass and impaired skeletal function. The most prevalent metabolic bone disease, it targets postmenopausal women and elderly individuals. It affects as many as 15 to 20 million people in the United States alone.[1] Osteoporotic fractures, including vertebral compression fractures, are estimated to occur in 33% of all North Americans in their lifetime.[2] The annual direct medical cost associated with osteoporotic fractures is approximately $13.8 billion. Furthermore, osteoporosis may contribute to numerous other spinal degenerative disorders further amplifying these costs.[3] The most common spinal complication related to osteoporotic bone is vertebral compression fractures, which have been shown to occur in as many as 50% of Caucasian females 85 years of age or older.[4]

Interbody fusion is a common surgical strategy used in spinal stabilization to provide an axial load-bearing structure to the ventral aspect of the injured spinal site. It is further utilized for a wide variety of degenerative spinal disorders. These include segmental lumbar instability, degenerative

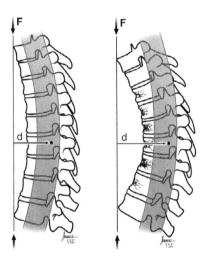

FIGURE 19.1 Illustration of (A) the natural kyphotic curvature and the neutral axis (the shaded area) of the thoracic spine and (B) a wedge compression fracture resulting from an induced ventral bending moment about the neutral axis of the spine. A wedge fracture will increase the ventral bending moment applied at the apical vertebra, thus increasing a kyphotic deformity.

disc disease, degenerative lumbar spondylolisthesis, and cervical spondylosis. Like osteoporosis, these are all conditions prevalent in the older spine. Thus, orthopaedic and neurologic surgeons must often manage patients whose degenerative spinal disease is complicated by the presence of osteoporosis. This can present a significant obstacle to achieving the goals of interbody fusion and stabilization in such patients. The decreased size and number of trabeculae indicative of the osteoporotic spine weaken the cancellous bone and may make it difficult to achieve adequate spinal fixation and fusion. There is value in understanding the biomechanics of the osteoporotic spine. Utilizing certain surgical strategies, such as multisegmental fixation, careful selection of graft type, adequate endplate preparation, optimal graft placement, and the use of laminar hooks or wires in place of or as an adjunct to pedicle screws, will improve the rate of successful fixation and interbody fusion.

A. OSTEOPOROSIS AND SPINAL FRACTURES

Osteoporosis-related spinal fractures consist of many types, including wedge compression fractures, crush fractures, and vertebral endplate fractures. Wedge compression fractures have a predilection for the thoracic spine due to its natural kyphotic curvature. They result from an induced ventral bending moment about the neutral axis of the thoracic spine, thereby creating a fracture with a loss of ventral vertebral height (Figure 19.1A and B). Progressive fracture leads to progressive loss of height of the ventral aspect of the vertebral body and may lead to a progressive kyphotic deformity.[5] Because of the natural kyphotic curvature of the thoracic spine, a kyphotic deformity that is not treated in a biomechanically sound manner with proper spinal instrumentation will further worsen the kyphosis. Hence, ventral support with an interbody graft, as well as posterior instrumentation with pedicle screws, hooks, or wires, is a common method of deformity correction.

A crush or collapse fracture is a uniform compressive fracture caused by a pure axial force at the neutral axis of the spine. These are more often seen in the lumbar region where forces can be distributed uniformly throughout the vertebral body. An endplate fracture may not involve a loss of ventral and dorsal height, but may result in a biconcave deformity due to a weakened trabecular core relative to the stronger periphery of bone at the cortical margin of the vertebrae. Lateral wedge

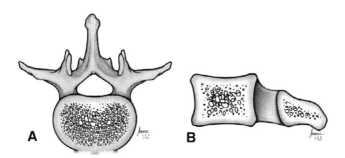

FIGURE 19.2 Illustration of the cortical shell surrounding a vertebral body: a transaxial view (A), and a sagittal view of a vertebral body (B). The cortical shell is the thickest at the margins of the vertebral body and provides significant compressive strength to the spine.

compression fractures may also occur. These often worsen a preexisting lateral deformity and progress to a symptomatic degenerative scoliosis.[6]

B. PATHOLOGIC CHANGES RELATED TO OSTEOPOROSIS AFFECT THE MECHANICAL BEHAVIOR

The spine is composed of many different types of viscoelastic tissues, including cortical bone, cancellous bone, ligamentous tissue, and the intervertebral disc. Viscoelasticity describes the mechanical characteristics of bone, ligaments, and other soft tissues relative to stress and strain.[7] This is a time-dependent and nonlinear response. In other words, the stress response of the bone or tissue is dependent on the rate at which it is deformed, i.e., strained. Furthermore, bone is an anisotropic material and applied stress will alter the bone integrity and healing rate.[8] According to the principles of Wolff's law, bone forms along the orientation of stresses and is resorbed where stress is not applied.[8]

Knowledge of the mechanical behavior related to the composite nature of the spinal column provides an understanding of the pathologic changes in the spinal elements (i.e., cortical bone, cancellous bone, intervertebral discs) that occur with aging. Morphologically, the vertebral body is a cylindrical mass consisting primarily of cancellous bone encased within a cortical shell, and the vertebral endplates are the boundaries to the vertebral bodies consisting of compact cancellous bone covered by a cartilaginous layer. Mechanically, the structural anisotropic nature of the trabeculae determines the mechanical behavior of cortical shell thickening.[7,9] The cortical shell surrounding cancellous bone contributes to the compressive strength of the spine. If the trabeculae are diminished, the central portion of the vertebral body is weakened and the cortical shell thickens in response to increased stress along the vertebral margins.[9] Edwards et al.[9] investigated the structural features and regional variations of the cortex and cancellous bone in the thoracolumbar spine. The study demonstrated a significantly greater cortical shell thickness ventrally when compared to the dorsal shell thickness along the lumbar spinal column (Figure 19.2A and B). They further discovered that a greater endplate thickness for the lumbar vertebrae was observed along the ventral and dorsal margins of the vertebral body, and was significantly thinner centrally. Endplate architecture is an important biomechanical feature to consider when choosing an interbody fusion device for placement into an osteoporotic spine.

Successful fixation and stabilization of the spine relies on the bone integrity and the biomechanical relationship at the bone–metal interface. Because bone is mechanically weaker than metal alloys, a symbiotic relationship between the two materials must exist. If the biomechanics of the host bone environment are not respected, the bone will fail, fracture, erode, wear, and resorb, causing implant loosening and eventual loss of fixation.

II. THE BIOMECHANICS OF SPINAL INSTRUMENTATION IN OSTEOPOROTIC BONE

Pedicle screw instrumentation is a common spinal stabilization procedure where rods and bone screws are placed on the dorsal portion of the spine. The instrumentation is used to reduce spinal deformities such as spondylolisthesis and scoliosis, as well as providing additional rigidity across a spinal motion segment to enhance bone fusion. Dorsal instrumentation is often implemented as supplemental fixation with interbody graft placements to help minimize micromotion across the fusion site, in turn, augmenting bony incorporation of the interbody graft. However, placement of pedicle screws into osteoporotic bone may lead to early instrumentation failure. Under repetitive cycling caused by spinal motion, screws can toggle loose out of the bone, causing loss of stabilization. Furthermore, the elastic modulus of bone is much weaker than that of metallic spinal implants, thus the transmission of force will follow the path of least resistance, causing the bone surrounding the screws to fail prior to implant breakage. This phenomenon of screw toggling and backing out of the bone results in excessive motion over the site of fixation and will lead to a pseudarthrosis. Employing interbody fusion devices or interbody bone grafts will minimize the motion across a destabilized motion segment, while providing axial load-bearing capabilities and structural support to the ventral aspect of the spine. Overall, placement of a bone graft or interbody device ventrally may alleviate the stress and the load-bearing duties of dorsally instrumented hooks and screws.

Numerous biomechanical studies have been conducted on cadaveric spines to compare spinal instrumentation and stabilization in normal and osteoporotic spines. Soshi et al.[10] performed pedicle screw pullout tests on normal and osteoporotic lumbar spines. Their data demonstrated a positive correlation between pullout force and bone mineral density (BMD). Additional studies have investigated the association between BMD and spinal fixation.[11-13] Linear positive correlations exist between BMD and screw purchase and pullout. Yamagata et al.[13] successfully exemplified a drastic reduction in implant fixation strength and screw purchase in the osteoporotic spine. Therefore, the ideal stabilizing situation for the osteoporotic spine is the question that currently needs to be addressed. Laminar hooks, as an alternative or adjunct to dorsal instrumentation, were shown to greatly improve fixation strength and pullout resistance in normal and osteoporotic spines.[12,14] Sublaminar hook fixation provided 50% greater pullout resistance than pedicle screw fixation.[14] When combined with pedicle screw fixation, the instrumentation stiffness obtained with both was significantly greater than with pedicle screws alone.[12] Therefore, an alternative for surgical stabilization in the osteoporotic spine would be the implantation of laminar hook fixation, with or without pedicle screws applied dorsally.

III. SURGICAL STRATEGIES FOR INTERBODY FUSION AND STABILIZATION IN THE OSTEOPOROTIC SPINE

A. INTERBODY GRAFT SELECTION

Ventral support through the use of an interbody graft composed of iliac crest autograft, allograft, or metal alloy provides resistance to axial forces and bending moments during spinal loading. The use of interbody grafts allows better resistance to flexion moments, minimizes motion across the spinal segment, restores disc height integrity to free neural compression, and provides a load-sharing environment between the ventral and dorsal instrumentation. In the unstable spine with a collapsed vertebral body, placement of a ventral graft provides axial support and shares the loads distributed through the vertebral bodies. In the patient with osteoporosis, the load transmitted through the spine to the graft should be shared with ventral or dorsal instrumentation due to the inability of the weakened bone to withstand such high loading parameters.

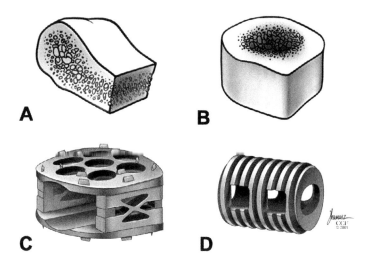

FIGURE 19.3 Types of interbody fusion grafts available: iliac crest autograft (A), femoral ring allograft (B), threaded interbody fusion cages (C), and flat-faced metallic cages (D).

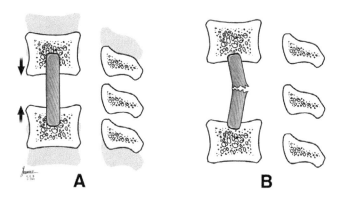

FIGURE 19.4 It is important to match the integrity of the host graft bed (vertebral body) with that of the bone graft. A bone graft that has a greater bone density than the vertebral body will have a tendency to piston its way through the endplate (A). Conversely, a bone graft that is less dense than the vertebral body will be likely to fracture (B).

Care should be taken when choosing the proper graft material. There are several types of interbody grafts, including autograft, allograft, metal-threaded interbody cages, synthetic grafts (ceramic), and flat-faced metallic or carbon fiber cages (Figure 19.3A, B, C, and D). For the osteoporotic spine, autograft usually provides the best chance for successful fusion. It is osteoinductive and osteoconductive and typically has a similar although slightly lower modulus of elasticity compared to the endplate and cancellous bone of the vertebral body. It is important to match the integrity of the bone graft bed (vertebral body) with that of the bone graft.[15] A bone graft with a significantly diminished BMD and lower modulus of elasticity may fracture or fail. Autograft taken from the iliac crest of a patient with osteoporosis may be too weak and result in early fracture after implantation. Conversely, a bone graft that is much denser than the vertebral body may piston its way through the vertebral body (Figure 19.4A and B).

If allograft is used, the elastic modulus of this bone (10 to 17 GPa) is often far greater than that of healthy cancellous bone (165 ± 110MPa) (Figure 19.3B). Therefore, the weakened bone of patients with osteoporosis may not resist the forces applied by the allograft, resulting in a pistoning of the graft through the vertebral endplates.[16] Threaded interbody fusion cages are typically composed of stainless steel (200 GPa) or titanium alloys (110 GPa) with a much greater modulus of elasticity than that of femoral ring allografts and autogenous grafts (Figure 19.3C and D). Furthermore, the cylindrical geometry of the fusion cage does not conform to the natural human curvature of the vertebral endplates, presenting limited surface area contact to the endplate for bony fusion exchange. The diminished surface area of contact creates a stress riser at the bone–cage interface. It is at this point that the force is distributed over a smaller surface area, thereby increasing the stress seen at this contact point and causing the stiffer implant to fracture through the endplate and subside within the cancellous bone. Their use in patients with osteoporosis may increase the chance of implant subsidence and fracture through the endplates due to the weakened nature of the bone, resulting in a fusion failure. Flat-faced metallic cages will perform slightly more favorably when compared with the cylindrical threaded interbody fusion cage. A larger surface area of contact is obtained with this design, distributing the load uniformly over this larger area, thus decreasing the stress at the endplates and reducing stress risers. However, a metallic implant with a significantly higher modulus of elasticity, either threaded or flat-faced in design, is not an ideal option in the osteoporotic spine. Carbon fiber cages are flat-faced cages that closely approximate the modulus of elasticity of the endplate and cancellous bone in patients with normal BMD.[17] The exchange of stress and strain at the bone–implant interface is much less than that at a metal interface. Although carbon fiber is gaining popularity in the spinal implant arena, its use in patients with osteoporosis has not been assessed.

Other types of interbody materials exist that are of a ceramic or of a polymer nature. Kaneda et al.[18] treated 22 patients with neurologic deficit due to delayed post-traumatic vertebral collapse after osteoporotic compression fractures of the thoracolumbar spine.[18] All patients underwent ventral reconstruction with a bioactive ceramic interbody graft and Kaneda instrumentation. No patients had postoperative neurologic deterioration and only one patient had graft subsidence into the vertebral body. Maintenance of kyphotic correction was superior to a similarly treated group of patients who underwent iliac crest strut graft placement.

B. INTERBODY GRAFT PLACEMENT

In general, it is best to place a ventral interbody bone graft within or slightly ventral to the neutral axis of the spine (Figure 19.5A and B).[15] The neutral axis is the longitudinal region of the spinal column that bears the axial load, where no elements ventral or dorsal to it significantly extend or compress during flexion or extension of the spine. It is usually located at the junction of the anterior and middle columns of Denis. Interbody graft placement here allows the sharing of axial loads between the ventral graft and the intact dorsal spinal elements, aiding in the prevention of spinal deformity.

Surface contact area is essential for a stable bone graft. The greater the cross-sectional area of a graft, the greater its "footprint" in the intervertebral space. This increases the area for which bony fusion can take place and distributes the axial loads over a larger surface area (Figure 19.5A and B). Since stress is a mathematical relationship between force and cross-sectional area, the greater the cross-sectional area of a graft, the smaller the stress seen over the entire graft. For this reason, relatively small diameter grafts such as fibular strut grafts, or cylindrical cages such as threaded interbody cages, may not provide an ample cross-sectional footprint to resist bending moments placed on the spine and may telescope through the endplates. Since graft subsidence is inversely proportional to the cross-sectional area of contact of the graft–vertebral body interface, maximization of the cross-sectional area of a graft will provide enhanced mechanical support and minimize the risk of subsidence.[15]

The cortical shell surrounding the cancellous bone of the vertebral body contributes greatly to the compressive strength of the spine. Cortical margining during interbody fusion refers to the attempt to place some portion of the graft toward the thicker and denser bone at the ventral portion of the vertebral endplates. A larger graft will encompass the cortical margin and provide increased stability with decreased risk of subsidence through the endplates. In the osteoporotic spine, this

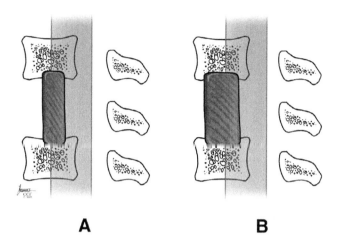

A   **B**

FIGURE 19.5 The neutral axis (the shaded area) of the spine is the region where axial loads are supported. Interbody bone grafts should be placed within or slightly ventral to the neutral axis in order to restore spinal stability (A and B). It is also important to consider the surface contact area of the bone graft. The greater the cross-sectional area of the graft, the greater the load-bearing capacity of the graft (B). Smaller diameter grafts may not provide enough surface area to distribute axial loads and will have an increased risk of subsidence (A).

potentially allows for the use of a bone graft as a spinal stabilizing device providing support and resistance to axial forces. The use of interbody fusion in the cervical spine using iliac crest bone is an excellent example of utilizing bone as a spinal implant for stabilization. These tricortical grafts can be placed with the outer cortical shell either toward the dorsal or the ventral aspect of the body when placed into the intervertebral disc space. However, if the outer cortical shell of the graft is placed ventrally, it will increase the resistance to bending moments and progressive kyphotic deformity, as well as take advantage of the boundary effect of the vertebral bodies.[19] The boundary effect is defined as the buttressing of an axial load provided by supporting a load at the edge of an inhomogeneous vertebral body that is denser at its periphery (Figure 19.6A and B).[17] Bone grafts and spinal instrumentation that take advantage of the denser bone toward these margins of the vertebral bodies will provide greater resistance to the axial forces of the spine.

Meticulous vertebral endplate preparation is essential for interbody fusion. It is important to remove as much of the disc material as possible to increase the surface area of contact and therefore promote fusion of the graft and the vertebral body. Conversely, if the host bed is compromised by overcuretting or fracturing of the endplate, there may be an increased risk of interbody subsidence. Lim et al.[20] assessed the effect of endplate thickness, endplate holes, and BMD of the vertebral body on the biomechanical strength of the endplate–graft interface in anterior interbody fusion in the cervical spine. Their study indicated that the load to failure decreased with incremental endplate removal. They also noted that load to failure of specimens with an intact endplate was significantly greater than that of specimens with no endplate.

C. MULTISEGMENTAL FIXATION

Fixation of the osteoporotic spine can be problematic. In general, interbody constructs are often enhanced with dorsal spinal instrumentation to augment the rate of fusion. One method of increasing the success of fusion and fixation in patients with osteoporosis is to utilize the concept of multi-segmental fixation.[21] Multisegmental fixation refers to the placement of additional points of fixation into the parent spine (i.e., pedicle screws, sublaminar wires) to decrease stresses seen at any one site. It uses the concept of load sharing, which is the distribution of an applied load among multiple components of an implant system.[20] This has been extensively studied in the Harrington distraction

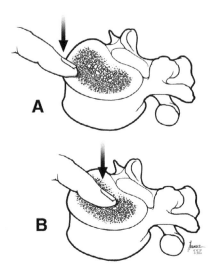

FIGURE 19.6 The dense cortical shell region of the vertebral body greatly increases the compressive strength of the spine resulting in a "boundary effect" provided by this bone. This means that the peripheral regions of the endplate are more resistant to axial loads (A). The less dense areas in the center of the vertebral body are not as effective at supporting axial loads (B).

rod (HDR) fixation. Augmentation of HDR fixation with multiple-level sublaminar wires has been shown to increase the stability and decrease the failure rate of HDR fixation.[22-25]

D. Use of Intralaminar Hooks

As mentioned previously, several biomechanical studies have shown a high correlation between bone mineral density and pedicle screw pullout resistance.[10,12,13] Studies that have assessed laminar hooks in osteoporotic spine have found that hooks greatly improve fixation and pullout resistance.[11,12,14] The dorsal laminae of the vertebral body possess a thicker cortical shell than the ventral aspect, which contributes to their success in the osteoporotic spine. The failure modes for laminar hooks were biomechanically compared to pedicle screws in the osteoporotic spine. The data showed that transpedicular screws failed predominantly by stripping the threads formed within the cancellous bone of the pedicle.[14] The laminar hooks failed mainly by breaking through the inner cortical table of the lamina, in effect, breaking the "ring" formed by the lamina, posterior vertebral body, and medial pedicle walls.[14] Ideally, if dorsal instrumentation is a necessity in the patient with osteoporosis, intralaminar hooks can be added at the distal ends of pedicle screw constructs to augment the pullout resistance of the screw and increase the chance of a successful stabilizing construct.

Whether it be hooks, wires, or screws, it is important that the instrumentation construct does not end at a kyphotic segment. This can lead to a junctional kyphosis and is a particular problem in patients with osteoporosis. Hu[6] recommends including more proximal segments in the construct to avoid this problem. This concept would increase the moment arm of the construct over the injured site to distribute the axial forces over a longer segment and reduce the stress concentration at the site of injury.

Despite the difficulties with the utilization of pedicle screws in the osteoporotic spine, often there is no other alternative to offer the patient. Particularly in the lumbar spine, decompression may be a necessary part of the surgical procedure and sublaminar wires or hooks will not provide adequate biomechanical stability.[6] Fortunately, the combination of hooks with pedicle screws and an interbody fusion device is a strategy that may optimize pedicle screw placement in the osteoporotic spine.

IV. USEFUL STRATEGIES FOR ENHANCED BIOMECHANICAL PERFORMANCE OF SPINAL INSTRUMENTATION DEVICES IN THE OSTEOPOROTIC SPINE

A. AVOIDING EXCESSIVE FORCES ON SPINAL INSTRUMENTATION PERIOPERATIVELY

Screw pullout is a significant concern in patients with osteoporosis. This usually occurs postoperatively when the patient is ambulatory and the spine is exposed to repetitive loading. However, it may also occur perioperatively while manipulating the instrumentation during insertion. Care should be taken not to expose hardware to excessive forces when pulling the rod to the screw or attempting long segment rod manipulation during deformity correction.[6] Stress risers placed on the spinal hardware during insertion will lead to early instrumentation failure.

B. TAPPING CONDITIONS FOR VERTEBRAL BONE

Cortical screws are placed after tapping to avoid microfracturing within the dense bony matrix of the cortical bone during screw insertions. Screw placement into cortical bone is often accompanied by high insertional torques representing optimal screw purchase, further contributing to increased pullout resistance. With respect to cancellous bone, tapping weakens the implant–bone interface by preventing pathologic bone compression around the screw threads and encouraging early screw toggling. Cancellous screws are commonly inserted without tapping so that the cancellous bone can be compressed during screw insertion, in turn increasing the density of bone between screw threads, which increases pullout resistance. The porous nature of cancellous bone lacks the need for tapping prior to screw insertion. Studies have demonstrated that tapping decreases pullout resistance in osteoporotic bone.[11,26] Furthermore, screw insertional torque is increased in cancellous bone if the area is devoid of tapping. The compressive effect of the bone surrounding the screw enhances the screw purchase, thus increasing the stabilizing effect of the spinal construct.

C. AUGMENTATION OF SPINAL HARDWARE PERFORMANCE WITH BONE CEMENT

Placing bone chips or polymethylmethacrylate (PMMA) into pedicle screw holes can be used to augment the integrity of the cancellous bone that may have undergone screw hole stripping intraoperatively.[26] Researchers have shown PMMA to be a feasible option for screw hole restoration when the PMMA is injected under pressure.[10,27] The addition of bone cement with pedicle screw placement into osteoporotic vertebrae led to a twofold stronger pullout force in comparison with that obtained without bone cement.

D. CROSS-FIXATION OF DORSAL SPINAL INSTRUMENTATION

Cross-fixation is the application of rigid fixation orthogonal to bilaterally placed dorsal instrumentation devices. The cross-fixation pieces are applied to the construct in a rigid or semirigid manner to make the construct perform effectively as a quadrilateral frame and eliminate the phenomenon of "parallelogramming" of the device (Figure 19.7A and B).[28] Substantially greater stiffness and stability is provided to a construct with cross-linking than those systems without, especially in torsion. Cross-fixation is a particularly advantageous addition to longer rod constructs as it prevents rods from telescoping.

E. TRIANGULATION OF SCREWS

Screw–bone interface failure may be minimized by careful choice of screw trajectory. Rigidly connecting diverging or converging screws (the concept of triangulation) provide increased pullout resistance due to the larger portions of bone that must be extracted with the implant.[26] This "triangulation effect" is optimal with the screws placed orthogonally to each other. Longer screw lengths require larger volumes of bone to be pulled, thus requiring greater pullout forces (Figure 19.8A, B, and C).

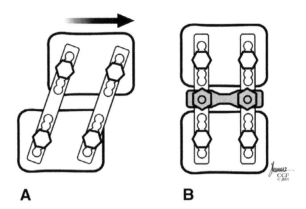

FIGURE 19.7 Cross-fixation of spinal instrumentation is needed to provide a quadrilateral frame for added spinal stability and to avoid a "parallelogramming" phenomenon of the spinal implant. If cross-fixation is not used, the construct will not be resistive to applied bending moments and translation may occur (A). Cross-fixation inhibits translational motion that may occur as a result of bending moments (B).

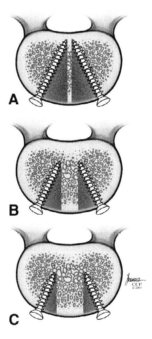

FIGURE 19.8 The triangulation effect is proportional to the bone incorporated by the screws, as indicated in the shaded areas (C). The shaded area can be increased by altering screw trajectory (B), or screw length (A), resulting in increased resistance to screw pullout.

F. EXPANDING TIP SCREWS

Expanding tip screws are screws that change configuration within the bone after insertion (Figure 19.9). The tip of the screw is allowed to expand, much like that of a wall anchoring screw found in a typical hardware store. These tips expand at angles much greater than the outer diameter of the screw, thereby increasing pullout resistance and screw performance, particularly in osteoporotic bone. [29,30]

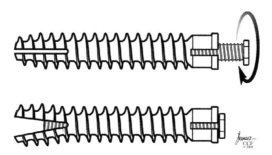

FIGURE 19.9 Illustration of an expanding tip screw. After insertion, the screw tip is expanded. This increases pullout resistance and screw performance.

G. VERTEBROPLASTY AND KYPHOPLASTY

Vertebroplasty and kyphoplasty represent newer, alternative methods of treatment for painful osteoporotic fractures. Vertebroplasty is the percutaneous injection of PMMA into a fractured vertebral body through bone biopsy needles. It is placed into the cancellous bone matrix under high pressures and allowed to cure. The modulus of elasticity of the PMMA is closer to that of bone than metal, allowing for a somewhat compatible biomechanical exchange between the bone and the PMMA. However, complications such as cement leakage and cement emboli do exist and are detrimental to the patient.[31] Kyphoplasty, a novel vertebral restoration procedure, uses current cement technology for injection into vertebral bodies; yet it involves the insertion of a balloon/bone tamp initially. The tamp creates a void in the osteoporotic bone, followed by insertion of a balloon that will inject PMMA with contrasting radiographic materials under lower pressure than vertebroplasty. Its major advantage is that it reduces the risk of cement migration by containing the material within the void and allows for correction of the kyphotic deformity. Both techniques have shown approximately a 95% improvement in pain with significant improvement in function following treatment. Kyphoplasty has been shown to improve kyphosis by over 50% in some studies.[31] Although these new techniques show promise, data obtained thus far have been from case reports and case series. Randomized clinical trials are lacking.

V. SUMMARY

In summary, the osteoporotic spine presents multiple challenges to the spine surgeon. Numerous surgical techniques may improve the rates of interbody fusion and decrease the rates of instrumentation failure in such patients, provided surgeons respect their biomechanical environment. Thorough consideration of graft type and graft placement, as well as meticulous endplate preparation, is essential for a successful interbody fusion. Other techniques, such as multisegmental fixation, the addition of laminar hooks or wires, and pedicle screw placement strategies using the concepts of screw triangulation and cross-fixation, may also increase the chance for a successful fusion. Understanding the biomechanics of the osteoporotic spine and the effects of instrumentation in osteoporotic bone may assist in the ultimate goals of successful interbody fusion and spinal fixation.

REFERENCES

1. "National Institutes of Health Consensus Development Conference: Statement on Osteoporosis," *J. Am. Med. Assoc.,* 252, 799, 1984.
2. Melton, L.J., III, "Epidemiology of vertebral fracture in women," *Am. J. Epidemiol.,* 129, 1000, 1989.
3. Wasnich, R.D., "Epidemiology of osteoporosis," in *Primer on the Metabolic Bone Diseases and Disorders of Mineral Metabolism*, 4th ed., Favus, M.J., Ed., Lippincott, Philadelphia, 1999, 257.
4. Melton, L.J., III, Lane, A.W., Cooper, C., et al., "Prevalence and incidence of vertebral deformities," *Osteoporos. Int.,* 3, 113, 1993.

5. Lane, J.M. and Bernstein, J., "Metabolic bone disorders of the spine," in *The Spine*, 4th ed., Herkowitz, H.N., Garfin, S.R., Balderston, R.A., et al., Eds., W.B. Saunders, Philadelphia, 1999, 1259.

6. Hu, S., "Internal fixation in the osteoporotic spine," *Spine*, 22, 43S, 1997.

7. Black, J., *Orthopaedic Biomaterials in Research and Practice*, Churchill Livingstone, New York, 1988.

8. Wolff, J., *Des Gesetz der Transformation der Knocken*, A. Hirschwald, Berlin, 1884.

9. Edwards, W.T., Zheng, Y., Ferrara, L.A., and Yuan, H.A., "Structural features and thickness of the vertebral cortex in the thoracolumbar spine," *Spine*, 26, 218, 2001.

10. Soshi, S., Shiba, R., Kondo, H., and Murota, K., "An experimental study on transpedicular screw fixation in relation to osteoporosis of the lumbar spine," *Spine*, 16, 1335, 1991.

11. Halvorson, T.L., Kelley, L.A., Thomas, K.A., et al., "Effects of bone mineral density on pedicle screw fixation," *Spine*, 19, 2415, 1994.

12. Hasegawa, K., Takahashi, H.E., Uchiyama, S., et al., "An experimental study of a combination method using a pedicle screw and laminar hook for the osteoporotic spine," *Spine* 22, 958, 1997.

13. Yamagata, M., Kitahara, H., Minami, S., et al., "Mechanical stability of the pedicle screw fixation systems for the lumbar spine," *Spine*, 17, S51, 1992.

14. Coe, J.D., Warden, K.E., Herzig, M.A., and McAfee, P.C., "Influence of bone mineral density on the fixation of thoracolumbar implants: a comparative study of transpedicular screws, laminar hooks, and spinous process wires," *Spine*, 15, 902, 1990.

15. Benzel, E.C., "Spinal fusion," in *Biomechanics of Spine Stabilization*, American Association of Neurologic Surgeons, Rolling Meadows, IL, 2001, 121.

16. Keaveny, T.M., Pinilla, T.P., Crawford, R.P., et al., "Systematic and random errors in compression testing of trabecular bone," *J. Orthop. Res.*, 15, 101, 1997.

17. Benzel, E.C., "Interbody constructs," in *Biomechanics of Spine Stabilization*, American Association of Neurologic Surgeons, Rolling Meadows, IL, 2001, 277.

18. Kaneda, K., Asano, S., Hashimoto, T., et al., "The treatment of osteoporotic post-traumatic vertebral collapse using the Kaneda device and a bioactive ceramic vertebral prosthesis," *Spine*, 17, 295S, 1992.

19. Benzel, E.C., "Subsidence and dynamic spine stabilization," in *Biomechanics of Spine Stabilization*, American Association of Neurologic Surgeons, Rolling Meadows, IL, 2001, 431.

20. Lim, T.H., Kwon, H., Jeon, C.H., et al., "Effect of end plate conditions and bone mineral conditions on the compressive strength of the graft–end plate interface in anterior cervical spinal fusion," *Spine*, 26, 951, 2001.

21. Benzel, E.C., "Qualitative attributes of spinal implants," in *Biomechanics of Spine Stabilization*, American Association of Neurologic Surgeons, Rolling Meadows, IL, 2001, 171,

22. Akbarnia, B.A. and Fogarty, J.P., "Contoured Harrington instrumentation in the treatment of unstable spinal fractures: the effect of supplementary sublaminar wires," *Clin. Orthop.*, 189, 186, 1984.

23. Akbarnia, B.A. and Fogarty, J.P., "New trends in surgical stabilization of thoraco-lumbar spinal fractures with emphasis for sublaminar wiring," *Paraplegia*, 23, 27, 1985.

24. Bryant, C.E. and Sullivan, J.A., "Management of thoracic and lumbar spine fractures with Harrington distraction rods supplemented with segmental wiring," *Spine*, 8, 532, 1983.

25. Munson, G. and Satterlee, C., "Experimental evaluation of Harrington rod fixation supplemented with sublaminar wires in stabilizing thoracolumbar fracture-dislocations," *Clin. Orthop.*, 189, 97, 1984.

26. Benzel, E.C., "Implant–bone interfaces," in *Biomechanics of Spine Stabilization*, American Association of Neurologic Surgeons, Rolling Meadows, IL, 2001, 155.

27. Zindrick, M.R. and Wiltse, L.L., "A biomechanical study of intrapedicular screw fixation in the lumbosacral spine," *Clin. Orthop.*, 203, 99, 1989.

28. Benzel, E.C., "Component–component interfaces," in *Biomechanics of Spine Stabilization*, American Association of Neurologic Surgeons, Rolling Meadows, IL, 2001, 143.

29. Cook, S.D. and Salkeld, S.L., "Biomechanical evaluation and preliminary clinical experience with an expansive pedicle screw design," *J. Spinal Disord.*, 7, 139, 2000.

30. Richter, M. and Wilke, H.J., "Biomechanical evaluation of a newly developed monocortical expansion screw for use in anterior internal fixation of the cervical spine: *in vitro* comparison with two established internal fixation systems," *Spine*, 24, 207, 1999.

31. Garfin, S.R., Yuan, H.A., and Reiley, M.A., "New technologies in the spine: kyphoplasty and verte-broplasty for the treatment of painful osteoporotic compression fractures," *Spine*, 26, 1511, 2001.

20 Investigations on Bone Cement for Vertebroplasty

Stephen M. Belkoff

CONTENTS

I. INTRODUCTION

Vertebroplasty is a procedure that introduces bone graft or some biomaterial, typically acrylic cement, into vertebral bodies (VBs) to augment their structural integrity.[1-10] Vertebroplasty was originally performed as an open technique to augment the purchase of pedicle screws for spinal instrumentation[11] and to fill voids resulting from tumor resection.[1,3,10,12] Percutaneous vertebroplasty (PVP), the process of injecting acrylic cement into VBs, was reportedly first performed in 1984 to stabilize a C2 vertebra invaded by an aggressive hemangioma.[13] The successful mechanical stabilization of the VB and the resulting pain relief experienced by the patient led investigators to adapt the procedure as a treatment for patients with painful vertebral compression fractures (VCFs) secondary to osteoporosis.[14] Although the procedure is being performed with increasing frequency, many basic questions regarding the efficacy and technical considerations of the procedure have only recently begun to be addressed scientifically. The results of those scientific investigations are summarized in this chapter.

II. MECHANISM OF PAIN RELIEF

Since the introduction of PVP, retrospective and prospective studies have reported pain relief in approximately 90% of patients treated for osteoporotic VCFs.[15,16] The mechanism of pain relief is currently unknown, but possible mechanisms include thermal, chemical, and mechanical interaction[17,18] with vertebral periosteal[19,20] or intraosseous pain receptors.[21]

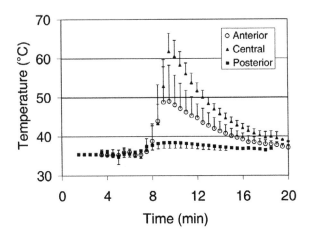

FIGURE 20.1 Average temperature increase measured by thermocouples placed at three locations in osteoporotic VBs after injection of 10 ml of PMMA cement.

A. THERMAL

When polymethylmethacrylate (PMMA) polymerizes, heat is generated in the exothermic polymerization reaction. It has been hypothesized that the heat of polymerization causes thermal necrosis of neural tissue and is therefore the mechanism responsible for pain relief.[17] Some investigators have reported temperatures as high as 122°C generated during polymerization, but the volumes of cement required to generate such temperatures are substantially greater than those typically used in PVP.[22] Thermal necrosis of osteoblasts occurs when temperatures are higher than 50°C for more than 1 min.[23,24] Neural tissue may be more sensitive to temperature than osteoblasts.[25] Thermal necrosis is governed by an Arrhenius relationship in which temperature and exposure time are factors. Thus, tissue exposed to lower temperatures, but for longer periods, may also become necrotic. A recent study has shown that osteoblasts exposed to 48°C for 10 min become apoptotic.[26] *In vivo* measurements of intravertebral temperatures during vertebroplasty are not currently available, but a recent *ex vivo* study has suggested that temperature is not a mechanism of pain relief.[27]

In that study, temperature was measured at three locations (inside the anterior cortex, centrally, and in the spinal canal) after concurrent bipedicular injection of 10 ml of PMMA cement. Although temperatures exceeded 50°C for more than 1 min at the center of the VB (Figure 20.1), the authors concluded that temperature was an unlikely mechanism of pain relief for several reasons. First, because the experiments were conducted on *ex vivo* VBs, the effect of active heat transfer due to blood perfusion was not included, as would be the case *in vivo* where perfusion would be expected to transfer much of the heat generated during cement polymerization. Second, the volume of cement injected was greater than that typically used for PVP.[28] And third, the cement was injected concurrently via both pedicles to maximize the thermal effect for experimental measurement. Clinically, it is injected more slowly.[18] Thus, the heat of polymerization from the initial injection would likely have diminished before the end of the procedure. For these reasons, it seems unlikely that temperature plays a role in pain relief. In addition, it has been reported that temperatures recorded in the spinal canal do not rise above 40°C;[27] therefore, the spinal cord appears to be at little risk of thermal injury as long as the cement is properly injected and contained within the VB.

B. CHEMICAL

It has also been suggested that the methylmethacrylate (MMA) monomer mixed with the PMMA cement is cytotoxic and is therefore a mechanism of pain relief.[17] Cell culture studies have shown that MMA monomer is toxic to leukocytes and endothelial cells when concentrations exceed 10 mg/ml,[29] but its effect on neural tissue remains unknown. During knee arthroplasty, blood serum levels immediately after cementation and tourniquet release have been measured as high as 120 µg/ml, but they are typically much lower (<2 µg/ml) and drop precipitously minutes after implantation.[30] Other investigators have reported blood serum concentration between 0.02 and 59 µg/ml during total hip replacement.[31] Considering that the volumes of cement used for total hip replacements and knee arthroplasty are two to three times greater than those typically used with PVP, and that monomer concentrations measured for those procedures are 10 to 100 times less than MMA concentrations reported to be cytotoxic to tissue cultures,[29] it seems unlikely that MMA toxicity is responsible for pain relief experienced with PVP. Even so, local serum monomer concentrations measured immediately after PVP are needed to determine definitively if MMA monomer cytotoxicity plays a role in pain relief.

C. MECHANICAL

Mechanical stabilization appears to be the most likely mechanism of pain relief. Pain associated with osteoporotic VCF is thought to be caused by motion at the fracture, which stimulates nociceptors concentrated in the periosteal region.[18] PVP stabilizes the fractured vertebral body,[32-34] minimizing micromotion, and thus preventing such nerve stimulation. By so doing, PVP achieves the goals of fracture stabilization consistent with those of other sites in the body, namely, to prevent painful micromotion and to provide a mechanically stable and biologically conducive environment in which fracture healing can occur. The mechanical stabilization provided by PVP is a function of the volume of cement injected and the material properties of the cement, but the optimal cement volume and material properties have not yet been determined. As with other types of fractures, stabilization depends on the bone material properties.

III. MECHANICAL STABILIZATION

A. VOLUME FILL

A recent *ex vivo* study reported that only 2 ml of PMMA was needed to restore strength in osteoporotic VBs (Figure 20.2), but that larger volumes (4 to 6 ml) were needed to restore stiffness.[35] These volumes are lower than what was previously thought to be necessary. Restoring initial strength would be expected to prevent refracture of the treated vertebra. If the spine were subjected to a load equal to that required to cause the original fracture, other vertebral levels would be expected to fracture before the repaired level refractured. Stiffness, not strength, is the mechanical parameter likely most closely linked with pain relief. Fixation stiffness also plays a large role in fracture healing,[36] yet restoring VB stiffness to prefracture levels may not be necessary or even desirable.[36] As with other fractures, the provision of some mechanical stability, even if less than that of the intact state, may be sufficient to allow healing. If the repair is too stiff, stress shielding may occur and may impede fracture healing. Furthermore, a repair resulting in greater stiffness than in adjacent levels hypothetically creates a stress concentration and may place those adjacent levels at risk of fracture. A preliminary clinical report has suggested that there is no higher incidence of fractures in adjacent levels than in remote levels.[37] On the other hand, if the repair is not stiff enough, excessive motion at the fracture site may occur and result in nonunion. For VCFs, the "internal splint" achieved by the injected cement may provide an appropriate mechanical environment in which healing can occur. The volume and material properties of cement needed to achieve "appropriate stabilization" have not yet been determined *in vivo*.

In one study, pain relief was experienced in 90% of patients (n = 29) whose VBs were injected with an average volume of 7.1 ml (2.2 to 11.0 ml) of PMMA.[15] In a recent clinical study, investigators

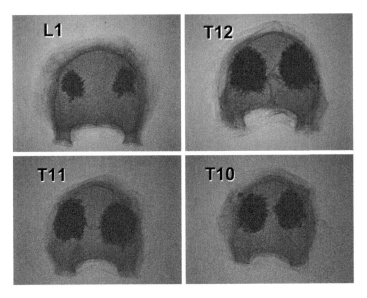

FIGURE 20.2 Radiograph of osteoporotic VBs injected with 4 ml (lower right T10), 6 ml (lower left T11), 8 ml (upper right T12), and 2 ml (upper left L1) to investigate the relationship between cement volume and restoration of mechanical properties.

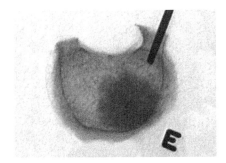

FIGURE 20.3 Unipedicular injection of 6 ml of PMMA cement into an osteoporotic VB.

reported that injection of 2 to 3 ml into the thoracic and 3 to 5 ml into the lumbar regions resulted in 97% moderate to complete pain relief.[38] These results suggest that pain relief may be achieved with volumes consistent with those needed to restore mechanical integrity *ex vivo*;[35] however, no correlation of level treated, volume injected, and clinical outcome has been explicitly reported. The volume of cement needed to produce a desired outcome still needs to be determined by a carefully controlled, prospective, randomized clinical study.

B. UNIPEDICULAR VS. BIPEDICULAR INJECTION

It may not be necessary to inject cement bipedicularly to achieve adequate stabilization. Tohmeh et al.[34] found that VB strength may be restored via a unipedicular cement injection of 6 ml without risk of VB collapse on the uninjected side (Figure 20.3). Unipedicular injection may result in reduced procedure time and risk associated with bilateral cannula placement. The unipedicular procedure has been performed on a limited number of patients, and the clinical outcomes have been encouraging.[38]

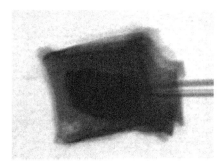

FIGURE 20.4 Inflatable bone tamp used to elevate collapsed VB end plates and create a void for subsequent fill.

C. Height Restoration

Height restoration has the potential benefit of reducing postfracture kyphosis and its associated sequelae.[19,39-42] There are no reports of height restoration subsequent to PVP *in vivo*. An *ex vivo* study of osteoporotic VBs that were compressed to create simulated fractures and were repaired with PVP suggested that half of the compressed height recovers elastically.[43] A similar phenomenon has been reported *in vivo*.[44] When the *ex vivo* specimens were repaired using PVP, approximately 30% of the permanent height loss was recovered.[43] A new device, the inflatable bone tamp (Figure 20.4), has been developed as a means of restoring height.[43,45] This tamp is placed inside the VB under fluoroscopic guidance via a percutaneously introduced cannula and is inflated, thereby compressing the cancellous bone, creating a void, and concurrently lifting the end plates in an *en masse* reduction. The void can be filled under lower pressure than that needed for PVP, thereby allowing alternative void fillers to be used. This procedure has been termed kyphoplasty. *Ex vivo* tests have suggested that the tamp treatment restores significantly more height than does standard PVP treatment, and yet it achieves similar mechanical restoration.[43,45] It is unknown if similar height restoration can be achieved *in vivo*.

IV. CEMENT CONSIDERATIONS

There is currently no commercially available cement specifically designed for PVP, and only Simplex P® (Stryker-Howmedica-Osteonics, Rutherford, NJ) has approval from the Food and Drug Administration (FDA) for use for pathologic fractures, including those of the spine. Clinicians routinely alter the composition of the cements by increasing the monomer-to-copolymer ratio to increase working time and decrease viscosity,[15,46-48] adding radiopacifiers to increase cement visualization under fluoroscopy,[15,46-48] and adding antibiotics.[15] These modifications make the cements more applicable to the practice of vertebroplasty but also void any FDA approval.

A. Monomer/Powder Ratio

Increasing the monomer-to-copolymer ratio decreases the compressive material properties of the cement[48-50] (Figure 20.5). Most PMMA cements are prepackaged for mixing 0.5 ml of monomer with 1 g of powder, or with a monomer-to-powder ratio of 0.5 ml/g. This mixture typically results in a cement with maximum compressive properties. Because $BaSO_4$ is often present in radiopaque cements (usually 10% by weight) as part of the powder, the ratio of monomer to copolymer is approximately 0.56 ml/g. When $BaSO_4$ is added to increase opacity for use in PVP, an equal mass of powder typically is removed and replaced with $BaSO_4$, thus altering the monomer-to-copolymer ratio. Usually, the monomer-to-copolymer ratio is increased to 0.72 ml/g. This increased monomer volume is needed to wet the powder, but not all of the extra monomer is involved in the polymerization

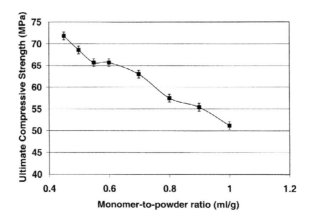

FIGURE 20.5 Increasing the monomer-to-polymer ratio decreases the material properties of the cement.

process. Thus, there is an increased amount of unbound monomer available to enter the circulatory system. Although the ratio of monomer to copolymer is greater, the quantity of cement injected (<10 ml) is smaller than that for hip arthrodesis (>40 ml).[30,31,51] For this reason, the actual blood serum concentration of monomer during PVP may be lower than that measured during total hip arthrodesis.

B. RADIOPACIFICATION

Altering the concentration of radiopacifiers affects the cement material properties, as does the combined alteration of monomer-to-powder ratio and opacification.[48] Although these modifications significantly alter the material properties of the cement,[48] there have been no reported clinical problems associated with cement material properties. In a recent study,[48] the cement composition exhibiting the minimum relative material properties was the composition that has been used clinically during the past decade in the United States with no complications associated with mechanical failure of the cement.[15] Thus, using a cement that can be injected easily and with proper opacification appears to take precedence over maintaining the ultimate material properties of the cement.

Proper fluoroscopic visualization during cement injection is essential for the safe practice of PVP (Figure 20.6). Extravasation of the cement is a risk of the procedure and may result in clinical complications.[15,52-54] As a general guide, approximately 30% of the dry cement component weight should be an opacifying agent to visualize the cement under fluoroscopy and to prevent extravasation.

C. ANTIBIOTICS

For immunocompromised patients, some clinicians routinely add antibiotics to the cement mixture.[15] The effect of adding antibiotics on the material properties of cement prepared for use in vertebroplasty is unknown, although it has been shown that adding antibiotics to PMMA cement used in arthroplasty does not affect its fatigue properties.[55] The efficacy of adding antibiotics to cement to reduce the risk of infection during PVP is unknown.

D. ALTERNATIVE CEMENTS

New types of cements and injection devices are being developed for use with vertebroplasty.[33,56-59] These cements are bioactive or bioresorbable,[56,58,60] are naturally radiopaque,[48,58] and have a non-existent exothermic reaction,[56,58] or one lower than that of PMMA cements.[27]

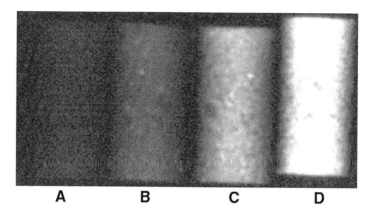

FIGURE 20.6 Optical density of PMMA cement (Simplex P) with 10% $BaSO_4$ (A), 20% $BaSO_4$ (B), and 30% $BaSO_4$ (C), and of Simplex P with 10% $BaSO_4$ and 18% tantalum powder (D).

The calcium-phosphate class of cements has proved difficult to inject,[56] although progress is being made in this area.[58] A recent study reported the successful injection of calcium carbonate (coral) into osteoporotic VBs. Details of the injection process were not given, nor were the mechanical effects of the augmentation with coral measured.[59] These more "biocompatible" cements may eliminate concerns about thermal necrosis and cytotoxicity and appear to result in mechanical stabilization of fractured VBs similar to that of PMMA.[58] Yet, if such mechanisms are determined to play a role in pain relief, then the non-PMMA cements may not be as effective. The bioresorbable cements are appealing for use in prophylactic augmentation because injected VBs would be mechanically augmented immediately and theoretically would provide an osteoconductive material for subsequent bone repair and remodeling.[59] It is unknown, however, whether the VB would once again be at risk of fracture after the cement is remodeled or resorbed. These issues are all topics worthy of investigation.

REFERENCES

1. Alleyne, C.H., Jr., Rodts, G.E., Jr., and Haid, R.W., "Corpectomy and stabilization with methylmethacrylate in patients with metastatic disease of the spine: a technical note," *J. Spinal Disord.*, 8, 439, 1995.
2. Cortet, B., Cotten, A., Deprez, X., et al., "[Value of vertebroplasty combined with surgical decompression in the treatment of aggressive spinal angioma. Apropos of 3 cases]," *Rev. Rhum. Ed. Fr.*, 61, 16, 1994.
3. Cybulski, G.R., "Methods of surgical stabilization for metastatic disease of the spine," *Neurosurgery*, 25, 240, 1989.
4. Harrington, K.D., Sim, F.H., Enis, J.E., et al., "Methylmethacrylate as an adjunct in internal fixation of pathologic fractures. Experience with three hundred and seventy-five cases," *J. Bone Joint Surg.*, 58A, 1047, 1976.
5. Harrington, K.D., "Anterior decompression and stabilization of the spine as a treatment for vertebral collapse and spinal cord compression from metastatic malignancy," *Clin. Orthop.*, 233, 177, 1988.
6. Knight, G., "Paraspinal acrylic inlays in the treatment of cervical and lumbar spondylosis and other conditions," *Lancet*, 2, 147, 1959.
7. Mavian, G.Z. and Okulski, C.J., "Double fixation of metastatic lesions of the lumbar and cervical vertebral bodies utilizing methylmethacrylate compound: report of a case and review of a series of cases," *J. Am. Osteopath. Assoc.*, 86, 153, 1986.
8. O'Donnell, R.J., Springfield, D.S., Motwani, H.K., et al., "Recurrence of giant-cell tumors of the long bones after curettage and packing with cement," *J. Bone Joint Surg.*, 76A, 1827, 1994.

9. Persson, B.M., Ekelund, L., Lovdahl, R., et al., "Favourable results of acrylic cementation for giant cell tumors," *Acta Orthop. Scand.*, 55, 209, 1984.

10. Sundaresan, N., Galicich, J.H., Lane, J.M., et al., "Treatment of neoplastic epidural cord compression by vertebral body resection and stabilization," *J. Neurosurg.*, 63, 676, 1985.

11. Kostuik, J.P., Errico, T.J., and Gleason, T.F., "Techniques of internal fixation for degenerative conditions of the lumbar spine," *Clin. Orthop.*, 203, 219, 1986.

12. Scoville, W.B., Palmer, A.H., Samra, K., et al., "The use of acrylic plastic for vertebral replacement or fixation in metastatic disease of the spine. Technical note," *J. Neurosurg.*, 27, 274, 1967.

13. Galibert, P., Deramond, H., Rosat, P., et al., "[Preliminary note on the treatment of vertebral angioma by percutaneous acrylic vertebroplasty]," *Neurochirurgie*, 33, 166, 1987.

14. Lapras, C., Mottolese, C., Deruty, R., et al., "[Percutaneous injection of methyl-metacrylate in osteoporosis and severe vertebral osteolysis (Galibert's technic)]," *Ann. Chir.*, 43, 371, 1989.

15. Jensen, M.E., Evans, A.J., Mathis, J.M., et al., "Percutaneous polymethylmethacrylate vertebroplasty in the treatment of osteoporotic vertebral body compression fractures: technical aspects," *Am. J. Neuroradiol.*, 18, 1897, 1997.

16. Cyteval, C., Sarrabere, M.P., Roux, J.O., et al., "Acute osteoporotic vertebral collapse: open study on percutaneous injection of acrylic surgical cement in 20 patients," *Am. J. Roentgenol.*, 173, 1685, 1999.

17. Bostrom, M.P.G. and Lane, J.M., "Future directions. Augmentation of osteoporotic vertebral bodies," *Spine*, 22, 38S, 1997.

18. Deramond, H., Depriester, C., Galibert, P., et al., "Percutaneous vertebroplasty with polymethylmethacrylate. Technique, indications, and results," *Radiol. Clin. North Am.*, 36, 533, 1998.

19. Silverman, S.L., "The clinical consequences of vertebral compression fracture," *Bone*, 13, S27, 1992.

20. Gennari, C., Agnusdei, D., and Camporeale, A., "Use of calcitonin in the treatment of bone pain associated with osteoporosis," *Calcif. Tissue Int.*, 49, S9, 1991.

21. Antonacci, M.D., Mody, D.R., and Heggeness, M.H., "Innervation of the human vertebral body: a histologic study," *J. Spinal Disord.*, 11, 526, 1998.

22. Jefferiss, C.D., Lee, A.J.C., and Ling, R.S.M., "Thermal aspects of self-curing polymethylmethacrylate," *J. Bone Joint Surg.*, 57B, 511, 1975.

23. Eriksson, R.A., Albrektsson, T., and Magnusson, B., "Assessment of bone viability after heat trauma. A histologic, histochemical and vital microscopic study in the rabbit," *Scand. J. Plast. Reconstr. Surg.*, 18, 261, 1984.

24. Rouiller, C. and Majno, G., "Morphologische und chemische Untersuchung an Knochen nach Hitzeeinwirkung," *Beitr. Pathol. Anat. Allg. Pathol.*, 113, 100, 1953.

25. De Vrind, H.H., Wondergem, J., and Haveman, J., "Hyperthermia-induced damage to rat sciatic nerve assessed *in vivo* with functional methods and with electrophysiology," *J. Neurosci. Methods*, 45, 165, 1992.

26. Li, S., Chien, S., and Branemark, P.I., "Heat shock-induced necrosis and apoptosis in osteoblasts," *J. Orthop. Res.*, 17, 891, 1999.

27. Deramond, H., Wright, N.T., and Belkoff, S.M., "Temperature elevation caused by bone cement polymerization during vertebroplasty," *Bone*, 25, 17S, 1999.

28. Cotten, A., Dewatre, F., Cortet, B., et al., "Percutaneous vertebroplasty for osteolytic metastases and myeloma: effects of the percentage of lesion filling and the leakage of methyl methacrylate at clinical follow-up," *Radiology*, 200, 525, 1996.

29. Dahl, O.E., Garvik, L.J., and Lyberg, T., "Toxic effects of methylmethacrylate monomer on leukocytes and endothelial cells *in vitro* [published erratum appears in *Acta Orthop. Scand.*, 66, 387, 1995]," *Acta Orthop. Scand.*, 65, 147, 1994.

30. Svartling, N., Pfaffli, P., and Tarkkanen, L., "Blood levels and half-life of methylmethacrylate after tourniquet release during knee arthroplasty," *Arch. Orthop. Trauma Surg.*, 105, 36, 1986.

31. Wenda, K., Scheuermann, H., Weitzel, E., et al., "Pharmacokinetics of methylmethacrylate monomer during total hip replacement in man," *Arch. Orthop. Trauma Surg.*, 107, 316, 1988.

32. Belkoff, S.M., Maroney, M., Fenton, D.C., et al., "An *in vitro* biomechanical evaluation of bone cements used in percutaneous vertebroplasty," *Bone*, 25, 23S, 1999.

33. Belkoff, S.M., Mathis, J.M., Erbe, E.M., et al., "Biomechanical evaluation of a new bone cement for use in vertebroplasty," *Spine*, 25, 1061, 2000.

34. Tohmeh, A.G., Mathis, J.M., Fenton, D.C., et al., "Biomechanical efficacy of unipedicular *versus* bipedicular vertebroplasty for the management of osteoporotic compression fractures," *Spine*, 24, 1772, 1999.

35. Belkoff, S.M., Mathis, J.M., Jasper, L.E., et al., "The biomechanics of vertebroplasty: the effect of cement volume on mechanical behavior," *Spine*, 26, 1537, 2001.

36. Terjesen, T. and Apalset, K., "The influence of different degrees of stiffness of fixation plates on experimental bone healing," *J. Orthop. Res.*, 6, 293, 1988.

37. Jensen, M.E., Kallmes, D.F., Short, J.G., et al., "Percutaneous vertebroplasty does not increase the risk of adjacent vertebral fracture — a retrospective study," presented at the 38th Annual Meeting of the American Society of Neuroradiology, Atlanta, April 3, 2000.

38. Barr, J.D., Barr, M.S., Lemley, T.J., et al., "Percutaneous vertebroplasty for pain relief and spinal stabilization," *Spine*, 25, 923, 2000.

39. Lyles, K.W., Gold, D.T., Shipp, K.M., et al., "Association of osteoporotic vertebral compression fractures with impaired functional status," *Am. J. Med.*, 94, 595, 1993.

40. Schlaich, C., Minne, H.W., Bruckner, T., et al., "Reduced pulmonary function in patients with spinal osteoporotic fractures," *Osteoporos. Int.*, 8, 261, 1998.

41. Leech, J.A., Dulberg, C., Kellie, S., et al., "Relationship of lung function to severity of osteoporosis in women," *Am. Rev. Respir. Dis.*, 141, 68, 1990.

42. Leidig-Bruckner, G., Minne, H.W., Schlaich, C., et al., "Clinical grading of spinal osteoporosis: quality of life components and spinal deformity in women with chronic low back pain and women with vertebral osteoporosis," *J. Bone Miner. Res.*, 12, 663, 1997.

43. Belkoff, S.M., Mathis, J.M., Fenton, D.C., et al., "An *ex vivo* biomechanical evaluation of an inflatable bone tamp used in the treatment of compression fracture," *Spine*, 26, 151, 2001.

44. Nelson, D.A., Kleerekoper, M., and Peterson, E.L., "Reversal of vertebral deformities in osteoporosis: measurement error or 'rebound'?" *J. Bone Miner. Res.*, 9, 977, 1994.

45. Wilson, D.R., Myers, E.R., Mathis, J.M., et al., "Effect of augmentation on the mechanics of vertebral wedge fractures," *Spine*, 25, 158, 2000.

46. Cotten, A., Boutry, N., Cortet, B., et al., "Percutaneous vertebroplasty: state of the art," *Radiographics*, 18, 311, 1998.

47. Deramond, H., Depriester, C., Toussaint, P., et al., "Percutaneous vertebroplasty," *Semin. Musculoskelet. Radiol.*, 1, 285, 1997.

48. Jasper, L.E., Deramond, H., Mathis, J.M., et al., "Material properties of various cements for use with vertebroplasty," *J. Mater. Sci. Mater. Med.*, 13, 1, 2002.

49. Jasper, L.E., Deramond, H., Mathis, J.M., et al., "The effect of monomer-to-powder ratio on the material properties of Cranioplastic," *Bone*, 25, 27S, 1999.

50. Belkoff, S.M. and Sanders, J.C., "The effect of the monomer/powder ratio on the mechanical properties of acrylic bone cement," *J. Biomed. Mater. Res.*, 63, 369, 2002.

51. Svartling, N., Pfaffli, P., and Tarkkanen, L., "Methylmethacrylate blood levels in patients with femoral neck fracture," *Arch. Orthop. Trauma Surg.*, 104, 242, 1985.

52. Padovani, B., Kasriel, O., Brunner, P., et al., "Pulmonary embolism caused by acrylic cement: a rare complication of percutaneous vertebroplasty," *Am. J. Neuroradiol.*, 20, 375, 1999.

53. Wilkes, R.A., MacKinnon, J.G., and Thomas, W.G., "Neurologic deterioration after cement injection into a vertebral body," *J. Bone Joint Surg.*, 76B, 155, 1994.

54. Perrin, C., Jullien, V., Padovani, B., et al., "[Percutaneous vertebroplasty complicated by pulmonary embolus of acrylic cement]," *Rev. Mal Respir.*, 16, 215, 1999.

55. Davies, J.P., O'Connor, D.O., Burke, D.W., et al., "Influence of antibiotic impregnation on the fatigue life of Simplex P and Palacos R acrylic bone cements, with and without centrifugation," *J. Biomed. Mater. Res.*, 23, 379, 1989.

56. Schildhauer, T.A., Bennett, A.P., Wright, T.M., et al., "Intravertebral body reconstruction with an injectable *in situ*-setting carbonated apatite: biomechanical evaluation of a minimally invasive technique," *J. Orthop. Res.*, 17, 67, 1999.

57. Mermelstein, L.E., McLain, R.F., and Yerby, S.A., "Reinforcement of thoracolumbar burst fractures with calcium phosphate cement. A biomechanical study," *Spine*, 23, 664, 1998.

58. Bai, B., Jazrawi, L.M., Kummer, F.J., et al., "The use of an injectable, biodegradable calcium phosphate bone substitute for the prophylactic augmentation of osteoporotic vertebrae and the management of vertebral compression fractures," *Spine*, 24, 1521, 1999.

59. Cunin, G., Boissonnet, H., Petite, H., et al., "Experimental vertebroplasty using osteoconductive granular material," *Spine*, 25, 1070, 2000.

60. Fujita, H., Nakamura, T., Tamura, J., et al., "Bioactive bone cement: effect of the amount of glass-ceramic powder on bone-bonding strength," *J. Biomed. Mater. Res.*, 40, 145, 1998.

21 Percutaneous Vertebroplasty — Therapy for Painful Osteoporotic Compression Fractures

John M. Mathis and Hervé Deramond

CONTENTS

I. INTRODUCTION

Vertebroplasty is a term that has for decades described a surgical procedure in which bone graft, cement, or metal implants are used to modify or reconstruct damaged or destroyed vertebra.[1-12] In such procedures, polymethylmethacrylate (PMMA) has been the cement most often used for reconstruction and augmentation of bone damaged by trauma or tumor invasion.[1,3,11,12]

Shortly after Galibert et al.[13] performed the first percutaneous vertebroplasty (PV) in 1984 by injecting PMMA into a C2 vertebra destroyed by an aggressive vertebral hemangioma (VH), Dusquenel adapted the procedure to treat pain from vertebral compression fractures (VCFs) associated with osteoporosis and malignancy.[14] In 1991, Debussche-Depriester et al.[15] published the results of a small series, reporting good pain relief in five patients whose osteoporotic VCFs had been treated with PV. Even though the procedure was known to be useful for osteoporotic VCFs, its early use in Europe was focused on the treatment for pain resulting from tumors of the spine.

The procedure was introduced into the United States in 1993 where investigators focused primarily on osteoporotic VCFs and subsequently provided the first clinical series for PV in the United States.[16] This report noted pain relief and increased mobility in 90% of patients treated for osteoporotic VCFs, a finding similar to that of early reports on PV in Europe. Since that time, the procedure has grown in popularity and is now becoming the standard of care for pain produced by osteoporotic VCFs.

The osteoporotic population at risk of fracture is huge, and more than 700,000 VCFs result each year from osteoporosis alone (Figure 21.1).[17] The incidence of VCFs exceeds that for hip fractures, and the annual number of all types of fractures secondary to osteoporosis is more than 1.5 million.[17,18] The incidence of osteoporosis is greatest in Caucasian, elderly women, and the

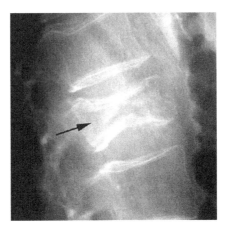

FIGURE 21.1 Radiograph of a compressed lumbar vertebra (arrow). This appearance is not unusual for an osteoporotic fracture. There is loss of height of the posterior wall in addition to the height loss in the anterior body. A simple fracture is defined as having preservation of the posterior wall but this part of a vertebra often fails too. There also is a central vertical fracture that will make this vertebra more prone to leak cement into the disc space during vertebroplasty.

number of affected individuals is growing yearly.[18,19] In addition, substantial numbers of fractures occur in men and in patients receiving steroids for conditions such as cancer, collagen vascular disease, immunosuppression in transplant therapy, and severe allergy or asthma.

PV is indicated for patients with pain from VCFs resulting from the weakening associated with bone mineral loss secondary to osteoporosis and who are not effectively treated by nonoperative therapy (i.e., analgesics, bed rest, external bracing, etc.).[16,20-28] Without PV, pain in such individuals typically lasts from 2 weeks to 3 months.[29] The chronic debilitation, limitation of activity, and decline in quality of life secondary to these fractures have been shown to result in depression and loss of self-esteem, as well as physical impairment. Recent data reveal that patients with VCFs have a higher mortality rate than age-matched controls.[30]

This chapter concentrates on the selection and treatment of patients with PV having presented with osteoporotic VCFs.

II. PATIENT WORKUP AND SELECTION

Some osteoporotic fractures may produce only mild pain or may demonstrate a rapid decrease in the initially severe pain after fracture. In either of these situations, PV is not usually indicated. However, persistent pain that limits the activities of daily living or requires narcotic analgesics (with or without hospitalization) may be rapidly improved with the use of PV. The time between fracture and therapy may vary because of failed attempts at nonoperative management or delayed referral. Patients with severe disability who require hospitalization and parenteral analgesics may be treated immediately. Others may present later with chronic, persistent pain and limitation of normal activity. There are no absolute exclusion criteria based on the time between fracture and PV. Old fractures are less likely to benefit from PV unless one can show signs of nonunion or instability with persistent fracture motion noted on fluoroscopy, osteonecrosis (Kummell disease), or persistent marrow edema on magnetic resonance (MR) images (which may indicate new or recurrent fracture). Preoperative augmentation of vertebra before instrumentation and routine prophylactic use of PV has not been validated for efficacy and should be used with extreme caution under investigational protocols.

On physical examination, the patient's pain should be appropriate to the fracture considered for treatment with PV, or the pain should be anatomically localized to (not remote from) the fracture

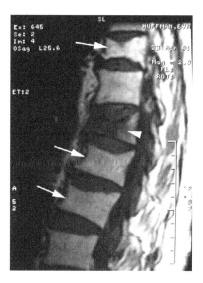

FIGURE 21.2 Sagittal MRI (T1 weighted) showing both acute and chronic compression fractures. The acute fracture (white arrowhead) shows loss of signal in the marrow space consistent with marrow edema. The chronic fractures (white arrows) show a normal signal to the marrow, similar to other noncompressed vertebra in this image. This information is vital for being able to select the appropriate level for vertebroplasty.

site. For example, a T10 fracture should have pain at this same level by patient description and local palpation of the posterior element of the spine or to local percussion. The pain should not be radicular, because such pain suggests nerve root compression. However, it is not uncommon to have referred pain (e.g., referred intercostal pain associated with a thoracic vertebral fracture or referred pelvic and hip pain associated with a lower lumbar fracture). These should not be considered a contraindication to treatment. Patients with simple physical findings that are well correlated with recent diagnostic images may be treated without additional complex studies such as MR imaging, computerize tomography (CT), or nuclear medicine.

Patients with previous fractures or nonfocal pain are often diagnostic dilemmas and require a more complex imaging evaluation. These patients should undergo MR imaging in addition to a standard radiographic evaluation. Acute fractures will be easily shown on T1-weighted sagittal images as having loss of signal in the affected vertebral marrow space (Figure 21.2). Short tau inversion recovery images with fat suppression are less routine but also offer high sensitivity for recent fracture and marrow edema (represented by abnormally bright signal in this sequence). Images made with T2 weighting only occasionally give additional information. On T1-weighted MR imaging sequences, normal marrow exhibits high (bright) signal, including vertebra that were previously compressed and that have undergone healing (Figure 21.2). One should be reluctant to perform PV for pain without being able to visualize an acute fracture or persistent marrow abnormality on MR images.

If MR imaging cannot be performed, then a nuclear medicine bone scan may be utilized. However, nuclear medicine may not be as useful as MR imaging for routine screening because it has poorer anatomic resolution and does not give information about associated conditions such as spinal stenosis or disc herniation. Also, abnormal activity on a bone scan may persist long after healing has been shown on an MR image. Such a positive scan may indicate only normal and continued healing and may mislead the physician about the possible benefit of PV.[31] However, there is a definite place for nuclear medicine in patient evaluation. For a patient who cannot tolerate MR imaging, nuclear medicine becomes the next best alternative. In the rare instance that information from the MR image is insufficient for accurately localizing an acute fracture, as usually occurs in a very inhomogeneous marrow (e.g., as a normal variation in elderly individuals or with conditions such as myeloma), nuclear medicine usually contributes sufficient information for identification of appropriate vertebra for PV.

CT offers high-quality anatomic information (as do standard radiographs) but is unable to distinguish acute from chronic fractures under most circumstances. Therefore, CT is not part of the routine initial patient workup. However, CT does have a potential pre- and postprocedural role in PV as it can demonstrate useful anatomic information and locate complications such as cement leaks outside the vertebral body.

The degree of compression does not necessarily correlate with the amount of local pain. Minimal compressions may be the cause of incapacitating pain in some individuals. In such cases there may be minimal radiographic evidence of deformity. However, acute fractures are easily identified on MR imaging because these vertebrae have local marrow edema. An MR image may also show more than one acute compression injury; in such a situation, therapy at each of the involved and painful levels is required. As the amount of compression increases, so does the degree of technical difficulty of performing PV. With complete or near-complete vertebral collapse, the likelihood of successful PV is reduced but not eliminated.[31] Before attempting PV in a near-complete collapse, an MR image should be obtained to rule out other possible sources of persistent pain. When attempting to treat these lesions, the patient should be made aware that there is a reduced chance of pain relief (compared with the results of a modestly compressed vertebral fracture) and a higher risk of complication.

The age of the VCF is not of great importance as long as there is local pain consistent with the site of compression and persistent marrow edema on MR imaging, as can be the case in VCFs that are months old. However, with a normal MR image or nuclear medicine scan, the chance of pain relief becomes very low, and the PV should be avoided except under unusual circumstances.

PV has been shown to be very durable. However, on rare occasions one may see a refracture with progressive height loss after PV. This scenario usually occurs in a patient who had a less than optimum fill during an initial treatment (even in the presence of initially good pain relief). Pain relief and cement filling are poorly correlated. The recurrence of pain, marrow edema, and additional vertebral collapse may indicate the need for repeat treatment.

Patients selected for PV should have normal coagulation test results and should not be taking coumadin. Coumadin may be discontinued and replaced with enoxaparin (Lovenox, Rhone-Poulenc Rorer, Collegeville, PA) and given once or twice per day on an outpatient basis. Coumadin may also be stopped and replaced with heparin, but this medication must be given intravenously, requiring hospital admission. Both enoxaparin and heparin can be reversed with protamine sulfate before PV and restarted postprocedure. Aspirin use is not a contraindication to the procedure. The procedure is not recommended in the patient with signs of an active infection, but elevated white counts clearly associated with medical conditions such as myeloma or secondary to steroid use are not contraindications.

III. CEMENT SELECTION AND PREPARATION

The first bone cement used for PV was the PMMA Simplex P® (Stryker-Howmedica-Osteonics, Rutherford, NJ). Although not specifically approved for PV, it is the only cement currently approved by the Food and Drug Administration (FDA) for use in the treatment of pathologic fractures in the spine. Many other PMMA cements have been used for PV and seem to have similar clinical results.[16,28,32,33] It is important to know that bone cement is not treated as a pharmaceutical by the FDA but, rather, as a device. Alterations in the composition are therefore equivalent to making a new (nonapproved) device. During PV, practitioners often alter the monomer-to-copolymer (liquid-to-powder) ratio or add other materials (opacification agents or antibiotics). The resulting material is no longer FDA approved. The clinician should inform the patient that such alterations in the cement are to be used and discuss the reasons for and consequences of those changes.

Inherent to performing PV safely is the need to monitor the injection of cement accurately in real time.[28] Such monitoring is usually accomplished with fluoroscopy, which requires that the cement be well opacified so that small quantities (as during introduction) may be adequately seen. It has been determined that barium sulfate (in quantities of 25 to 30% by weight) mixed with the PMMA provides an appropriate level of opacification.[28,32,34] Simplex P contains only 10% by weight of barium sulfate; thus, additional barium sulfate must be added to obtain an adequate mix for visualization. *In vitro* biomechanical evaluations have shown that this level of change in the barium sulfate content minimally alters the handling and mechanical properties of the cement. Changes in the liquid-to-powder ratio result in significant mechanical alterations.[32,34,35] Nevertheless, clinical studies using the modified cements have reported uniformly positive results.[16,21,25,28] No untoward results related to cement alterations have been reported clinically.

Some investigators routinely add antibiotics to PMMA before injection; the most common is tobramycin.[16,28] However, the infection rate with PV is very low and the efficacy of adding antibiotics to the cement has not been scientifically substantiated in normal, uninfected patients. One report in the orthopaedic literature did show reduced infection rates in cement containing antibiotics in immunosuppressed patients.[36] Therefore, the addition of antibiotics to cements is not recommended except in situations of immunocompromise.

Adequate precautions should be given to cement mixing to maintain sterility. Open mixing should be avoided whenever possible because it increases the risk of cement contamination, reduces the cement strength by the inclusion of air bubbles, and may produce inhomogeneous mixing of opacifiers with the cement. A sterile environment should be maintained by using the closed vacuum kit provided by the cement manufacturers.

IV. PERCUTANEOUS VERTEBROPLASTY TECHNIQUE

This procedure must be performed using sterile technique, with sterile skin preparation and drapes. Unnecessary traffic in the procedure room is restricted, and all personnel are required to wear surgical scrubs, caps, and masks. The patient receives intravenous antibiotics 30 min before the procedure (a commonly used antibiotic is 1 g of cephazolin).

Every effort is made to make the patient comfortable on the operative or radiographic table. Because most procedures are performed with local anesthesia and conscious sedation, poor table padding will result in early patient fatigue and produce unacceptable patient motion. Therefore, the amount of padding normally found on most angiographic tables should be augmented and extremity supports should be used as needed.

Once the patient is positioned and the surgical area has been prepared and draped, the area to be treated is identified fluoroscopically. Local anesthesia is introduced into the skin, subcutaneous tissues, and periosteum of the posterior elements of the fractured vertebra. Conscious sedation, such as intravenous fentanyl and Versed, are given as needed. After determining the intended trajectory of the introductory trocar and cannula, a skin incision is made with a #11 scalpel blade. Using fluoroscopic guidance, a trocar and cannula (typically, 11 gauge) are advanced through the soft tissues to the margin of the bone. By advancing the cannula farther, a small osteotomy is made in the posterior element of the vertebra. The trocar and cannula are then passed transpedicularly into the vertebral body until the tip rests anterior to the midline of the vertebral body, as viewed from the lateral projection (Figure 21.3). This transpedicular route, the classic approach to the vertebral body, has proved exceedingly safe and dependable for PV as well as for intrabody bone biopsies. The 11-gauge device offers a good size compromise: it is not too large for most pedicles, and it allows reasonable cement introduction pressures. For smaller pedicles, a 13-gauge system will work, but it may increase the difficulty of cement injection.

A parapedicular approach (passing just lateral to the outer margin of the pedicle) is also gaining favor and is commonly used as a method to avoid small pedicles and to gain access to the middle

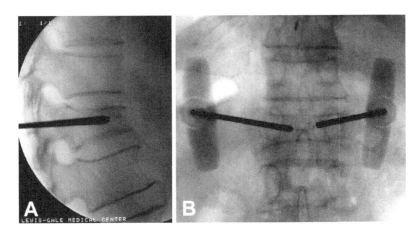

FIGURE 21.3 (A) Lateral radiograph showing two cannulas (partially overlapping) in place for vertebroplasty. The tips of both cannulas are in the anterior vertebral body which will help protect against cement leaks into the epidural space. (B) Anterioposterior radiograph of the same vertebra shows two cannulas in place via a transpedicular approach.

of the vertebra for a bilateral fill by means of a single injection. The entry point into the bone is lateral to the pedicle and not below the pedicle. A lower entry approach commonly puts the exiting nerve root at risk of injury.

We do not believe that venography contributes substantially to PV, and do not perform it as part of routine PVs.

Only after all needle placements are accomplished is the cement prepared (with appropriate opacification) and injected using small syringes (typically, 1 ml). This small syringe size allows easy control of the injected cement quantity and pressure. The cement should be monitored in real time during the injection, or small quantities (i.e., 0.1 to 0.2 ml) should be injected and the result should be visualized before additional cement is introduced. This latter approach allows monitoring while minimizing radiographic exposure for the practitioner. Any cement leak outside the vertebral body is an indication to terminate the injection at that site. Subsequent injections may be safely attempted from a different needle position after the original cement has polymerized.

The amount of cement needed to produce pain relief has not been accurately determined in published clinical reports. An *ex vivo* study reported the amount of cement needed to restore prefracture strength and stiffness to fractured vertebral bodies.[37] It is interesting to note that relatively small amounts of cement (4 to 8 ml) were needed to restore biomechanical integrity. A recent study has also shown that a unipedicular injection that results in cement filling across the midline of the vertebral body provides a significant increase in vertebral body strength.[38] This finding suggests that unipedicular fills that achieve adequate cement volumes clinically are likely to be successful at achieving pain relief.

After adequate vertebral filling has been achieved (Figure 21.4), the needle is removed. Occasionally, venous bleeding is experienced at the needle entry site. Hemostasis is easily achieved with local pressure for 5 min. The entry site is dressed with Betadine ointment and a sterile bandage. The patient is maintained recumbent for 1 to 2 hours after the procedure and monitored for changes in neurologic function or for signs of any other clinical change or side effects. Any sign of adverse events should trigger a search for an explanatory cause using appropriate imaging modalities (usually CT). It is well known that 1 to 2% of patients will have a transient period of benign increase in local pain after PV. However, this is a diagnosis of exclusion and should prompt extended monitoring (or hospitalization if the pain is severe and requires aggressive therapy) and imaging evaluation to exclude other causes for the pain (such as cement extravasation). Pain alone will usually be adequately treated with analgesics, nonsteroidal anti-inflammatory medications, or local

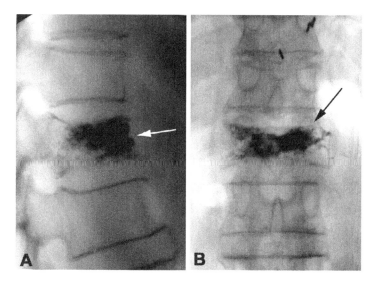

FIGURE 21.4 (A) Lateral radiograph showing the vertebra containing radiopaque PMMA after vertebroplasty (white arrow). (B) Anterioposterior radiograph of the same vertebra (black arrow).

steroid injections adjacent to affected nerve roots or in the epidural space. Neurologic dysfunction should prompt an immediate surgical consultation.

PV is easily performed on an outpatient basis, with the patient discharged after 1 to 2 hours of uneventful recovery. Follow-up is indicated to monitor the results of therapy and should be incorporated into a quality management program. A record of results and complications should be maintained for the facility as well as for each individual provider.

V. RESULTS AND COMPLICATIONS

To date there are no published prospective, randomized trials evaluating PV. Several retrospective series have uniformly reported good pain relief and reduced requirements for analgesics after PV compared with preprocedure levels.[16,21,25,39,40] This finding is especially true with regard to pain related to VCFs produced by osteoporosis. Additional fractures can occur at other levels. Once an osteoporotic VCF occurs, every effort to minimize future bone loss medically should be made. Also, modifications in lifestyle should be attempted to minimize mechanical stress on the spine and thereby lessen the risk of additional fractures.

The initial low incidence of complications associated with PV appears to be increasing as more physicians attempt the procedure without adequate image guidance, cement opacification, or sufficient knowledge to perform the procedure safely. Appropriate training needs to be completed before attempting the procedure.

In osteoporosis-induced vertebral fractures, the incidence of clinical complications is approximately 1%.[16,21,25,39,41] Many of these complications are transient and include increased local pain after cement introduction (nonradicular and not associated with neurologic deficit), which is often successfully treated with nonsteroidal anti-inflammatory medications for 24 to 48 hours. Cement leaking from the vertebra adjacent to a nerve root uncommonly produces radicular pain. Analgesics combined with local steroid and anesthetic injections usually provide adequate relief. A trial of this type of therapy is warranted as long as there are no associated motor deficits. The discovery of a motor deficit (or bowel or bladder dysfunction) should initiate an immediate surgical consult.

Cement leaks have also been implicated in producing pulmonary emboli.[16] These emboli are usually not symptomatic but have on rare occasions produced the clinical symptoms of pulmonary infarct.

Similarly, infection has been rare.

It has been suggested that PV may contribute to a higher risk of VCFs in vertebrae adjacent to the treated one. However, a retrospective review of cases at the University of Virginia revealed no higher incidence of fractures in adjacent vs. nonadjacent fracture sites.[42] There has also been discussion in the medical community about cement leaks into the disc space predisposing patients to an increased risk of adjacent fractures. To date, this information remains anecdotal; there are no supportive data. Therefore, our current opinion is that this situation does not predispose to adjacent fractures.

The overall complication rate after treating VCFs secondary to malignant tumors is considerably higher than that for osteoporotic VCFs.[21,24,43,44] This finding may occur because there are frequently lytic areas involving the vertebral cortex and, therefore, a greater propensity for cement leaking into the surrounding tissues or vessels. Significant cement leaks in this setting occur in up to 10% of patients.

The "safe" number of vertebrae to be treated at one time has yet to be established. Mathis et al.[45] reported treating seven vertebrae in a 35-year-old patient who had multiple fractures associated with steroid use for lupus. This patient's therapy occurred in three treatment sessions, 2 to 3 weeks apart. Because the introduction of cement is a hydraulic event with as much marrow pushed out of the trabecular space as cement injected, there is concern about fat emboli in large-volume cement injections. For reasons described above, we recommend treating no more than three vertebrae in any one session. Additionally, there are no data that support the prophylactic use of PV to treat vertebrae believed to be at risk of fracture. Except for prophylactic use, there is little conceivable reason to perform PV on large numbers of vertebrae at one time.

Any deviation from an expected good result (such as increased pain or neurologic compromise) should initiate immediate imaging with CT to search for a cause of the clinical change. Unremitting or progressive symptoms may require surgical or aggressive medical intervention, and outpatients should be hospitalized and monitored.

VI. SUMMARY

PV has been shown to be very effective at relieving the pain associated with VCFs of vertebra caused by both primary (age-related) and secondary (steroid-induced) osteoporosis. Indeed, PV is rapidly becoming the standard of care for VCF pain not responding to nonoperative therapy. However, this simple procedure must be treated with respect because its application, without appropriate preparation and physician experience, can quickly produce increased pain, permanent neurologic injury, and even death.

REFERENCES

1. Alleyne, C.H., Jr., Rodts, G.E., Jr., and Haid, R.W., "Corpectomy and stabilization with methylmethacrylate in patients with metastatic disease of the spine: a technical note," *J. Spinal Disord.,* 8, 439, 1995.
2. Cortet, B., Cotton, A., Deprez, X., et al., "[Value of vertebroplasty combined with surgical decompression in the treatment of aggressive spinal angioma. Apropos of 3 cases]," *Rev. Rhum. Ed. Fr.,* 61, 16, 1994.
3. Cybulski, G.R., "Methods of surgical stabilization for metastatic disease of the spine," *Neurosurgery,* 25, 240, 1989.
4. Harrington, K.D., "Anterior decompression and stabilization of the spine as a treatment for vertebral collapse and spinal cord compression from metastatic malignancy," *Clin. Orthop.,* 233, 177, 1988.

5. Harrington, K.D., Sim, F.H., Enis, J.E., et al., "Methylmethacrylate as an adjunct in internal fixation of pathologic fractures. Experience with three hundred and seventy-five cases," *J. Bone Joint Surg.*, 58A, 1047, 1976.

6. Knight, G., "Paraspinal acrylic inlays in the treatment of cervical and lumbar spondylosis and other conditions," *Lancet*, 2, 147, 1959.

7. Kostuik, J.P., Errico, T.J., and Gleason, T.F., "Techniques of internal fixation for degenerative conditions of the lumbar spine," *Clin. Orthop.*, 203, 219, 1986.

8. Mavian, G.Z. and Okulski, C.J., "Double fixation of metastatic lesions of the lumbar and cervical vertebral bodies utilizing methylmethacrylate compound: report of a case and review of a series of cases," *J. Am. Osteopath. Assoc.*, 86, 153, 1986.

9. O'Donnell, R.J., Springfield, D.S., Motwani, H.K., et al., "Recurrence of giant-cell tumors of the long bones after curettage and packing with cement," *J. Bone Joint Surg.*, 76A, 1827, 1994.

10. Persson, B.M., Ekelund, L., Lovdahl, R., and Gunterberg, B., "Favourable results of acrylic cementation for giant cell tumors," *Acta Orthop. Scand.*, 55, 209, 1984.

11. Scoville, W.B., Palmer, A.H., Samra, K., and Chong G., "The use of acrylic plastic for vertebral replacement or fixation in metastatic disease of the spine. Technical note," *J. Neurosurg.*, 27, 274, 1967.

12. Sundaresan, N., Galicich, J.H., Lane, J.M., and Greenberg, H.S., "Treatment of odontoid fractures in cancer patients," *J. Neurosurg.*, 54, 187, 1981.

13. Galibert, P., Deramond, H., Rosat, P., and Le Gars, D., "[Preliminary note on the treatment of vertebral angioma by percutaneous acrylic vertebroplasty]," *Neurochirurgie*, 33, 166, 1987.

14. Lapras, C., Mottolese, C., Deruty, R., et al., "[Percutaneous injection of methyl-metacrylate in osteoporosis and severe vertebral osteolysis (Galibert's technic)]," *Ann. Chir.*, 43, 371, 1989.

15. Debussche-Depriester, C., Deramond, H., Fardellone, P., et al., "Percutaneous vertebroplasty with acrylic cement in the treatment of osteoporotic vertebral crush fracture syndrome," *Neuroradiology*, 33, 149, 1991.

16. Jensen, M.E., Evans, A.J., Mathis, J.M., et al., "Percutaneous polymethylmethacrylate vertebroplasty in the treatment of osteoporotic vertebral body compression fractures: technical aspects," *Am. J. Neuroradiol.*, 18, 1897, 1997.

17. Riggs, B.L. and Melton, L.J., III, "The worldwide problem of osteoporosis: insights afforded by epidemiology," *Bone*, 17, 505S, 1995.

18. Cooper, C., Atkinson, E.J., O'Fallon, W.M., and Melton, L.J., III, "Incidence of clinically diagnosed vertebral fractures: a population-based study in Rochester, Minnesota, 1985–1989," *J. Bone Miner. Res.*, 7, 221, 1992.

19. Cooper, C., Atkinson, E.J., Jacobsen, S.J., et al., "Population-based study of survival after osteoporotic fractures," *Am. J. Epidemiol.*, 137, 1001, 1993.

20. Bostrom, M.P. and Lane, J.M., "Future directions. Augmentation of osteoporotic vertebral bodies," *Spine*, 22, 38S, 1997.

21. Chiras, J., Depriester, C., Weill, A., et al., "[Percutaneous vertebral surgery. Technics and indications]," *J. Neuroradiol.*, 24, 45, 1997.

22. Cotton, A., Boutry, N., Cortet, B., et al., "Percutaneous vertebroplasty: state of the art," *Radiographics*, 18, 311, 1998.

23. Cotton, A., Deramond, H., Cortet, B., et al., "Preoperative percutaneous injection of methyl methacrylate and N-butyl cyanoacrylate in vertebral hemangiomas," *Am. J. Neuroradiol.*, 17, 137, 1996.

24. Cotton, A., Dewatre, F., Cortet B., et al., "Percutaneous vertebroplasty for osteolytic metastases and myeloma: effects of the percentage of lesion filling and the leakage of methyl methacrylate at clinical follow-up," *Radiology*, 200, 525, 1996.

25. Deramond, H., Depriester, C., Galibert, P., and Le Gars, D., "Percutaneous vertebroplasty with polymethylmethacrylate. Technique, indications, and results," *Radiol. Clin. North Am.*, 36, 533, 1998.

26. Deramond, H., Galibert, P., Debussche, C., et al., "Percutaneous vertebroplasty with methylmethacrylate: technique, method, results [abstr]," *Radiology*, 177P, 352, 1990.

27. Dousset, V., Mousselard, H., de Monck d'User, L., et al., "Asymptomatic cervical haemangioma treated by percutaneous vertebroplasty," *Neuroradiology*, 38, 392, 1996.

28. Mathis, J.M., Eckel, T.S., Belkoff, S.M., and Deramond, H., "Percutaneous vertebroplasty: a therapeutic option for pain associated with vertebral compression fracture," *J. Back Musculoskel. Rehabil.*, 13, 11, 1999.

29. Silverman, S.L., "The clinical consequences of vertebral compression fracture," *Bone*, 13, S27, 1992.

30. Kado, D.M., Browner, W.S., Palermo L., et al., "Vertebral fractures and mortality in older women: a prospective study. Study of Osteoporotic Fractures Research Group," *Arch. Intern. Med.,* 159, 1215, 1999.

31. Maynard, A.S., Jensen, M.E., Schweickert, P.A., et al., "Value of bone scan imaging in predicting pain relief from percutaneous vertebroplasty in osteoporotic vertebral fractures," *Am. J. Neuroradiol.,* 21, 1807, 2000.

32. Belkoff, S.M., Maroney, M., Fenton, D.C., and Mathis, J.M., "An *in vitro* biomechanical evaluation of bone cements used in percutaneous vertebroplasty," *Bone,* 25, 23S, 1999.

33. Jensen, M.E. and Dion, J.E., "Percutaneous vertebroplasty in the treatment of osteoporotic compression fractures," *Neuroimaging Clin. North Am.,* 10, 547, 2000.

34. Jasper, L., Deramond, H., Mathis, J.M., and Belkoff, S.M., "Evaluation of PMMA cements altered for use in vertebroplasty," presented at 10th Interdisciplinary Research Conference on Injectible Biomaterials, Amiens, France, March 14–15, 2000.

35. Jasper, L.E., Deramond, H., Mathis, J.M., and Belkoff, S.M., "The effect of monomer-to-powder ratio on the material properties of Cranioplastic," *Bone,* 25, 27S, 1999.

36. Norden, C.W., "Antibiotic prophylaxis in orthopaedic surgery," *Rev. Infect. Dis.,* 13, S842, 1991.

37. Belkoff, S., Deramond, H., Mathis, J., and Jasper, L., "Vertebroplasty: the biomechanical effect of cement volume," presented at 46th Annual Meeting of the Orthopaedic Research Society, Orlando, FL, March 13, 2000.

38. Tohmeh, A.G., Mathis, J.M., Fenton, D.C., et al., "Biomechanical efficacy of unipedicular vs. bipedicular vertebroplasty for the management of osteoporotic compression fractures," *Spine,* 24, 1772, 1999.

39. Cyteval, C., Sarrabere, M.P., Roux, J.O., et al., "Acute osteoporotic vertebral collapse: open study on percutaneous injection of acrylic surgical cement in 20 patients," *Am. J. Roentgenol.,* 173, 1685, 1999.

40. Barr, J.D., Barr, M.S., Lemley, T.J., and McCann, R.M., "Percutaneous vertebroplasty for pain relief and spinal stabilization," *Spine,* 25, 923, 2000.

41. Cortet, B., Cotton, A., Boutry, N., et al., "Percutaneous vertebroplasty in the treatment of osteoporotic vertebral compression fractures: an open prospective study," *J. Rheumatol.,* 26, 2222, 1999.

42. Jensen, M.E., Kallmes, D.F., Short, J.G., et al., "Percutaneous vertebroplasty does not increase the risk of adjacent vertebral fracture — a retrospective study," presented at 38th Annual Meeting of the American Society of Neuroradiology, Atlanta, GA, April 3, 2000.

43. Deramond, H., Depriester, C., and Toussaint P., "[Vertebroplasty and percutaneous interventional radiology in bone metastases: techniques, indications, contra-indications]," *Bull. Cancer Radiother.,* 83, 277, 1996.

44. Weill, A., Chiras, J., Simon, J.M., et al., "Spinal metastases: indications for and results of percutaneous injection of acrylic surgical cement," *Radiology,* 199, 241, 1996.

45. Mathis, J.M., Petri, M., and Naff, N., "Percutaneous vertebroplasty treatment of steroid-induced osteoporotic compression fractures," *Arthritis Rheum.,* 41, 171, 1998.

Part V

Joint Prosthesis and Osteoporosis

22 Joint Replacement in Osteoporotic Bone

Christopher V. Bensen and H. Del Schutte, Jr.

CONTENTS

I. INTRODUCTION

Total joint replacement remains one of the most commonly performed and successful procedures in modern orthopaedic surgery. Reported long-term success rates above 95% in many large case series have led to a steady increase in popularity with more than 1 million joint replacement procedures performed annually worldwide.[1] Considering the aging population, this number should continue to increase as most joint replacements are performed in patients over 65 years of age. Numerous outcome studies have documented the utility of joint replacement by significant improvements in both functional status and quality of life.

Despite this remarkable success and ever-advancing technology in this field of orthopaedics, certain problems and complications still exist that limit even greater success of these procedures. The fundamental challenge in total joint arthroplasty lies in the fixation of an inert, metal prosthesis to a constantly changing, living tissue. Failure of this fixation remains a significant mechanical problem facing the joint replacement surgeon with respect to long-term stability of the implant. Current strategies for fixation rely on one of two basic methods of fixation: ingrowth or outgrowth of the host bone to a porous-surfaced prosthesis, termed *osseointegration,* or the use of poly-methylmethacrylate (PMMA) bone cement. Stable fixation of an implant depends on (1) implant factors including size, shape, design, and degree and type of porous coating; (2) surgeon factors including preparation of the host bone surface, positioning of the implant, and cement technique; and (3) patient factors including weight, habitus, activity level, underlying disease, and quantity and quality of bone. The last factor is perhaps the most important as the status of the host bone has profound influence on the long-term success of total joint arthroplasty.

Osteoporotic bone has several important effects on total joint arthroplasty. In this chapter, we will address the difficulties associated with joint replacement in osteoporotic bone including altered loading mechanics, implant fixation, perioperative risk factors, mechanisms of postoperative bone loss, implant loosening, and clinical strategies and results.

II. LOADING MECHANICS IN OSTEOPOROTIC BONE

The forces exerted on intact metaphyseal bone are normally distributed by both cortical and trabecular structures. Removal of bone at the time of total joint arthroplasty creates stress concentration on the remaining bony structures. This may also be compounded by an inserted implant that distributes stress differently than intact bone. The circumferential "hoop stresses" produced and consequent torsional loads have been purported as a major cause of mechanical loosening and ultimate failure of femoral components.[2,3] It would be logical that disruption of the bony trabeculae that occurs in osteoporosis might compound this problem. Otani et al.[4] investigated the pattern of load transfer in the intact proximal femur using human cadaveric femora with varying degrees of osteoporosis. They found Singh classification strongly affected proximal longitudinal strain in response to axial load. Femora with Singh Grades III and IV showed significantly greater circumferential strain than those of Grades V or VI both in the proximal metaphyseal and diaphyseal regions.[4] The authors concluded that femoral implants that rely on high hoop stresses in the proximal femur for early fixation are more likely to fracture the femur during insertion or loosen in the early postoperative period. This problem is potentially compounded in the presence of osteoporotic bone, and changes in the mechanical behavior of the femur following hemiarthroplasty have been documented.[5]

III. IMPLANT FIXATION IN OSTEOPOROTIC BONE

During the last three decades, there has been extensive research and development of porous-coated components for use in total joint arthroplasty. The concept of biological fixation through osseointegration of orthopaedic implants as an alternative to cemented fixation offers several potential advantages; however, it is generally accepted that requisite factors of osseointegration include an adequate bony structure in the host, close initial bone–implant apposition, and minimal or no movement between the implant and the bone.[6-9]

For several reasons, the patient with osteoporosis presents significant challenges with respect to the first two of these requisites. First, the deficient bony bed allows less than optimal contact between bone and the porous surfaces of the component. Many authors have reported that bone ingrowth occurs only to a limited extent involving small percentages of the total surface area of the implant. Cook and colleagues[10] analyzed 90 retrieved uncemented porous-coated total joint components recovered from 58 patients. More than 90% of the components had been *in situ* at least 6 weeks and a majority had been functional for at least 9 months. In no case was the implant removed due to clinically or radiographically apparent loosening. Remarkably, the authors found no bone ingrowth or apposition in one third of the implants, with none having greater than 10% of the available porous surface ingrown with bone. Instead, a majority of the pores were filled with fibrous tissue. They concluded that a combination of limited bone ingrowth with extensive fibrous tissue ingrowth was adequate for stable implant fixation.[10]

It is conceivable that, as an osteoporotic host bone bed would provide a smaller quantity of bone available for ingrowth of porous-coated components, the degree of osseointegration might be reduced and, consequently, the performance of the implant compromised. Although numerous basic and clinical studies have been carried out to address this question, it remains largely unanswered. Nonetheless, many surgeons have advised caution with the use of ingrowth implants and some have advocated the use of cemented components in individuals with osteoporosis because of concern about poor ingrowth with the use of porous-coated prostheses.[11,12]

Fini et al.[13] evaluated bone ingrowth to titanium and hydroxyapatite rods in both normal and ovariectomized osteopenic rats. Affinity indices were calculated for each implant based on the percentage of available implant surface area in contact with bone. The authors found a decrease in the affinity index for both implants in osteoporotic bone when compared with normal bone; however, the difference was statistically significant only in the hydroxyapatite implants (Figure 22.1).[13]

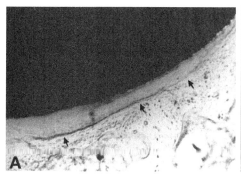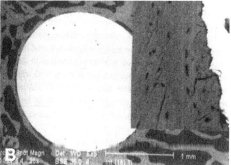

FIGURE 22.1 (A) Titanium rod implanted in an osteopenic rat. Note the presence of fibrous tissue wall between the trabecular bone and the implant (arrow). (B) Titanium rod inserted in normal bone with absence of a fibrous rim. (From Fini, M. et al., *Int. J. Artif. Org.*, 20, 291, 1997. With permission.)

In another study from the same group, titanium and ceramic materials were implanted in both healthy and osteoporotic rat femora. At 2 months, there was significantly less osseointegration in osteopenic bone. In addition, one of the ceramic materials osseointegrated only in normal bone.[14]

Numerous animal studies have been conducted on dental and prosthodontic implants in osteoporotic bone with conflicting conclusions. Several authors found significantly decreased osseointegration in osteoporotic bone while others found no compelling evidence to conclude that osteoporosis was a risk factor for osseointegration of dental implants.[15-19]

Several clinical studies have also been carried out to examine the relationship between osteoporosis and bone ingrowth. Moreland and Bernstein[20] retrospectively reviewed 175 femoral revision procedures using cementless porous-coated implants. They found a significant correlation between preoperative osteoporosis and degree of bony ingrowth using Engh's radiographic criteria. Of the 43 patients with minimal femoral bone stock deficiency, 97.7% achieved bone ingrowth compared to 76.5% in those with severe preoperative bone stock deficiency.[20]

Several strategies have been investigated to increase osseointegration into porous-coated implants including bone grafting, demineralized bone matrix, hydroxyapatite coating, and the use of growth factors such as bone morphogenic protein. Further discussion on these strategies and the effects of osteoporosis on bone ingrowth to prosthetic surfaces can be found in Chapter 24.

IV. PERIOPERATIVE RISK FACTORS

Several perioperative complications may occur in total joint arthroplasty that could potentially be exacerbated by the presence of osteoporotic bone. These include intraoperative bony fracture, postoperative periprosthetic fracture, implant fracture, and nonunion of trochanteric osteotomy.

Several steps in joint arthroplasty procedures predispose the host bone to fracture. During hip arthroplasty, dislocation of the femoral head from the acetabulum creates significant rotational forces that can cause spiral fractures of the neck and shaft of the femur. Broaching the proximal femur and insertion of press-fit femoral components both exert tremendous circumferential hoop stress forces on the proximal femur. Consequently, fractures of the femoral calcar can occur. Fractures can often be avoided simply by careful handling of instruments and controlled, properly sequenced dislocation maneuvers. In revision cases, excision of heterotopic bone, tenotomy of the psoas tendon, and trochanteric osteotomy may all be helpful in avoiding fractures during dislocation.[21]

Postoperative periprosthetic fractures are infrequent complications in total joint arthroplasty. However, several series of femoral shaft and supracondylar fractures have been reported with some surgeons attributing the etiology largely to osteoporotic bone (Figure 22.2).[22]

Osteotomy of the greater trochanter for exposure of the hip joint was introduced by Charnley to avoid damage to the abductor mechanism. Although many surgeons favor other alternatives for

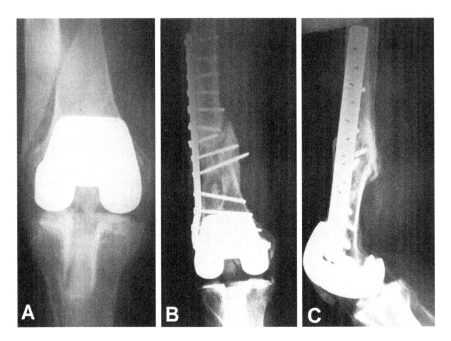

FIGURE 22.2 Radiographs of a periprosthetic supracondylar femur fracture following total knee replacement in an 80-year-old female osteoporotic patient (A). The fracture was managed successfully with a condylar blade plate (B and C). (From Rand, J.A., in *Joint Replacement Arthroplasty*, Morrey, B.F., Ed., Churchill Livingstone, New York, 1991, 1081. With permission.)

primary cases, trochanteric osteotomy may still be the safest method under certain conditions including revision cases, stiff hips, severe protrusio acetabuli, and osteoporosis.[21] One potential complication of trochanteric osteotomy is delayed union or nonunion. Although no specific defect in fracture healing has been identified in patients with osteoporosis, some studies suggest an increased incidence of nonunion in such patients.[21]

V. POSTOPERATIVE BONE LOSS AND IMPLANT LOOSENING

Periprosthetic bone loss during the postoperative period following total joint arthroplasty occurs by several means including disuse, stress shielding, natural aging, and as a consequence of particulate debris. It has long been recognized that disuse, immobilization, and reduced weight bearing lead to decreased bone mineral density.[23-26] Some examples in which this phenomenon has been implicated include casting, paraplegia, prolonged bed rest, decreased physical activity, and spaceflight. A certain degree of reduced activity and extremity loading in the preoperative and immediate postoperative period due to pain and muscle weakness is expected and largely unavoidable. Furthermore, many patients with total joint replacement are subjected to a variable period of bed rest and/or relative inactivity, especially in the face of perioperative complications such as deep venous thrombosis. Finally, with porous-ingrowth prostheses, some surgeons have recommended a period of partial weight bearing to facilitate osseointegration of the implant. Consequently, in light of these factors, one might expect these patients to have a higher risk of localized disuse osteoporosis with the potential for loosening and poor clinical results. Indeed, some authors have warned that periprosthetic bone loss is the single most important factor limiting implant longevity and it was responsible for approximately 70% of implant failures in one large series.[1]

Using quantitative computed tomography, Rüegsegger et al.[27] examined the bone density of both the operated and contralateral tibiae of patients undergoing total hip arthroplasty. They found a slight but significant bone loss (average 1%, range 0 to 4%) in both legs, which they attributed to immobilization and reduced activity during the first 6 months postoperatively. However, this loss was transient with the majority of patients having bone densities at 1 year postoperatively not significantly lower than initial values. The authors reported a drastic variation in activity from sedentary to intensive sports activities but found no correlation between activity and bone loss.[27] Conversely, Dubs and colleagues[28] followed a group of young male patients after total hip arthroplasty and found a significantly lower rate of implant loosening in those patients engaged in sports activities (1.6 vs. 14.3%).

Several authors have reported changes in bone density beneath tibial components following total knee arthroplasty.[29-31] Levitz et al.[31] measured bone density with dual photon absorptiometry and dual X ray absorptiometry (DEXA) under the medial and lateral plateaus and central peg of tibial components from 1 week to 8 years postoperatively. Concurrent with several previous studies, they reported an initial decline in bone density with normalization at 1 year. However, at the 8-year follow-up, there was a 36.4% average decrease in bone mineral density. Interestingly, they found similar rates of bone loss in male and female patients despite significantly higher initial bone density in the male patients.[31] The authors of this and other studies have concluded that failure of tibial components may be related to changes in the quality of bone over time.[31,32]

In addition to localized, periprosthetic bone loss, it is conceivable that a more generalized loss of bone density might also result from a postoperative decrease in activity level. This theory was confirmed by Black et al.[33] who compared vertebral bone density in patients who had undergone total hip replacement with both preoperative patients as well as age-matched controls. They found no statistical difference between postoperative patients with good activity and either control or preoperative patients. In contrast, postoperative patients with poor activity had significantly lower vertebral bone density than both preoperative patients and controls. The authors concluded that postoperative total hip arthroplasty patients maintain their axial bone stock if activity level is restored. Likewise, significant bone loss may occur if activity level is not restored.[33]

The second means of bone loss in the perioperative period is that of adaptive bone remodeling as a result of "stress shielding." The stiffness disparity between implant and bone as well as osseointegration in the case of porous-coated implants causes redistribution of stress transfer in the proximal femur. This ultimately results in resorption of bone that is greatest in the proximal medial femur (Figure 22.3).

Implant size, geometry, and material stiffness, as well as extent and pattern of porous coating, have all been shown to affect the degree of stress shielding.[34,35] Although the radiographic appearance is often quite impressive, the clinical consequences of this phenomenon and its effect on stability of total joint components are not fully understood.

One concern, however, is the potential susceptibility of stress-shielded osteoporotic bone to macrophage-mediated osteolysis secondary to particulate wear debris.[36] This is perhaps the most important and significant mode of bone loss that has been well documented in clinical and histologic studies over the past two decades. Furthermore, many surgeons believe this osteolytic process is accelerated in osteoporotic bone. A full discussion of this problem is beyond the scope of this chapter and excellent discussions can be found in other texts.

A final possible mode of bone loss in the postoperative period is that of natural aging. As approximately 25% of bone mineral density is lost from the proximal femur between age 40 and 70, there is concern for loss of support and ultimate loosening of the femoral component.[37,38] Jasty et al.[39] reported cancellous bone remodeling around well-fixed cemented stems implanted for extended periods of time and concluded that normal age-related bone loss did not pose a threat to the integrity of femoral component stability. Other investigators have agreed that preoperative osteoporosis does not predispose the femoral component to early loosening.[40,41]

The problems described above may be compounded by implant fixation to preexisting osteoporotic bone. Engh et al.[42] analyzed paired postmortem femoral specimens retrieved from patients who had undergone unilateral total hip arthroplasty. They performed DEXA and demonstrated a 5 to 52% loss of periprosthetic bone mineral content. A strong correlation was found

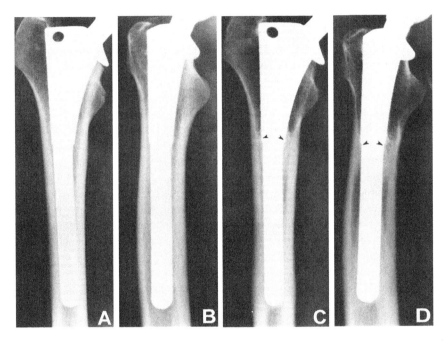

FIGURE 22.3 Immediate (A, B) and 1-year (C, D) postoperative radiographs demonstrating progressive bone resorption or "stress shielding" in the proximal femur following total hip arthroplasty. The most significant loss is seen in the proximal medial cortex. Arrows denote extensive new bone formation or "spot welds" at the junction of the porous and smooth surfaces of the implant suggesting localized stress transfer. (From Engh, C.A. and Bobyn, J.D., *Clin. Orthop.*, 231, 7, 1988. With permission.)

between the extent of this bone loss and the bone mineral content of the contralateral femur, suggesting the extent of resorptive changes is closely related to preoperative osteoporosis.[42]

To date, few clinical strategies have been employed to reduce the degree of postoperative bone loss. However, several recent studies have investigated the use of bisphosphonates that have previously been used in the treatment of bone loss associated with postmenopausal osteoporosis, Paget's disease, and other conditions.[43-45] To investigate the effect of pamidronate in preventing postoperative bone loss, Wilkinson et al.[46] performed a 26-week prospective, randomized, double-blind clinical trial in 47 patients undergoing total hip arthroplasty. Patients were given a single-dose infusion of 90 mg of pamidronate on the fifth postoperative day and evaluated with bone mineral density measurements and biochemical markers of bone turnover. Patients receiving pamidronate had a significant reduction in bone loss and suppression of biochemical markers compared with controls. The therapy was well tolerated and there were no significant adverse effects or interference with bone ingrowth. The authors concluded that the acute bone loss that occurs after total hip arthroplasty can be markedly attenuated by a single infusion of pamidronate.[46]

These and other data are certainly promising and warrant further investigation in large-scale clinical trials. Strategies for prevention of periprosthetic osteopenia are further discussed in Chapter 26.

VI. CLINICAL RESULTS OF TOTAL JOINT ARTHROPLASTY IN PATIENTS WITH OSTEOPOROSIS

Numerous animal and preclinical studies have made significant contributions toward the understanding of the aforementioned problems. However, it is ultimately the clinical performance of joint replacement procedures in individuals with osteoporosis that is of paramount importance.

Numerous clinical studies have been conducted on elderly patients who, on average, are assumed to have some degree of osteoporosis. Many of these studies have reported excellent results with both cemented and uncemented components.[47-50] However, surprisingly few series that document a uniform preoperative state of postmenopausal osteoporosis have been published.

Kligman and Kirsh[51] prospectively reviewed 22 patients with osteoporosis (Singh index 1 to 3) who underwent total hip arthroplasty with hydroxyapatite-coated implants and compared the results to a control group of 45 patients with normal bone (Singh index 4 to 6). Preoperative Harris hip scores and diagnoses were similar for both groups. At a mean follow-up of 5 years (range 2 to 7), there was no significant difference in average Harris hip score or radiographically determined bone ingrowth between the two groups. Based on their results, the authors concluded that osteoporosis does not compromise the early results of uncemented total hip replacement.[51]

Several studies have been carried out in renal transplant recipients who have undergone total hip arthroplasty. Although the primary indication for the vast majority of these patients was osteonecrosis of the femoral head, steroid-induced osteoporosis was documented in one series and can be assumed to be present in nearly all these patients. This is clearly a very different population than postmenopausal patients with degenerative joint disease. However, these studies represent the vast majority of series patients with documented preoperative osteoporosis of undergoing total joint arthroplasty.

Bradford et al.[52] evaluated 39 renal transplant recipients who had undergone 60 total hip arthroplasties at an average follow-up period of 44 months. Although they had a relatively high rate of dislocation, femoral component loosening requiring revision occurred in only one case, and that was successfully revised. The authors believed the reasons for these dislocations were multifactorial and recommended total hip arthroplasty as the treatment of choice for renal transplant patients with osteonecrosis of the femoral head.[52] Other authors have reported similar clinical success with joint arthroplasty in renal transplant patients.[53-55]

Other studies have demonstrated less satisfactory results. Devlin and colleagues[56] reviewed 36 total hip arthroplasties in 22 patients who had previously undergone renal transplantation. A subset of 7 patients with 11 arthroplasties had ipsilateral transilial bone biopsy performed at the time of arthroplasty. All but 1 of these 7 patients had active osteoporosis documented by histologic evaluation. The patients were reevaluated at a mean follow-up of 86 months and the authors reported an overall failure rate of 25%, significantly higher than that of total hip arthroplasty in the general population. They concluded that the presence of preexisting renal osteodystrophy and steroid-induced osteoporosis posed a significant threat to the long-term survival of total hip implants.[56] Another study by Karas et al.[57] also reported less than satisfactory results in this population with longer follow-up.

Although these authors may disagree on the relative success of total hip arthroplasty in renal transplant patients, most suggest a multifactorial etiology of the failures and, more importantly, do not directly attribute them to the presence of osteoporotic bone.

VII. SUMMARY

The patient with osteoporosis presents several challenges to the joint replacement surgeon. Osseointegration, perioperative complications, postoperative bone loss, component loosening, and implant failure may all potentially be affected by the presence of osteoporotic bone. Several relatively new strategies for improving the performance of total joint arthroplasty in patients with osteoporosis have been described. These include growth factors and chemical coatings to improve osseointegration and the use of bisphosphonates to reduce postoperative bone loss. Such developments are encouraging and certainly warrant further investigation. The relative paucity of clinical studies on total joint arthroplasty in patients with osteoporosis makes it difficult for any meaningful conclusions to be drawn. Further long-term studies are clearly needed to better delineate and quantify the risk factors in these patients as well as the most appropriate techniques and clinical strategies to address them.

REFERENCES

1. Malchau, H., Herberts, P., and Ahnfelt, L., "Prognosis of total hip replacement in Sweden. Follow up of 92,675 operations performed 1978–1990," *Acta Orthop. Scand.*, 64, 497, 1993.
2. Charnley, J., "Fracture of the femoral prosthesis in total hip replacement: a clinical study," *Clin. Orthop.*, 11, 105, 1975.
3. Wroblewski, B.M., "The mechanism of fracture of the femoral prosthesis in total hip replacement," *Orthop. Int.*, 3, 137, 1979.
4. Otani, T., Whiteside, L.A., and White, S.E., "The effect of axial and torsional loading on strain distribution in the proximal femur as related to cementless total hip arthroplasty," *Clin. Orthop.*, 292, 376, 1993.
5. Cook, S.D., Skinner, H.B., Weinstein, A.M., et al., "The mechanical behavior of normal and osteoporotic canine femora before and after hemiarthroplasty," *Clin. Orthop.*, 170, 303, 1982.
6. Chen, P.Q., Turner, T.M., Ronnigen, H., et al., "A canine cementless total hip prosthesis model," *Clin. Orthop.*, 176, 24, 1983.
7. Harris, W.H., "The first 32 years of total hip arthroplasty: one surgeon's perspective," *Clin. Orthop.*, 274, 6, 1992.
8. Harris, W.H. and Jasty, M., "Bone ingrowth into porous coated canine acetabular replacements: the effect of pore size, apposition and dislocation," in *The Hip: Proceedings of the Thirteenth Open Scientific Meeting of The Hip Society*, C.V. Mosby, St. Louis, MO, 1985, 214.
9. Jasty, M., Bragdon, C., Burke, D., et al., "*In vivo* skeletal responses to porous-surfaced implants subjected to small induced motions," *J. Bone Joint Surg.*, 79A, 707, 1997.
10. Cook, S.D., Thomas, K.A., and Haddad, R.J., "Histologic analysis of retrieved human porous-coated total joint components," *Clin. Orthop.*, 234, 90, 1988.
11. Dorr, L.D., Arnala, I., Faugere, M.C., and Malluche, H.H., "Five year postoperative results of cemented femoral arthroplasty in patients with systemic bone disease," *Clin. Orthop.*, 259, 114, 1990.
12. Fitzgerald, R.H., Ed., *Non-Cemented Total Hip Arthroplasty*, Lippincott-Raven, Philadelphia, 1988.
13. Fini, M., Aldini, N.N., Gandolfi, M.G., et al., "Biomaterials for orthopaedic surgery in osteoporotic bone: a comparative study in rats," *Int. J. Artif. Org.*, 20, 291, 1997.
14. Fini, M., Giavaresi, G., Torricelli, P., et al., "Biocompatability and osseointegration in osteoporotic bone: a preliminary *in vitro* and *in vivo* study," *J. Bone Joint Surg.*, 83B, 139, 2001.
15. Fujimoto, T., Niimi, A., Sawai, T., and Ueda, M., "Osseointegrated implants in a patient with osteoporosis: a case report," *Int. J. Oral Maxillofac. Impl.*, 11, 539, 1996.
16. Fujimoto, T., Niimi, A., Sawai, T., and Ueda, M., "Effects of steroid-induced osteoporosis on osseointegration of titanium implants," *Int. J. Oral Maxillofac. Impl.*, 13, 183, 1998.
17. Mori, H., Manabe, M., Kurachi, Y., and Nagumo, M., "Osseointegration of dental implants in rabbit bone with low mineral density," *J. Oral Maxillofac Surg.*, 55, 351, 1997.
18. Starck, W.J. and Epker, B.N., "Failure of osseointegrated dental implants after diphosphonate therapy for osteoporosis: a case report," *Int. J. Oral Maxillofac. Impl.*, 10, 74, 1995.
19. Dao, T.T., Anderson, J.D., and Zarb, G.A., "Is osteoporosis a risk factor for osseointegration of dental implants?" *Int. J. Oral Maxillofac. Impl.*, 8, 137, 1993.
20. Moreland, J.R. and Bernstein, M.L., "Femoral revision hip arthroplasty with uncemented, porous-coated stems," *Clin. Orthop.*, 319, 141, 1995.
21. Eftekhar, N.S., *Total Hip Arthroplasty*, Mosby Year Book, St. Louis, MO, 1993.
22. Sim, F.H. and Cabenela, M.E., "Proximal femoral fracture," in *Joint Replacement Arthroplasty*, Morrey, B.F., Ed., Churchill Livingstone, New York, 1991.
23. Donaldson, C.L., Hulley, S.B., Vogel, J.M., et al., "Effect of prolonged bed rest on bone mineral," *Metabolism*, 19, 1071, 1970.
24. Minaire, P., Meunier, P., Edouard, B., et al., "Quantitative histologic data on disuse osteoporosis," *Calcif. Tissue Res.*, 17, 57, 1974.
25. Exner, G.U., Prader, A., Elsasser, U., et al., "Bone densitometry using computed tomography, Parts I and II," *Br. J. Radiol.*, 52, 14, 1979.
26. Worley, R.J., "Age, estrogen, and bone density," *Clin. Obstet. Gynecol.*, 24, 203, 1981.
27. Rüegsegger, P., Seitz, P., Gschwend, N., and Dubs, L., "Disuse osteoporosis in patients with total hip prostheses," *Arch. Orthop. Trauma Surg.*, 105, 268, 1986.

28. Dubs, L., Gschwend, N., and Minzinger, U., "Sport after total hip arthroplasty," *Arch. Orthop. Trauma Surg.*, 101, 16, 1983.

29. Bohr, H.H. and Lund, B., "Bone mineral density of the proximal tibia following uncemented arthroplasty," *J. Arthroplasty*, 2, 309, 1987.

30. Seitz, P., Rüegsegger, P., Gschwend, N., and Dubs, L., "Changes in local bone density after total knee replacement," *J. Bone Joint Surg.*, 69B, 407, 1987.

31. Levitz, C.L., Lotke, P.A., and Karp, J.S., "Long-term changes in bone mineral density following total knee replacement," *Clin. Orthop.*, 321, 68, 1995.

32. Windsor, R.E., Scuderi, G.R., Moran, M., and Insall, J.N., "Mechanisms of failure of the femoral and tibial components in total knee arthroplasty," *Clin. Orthop.*, 248, 15, 1989.

33. Black, D.M., Daniels, A.U., Dunn, H.K., and Kruger, R.A., "Computerized tomographic determination of vertebral density after total hip arthroplasty," *Clin. Orthop.*, 198, 259, 1985.

34. Bobyn, J.D., Glassman, A.H., Goto, H., et al., "The effect of stem stiffness on femoral bone resorption after canine porous-coated total hip arthroplasty," *Clin. Orthop.*, 261, 196, 1990.

35. Engh, C.A. and Bobyn, J.D., "The influence of stem size and extent of porous coating on femoral bone resorption after primary cementless hip arthroplasty," *Clin. Orthop.*, 231, 7, 1988.

36. Rubash, H.E., Sinha, R.K., Shanbhag, A.S., and Kim, S.Y., "Pathogenesis of bone loss after total hip arthroplasty," *Orthop. Clin. North Am.*, 29, 173, 1998.

37. Bobyn, J.D., Mortimer, E.S., Glassman, A.H., et al., "Producing and avoiding stress shielding: laboratory and clinical observations of noncemented total hip arthroplasty," *Clin. Orthop.*, 274, 79, 1992.

38. Comadoll, J.L., Sherman, R.E., Gustilo, R.B., et al., "Radiographic changes in bone dimensions in asymptomatic cemented total hip arthroplasties: results of nine to thirteen year follow-up," *J. Bone Joint Surg.*, 70A, 433, 1988.

39. Jasty, M., Maloney, W.J., Bragdon, C.R., et al., "Histomorphologic studies of the long-term skeletal responses to well fixed cemented femoral components," *J. Bone Joint Surg.*, 72A, 1220, 1990.

40. Hierton, C., Blomgren, G., and Lindgren, U., "Factors associated with early loosening of cemented total hip prostheses," *Acta Orthop. Scand.*, 54, 168, 1983.

41. Carlsson, A.S. and Nilsson, B.E., "The relationship of bone mass and loosening of the femoral component in total hip replacement," *Acta Orthop. Scand.*, 51, 285, 1980.

42. Engh, C.A., Hooten, J.P., Zettl-Schaffer, K.F., et al., "Porous-coated total hip replacement," *Clin. Orthop.*, 298, 89, 1994.

43. Reid, I.R., Wattie, D.J., Evans, M.C., et al., "Continuous therapy with pamidronate, a potent bisphosphonate, in postmenopausal osteoporosis," *J. Clin. Endocrinol. Metab.*, 79, 1595, 1994.

44. Frijlink, W.B., Bijvoet, O.L., te Velde, J., and Heynen, G., "Treatment of Paget's disease with (3-amino-1-hydroxypropylidene)-1,1-bisphosphonate (A.P.D.)," *Lancet*, 1, 799, 1979.

45. Berenson, J.R., Lichtenstein, A., Porter, L., et al., "Efficacy of pamidronate in reducing skeletal events in patients with advanced multiple myeloma. Myeloma Aredia Study Group," *N. Engl. J. Med.*, 334, 488, 1996.

46. Wilkinson, J.M., Stockley, I., Peel, N.F.A., et al., "Effect of pamidronate in preventing local bone loss after total hip arthroplasty: a randomized, double-blind, controlled trial," *J. Bone Miner. Res.*, 16, 556, 2001.

47. Keisu, K.S., Orozco, F., Sharkey, P.F., et al., "Primary cementless total hip arthroplasty in octogenarians. Two to eleven year follow-up," *J. Bone Joint Surg.*, 83A, 359, 2001.

48. Konstantoulakis, C., Anastopoulos, G., Papaeliou, A., et al., "Uncemented total hip arthroplasty in the elderly," *Int. Orthop.*, 23, 334, 1999.

49. Laskin, R.S., "Total knee replacement in patients older than 85 years," *Clin. Orthop.*, 367, 43, 1999.

50. Brander, V.A., Malhotra, S., Jet, J., et al., "Outcome of hip and knee arthroplasty in persons aged 80 years and older," *Clin. Orthop.*, 345, 67, 1997.

51. Kligman, M. and Kirsh, G., "Hydroxyapatite-coated total hip arthroplasty in osteoporotic patients," *Bull. Hosp. Joint Dis.*, 59, 136, 2000.

52. Bradford, D.S., Janes, P.C., Simmons, R.S., and Najarian, J.S., "Total hip arthroplasty in renal transplant recipients," *Clin. Orthop.*, 181, 107, 1983.

53. Kenzora, J.E. and Sledge, C.B., "Hip arthroplasty and the renal transplant patient," in *Proceedings of The Hip Society*, C.V. Mosby, St. Louis, MO, 1975, 35.

54. Ibels, L.S., Alfrey, A.C., Huffer, W.E., et al., "Aseptic necrosis of bone following renal transplantation: experience in 194 transplant recipients and review of the literature," *Medicine*, 57, 25, 1975.

55. Gustafsson, L.A., Meyers, M.H., and Berne, T.V., "Total hip replacement in renal transplant recipients with aseptic necrosis of the femoral head," *Lancet*, 2, 606, 1976.

56. Devlin, V.J., Einhorn, T.A., Gordon, S.L., et al., "Total hip arthroplasty after renal transplantation: long term follow-up study and assessment of metabolic bone status," *J. Arthroplasty*, 3, 205, 1988.

57. Karas, S.E., Gebhardt, E.M., Kenzora, J.E., and Thornhill, T.S., "Total hip arthroplasty for osteonecrosis following renal transplantation," *Orthop. Trans.*, 8, 379, 1984.

23 Transient Osteoporosis — A Regional Osteoporosis in the Clinic

Paul I. Wuisman and Onno G. Meijer

CONTENTS

I. INTRODUCTION

Transient osteoporosis is now a well-recognized syndrome characterized by a symptomatic, regional osteoporosis. The syndrome-related problems and complications frequently interfere with the activities of daily life. Increasing numbers of patients will appear, so it is likely that total treatment, aiming to shorten the duration of the disease, avoid potential hazardous complications, and achieve rapid and full, uncomplicated return to previous levels of activities, will be required.

The term *osteoporosis* was used by Albright and Reifenstein[1] to describe a fracture syndrome resulting from reduced bone mass. A World Health Organization (WHO) commission defined osteoporosis as a bone mineral density or content 2.5 standard deviations or more below comparable

TABLE 23.1
Proposed Etiopathogenesis of Transient Osteoporosis

Genetic	Genetic predisposition
	Osteogenesis imperfecta
Trauma	Microfracture
	Microfracture because of fetal movements
Chemical and hormonal mechanism	Chemical and hormonal factors associated with pregnancy
	Phosphate depletion
	Association with liver cirrhosis
	Disorder of increased bone turnover
	Association with hypercalciuric osteoporosis
Vascular mechanism	Ischemia of the small vessels proximal to the nerve roots
	Obstruction of venous return
	Transient ischemia, as in myocardial infarction
	Early phase of avascular femoral head necrosis
Neural mechanism	Form frustes of reflex sympathetic dystrophy
	Associated with hyperlipoproteinemia Type IV
	Pathology of peripheral nerves
	Compression of obturator nerve
	Irritation of or compression of pelvic nerves

norms.[2] Although fracture is the most important complication, osteoporosis is at present defined as a disease characterized by low bone mass (microarchitectural deterioration of bone tissue with about 65 to 80% of the bone mass affected[3]), which can be measured accurately and noninvasively by recently developed techniques. Osteoporosis therefore varies in degree of severity, and can be regional, as in transient osteoporosis.

The term *transient demineralization of the hip* was introduced by Curtiss and Kincaid[4] and refers to a rapidly developing, painful local osteoporosis of limited nature and unexplained pathophysiology.[5-15] The syndrome was later termed *transient osteoporosis* of the hip by Lequesne in 1968.[10] Because of the rarity of the disease and the uncertainty of the underlying etiology, transient osteoporosis may be confused with a variety of other conditions, with avascular necrosis perhaps the most common misdiagnosis. Numerous synonyms exist such as algodystrophy, bone-marrow-edema syndrome, and transient marrow edema syndrome.[16-19]

II. DEMOGRAPHIC AND CLINICAL DATA

Transient osteoporosis can occur at any age and in either sex, but most often it occurs in women in the third trimester of pregnancy and in middle-aged men.[6,20] Rare cases of transient osteoporosis have been reported in woman during the second trimester of pregnancy,[21] after childbirth,[22] and in children.[23,24] There are no known predisposing factors except pregnancy. In addition, the risk of acquiring transient osteoporosis is much higher in patients with osteogenesis imperfecta than in the general population.[12,25] Other suggested etiopathogenic mechanisms are listed in Table 23.1.

Transient osteoporosis mostly affects a single joint, most often the hip, but there may be a local recurrence in the same or contralateral hip.[21] Simultaneous involvement of both hips is rare and has been only reported in pregnant women.[6,21,26] In addition, there have been reports of a radial form of the disease that involves one or two rays of the hand or foot, and a zonal form that affects a quadrant of a joint.[27,28] Clinically, sequential involvement of additional joints may occur, causing a migratory pattern.[12,29] Regional migratory osteoporosis is thought to be a variant of transient osteoporosis. The migratory pattern is not restricted to the contralateral hip, but commonly affects the foot and ankle and is associated with swelling of the affected part (Figures 23.1 through 23.4).

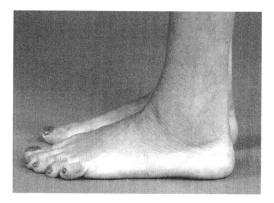

FIGURE 23.1 Clinical picture demonstrating swelling of the left ankle joint.

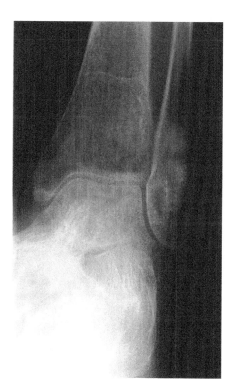

FIGURE 23.2 Radiograph of the left ankle joint demonstrating periarticular osteopenia of the distal tibia and talus.

The clinical diagnosis can be elusive, and the symptoms are often initially misinterpreted. Misdiagnosis as symphysiolysis, tuberculosis, avascular necrosis, stress fracture of the femoral neck, a malignant lesion, synovial chondromatosis, or vilonodular synovitis has led to unnecessary tests and morbidity.[30] Usually patients report an acute onset of (mild) pain in the affected area that progresses for several weeks to months to severe pain or disability. In case of hip involvement, the pain is usually localized to the trochanter, groin, and anterior part of the thigh.[6] The pain is usually worse during weight bearing and mild or absent during rest. Only rarely is there pain at night. During the period of maximum symptoms, there is a disproportionate functional disability as described by Lequesne.[10]

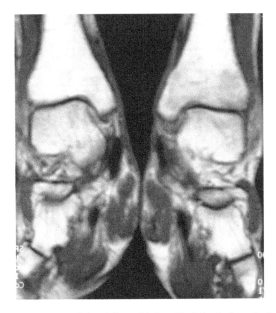

FIGURE 23.3 T1-weighted MR image of the right and left ankle joint in lateral view demonstrating irregular areas of decreased signal intensity of the left distal tibia and talus.

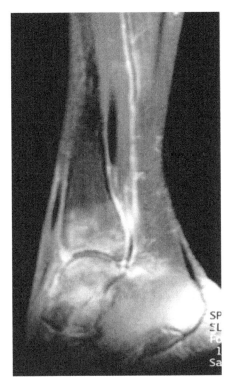

FIGURE 23.4 T2-weighted fat suppressed (STIR) MR image of the same joint in lateral view demonstrating high signal intensity in the area corresponding to the regions of low signal intensity of Figure 23.3.

Physical examination shows minimal restriction of joint movement, but pain often is elicited at the limits of motion.[6,30,31] In the case of hip involvement, an antalgic limb can be observed and thigh atrophy may occasionally be seen but is never marked and recovers as pain lessens. The discrepancy between the disability and the minimal abnormalities on examination is characteristic and provides help in the differential diagnosis. In pregnant women the condition is often first diagnosed as symphysiolysis of the pubis, but there is no tenderness over the symphysis or adductor muscle origins and abduction is not limited by adductor spasm.

Three distinctive phases of clinical involvement (rapid aggravation, maximal intensity, and regression) are described in transient osteoporosis.[32] The initial phase is characterized by a rapid progression of pain resulting in functional disability, followed by a second phase in which the symptoms reach a plateau in intensity. Finally, the symptoms subside until complete clinical resolution.

III. ETIOPATHOGENESIS

The etiology of transient osteoporosis is uncertain, and the proposed hypotheses are only speculative (see Table 23.1).

In 1968, Lequesne reported on ten cases and suggested that transient osteoporosis was a nontraumatic variety of sympathetic reflex dystrophy.[10] However, the absence of classical signs that are usually diagnostic of sympathetic reflex dystrophy does not support that pathophysiologic mechanism. Nevertheless, many authors have theorized that focal transient osteoporosis syndromes are forms of reflex sympathetic dystrophy.

Curtiss and Kincaid[4] suggested the possibility of intermittent mechanical compression of the mother's obturator nerve by the child's head. However, neither experimental compression nor obturatorius neurectomy produced osteopenia of the hip in dogs.[4] Compression of the pelvic nerves has also been mentioned but has never been confirmed by other authors.[33]

McCord et al.[34] reported positive electromyographic findings (denervation potentials), but other investigators have obtained normal electromyographic data from individual patients experiencing transient osteoporosis.

Impairment of venous return has been suggested,[35] while Hunder and Kelly[25] pointed out that the bone demineralization is unlikely to be due to disuse because normal density is restored despite restricted weight bearing. Both the development of edema of the bone marrow and the increased intramedullary pressure suggest that the cause of transient osteoporosis may be disturbed venous outflow, rather than an interrupted arterial supply.[18]

Other authors have postulated that a transient ischemic insult to the bone may be responsible for transient osteoporosis.[18,36,37] Accordingly, the ischemic insult results in a limited cell death involving only the hematopoietic and fatty elements.

Most often transient osteoporosis develops spontaneously, but it might occur after overexertion or mild trauma, lending support to the microfracture hypothesis.[31] The similarity of idiopathic transient osteoporosis of the hip and regional osteoporosis elsewhere in the skeleton[29,38] suggests a common etiology, and Frost[39] has classified the latter as a disorder of increased bone turnover. It is proposed that, in idiopathic transient osteoporosis, an unknown stimulus activates a large number of bone turnover foci, initiating intensive osteoclast resorption. Later in the cycle, osteoid is laid down, mineralized, and remodeled, but during the hiatus between resorption and formation, significant loss of bone tissue is manifested by decreased radiographic density. During this interval the bone is weak and vulnerable to microfractures, which we consider to be the cause of pain in the absence of weight bearing. The periosteal reaction occasionally observed along the femoral neck is further evidence, and if healing of microfractures is inadequate a stress fracture may occur.

There is a lack of evidence for the primary role of synovial inflammation in the etiopathogenesis of transient osteoporosis.

TABLE 23.2
Putative Risk Factors for Osteoporosis

Genetic factors
Age
Gender
Menopausal state
Body weight
Calcium intake
Caffeine intake
Smoking
Alcohol consumption
Physical activity
Vitamin D status
Medication

TABLE 23.3
Risk Factors for Osteoporosis
Common in Elderly Individuals

Postmenopausal status
Declining physical activity
Immobilization
Deficient nutrition
Declining body weight
Declining calcium consumption
Vitamin D deficiency
Use of medication

IV. RISK FACTORS

Bone mass is the result of the peak bone mass, attained during early adulthood, and subsequent bone loss.[40] Many risk factors for osteoporosis have been proposed, but it is unknown whether these factors are important in cases of transient osteoporosis (Table 23.2). Risk factors in elderly individuals are, in principle, not different from those in younger groups. The prevalence of some risk factors, however, increases dramatically with age, as shown in Table 23.3.

A. Aging

Aging is associated with increased morbidity, resulting in decreased activity, immobilization, poor vitamin D status, decrease in calcium absorption, and more frequent use of harmful medicines such as corticosteroids.[40] These factors account much for the age-related generalized bone loss. To what extent the aging process itself is responsible for transient bone loss is unclear. Transient osteoporosis occurs in middle-aged men and there are no known risk factors for this group.

B. Gender

An accepted risk factor in the development of transient osteoporosis in pregnant women in the third trimester of pregnancy.[6,20] To date, only cases of involvement of the hip joint have been described in pregnant women and other joints seem not to be affected.

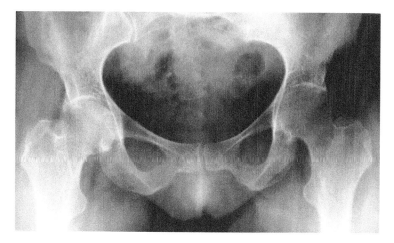

FIGURE 23.5 Radiograph of the pelvis demonstrating diffuse demineralization of the left femoral head and neck. The joint space is preserved.

C. GENETICS

The risk of acquiring transient osteoporosis is much higher in patients with osteogenesis imperfecta than in the general population.[12] It is not known if the increased risk is due to the genetic disorder itself or due to the increased risk of developing microfractures in patients with osteogenesis imperfecta.

D. OTHER RISK FACTORS

Usually patients with transient osteoporosis do not have any disease definitely associated with osteoporosis or with osteonecrosis. However, patients with transient osteoporosis may have risk factors associated with avascular necrosis such as alcohol abuse, nicotine consumption, or hyperuricemia.[5] In addition, rarely, transient osteoporosis has been described in association with diseases like hyperlipoproteinemia Type IV[13] and liver cirrhosis.[41]

V. DIAGNOSIS

A. LABORATORY TESTS

Laboratory values usually are within normal limits, but elevated erythrocyte sedimentation rate and increased level of urinary hydroxyproline can be found, usually during the third trimester of pregnancy.[6,20,21] Other hematologic and biochemical studies are usually within normal limits. Serologic and specific tests including rheumatoid factor, antinuclear antibodies, and HLA B-27 antigen are all negative. Cultures for aerobic, anaerobic acid-fast, and fungal organisms are negative.

B. RADIOLOGIC EVALUATION

Conventional roentgenographs usually show regional periarticular osteoporosis of the hip, particular of the femoral head, with thinning and obscuration of the subchondral plate, and with preservation of the joint space (Figure 23.5).[42] Changes are seen on radiographs approximately 4 to 8 weeks after the onset of clinical symptoms and are best seen by comparison with a radiograph of the asymptomatic hip.[35,42,43] The cortical outline of the involved area thins, with blurring of its margins and mottling. This may progress to complete effacement of the subchondral cortex and, in patients who have severe disease, to nearly total disappearance of the osseous architecture, which creates

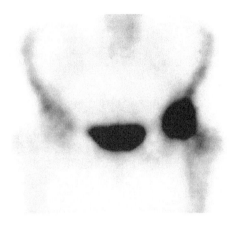

FIGURE 23.6 Bone scan demonstrating homogeneous increased uptake of tracer in the left femoral neck and head.

an optical void and a so-called phantom appearance. Rarely, the trochanters, the acetabula, and even the iliac wings and the ischiopubic rami may be affected. There may be periosteal reaction. Thus, radiographs taken during the early phase of transient osteoporosis reveal normal findings, the so-called window period. An indistinct femoral head in association with a normal cartilage space is sometimes difficult to differentiate from radiographic images of early stages of low-grade infection, rheumatic arthritis, or Wilson's disease.[6,44]

Bone scintigraphy shows intense, homogeneous uptake, even before radiographic changes appear (Figure 23.6).[43,45] The change seen on the bone scan most often is homogeneously intense, involving the affected area. Extension of the increased uptake into the diaphysis of the femur occurs in more than half of the patients with transient osteoporosis of the hip.[45] The bone scan abnormalities gradually decrease, heralding a normal background appearance and paralleling the clinical course.[46] As an isotope scan lacks specificity, additional investigations (computerized tomography, or CT; magnetic resonance imaging, or MRI) should be performed to confirm the diagnosis or help to exclude other disease processes.

Bone mineral measurements determine quantitatively the amount of calcium in the skeleton by measuring the attenuation of photons from a radioisotope source or an X-tube. Its application for screening for osteoporosis is still being debated.[47] The technique can be used to identify those patients at risk for fracture to monitor the efficacy of treatment, and to improve therapy compliance.[48] The attenuation is usually transformed to bone mineral content (BMC, in grams) or, when projected for the specific bone area to bone mineral density (BMD, in g/m^2). Several techniques are available, such as single-photon absorptiometry, dual energy X-ray absorptiometry (DXA), and quantitative CT. This last technique is expensive and has a very much higher radiation dose equivalent, which makes it unsuitable for routine use.[49] Dual energy X-ray absorption can confirm the local osteopenia in transient osteoporosis and can be used to monitor pharmaceutical treatment.[12]

CT and MRI help to exclude other diseases.[16,17,42,50,51] CT studies usually demonstrate a homogeneous decrease in bone density. MRI may show altered signal changes within 48 hours after the onset of transient osteoporosis and, especially in the early phase, the distinction between transient osteoporosis and avascular necrosis can be subtle.[43] Findings on MRI include a diffuse bone-marrow-edema pattern signal with ill-defined area of decreased intensity on T1-weighted images (Figure 23.7) with a matching area of increased signal intensity on T2-weighted images (Figure 23.8).[16,51]

However, the precise distribution of areas of abnormal bone marrow may vary from patient to patient. Wilson et al.[52] attributed these signal abnormalities to bone marrow edema, as the characteristics of the signal intensity are consistent with free water or edema within the normal fatty

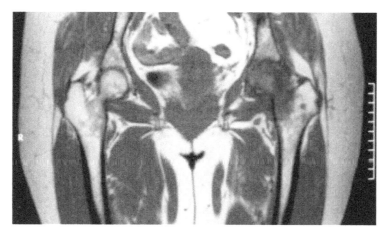

FIGURE 23.7 T1-weighted MR image of both hips demonstrating irregular areas of decreased signal intensity in the acetabulum, and head, neck, and intertrochanter region of the left femur.

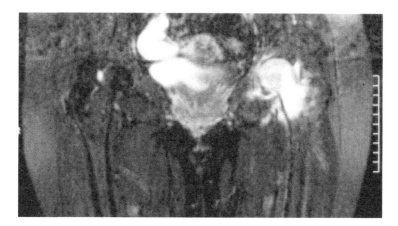

FIGURE 23.8 T2-weighted fat suppressed (STIR) MR image in the coronal plane demonstrating irregular high signal intensity in the area corresponding to the regions of low signal intensity of Figure 23.7. There is marked joint effusion.

marrow of the involved area. On MRI images, the loss of signal intensity is usually much more diffuse in patients who have transient osteoporosis of the hip than in patients with osteonecrosis of the femoral head. In patients who have transient osteoporosis, the alteration of the signal typically extends into the femoral neck and sometimes into the acetabulum (Figure 23.8). On T2-weighted images a variable degree of joint effusion can be demonstrated, as defined by the Mitchell classification (Figure 23.8).[53]

Bloem[16] has stated that the signal intensity changes in transient osteoporosis can be differentiated from those encountered in neoplasms[54] and osteomyelitis[55] in a proper clinical setting. Differentiation of the signal intensities changes between septic arthritis, complicated by osteomyelitis or by noninfective inflammatory reaction of bone marrow, and transient osteoporosis is probably impossible; therefore, cultures of synovial fluid should be taken. However, these conditions may be excluded by clinical history and laboratory findings in differential diagnosis.

Follow-up MRI images at time of convalescence may still demonstrate reduced areas of abnormalities of the bone marrow (Figure 23.9).[51] Thus, the recovery of clinical symptoms seems to precede remission of the MRI abnormalities. Joint effusion reduces simultaneously with the MRI

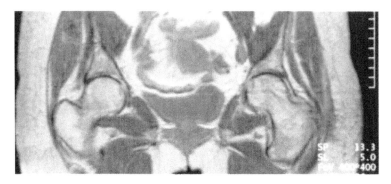

FIGURE 23.9 T1-weighted MR images in the coronal plane 5 months after starting coxalgia demonstrating improvement of the decreased signal intensity.

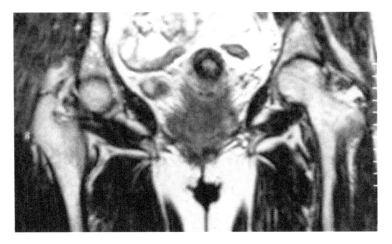

FIGURE 23.10 T1-weighted MR images in the coronal plane 1 year after core decompression of the left hip demonstrating completely normal signal intensity in comparison to the right site.

abnormalities. MRI monitoring over long intervals has shown complete disappearance of all marrow abnormalities (Figure 23.10).

C. HISTOLOGY

Invasive techniques usually are not helpful in diagnosing transient osteoporosis. While opening the joint space, increased synovial fluid and macroscopically abnormal synovium can be observed. In addition to normal histologic findings, evidence of osteoporosis (slender trabeculae), increased bone turnover, focal necrosis, partial fibrotic bone marrow, and mild inflammatory changes can be found in transient osteoporosis (Figure 23.11).[12,25,29,56] There are fragmented necrotic fat cells and the remnants of hemopoietic marrow show necrosis. In some areas hemopoietic or fatty marrow has been replaced by fibroblastic proliferation, a fibrous matrix, and new dilated vessels, suggesting an active repair process. The bone of the trabeculae appears to be viable except in some areas in the central portions of enlarged trabeculae in which there can be empty osteocyte lacunae. Usually extended osteoid seams can be demonstrated, mostly covered by active osteoblasts around the trabeculae. Osteoclastic resorption is rarely found. The decreased signal intensity on T1-weighted images and a corresponding increased signal intensity on T2-weighted images suggest an increase of water content in the bone marrow rather than bone marrow replacement.[53] However, ordinary processing of histologic preparations includes complete dehydration, and therefore it is almost

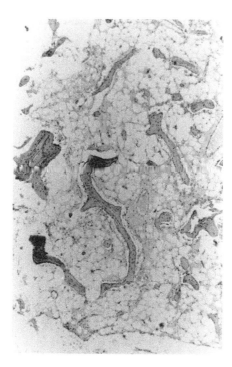

FIGURE 23.11 Core decompression biopsy of the left hip demonstrating areas of bone marrow edema and a reduced number of slender trabecula, lined with osteoblasts (hematoxylin and eosin; original magnification × 80).

impossible to detect the evidence of increased water content in biopsy or core decompression specimens. In undecalcified sections, however, this problem can be avoided and an increased interstitial fluid in bone marrow spaces has been demonstrated.[18]

Bone trabeculae show normal volume density and no sign of "osteoporosis." Quantitative microradiographs, however, can demonstrate a distinct loss of hydroxyapatite content, as compared to healthy, age-matched control femoral heads.[18] The abundant osteoid seams, the mineral loss detected by quantitative microradiography, and the marrow changes may be responsible for the focal loss of radiodensity.[18]

Aspirates of synovial fluid are sterile,[6] and microscopically synovial biopsies may show normal tissue or mild, chronic inflammation changes.[29]

D. DIFFERENTIAL DIAGNOSIS

The diagnosis of transient osteoporosis usually is made after exclusion of other abnormalities (Table 23.4). It is necessary to exclude other diseases, because effective prevention and treatment depends on it. In a "true transient osteoporosis," local bone fragility may increase to such an extent that normal activity can cause a regional pain syndrome and/or a spontaneous fracture, mainly affecting the involved joint. However, falls could also cause other extremity bone fractures. In a "true transient osteoporosis," reduced bone strength and "mass" would fit correspondingly reduced physical activities and muscle strength so well that fractures would not happen without falls or other injuries.

1. Osteonecrosis

The distinction between osteonecrosis and transient osteoporosis is important because the disorders may have distinct natural histories with respect to etiopathology, presentation, radiographic characteristics, and course. However, there is still controversy whether transient osteoporosis of a joint

TABLE 23.4
Differential Features between Transient Osteoporosis, Avascular Necrosis, and Sympathetic Reflex Dystrophy

	Transient Osteoporosis	Avascular Necrosis	Sympathetic Reflex Dystrophy
Gender	Female predominant	Equal	Female predominant
Age	Men 40–50 years old Female during last trimester of pregnancy	20–40 years old	Female 40–70 years old
Risk factors	Pregnancy, osteogenesis imperfecta	Steriods, alcohol, systemic lupus erythematosus, sickle cell disease, others	Hyperlipidemia, diabetes mellitus, hemiplegia, alcoholism, psychosocial factors
Etiology	Unknown	Circulation disturbance	Unknown
Onset	Acute	Insidious	Acute
Location	One joint, most often hip, most often one side	One joint, most often hip, 30% bilateral involvement	Limb, one or more joints, unilateral involvement
Symptoms	Pain with weight-bearing, normal soft tissues	Pain at rest, normal soft tissues	Pain during rest and with weight-bearing, abnormal soft tissue reaction
Motion joint	Minimal limited	Late phase limited	Limited
Muscle force	Normal	Normal	Limited
Roentgenogram	Osteopenia at 4–6 weeks, joint space preserved	Mottled radiolucency, sclerosis, crescent sign, collapse	Endosteal, cortical, subperiosteal resorption, subchondral erosion, preservation of joint space
Bone scan	Diffuse increased uptake	Focal increased uptake	Diffuse increased uptake
MRI	Diffuse bone marrow edema, T-1 decreased uptake, T-2 increased uptake	Focalized lesions, sometimes with some bone marrow edema	Most often normal bone marrow signal intensities
Treatment	Avoidance of weight bearing, pain relief, bisphosphonates	Core decompression, osteotomy, (non)vascularized graft, arthroplasty	Physiotherapy, drugs local and systemic, blocks, neurosurgical procedures, miscellaneous
Complication	Fracture	Collapse joint	Collapse, ankylosis
Prognosis	Excellent, complete recovery within 3–6 months	In 70–80%, progression to collapse resulting in degenerative joint disease	Recovery in 60–70%, frequent severe disability

represents a distinct self-limiting disease, or reflects only an early, reversible subtype of nontraumatic osteonecrosis.[19,57]

The etiology of osteonecrosis is myriad and may involve mechanical, hormonal, and coagulation factors,[58] with a perceived common final pathway resulting in the disruption of the circulation to the femoral head. Symptoms tend to include non-activity-related aching, with the development of limb changes only late in the course of the disease. Pain is typically exacerbated by weight bearing, but also is often present at rest. Limb changes and an antalgic gait are typically late findings, and the functional disability is proportional to the level of pain. Usually, the pain becomes severe as fragmentation and collapse of the femoral head take place.

As in transient osteoporosis, radiographs taken during the early phase of avascular necrosis reveal normal findings, so there is a so-called diagnostic window period in which symptoms are present without objective radiographic findings (Figure 23.12). In more advanced stages, radiographs reveal sclerosis, mottled radiolucency, subchondral radiolucency (the crescent line), and collapse. In later stages, a radiolucent so-called crescent sign may develop just distal to the articular

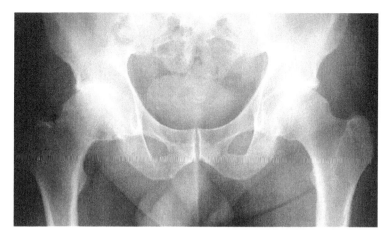

FIGURE 23.12 Radiograph of the pelvis demonstrating slightly decreased mineralization of the right femoral head with slightly reduced joint space compared to a normal left femoral head and hip joint.

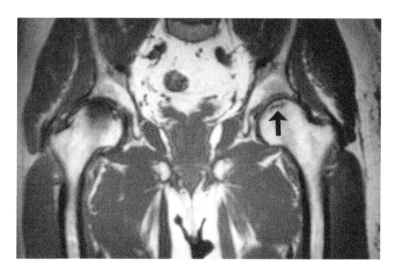

FIGURE 23.13 T1-weighted MR image of both hips demonstrating, at right, diffuse irregular areas of decreased signal intensity of the head and neck. In addition, there is a focal lesion specific for avascular necrosis at left (arrow).

surface and still later collapse of the femoral head and degenerative joint disease may become apparent.

Bone scans reveal focal areas of increased uptake within the femoral head.[43]

The advent of MRI has aided in the early diagnosis of osteonecrosis. Osteonecrosis results in focal lesions typically in the anterolateral aspect of the femoral head. These lesions demonstrate decreased signal intensity on both T1- and T2-weighted images, with a frequent finding of a double-density signal surrounding the lesion.[53,59] However, MRI images of patients who have early avascular necrosis occasionally demonstrate focal changes that are consistent with a diagnosis of avascular necrosis, accompanied by a surrounding pattern of bone marrow edema (Figures 23.13 and 23.14).[53,60] Thus, the distinction between these two entities early in their respective courses based on imaging studies alone is subtle.

In contrast to transient osteoporosis, osteonecrosis most often is progressive, and the outcome may include the collapse of the articular surface and the development of degenerative joint disease

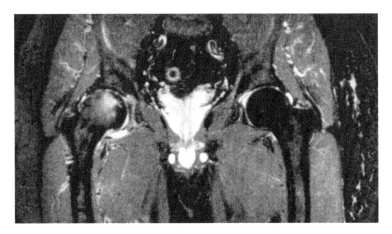

FIGURE 23.14 T2-weighted fat suppressed (STIR) MR image in the coronal plane demonstrating irregular high signal intensity in the area corresponding to the region of low signal intensity of the right and left hip.

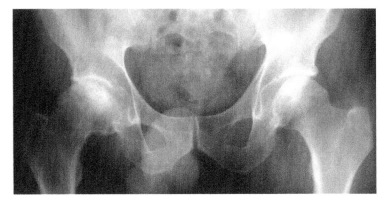

FIGURE 23.15 Radiograph of the pelvis 1 year after core decompression demonstrating early features of collapse of the right femoral head and an unchanged normal left femoral head.

(Figure 23.15). However, the potential for spontaneous healing of osteonecrosis has been clearly demonstrated in nontraumatic osteonecrosis of the femoral head that was diagnosed with MRI before any changes were visible on plain radiographs as well as in devascularized femoral heads after fracture of the femoral neck or dislocation.[61,62] The probability of progression to collapse is thought to increase after the development of an abnormality, i.e., the so-called crescent sign that can be seen on radiographs and that is indicative of a subchondral fracture. Ficat and Arlet[63] defined the appearance of the crescent sign as a transitional stage between a spherical and a flattened femoral head. It is widely agreed that after development of a crescent sign a progressive collapse occurs. However, the precise details of progression and the course of collapse are unknown and may be highly variable. Nevertheless, the often poor prognosis of osteonecrosis justifies the consideration of more invasive treatment options for this disease including osteotomy,[64,65] use of a nonvascularized structural graft,[66,67] core decompression,[68-70] and use of a vascularized graft.[62,71] The use of a free vascularized graft may provide a better outcome than core decompression in terms of avoiding or delaying the need for a total hip arthroplasty.[58] Bone regeneration in the necrotic area of avascular necrosis, however, is extremely slow, and the progression of collapse of the necrotic area cannot be prevented entirely, regardless of the intervention used (Figure 23.16).[72]

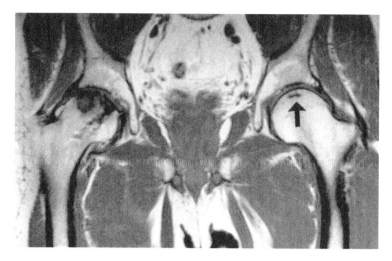

FIGURE 23.16 T1-weighted MR image of both hips 1 year after core decompression of the right femoral head demonstrating decreased signal intensity with early features of collapse. The core track is still visible. On the left unchanged increased signal intensity (arrow).

2. Sympathetic Reflex Dystrophy

Sympathetic reflex dystrophy is a complex regional pain syndrome for which numerous synonyms exist.[73] Most synonyms are related to a supposed pathogenesis, to the clinical signs, to diagnostic findings like those on radiographs, or to the inciting event.[74,75] Over the years, thoughts about the pathogenesis, definitions, and therapies have changed and they are still changing.

The causative events of sympathetic reflex dystrophy may vary considerably, including a minor strain, a contusion, a fracture, frostbite, myocardial infarction, and cancer. Sometimes it arises spontaneously or the causative event was so minor that the patient cannot remember it.

Risk factors for sympathetic reflex dystrophy are coexisting diseases including hyperlipidemia, diabetes mellitus, hemiplegia, or alcoholism. Women between the ages of 40 and 70 are more at risk than others.

In the pathogenesis of sympathetic reflex dystrophy two main theories exist: involvement of the sympathetic nerve system or an abnormal inflammatory reaction.[76] The involvement of the sympathetic system is assumed to be overactivity in the affected limb.[77] A theory of abnormal inflammation tissue reaction was described in 1982 by Fantone and Ward.[78] Excessive production of radicals produced by activated phagocytes or by ischemia induces an inflammatory process that leads to destruction of healthy tissues, which may lead to sympathetic reflex dystrophy. Positive results of treatment with scavengers substantiate this theory.[75,76]

The diagnosis is made mostly on the basis of clinical criteria, but no uniformly defined criteria exist.[79] Many physicians believe that the diagnosis of sympathetic reflex dystrophy can be made only when additional investigations have been made, such as a bone scan, thermography, testing of the sympathetic system, or radiography. Evidence for this belief is lacking, however.

Clinically, reflex sympathetic dystrophy may manifest within the first 6 weeks or so after injury by pain, edema, discoloration, hyperemia, hyperhydrosis, etc.[75] The intensity of the pain is disproportional to the causative event and shows a nonanatomic distribution. This suggests a behavioral or psychologic component. The typical cutaneous vasomotor signs and trophic changes and the high percentage of permanent disability are signs usually not seen in transient osteoporosis.[21]

Unlike findings at physical examination in transient osteoporosis, patients with sympathetic reflex dystrophy may show striking painful limitation of motion or joint stiffness.[75,80] One of the

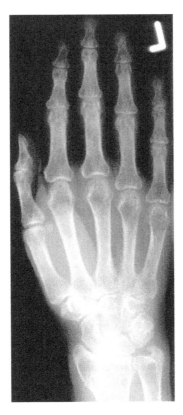

FIGURE 23.17 Radiograph of the left hand of a patient with sympathetic reflex dystrophy demonstrating diffuse periarticular osteoporosis.

earliest helpful signs of early sympathetic reflex dystrophy is intolerance to cold. In addition, in long-standing cases there are trophic changes (dystrophic, smooth, shiny skin, osteoporosis, fast-growing and brittle nails, hypertrichosis), a significant reduction in muscle force, and subcutaneous atrophy, findings not seen in transient osteoporosis.

Roentgenographs may show a variety of changes like resorption of cancellous or trabecular bone in the metaphyseal region leading to patchy or periarticular osteoporosis, subperiosteal bone resorption, intracortical bone resorption, endosteal bone resorption, and subchondral and juxta-articular erosion (Figure 23.17). The absence of significant intra-articular erosions and joint space loss usually allows accurate differentiation of reflex sympathetic dystrophy from various arthritides.

Bone scans usually show a diffuse, juxta-articular tracer uptake. Rarely, normal or decreased accumulation of the radionuclide on bone scans is observed, a finding that may be seen more frequently in children.

MRI studies show a periarticular marrow edema in all patients with the warm form of sympathetic reflex dystrophy, best seen on T2-weighted images, especially when fat suppression is used.[81] In addition, enhancement is noted on postgadolinium sequences. Other findings including soft tissue edema and thickening, joint effusion, and fissures are commonly noted but their absence does not exclude a diagnosis of sympathetic reflex dystrophy. Patients with the cold form of reflex sympathetic dystrophy have no abnormality of signal at MRI and this can be used to differentiate both forms. The main pitfall of using MRI, however, remains the lack of specificity for diagnosis of sympathetic reflex dystrophy.

A variety of treatment modalities have been proposed including physical therapy, drugs applied to the skin (DMSO), drugs administered regionally (guanethidine), drugs administered systemically, drugs administered at the level of the spinal cord (opiates), nerve blocks with local anesthetics, surgical procedures, neurosurgical procedures (thalamotomy), electrical neurostimulation, and other methods (radiation therapy, acupuncture).[74]

In contrast to the favorable prognosis of transient osteoporosis, successful cure rates of sympathetic reflex dystrophy are about 60 to 70%.[73,82,83] This claim, however, conflicts with the finding that a number of patients go medical-shopping, including physicians. In persistent cases, sympathetic reflex dystrophy may lead to chronic invalidism or even to amputation of the involved limb.

3. Disuse Osteoporosis

Osteoporosis confined to a region or segment of the skeleton can also develop in association with immobilization of a limb or portion of a limb. Disuse osteoporosis occurs subsequent to localized or generalized conditions, of which immobilization is a direct sequel. Many traumatic and non-traumatic conditions can lead to BMD loss associated with disuse osteoporosis, including extremity fracture, soft tissue injury, paralysis, long-term bed immobilization, and weightlessness. The resultant loss in BMD weakens the affected bone and predisposes that site to increased fracture risk.[84,85]

Disuse osteoporosis can develop at any age and in either sex, but most often it occurs in the immobilized regions of patients with fractures, motor paralysis due to central nerve disease or trauma, and bone and joint inflammation.

Pathogenetically, immobilization is associated with a significant increase in bone resorption; however, bone formation may be either slightly increased or decreased.[29,86] The initial active phase is characterized by a rapid loss of bone mineral content within the first 6 months of immobilization. The bone loss may include trabecular and cortical bone mass.[86] The inactive phase begins approximately 6 months after immobilization, and then bone loss reaches its nadir and less bone mass is maintained.[87] The development of a disuse osteoporosis depends on many factors including the age of the patient (in patients younger than 20 years or older than 50 years the osteoporosis develops sooner), and the extent and duration of the immobilization. Generally, after paralysis the osteoporosis appears within 2 to 3 months and within 8 weeks after immobilization.

Radiographically, a variable pattern of bone resorption can be observed, which may appear very aggressively. These findings include uniform osteoporosis (diffuse osteoporosis), speckled or spotty osteoporosis (a permeative pattern of bone destruction), bandlike osteoporosis, and lamellation and scalloping of the endosteal and or periosteal surface of the cortex (Figure 23.18).[29,88] Sometimes a generalized or scattered pattern can be observed. Furthermore, stress fractures or even true fractures may occur.

Both single-energy X-ray absorptiometry and dual absorptiometry have been proven reliable indicators monitoring the decrease of BMD and the recovery under treatment.[86,89]

In the acute phase increased calcium and phosphorus concentration can be measured in the urine; this is not compensated for by increase in intestinal calcium absorption. Thus, disuse osteoporosis is a high turnover osteoporosis.

In the course of the disease intra-articular alterations may develop as a result of cartilage fibrillation, erosion, denudation, and atrophy, and subchondral bone abnormalities including cysts are additional recognized findings. This and soft tissue changes may result in joint stiffness and sometimes even in ankylosis.

Evidence indicates that reversal of bone loss depends on return of mobilization during the active phase, before long-term bone has been established during the inactive phase.[90,91] However, the loss of BMD may continue after remobilization and after long-term immobilization losses in bone mass may never be recovered.[86,92,93]

4. Transient Regional Osteoporosis around Implants

Bone remodeling after insertion of plates/screws or a joint implant is a well-known phenomenon caused by (focal) reduction of bone stress (stress shielding) beneath a plate or along a joint implant.

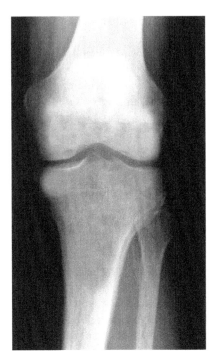

FIGURE 23.18 Radiograph of the left knee joint demonstrating speckled osteoporosis of the distal femur toward diffuse osteoporosis of the proximal tibia.

TABLE 23.5
Bone Loss around Implants Secondary
to Adaptive Bone Remodeling

Cemented vs. uncemented
Stem diameter
Cross-sectional geometry
Alloy
Porous coating
Pore geometry
Bone loss secondary to particle debris
Bone loss as a natural consequence of aging

The complex interaction among materials, design, fixation, surgical method, and bone makes selection of the most appropriate material difficult. This is further complicated by the uncertain role of other as yet unidentified factors, either alone or in combination with factors that contribute to continuous and temporarily focal bone loss (Table 23.5).

Continuous bone remodeling may play an important factor in both the development of regional osteoporosis around joint implants and as a mechanism of loosening.[94] Poss[95] measured a mean rate of cortical expansion of 0.33 mm per year and an average bone loss of cortical bone of 0.15 mm per year at a mean of 11.5 years after cemented femoral replacements. Although Comadoll et al.[96] have suggested that this decrease in cortical thickness and increase in canal enlargement with time may lead to loss of support and loosening of the femoral prosthesis, its role in femoral component loosening is not well established. Jasty et al.[97] found evidence of periprosthetic cancellous bone remodeling around well-fixed cemented stems that had been implanted for long periods. They

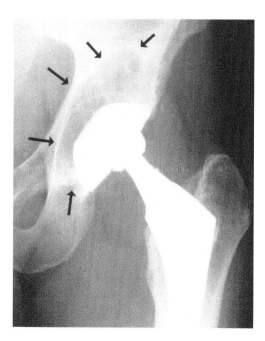

FIGURE 23.19 Radiograph taken 5 years after surgery with a 5 × 2 cm osteolytic lesion. The arrows point to the boundaries of the acetabular osteolytic lesion.

concluded that the aging process does not represent a threat to the mechanical stability of cemented femoral components.[97,98] The remodeling changes after inserting a cemented femoral stem drastically differ from the normal patterns of endosteal enlargement and thinning of the original cortex with age; a neocortex develops around the cement mantle. This occurs in the form of dense trabecular bone and, in some areas, the transformation into cortical structures that grow surrounding the cement mantle. Therefore, the implants can remain rigidly fixed. Similar intramedullary remodeling is likely to occur around uncemented stems.

Not only has continuous bone loss around implants been observed, but also, superimposed on localized bone resorption in the vicinity of an implant, a disuse osteoporosis may develop.[99] Prior to operative intervention in patients having osteoarthrosis and in the first few months after implantation of a total hip or knee prosthesis a decreased BMC has been measured.[100] The bone loss can be attributed in part to the unloading of the osteoarthrotic leg, the operative intervention, and the reduced activity in the first few months. After successful operation, the disuse osteoporosis comes to a complete halt and normalizes after 1 year.[100]

Continuous and temporary bone loss around joint implants should be differentiated from increased regional bone loss due to osteolysis (Figure 23.19).[101,102] The terms *osteolysis* and *aseptic loosening,* although appearing to refer to distinct clinical entities, actually represent a similar disease process with the same basic mechanisms. Today, the pathogenesis of osteolysis is called "particle disease." Factors that are involved are metal debris[103-105] and particulate debris of PMMA as a result of cement mantle defects and of ultra-high-molecular-weight polyethylene (UHMWPE).[106,107] Also, specific design features of a prosthesis can affect the adaptive remodeling patterns. Cemented femoral stems are generally more flexible and create less stress shielding than uncemented stems.[108] The critical factor governing bone loss is not just the absolute stem stiffness but also its stiffness relative to the femur. This relationship depends on the cross-sectional geometry and the material properties of the stem of the femur. Differences in stiffness between the stem and the femur are greatest in the metaphysis for all stem sizes, owing to the triangular proximal implant shape. The proximal stiffness disparity between the implant and the femur may explain the general tendency for the most bone loss and the fastest rate of bone loss to occur in the metaphysis that may be altered by increased stem flexibility.[109] However, increased stem flexibility may enhance relative motion between the stem and the endosteal bone surface, which more readily leads to abrasion and formation of particulate debris. Thus, the material of the implant affects the loading features of the femur and the ultimate remodeling of the femur.

In addition, various types of porous coatings have different pore geometries, mechanical properties, and patterns of bone ingrowth. These may affect stress transfer mechanisms and, in turn, influence the bone remodeling processes.[110] Thus, the extent of stem coverage by the porous coating is another important variable. Extensive coating of femoral stems may encourage distal fixation and thereby promote transfer of load distally, which would tend to reduce strains in the proximal cortex and ultimately lead to a net loss of bone proximally.[111] Proximally coated stems reduce the loss of bone relative to fully coated stems regardless of size and may have a beneficial long-term effect on femoral integrity.[112] Thus, patterns of stress shielding also are influenced by the nature of the porous coating in cementless femoral components.

Osteonecrosis is a rare but dramatic cause of focal bone loss following joint arthroplasty. Patellar osteonecrosis[113] and even a stress fracture of a lateral femoral condyle,[114] both following total knee arthroplasty, have been described.

Reliable quantitative information concerning bone remodeling is difficult to obtain from plain radiographs. DEXA studies are in this respect superior and usually demonstrate a reduction in BMD in the region of the calcar and an increase in BMD in the femoral shaft distal to the tip of the implant after cemented total hip arthroplasty.[115] The greatest decrease in BMD has been observed in the proximal medial femoral cortex after cementless total hip arthroplasty (THA).[116] However, the proximal medial cortex still represents the specific region of maximal bone loss after both types of implant fixation.

It should be emphasized that few clinical problems have arisen from pronounced stress-related bone resorption, and patients with well-fixed bone-ingrowth prostheses typically have excellent clinical results. However, the concern of stress shielding and bone loss is not trivial, especially at the time of revision. The identification of specific biologic pathways important in initiating (temporary) regional bone loss and/or inflammation as a result of the implant and of operative intervention and rehabilitation has the potential to lead to the development of improvement in implant material, design, and operative method and even pharmacologic interventions designed to reduce or reverse focal osteolysis. This last, however, remains a future hope rather than a close reality.

5. Transient Regional Osteoporosis and Osteoarthrosis

The incidence of patients with transient osteoporosis and osteoarthrosis is not known. There may be significant errors regarding the true incidence because the sampling rate is not accurate and the selection of the patient has not been performed by proper standards. There may be patients who have osteoarthrosis and who have no symptoms despite development of (transient) osteoporosis. In addition, radiography or other imaging modalities may not be able to identify osteoporosis accurately.

Clinical studies have shown that the two most common musculoskeletal disorders, osteoporosis and osteoarthrosis, are rarely present together in the same patient and that the presence of one may be protective against the other.[117-119] Pogrund et al.[120] found the prevalence of osteoporosis and osteoarthrosis in 641 pelvic radiographs separately was 16.1 and 4.1%, but in only 0.5% did osteoarthrosis and osteoporosis coexist in the same individual. Hip fractures in patients with osteoporosis and osteoarthrosis, therefore, are rare (Figure 23.20). Osteoporosis was more prevalent in an ethnic subpopulation, whereas osteoarthrosis appeared to have no relationship to ethnic origin.

Epidemiological surveys have suggested a negative association between the osteoarthrosis and osteoporosis and support the hypothesis that the two conditions are two distinct diseases and not phenomena related to aging.[120,121] However, it has not been established whether this apparent lack of association occurs by chance or whether there are underlying causal factors.

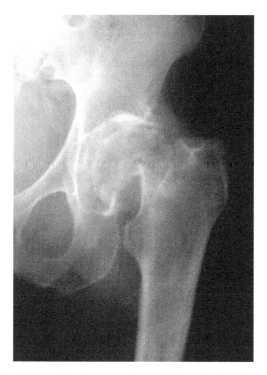

FIGURE 23.20 Radiograph of the pelvis demonstrating a displaced subcapital fracture of the left femoral neck with features of osteoarthrosis and regional osteoporosis.

Probably the most marked difference between osteoporosis and osteoarthrosis is the quantity of bone present. The presence of plentiful trabecular bone in osteoarthrosis may alter stress distribution within the femoral neck and provides additional strength in regions of high stress engendered by a fall. In osteoarthrotic bone, trabecular bone does have an increased density but a reduced material density, apparently as a consequence of a reduced mineral content, whereas the calcar bone shows small, but significant, increase in mineral content compared to osteoporosis.[122] Radin and Paul[123] produced evidence that loss of resilience of subchondral bone may predispose to osteoarthrosis. This loss of resilience allows easier compression of articular cartilage, thereby interfering with nutrition and contributing to the so-called compression necrosis of Salter and Field.[124]

It is difficult to reconcile the theory outlined above with the reality of osteoporosis. With decreasing numbers of trabeculae in osteoporotic bone, together with marked thinning of those remaining, it would appear that so-called resilience and subchondral bone support cannot possibly be retained. A study of trabecular bone from sites all over the femoral head showed there was a significant loss of stiffness and strength in an osteoporosis group and that this was largely due to an 18% loss in bone volume.[125] Both calcar and trabecular bone show a reduction of density due to loss of bone; however, composition and material do not change when compared with normal individuals.[122]

VI. COMPLICATIONS

A pathologic fracture is considered to be the most serious complication of transient osteoporosis; however, this happens only in the minority of cases and has only been described in patients with transient osteoporosis of the hip.[4,6,43,126] In all cases there was a delay between establishing the diagnosis and the onset of symptoms. Especially in pregnant women there may be a delay in diagnosis due to the fear of using radiography.[31,127] In some cases the symptoms were interpreted to be consistent with peripelvic pain syndrome, others were thought to be sciatica,[126,128] while in other cases only retrospectively was an impacted, healed subcapital fracture of the involved femur diagnosed.[4,31] In the presented cases, minimum to severe displacement of a subcapital fracture of the hip was found.[31,126-128] Subsequent to a transient osteoporosis of the proximal femur with a subcapital stress fracture, the development of a transient, multifocal transient osteoporosis of the knee, ankle, foot, and spine has been reported.[31] In case of displacement, conservative (non-weight-bearing, casting) and operative (cannulated screws) interventions had been performed. In all cases, follow-up radiographs showed increased mineralization of the osteopenic part of the proximal femur, healing of the fracture, and excellent hip function. Shifrin et al.[31] also noted radiographic evidence of new periosteal bone formation along the femoral neck, consistent with healing microfractures. Apparently, in transient osteoporosis the osteopenic bone has excellent healing potential and operative intervention of a displaced fracture can lead to a successful outcome.

Contractures may develop and therefore additional physical therapy may be necessary.

VII. TREATMENT

Transient osteoporosis is thought to be a self-limiting disorder. Many modes of treatment have been proposed and tried. Conservative treatment includes bed rest,[22] traction,[26,35] and physical therapy.[22,35] At present, protected weight bearing or avoidance of weight bearing is the preferred treatment for pain relief and prevention of pathologic fractures.[6,43,126] Active and passive range-of-motion exercises under physiotherapeutic guidance may be necessary to support balance and to prevent contractures when the course of the disorder is prolonged.[6] Surgical treatment of a fracture during pregnancy is problematic and some authors propose even to postpone the intervention until after delivery because of the risk inevitably linked with an anesthetic and operative measures.[128]

The issue of treating these patients with newer pharmaceuticals has attracted little interest until recently, because of the difficulty of treating these patients effectively and of the overall excellent prognosis even without treatment. However, since effective drugs to treat osteoporosis are becoming available and it has become clear that the lengthy period of symptoms with impairment and the possibility of serious complications of transient osteoporosis interfere with active return to or participation in society, efforts should be made to treat these patients more effectively. There are reports of benefit of analgesics for pain relief, but other medications (corticosteroids, nonsteroidal anti-inflammatory agents, and calcitonin) seem to have little benefit.[10,14,22,129] Even sympathetic blocks have been tried,[10] but none of the treatment regimes seems to alter the natural benign course of the disease. However, pharmaceutical intervention to prevent or halt the progression of transient osteoporosis should still be considered. Many cytokines may have multiple, overlapping activities, regulate each other, and may interfere with receptor expression and activation of certain bone resorbing agents, such as metalloproteinases and cyclooxygenases. Tissue inhibitors of metalloproteinases or anticytokine antibodies may be a therapeutic option. In addition, the clinical application of bisphosphonates in appropriate doses and time schedule, which now are widely used in the treatment of generalized osteoporosis, should be investigated as well for prevention or treatment of transient osteoporosis (Table 23.6). To underline this rationale, it has been shown that bisphosphonates can prevent the development of osteolysis significantly in a canine osteolysis model.[130]

Because low-grade infection can present similar findings, joint aspiration and culture should be considered. Core decompression is suggested to increase clinical improvement,[18] but the benefit of this procedure is doubtful.

VIII. PROGNOSIS

Usually transient osteoporosis resolves spontaneously after 3 to 8 months.[20,43] However, recurrences of transient osteoporosis in the same or another joint have been reported in as many as 41%.[21] Serial MRI can be performed to monitor the progress of the disorder and to distinguish, at an early

TABLE 23.6
Various Bisphosphonates

Bisphosphonate	Labeled use
Alendrolate	Glucosteroid-induced osteoporosis
	Osteoporosis prevention
	Paget's disease
Pamidronate	Bone metastasis
	Hypercalcemia of malignancy
	Osteolytic bone metastasis
	Paget's disease
Etidronate	Heterotopic ossification
	Hypercalcemia of malignancy
	Osteolytic bone metastasis
	Paget's disease
Risedronate	Primary hyperparathroidysm
	Paget's disease
Tiludronate	Paget's disease

stage, transient osteoporosis from avascular necrosis of the hip.[43] Transient osteoporosis in pregnancy deserves special attention, while traumatic fractures of the femoral neck and stress fractures have been described only in pregnant women.[128] Conservative and operative interventions in the case of a fracture have an excellent prognosis. Recurrences with later pregnancies have been described.[31] In addition, patients with osteogenesis imperfecta should be followed carefully to exclude (micro) fractures and to monitor migration pattern.

IX. FUTURE DEVELOPMENTS

The assessment of biochemical markers for the diagnosis and monitoring of osteoporosis is a recently used strategy, but to our knowledge, has not yet been used in cases of regional osteoporosis. The mark of resorption is the breakdown of collagen and the release of nondegradable collagen fragments measurable in either the serum or urine.

The rate of formation and degradation of bone can be established by measuring the spillover in blood enzymatic activity of bone-forming and bone-resorbing cells, or by measuring bone matrix components that are released into the circulation during formation and resorption. These markers are useful in determining the rate of turnover and in monitoring the effect of therapy.

There is a great variation in specificity and sensitivity between the markers.[131,132] The best-known marker of bone formation is the enzyme alkaline phosphatase (Aph), which is released by osteoblasts during bone formation. Aph can be very high when there is a disturbance in mineralization, e.g., in case of osteomalacia. As only a part of the Aph originates from the bone, the poor specificity can be enhanced by determining the bone specific fraction.[133] Osteocalcin also reflects bone formation. It is a small vitamin K–dependent, calcium-binding protein, specific for bone and dentine, which is embedded in the matrix after its production of the osteoblast. Some osteocalcin, however, will be released into the bloodstream during bone resorption as well.[134] Hydroxyproline, measured in a fasting morning sample of urine, can serve as a marker for bone resorption,[135] because about 50% of the collagen is located in bone, and about 13% of the collagen amino acid content is hydroxyproline. Nevertheless, the correlation between urine hydroxyproline and bone resorption as measured by other methods is small. The kidney excretes only about 10%, and significant amounts of collagen and hydroxyproline can be found in other tissues, which causes poor sensitivity and specificity.[132] Other promising markers for bone resorption are cross-linked N-telopeptide, pyridoline, and deoxypyridoline measured in urine and cross-linked carboxyterminal telopeptide of type I collagen measured in blood. These are, like hydroxyproline, freed during degradation of collagen. They have the advantage of being more specific to bone, and are excreted in urine without further metabolism.[132,136,137]

Biochemical markers as a method of evaluation, however, cannot be recommended strongly at this time for the diagnosis of resorption, but the sequential determination of bone resorption markers may be useful for ongoing and future treatment effects and for assessing treatment protocols.

It is not yet clear, however, if second- and third-generation bisphosphonates already in use for diverse bone diseases seem to offer a successful medical strategy to combat transient osteoporosis and other disorders with regional osteoporosis.

In conclusion, the diagnosis of transient osteoporosis is by exclusion of other diseases in addition to the typical findings described. Treatment is based on the premise that the condition is benign and self-limiting, requiring a conservative treatment. This means that the diagnosis cannot be absolutely certain until the patient has made a complete recovery.

REFERENCES

1. Albright, F. and Reifenstein, E.C., *The Parathyroid Glands and Metabolic Bone Disease*, Williams & Wilkins, Baltimore, MD, 2001.
2. Kanis, J.A., "Assessment of fracture risk and its application to screening for postmenopausal osteoporosis: synopsis of a WHO report. WHO Study Group," *Osteoporos. Int.*, 4, 368, 1994.
3. Shah, K.M., Goh, J., and Bose, K., "The relationship between femoral neck strength, bone mineral content and fracture fixation strength: an *in vitro* study," *Osteoporos. Int.*, 3, 51, 1993.
4. Curtiss, P.H. and Kincaid, W.E., "Transitory demineralization of the hip in pregnancy: a report of three cases," *J. Bone Joint Surg.*, 41A, 1327, 1959.
5. Banas, M.P., Kaplan, F.S., Fallon, M.D., and Haddad, J.G., "Regional migratory osteoporosis. A case report and review of the literature," *Clin. Orthop.*, 250, 303, 1990.
6. Bramlett, K.W., Killian, J.T., Nasca, R.J., and Daniel, W.W., "Transient osteoporosis," *Clin. Orthop.*, 222, 197, 1987.
7. Chigira, M., Watanabe, H., and Udagawa, E., "Transient osteoporosis of the hip in the first trimester of pregnancy. A case report and review of Japanese literature," *Arch. Orthop. Trauma Surg.*, 107, 178, 1988.
8. Dihlmann, W. and Delling, G., "Ist die transitorische Huftosteoporose eine transitorische Osteonekrose?" *Z. Rheumatol.*, 44, 82, 1985.
9. Gerster, J.C., Jaeger, P., Gobelet, C., and Boivin, G., "Adult sporadic hypophosphatemic osteomalacia presenting as regional migratory osteoporosis," *Arthritis Rheum.*, 29, 688, 1986.
10. Lequesne, M., "Transient osteoporosis of the hip. A nontraumatic variety of Sudeck's atrophy," *Ann. Rheum. Dis.*, 27, 463, 1968.
11. McCord, W.C., Nies, K.M., Campion, D.S., and Louie, J.S., "Regional migratory osteoporosis. A denervation disease," *Arthritis Rheum.*, 21, 834, 1978.
12. Noorda, R.J., van der Aa, J.P., Wuisman, P., et al., "Transient osteoporosis and osteogenesis imperfecta. A case report," *Clin. Orthop.*, 337, 249, 1997.
13. Pinals, R.S. and Jabbs, J.M., "Type-IV hyperlipoproteinaemia and transient osteoporosis," *Lancet*, 2, 929, 1972.
14. Scheinberg, M.A., Aristides, R.S., and Svartman, C., "Transient regional osteoporosis of the hip treated with calcitonin," *J. Rheumatol.*, 5, 236, 1978.
15. Steinberg, M.E., Hayken, G.D., and Steinberg, D.R., "A quantitative system for staging avascular necrosis," *J. Bone Joint Surg.*, 77B, 34, 1995.
16. Bloem, J.L., "Transient osteoporosis of the hip: MR imaging," *Radiology*, 167, 753, 1988.
17. Grimm, J., Higer, H.P., Benning, R., and Meairs, S., "MRI of transient osteoporosis of the hip," *Arch. Orthop. Trauma Surg.*, 110, 98, 1991.
18. Hofmann, S., Engel, A., Neuhold, A., et al., "Bone-marrow oedema syndrome and transient osteoporosis of the hip. An MRI-controlled study of treatment by core decompression," *J. Bone Joint Surg.*, 75B, 210, 1993.

19. Hofmann, S., Schneider, W., Breitenseher, M., et al., "Die 'transiente Osteoporose' als reversible Sonderform der Huftkopfnekrose," *Orthopäde*, 29, 411, 2000.
20. Schapira, D., "Transient osteoporosis of the hip," *Semin. Arthritis Rheum.*, 22, 98, 1992.
21. Lakhanpal, S., Ginsburg, W.W., Luthra, H.S., and Hunder, G.G., "Transient regional osteoporosis. A study of 56 cases and review of the literature," *Ann. Intern. Med.*, 106, 444, 1987.
22. Valenzuela, F., Aris, H., and Jacobelli, S., "Transient osteoporosis of the hip," *J. Rheumatol.*, 4, 59, 1977.
23. Nicol, R.O., Williams, P.F., and Hill, D.J., "Transient osteopaenia of the hip in children," *J. Pediatr. Orthop.*, 4, 590, 1984.
24. Nishiyama, K. and Sakamaki, T., "Transient osteopenia of the hip joint in children," *Clin. Orthop.*, 275, 199, 1992.
25. Hunder, G.G. and Kelly, P.J., "Roentgenologic transient osteoporosis of the hip. A clinical syndrome?" *Ann. Intern. Med.*, 68, 539, 1968.
26. Beaulieu, J.G., Razzano, C.D., and Levine, R.B., "Transient osteoporosis of the hip in pregnancy," *Clin. Orthop.*, 115, 165, 1976.
27. Swezey, R.L., "Transient osteoporosis of the hip, foot and knee," *Arthritis Rheum.*, 13, 858, 1970.
28. Bianchi, S., Abdelwahab, I.F., and Garcia, J., "Partial transient osteoporosis of the hand," *Skeletal Radiol.*, 28, 324, 1999.
29. Arnstein, A., "Regional osteoporosis," *Orthop. Clin. North Am.*, 3, 585, 1972.
30. Kaplan, S.S. and Stegman, C.J., "Transient osteoporosis of the hip. A case report and review of the literature," *J. Bone Joint Surg.*, 67A, 490, 1985.
31. Shifrin, L.Z., Reis, N.D., Zinman, H., and Besser, M.I., "Idiopathic transient osteoporosis of the hip," *J. Bone Joint Surg.*, 69B, 769, 1987.
32. Lequesne, M. and Mauger, B., "Cent algodystrophies decalcifiantes de la hanche chez 74 malades," *Rev. Rhum. Mal. Osteoartic.*, 49, 787, 1982.
33. Cayla, J., Chaouat, D., Rondier, J., et al., "Les algodystrophies reflexes des membres inferieurs au cours de la grossesse," *Rev. Rhum. Mal. Osteoartic.*, 45, 89, 1978.
34. McCord, W.C., Nies, K.M., Campion, D.S., and Louie, J.S., "Regional migratory osteoporosis: a denervation disease," *Arthritis Rheum.*, 21, 7, 834.
35. Rosen, R.A., "Transitory demineralization of the femoral head," *Radiology*, 94, 509, 1970.
36. Dunstan, C.R., Evans, R.A., and Somers, N.M., "Bone death in transient regional osteoporosis," *Bone*, 13, 161, 1992.
37. Hayes, C.W., Conway, W.F., and Daniel, W.W., "MR imaging of bone marrow edema pattern: transient osteoporosis, transient bone marrow edema syndrome, or osteonecrosis," *Radiographics*, 13, 1001, 1993.
38. Duncan, H., Frame, B., Frost, H.M., and Arnstein, A.R., "Migratory osteolysis of the lower extremities," *Ann. Intern. Med.*, 66, 1165, 1967.
39. Frost, H.M., "Osteoporosis and osteomalacias in spinal surgery," in *Spinal Disorders: Diagnosis and Treatment*, Ruge, D. and Wiltse, L.L., Eds., Lea & Febiger, Philadelphia, 1977, 87.
40. Lips, P. and Obrant, K.J., "The pathogenesis and treatment of hip fractures," *Osteoporos. Int.*, 1, 218, 1991.
41. Rozenbaum, M., Zinman, C., Nagler, A., and Pollak, S., "Transient osteoporosis of hip joint with liver cirrhosis," *J. Rheumatol.*, 11, 241, 1984.
42. Resnick, D. and Niwayama, G., "Transient osteoporosis of the hip," in *Diagnosis of Bone and Joint Disorders*, Resnick, D., Ed., W.B. Saunders, Philadelphia, 1995, 1802.
43. Guerra, J.J. and Steinberg, M.E., "Distinguishing transient osteoporosis from avascular necrosis of the hip," *J. Bone Joint Surg.*, 77A, 616, 1995.
44. Feller, E.R. and Schumacher, H.R., "Osteoarticular changes in Wilson's disease," *Arthritis Rheum.*, 15, 259, 1972.
45. Gaucher, A., Colomb, J.N., Naoun, A., et al., "The diagnostic value of 99m Tc-diphosphonate bone imaging in transient osteoporosis of the hip," *J. Rheumatol.*, 6, 574, 1979.
46. O'Mara, R.E. and Pinals, R.S., "Bone scanning in regional migratory osteoporosis. Case report," *Radiology*, 97, 579, 1970.
47. Melton, L.J., III, Eddy, D.M., and Johnston, C.C., "Screening for osteoporosis," *Ann. Intern. Med.*, 112, 516, 1990.

48. Ross, P.D., Heilbrun, L.K., Wasnich, R.D., et al., "Perspectives: methodologic issues in evaluating risk factors for osteoporotic fractures," *J. Bone Miner. Res.*, 4, 649, 1989.

49. Genant, H.K., Faulkner, K.G., Gluer, C.C., and Engelke, K., "Bone densitometry: current assessment," *Osteoporos. Int.*, 3, 91, 1993.

50. Daniel, W.W., Sanders, P.C., and Alarcon, G.S., "The early diagnosis of transient osteoporosis by magnetic resonance imaging. A case report," *J. Bone Joint Surg.*, 74A, 1262, 1992.

51. Takatori, Y., Kokubo, T., Ninomiya, S., et al., "Transient osteoporosis of the hip. Magnetic resonance imaging," *Clin. Orthop.*, 271, 190, 1991.

52. Wilson, A.J., Murphy, W.A., Hardy, D.C., and Totty, W.G., "Transient osteoporosis: transient bone marrow edema?" *Radiology*, 167, 757, 1988.

53. Mitchell, D.G., Rao, V., Dalinka, M., et al., "MRI of joint fluid in the normal and ischemic hip," *Am. J. Roentgenol.*, 146, 1215, 1986.

54. Richardson, M.L., Kilcoyne, R.F., Gillespy, T., et al., "Magnetic resonance imaging of musculoskeletal neoplasms," *Radiol. Clin. North Am.*, 24, 259, 1986.

55. Unger, E., Moldofsky, P., Gatenby, R., et al., "Diagnosis of osteomyelitis by MR imaging," *Am. J. Roentgenol.*, 150, 605, 1988.

56. Bruinsma, B.J. and LaBan, M.M., "The ghost joint: transient osteoporosis of the hip," *Arch. Phys. Med. Rehabil.*, 71, 295, 1990.

57. Solomon, L., "Bone-marrow oedema syndrome," *J. Bone Joint Surg.*, 75B, 175, 1993.

58. Montella, B.J., Nunley, J.A., and Urbaniak, J.R., "Osteonecrosis of the femoral head associated with pregnancy. A preliminary report," *J. Bone Joint Surg.*, 81A, 790, 1999.

59. Mitchell, D.G., Burk, D.L., Vinitski, S., and Rifkin, M.D., "The biophysical basis of tissue contrast in extracranial MR imaging," *Am. J. Roentgenol.*, 149, 831, 1987.

60. Turner, D.A., Templeton, A.C., Selzer, P.M., et al., "Femoral capital osteonecrosis: MR finding of diffuse marrow abnormalities without focal lesions," *Radiology*, 171, 135, 1989.

61. Catto, M., "A histologic study of avascular necrosis of the femoral head after transcervical fracture," *J. Bone Joint Surg.*, 47B, 749, 1965.

62. Urbaniak, J.R., Coogan, P.G., Gunneson, E.B., and Nunley, J.A., "Treatment of osteonecrosis of the femoral head with free vascularized fibular grafting. A long-term follow-up study of one hundred and three hips," *J. Bone Joint Surg.*, 77A, 681, 1995.

63. Ficat, R.P. and Arlet, J., *Ischemia and Necrosis of Bone*, Williams & Wilkins, Baltimore, MD, 1980.

64. Scher, M.A. and Jakim, I., "Intertrochanteric osteotomy and autogenous bone-grafting for avascular necrosis of the femoral head," *J. Bone Joint Surg.*, 75A, 1119, 1993.

65. Sugioka, Y., Hotokebuchi, T., and Tsutsui, H., "Transtrochanteric anterior rotational osteotomy for idiopathic and steroid-induced necrosis of the femoral head. Indications and long-term results," *Clin. Orthop.*, 277, 111, 1992.

66. Buckley, P.D., Gearen, P.F., and Petty, R.W., "Structural bone-grafting for early atraumatic avascular necrosis of the femoral head," *J. Bone Joint Surg.*, 73A, 1357, 1991.

67. Boettcher, W.G., Bonfiglio, M., and Smith, K., "Nontraumatic necrosis of the femoral head. II. Experiences in treatment," *J. Bone Joint Surg.*, 52A, 322, 1970.

68. Fairbank, A.C., Bhatia, D., Jinnah, R.H., and Hungerford, D.S., "Long-term results of core decompression for ischaemic necrosis of the femoral head," *J. Bone Joint Surg.*, 77B, 42, 1995.

69. Markel, D.C., Miskovsky, C., Sculco, T.P., et al., "Core decompression for osteonecrosis of the femoral head," *Clin. Orthop.*, 323, 226, 1996.

70. Mont, M.A., Carbone, J.J., and Fairbank, A.C., "Core decompression vs. nonoperative management for osteonecrosis of the hip," *Clin. Orthop.*, 324, 169, 1996.

71. Wassenaar, R.P., Verburg, H., Taconis, W.K., and van der Eijken, J.W., "Avascular osteonecrosis of the femoral head treated with a vascularized iliac bone graft: preliminary results and follow-up with radiography and MR imaging," *Radiographics*, 16, 585, 1996.

72. Yasunaga, Y., Hisatome, T., Ikuta, Y., and Nakamura, S., "A histologic study of the necrotic area after transtrochanteric anterior rotational osteotomy for osteonecrosis of the femoral head," *J. Bone Joint Surg.*, 83B, 167, 2001.

73. Atkins, R.M., Duckworth, T., and Kanis, J.A., "Features of algodystrophy after Colles' fracture," *J. Bone Joint Surg.*, 72B, 105, 1990.

74. Kurvers, H.A.J.M., Reflex Sympathetic Dystrophy: A Clinical and Experimental Study, Ph.D. thesis, University of Maastricht, Maastricht, the Netherlands, 1997.

75. Veldman, P.H.J.M., Clinical Aspects of Reflex Sympathetic Dystrophy, Ph.D. thesis, University of Nijmegen, Nijmegen, the Netherlands, 1995.

76. Goris, R.J., "Treatment of reflex sympathetic dystrophy with hydroxyl radical scavengers," *Unfallchirurg.*, 88, 330, 1985.

77. Bonica, J.J., "Causalgia and other reflex sympathetic dystrophies," in *Advances in Pain Research And Therapy*, Bonica, J.J., Liebeskind, J.C., and Albe-Fessard, D.G., Eds., Raven Press, New York, 1990, 220.

78. Fantone, J.C. and Ward, P.A., "Role of oxygen-derived free radicals and metabolites in leukocyte-dependent inflammatory reactions," *Am. J. Pathol.*, 107, 395, 1982.

79. Amadio, P.C., Mackinnon, S.E., Merritt, W.H., et al., "Reflex sympathetic dystrophy syndrome. consensus report of an ad hoc committee of the American Association for Hand Surgery on the definition of reflex sympathetic dystrophy syndrome," *Plast. Reconstr. Surg.*, 87, 371, 1991.

80. Geertzen, J.H., de Bruijn, H., de Bruijn-Kofman, A.T., and Arendzen, J.H., "Reflex sympathetic dystrophy: early treatment and psychologic aspects," *Arch. Phys. Med. Rehabil.*, 75, 442, 1994.

81. Darbois, H., Boyer, B., Dubayle, P., et al., "Semeiologie IRM de l'algodystrophie du pied," *J. Radiol.*, 80, 849, 1999.

82. Field, J., Warwick, D., and Bannister, G.C., "Features of algodystrophy ten years after Colles' fracture," *J. Hand Surg. Br.*, 17, 318, 1992.

83. Subbarao, J. and Stillwell, G.K., "Reflex sympathetic dystrophy syndrome of the upper extremity: analysis of total outcome of management of 125 cases," *Arch. Phys. Med. Rehabil.*, 62, 549, 1981.

84. Finsen, V., Haave, O., and Benum, P., "Fracture interaction in the extremities. The possible relevance of post-traumatic osteopenia," *Clin. Orthop.*, 240, 244, 1989.

85. Ragnarsson, K.T. and Sell, G.H., "Lower extremity fractures after spinal cord injury: a retrospective study," *Arch. Phys. Med. Rehabil.*, 62, 418, 1981.

86. Houde, J.P., Schulz, L.A., Morgan, W.J., et al., "Bone mineral density changes in the forearm after immobilization," *Clin. Orthop.*, 317, 199, 1995.

87. Minaire, P., "Immobilization osteoporosis: a review," *Clin. Rheumatol.*, 8, 95, 1989.

88. Jones, G., "Radiologic appearances of disuse osteoporosis," *Clin. Radiol.*, 20, 345, 1969.

89. Nieves, J.W., Cosman, F., Mars, C., and Lindsay, R., "Comparative assessment of bone mineral density of the forearm using single photon and dual X-ray absorptiometry," *Calcif. Tissue Int.*, 51, 352, 1992.

90. Jaworski, Z.F. and Uhthoff, H.K., "Reversibility of nontraumatic disuse osteoporosis during its active phase," *Bone*, 7, 431, 1986.

91. Mattsson, S., "The reversibility of disuse osteoporosis. Experimental studies in the adult rat," *Acta Orthop. Scand. Suppl.*, 144, 11, 1972.

92. Nilsson, B.E. and Westlin, N.E., "Long-term observations on the loss of bone mineral following Colles' fracture," *Acta Orthop. Scand.*, 46, 61, 1975.

93. Westlin, N.E., "Loss of bone mineral after Colles' fracture," *Clin. Orthop.*, 102, 194, 1974.

94. Turner, R.T., "The skeletal response to arthroplasty," in *Joint Replacement Arthroplasty*, Morrey, B.F., Ed., Churchill Livingstone, New York, 1991, 81.

95. Poss, R., "Natural factors that affect the shape and strength of the aging human femur," *Clin. Orthop.*, 274, 194, 1992.

96. Comadoll, J.L., Sherman, R.E., Gustilo, R.B., and Bechtold, J.E., "Radiographic changes in bone dimensions in asymptomatic cemented total hip arthroplasties. Results of nine- to thirteen-year follow-up," *J. Bone Joint Surg.*, 70A, 433, 1988.

97. Jasty, M., Maloney, W.J., Bragdon, C.R., et al., "Histomorphologic studies of the long-term skeletal responses to well fixed cemented femoral components," *J. Bone Joint Surg.*, 72A, 1220, 1990.

98. Wixson, R.L., Stulberg, S.D., and Mehlhoff, M.A., "A comparison of the bone remodeling and radiographic changes between cemented and cementless total hip replacements," presented at 56th Annual Meeting American Academy of Orthopaedic Surgeons, Las Vegas, NV, 1989.

99. Rüegsegger, P., Seitz, P., Gschwend, N., and Dubs, L., "Disuse osteoporosis in patients with total hip prostheses," *Arch. Orthop. Trauma Surg.*, 105, 268, 1986.

100. Seitz, P., Rüegsegger, P., Gschwend, N., and Dubs, L., "Changes in local bone density after knee arthroplasty. The use of quantitative computed tomography," *J. Bone Joint Surg.*, 69B, 407, 1987.

101. Rubash, H.E., Sinha, R.K., Shanbhag, A.S., and Kim, S.Y., "Pathogenesis of bone loss after total hip arthroplasty," *Orthop. Clin. North Am.*, 29, 173, 1998.

102. Lewis, P.L., Brewster, N., and Graves, S.E., "The pathogenesis of bone loss following total knee arthroplasty," *Orthop. Clin. North Am.*, 29, 187, 1998.

103. Martell, J.M., Pierson, R.H., Jacobs, J.J., et al., "Primary total hip reconstruction with a titanium fiber-coated prosthesis inserted without cement," *J. Bone Joint Surg.*, 75A, 554, 1993.

104. Nasser, S., Campbell, P.A., Kilgus, D., et al., "Cementless total joint arthroplasty prostheses with titanium-alloy articular surfaces. A human retrieval analysis," *Clin. Orthop.*, 261, 171, 1990.

105. Willert, H.G., "Reactions of the articular capsule to wear products of artificial joint prostheses," *J. Biomed. Mater. Res.*, 11, 157, 1977.

106. Jasty, M., Maloney, W.J., Bragdon, C.R., et al., "The initiation of failure in cemented femoral components of hip arthroplasties," *J. Bone Joint Surg.*, 73B, 551, 1991.

107. Maloney, W.J., Jasty, M., Harris, W.H., et al., "Endosteal erosion in association with stable uncemented femoral components," *J. Bone Joint Surg.*, 72A, 1025, 1990.

108. Huiskes, R., "The various stress patterns of press-fit, ingrown, and cemented femoral stems," *Clin. Orthop.*, 261, 27, 1990.

109. Skinner, H.B. and Curlin, F.J., "Decreased pain with lower flexural rigidity of uncemented femoral prostheses," *Orthopaedics*, 13, 1223, 1990.

110. Turner, T.M., Sumner, D.R., Urban, R.M., et al., "A comparative study of porous coatings in a weight-bearing total hip-arthroplasty model," *J. Bone Joint Surg.*, 68A, 1396, 1986.

111. Engh, C.A., Bobyn, J.D., and Glassman, A.H., "Porous-coated hip replacement. The factors governing bone ingrowth, stress shielding, and clinical results," *J. Bone Joint Surg.*, 69B, 45, 1987.

112. Bobyn, J.D., Glassman, A.H., Goto, H., et al., "The effect of stem stiffness on femoral bone resorption after canine porous-coated total hip arthroplasty," *Clin. Orthop.*, 261, 196, 1990.

113. Holtby, R.M. and Grosso, P., "Osteonecrosis and resorption of the patella after total knee replacement: a case report," *Clin. Orthop.*, 328, 155, 1996.

114. Insall, J.N. and Haas, S.B., "Complications of total knee arthroplasty," in *Surgery of the Knee*, Insall, J.N., Ed., Churchill Livingstone, New York, 1993, 891.

115. Cohen, B. and Rushton, N., "Bone remodeling in the proximal femur after Charnley total hip arthroplasty," *J. Bone Joint Surg.*, 77B, 815, 1995.

116. Kilgus, D.J., Shimaoka, E.E., Tipton, J.S., and Eberle, R.W., "Dual-energy X-ray absorptiometry measurement of bone mineral density around porous-coated cementless femoral implants. Methods and preliminary results," *J. Bone Joint Surg.*, 75B, 279, 1993.

117. Byers, P.D., Contepomi, C.A., and Farkas, T.A., "A postmortem study of the hip joint. Including the prevalence of the features of the right side," *Ann. Rheum. Dis.*, 29, 15, 1970.

118. Solomon, L., Schnitzler, C.M., and Browett, J.P., "Osteoarthritis of the hip: the patient behind the disease," *Ann. Rheum. Dis.*, 41, 118, 1982.

119. Cooper, C., Cook, P.L., Osmond, C., et al., "Osteoarthritis of the hip and osteoporosis of the proximal femur," *Ann. Rheum. Dis.*, 50, 540, 1991.

120. Pogrund, H., Rutenberg, M., Makin, M., et al., "Osteoarthritis of the hip joint and osteoporosis: a radiologic study in a random population sample in Jerusalem," *Clin. Orthop.*, 164, 130, 1982.

121. Dequeker, J. and Johnell, O., "Osteoarthritis protects against femoral neck fracture: the MEDOS study experience," *Bone*, 14, S51, 1993.

122. Li, B. and Aspden, R.M., "Material properties of bone from the femoral neck and calcar femorale of patients with osteoporosis or osteoarthritis," *Osteoporos. Int.*, 7, 450, 1997.

123. Radin, E.L. and Paul, I.L., "Does cartilage compliance reduce skeletal impact loads? The relative force-attenuating properties of articular cartilage, synovial fluid, periarticular soft tissues and bone," *Arthritis Rheum.*, 13, 139, 1970.

124. Salter, R.B. and Field, P., "The effects of continuous compression on living articular cartilage: an experimental investigation," *J. Bone Joint Surg.*, 42A, 31, 1960.

125. Li, B. and Aspden, R.M., "Composition and mechanical properties of cancellous bone from the femoral head of patients with osteoporosis or osteoarthritis," *J. Bone Miner. Res.*, 12, 641, 1997.

126. Fingeroth, R.J., "Successful operative treatment of a displaced subcapital fracture of the hip in transient osteoporosis of pregnancy. A case report and review of the literature," *J. Bone Joint Surg.*, 77A, 127, 1995.

127. Brodell, J.D., Burns, J.E., and Heiple, K.G., "Transient osteoporosis of the hip of pregnancy. Two cases complicated by pathologic fracture," *J. Bone Joint Surg.,* 71A, 1252, 1989.

128. Junk, S., Ostrowski, M., and Kokoszczynski, L., "Transient osteoporosis of the hip in pregnancy complicated by femoral neck fracture: a case report," *Acta Orthop. Scand.,* 67, 69, 1996.

129. Laroche, M., Dromer, C., Jacquemier, J.M., et al., "Association algodystrophie et maladie de Lobstein. Interet eventuel du traitement par l'acide 3 amino 1 hydroxy-propane 1-1-biphosphonique," *Rev. Rhum. Mal. Osteoartic.,* 57, 221, 1990.

130. Shanbhag, A.S., Hasselman, C.T., and Rubash, H.E., "The John Charnley Award. Inhibition of wear debris mediated osteolysis in a canine total hip arthroplasty model," *Clin. Orthop.,* 344, 33, 1997.

131. Kotowicz, M.A., Melton, L.J., Cedel, S.L., et al., "Effect of age on variables relating to calcium and phosphorus metabolism in women," *J. Bone Miner. Res.,* 5, 345, 1990.

132. Delmas, P.D., "Biochemical markers of bone turnover for the clinical investigation of osteoporosis," *Osteoporos. Int.,* 3(Suppl. 1), 81, 1993.

133. Brixen, K., Nielsen, H.K., Eriksen, E.F., et al., "Efficacy of wheat germ lectin-precipitated alkaline phosphatase in serum as an estimator of bone mineralization rate: comparison to serum total alkaline phosphatase and serum bone Gla-protein," *Calcif. Tissue Int.,* 44, 93, 1989.

134. Knapen, M.H., Jie, K.S., Hamulyak, K., and Vermeer, C., "Vitamin K-induced changes in markers for osteoblast activity and urinary calcium loss," *Calcif. Tissue Int.,* 53, 81, 1993.

135. Dempster, D.W. and Lindsay, R., "Pathogenesis of osteoporosis," *Lancet,* 341, 797, 1993.

136. Branca, F., Robins, S.P., Ferro-Luzzi, A., and Golden, M.H., "Bone turnover in malnourished children," *Lancet,* 340, 1493, 1992.

137. Hanson, D.A., Weis, M.A., Bollen, A.M., et al., "A specific immunoassay for monitoring human bone resorption: quantitation of type I collagen cross-linked N-telopeptides in urine," *J. Bone Miner. Res.,* 7, 1251, 1992.

24 Bone Ingrowth to Prosthetic Surfaces in Osteoporotic Bone

Donald G. Eckhoff

CONTENTS

I. INTRODUCTION

Studies of biologic fixation have traditionally ignored or poorly documented the effect of osteoporosis on the quality and quantity of bone formed around orthopaedic implants. In the clinical setting, most orthopaedic implants are placed in aged, osteoporotic skeletons. It is a paradox that most studies of biologic fixation traditionally have used young, non-osteoporotic animals to demonstrate the osseointegration of an implant. The argument may be raised that biologic fixation has been reserved for young individuals, therefore justifying testing in young, non-osteoporotic bone. However, the clinical indications for biologic fixation have expanded to include old as well as young candidates for cementless implants. Despite the broadening indications to include old, osteoporotic candidates, the effect of osteoporosis on the quality and quantity of biologic fixation of an implant has, with few exceptions, been ignored. Furthermore, studies of adjunctive coatings have been conducted with little concern for the confounding effect of bone characteristics on the quality and quantity of bone formed around the implant. The purpose of this chapter is to review the limited information available on the impact of osteoporosis on implant fixation and speculate on the role further study may play on refining this topic in the future.

II. FIXATION STUDIES

A. HOST FACTORS AFFECTING BIOLOGIC FIXATION

1. Historical Background

Biologic fixation with a porous implant was first reported in 1951 by Grindlay and Waugh.[1] The device they studied and reported was a polyvinyl sponge material for the filling and repair of soft tissue defects found in plastic surgery. Struthers[2] appreciated the fact that "new bone from skeletal structures might grow into the scaffolding offered by polyvinyl sponge" and suggested in 1955 the first use of a porous implant to fill a bone defect. Early investigations of porous material focused on ceramics and polymers for non-load-bearing applications. Because ceramic and polymer implants were unsuited to load-bearing orthopaedic and dental applications, later investigation turned to porous-coated metallic implants. Models developed to study the early, nonloaded ceramic and polymer implants in normal, non-osteoporotic bone were adopted to study the new porous-coated metallic implants. Biologic fixation was extensively studied in young, non-osteoporotic animals (rats, rabbits, dogs), where ingrowth of bone on the new porous-coated, metallic implants approached 100% of the implant surface.[3,4]

Based on the success of porous-coated, metallic implants in animal research, devices designed to treat the fractured hip were enthusiastically embraced for clinical trial. However, clinical retrieval studies of uncemented metal porous-coated prostheses failed to support the early enthusiasm generated by the animal models. Unlike the excellent results seen in animal studies, clinical retrievals revealed that many of the components were fixed to the skeleton by fibrous tissue ingrowth instead of bony ingrowth. The best clinical results in human subjects approached 50% of the implant surface covered with ingrowth of bone.[5,6] A majority of human clinical retrievals revealed less than 10% of the implant surface covered by ingrowth of bone.[7-11] Suspicion began to grow that the non-osteopenic animal model did not reflect the conditions found around the adult human implant.

2. Senile Osteoporosis

Few studies, whether animal or human, have addressed the issue of bone quality and quantity at the site of implantation of porous-coated, load-bearing orthopaedic implants. Magee et al.[12] attempted to address the issue of the quality of implant fixation in senile osteoporotic bone in a study of osseointegrated, transcortical, porous-coated plugs in old (6.6 years) and young (2.3 years) greyhounds. Their study documented a decrease in interface shear stress in the older animals, but several aspects of this study make the data difficult to interpret. The age of these animals was well documented, because accurate records are kept for racing animals. However, both genders were used in the study, and the integrity of the ovaries of the females was not documented. Gender influences the percentage of bone volume, a well-documented fact in humans.[13,14] Ovarian function influences bone metabolism, a fact well established in studies of osteopenia in the beagle.[15] If not ovariectomized, greyhounds experience the stress of training and racing that causes a cessation of ovarian function, much like amenorrhea in the female human athlete. Unovariectomized greyhound bitches often are subjected to long-term testosterone therapy to suppress estrus while racing, which would have a bone-sparing effect. The impact of these endogenous and exogenous hormones on biologic fixation in the greyhound is unclear. Therefore, the low-interface shear stress identified in the older animals in this study may reflect hormonal effects on the bone–implant interface or they may reflect, as suggested by the authors, a decreased capacity of senile, osteoporotic bone to form a strong bone–implant interface.

Nakajima et al.[16] studied implant fixation in the mid-diaphysis in young and old mongrel dogs. Age was loosely defined by the "degree of teeth wear and the color of the muzzle." Gender and reproductive status were not mentioned. Notwithstanding these significant limitations, they showed that the percentage of callus formation and callus quality around the mid-diaphyseal implant was significantly inferior in the old dogs during the early postoperative period (3 and 6 weeks). New bone formation occurred faster in the young dogs. In histologic sections, bone ingrowth increased in the young dogs more than in the old dogs. Other histomorphometric and biomechanical measurements were found not to differ significantly between the two age groups. Factors making interpretation of this study difficult are the poor documentation of age, gender, and reproductive status. Also, the diaphyseal location of the implant did not reflect the response of bone to an implant placed in a metaphyseal location, the location of most human clinical applications.

These two studies[12,16] are the only entries identified in either the animal or the human literature that support the intuitive notion that osseointegration of implants is age dependent, with old animals showing less capacity to produce a strong bone–ingrowth interface.

Eckhoff et al.[17] found no difference between old and young animals in their capacity to undergo osseointegration of a porous-coated implant. They studied sheep of known age and reproductive status. Functioning ovaries were identified histologically. The results of histomorphometric studies of the iliac crest in this study clearly demonstrated age-related decline in bone volume in the older sheep. Despite this aging effect of bone, the older animals showed no statistical difference in the interface shear stress for either an uncoated or a hydroxyapatite-coated implant when compared with the younger animals. In other words, there was no effect of age as an isolated variable on implant osseointegration in this study. The conventional wisdom that aging alone adversely affects biologic fixation must be challenged on the basis of this work.

Clinical studies of human implants further challenge the conventional wisdom that aging alone adversely affects implant osseointegration. In a study by Shaw et al.[18] reviewing the success of 178 AML porous-coated hip implants, bony ingrowth was achieved in all age groups with equal frequency. In a survey of patients in the Toronto Implant Study, Dao et al.[19] found patients at risk for osteoporosis were not at risk for implant failure. There were opposite age trends observed in the implant failure rate (a decrease with age) and the prevalence of osteoporosis (an increase with age), suggesting that it is unlikely that osteoporosis had any influence on implant failure in the clinical setting. Also, the rate of implant failure was not correlated with sex. These observations are consistent with data reported by Kondell et al.[20] in another clinical study that documents that age alone does not correlate with successful osseointegration of a porous-coated implant.

3. Menopause and Other Sources of Osteoporosis

If age and its associated senile osteoporosis do not bear a statistically significant relationship to the quality and quantity of osseointegration, do other sources of osteoporosis in the human skeleton have any effect? In animal models of estrogen deficiency induced by ovariectomy, osteoporosis has been clearly documented, but decreased osseointegration has not been found.[21-23] One of these investigations[23] did identify a slower rate of biologic fixation, without a difference in the final amount of osseointegration. This delay in osseointegration associated with estrogen deficiency may account for the results of the two studies[12,16] reported above where the authors believed they were observing a correlation between early interface strength and aging. Another study[21] demonstrated no difference in the amount of ingrowth of bone, but there was a significant increase in the amount of fibrous connective tissue within the pores. The push-out strength of the implants from the ovariectomized dogs was 31% less than in the control animals, suggesting that fibrous tissue plays an important role in bone–implant fixation. From a clinical perspective, however, a case report from a patient with documented postmenopausal osteoporosis demonstrated no decrease in bone ingrowth around a porous-coated implant.[24]

There are a number of studies documenting osteoporosis in association with renal disease[26] and kidney transplant,[27,28] but no animal or clinical studies could be found that addressed the effect of renal osteoporosis on the osseointegration of porous-coated implants. Several models of disuse osteoporosis have been developed that show osteoporosis forming after amputation,[29] casting,[30,31] and sciatic nerve transection.[32-34] Only the last model, osteoporosis induced by sciatic nerve transection, has been used to investigate the impact of disuse osteopenia on biologic fixation in the rat. The conclusion of this study was that osseointegration was improved with hydroxyapatite coating on the implant,[34] but the question whether disuse osteoporosis itself had any effect on biologic fixation was not addressed. No clinical studies of disuse osteoporosis are available to address the relationship between activity and biologic fixation.

There has been considerable interest in the osteoporosis associated with arthritis and its effect on the osseointegration of implants. The model most investigated in this regard has been the dog following intra-articular injection of Carragheenin.[35-37] The shear strength of titanium-coated (Ti) implants in Carragheenin-induced osteopenic bone was significantly reduced compared with the control bone ($p < 0.01$).[36,37] With the addition of hydroxyapatite-coating (HA) to the implants, no differences between the osteopenic bone and control bone were found. In the control bone, the ultimate shear strength of the Ti implants was significantly higher, compared to that of the HA implants ($p < 0.01$), whereas no difference was found between HA and Ti implants in osteopenic bone. These results agree with the observations of studies already quoted,[16,24] but issues raised with respect to the confounding effects of hormones and fibrous tissue ingrowth were not addressed. It is again unclear whether the change in observed shear strength is a reflection of impaired bone ingrowth associated with arthritis-induced osteopenia, or the presence of increased fibrous tissue associated with hormonal changes in the model. There are no clinical studies of arthritic osteoporosis and osseintegration to support these findings.

Numerous medications (steroids, nonsteroidal anti-inflammatory drugs, diphosphonate, methotrexate, Coumadin) have also been implicated as a source of osteoporosis as well as a potential source of failure of biologic fixation. Steroids have been a mainstay of therapy for rheumatoid arthritis and other less prevalent forms of inflammatory arthropathy. Their effects, including the induction of osteoporosis, are well documented.[38] The relative impact of steroid-induced osteopenia on osseointegration is not entirely clear, however. Some work suggests there is no effect on the quality or quantity of bone ingrowth,[39] while other work suggests that there are regional effects that make bone ingrowth dependent on the implant location.[40] The issue of regional variation in osteoporosis will be addressed in greater detail shortly. There appears to be more consensus on the effect of nonsteroidal anti-inflammatory medication, with several studies documenting inhibition of bone formation around porous-coated implants in the presence of indomethacin.[41,42] However, it is not clear that all medications in the nonsteroidal class of drugs have the same effect.[43] Methotrexate, a drug with wide acceptance in the treatment of recalcitrant arthritis and as a chemotherapeutic agent in the treatment of cancer, and sodium warfarin (Coumadin) have also been documented to inhibit bone formation around an orthopaedic implant.[44] An interesting, if not paradoxical, effect of a drug used to treat osteoporosis, disodium etidronate (EHDP), is that it also inhibits osseointegration and can lead to late failure of well-integrated implants in patients being treated for their osteoporosis.[45,46] The case for a negative correlation between these medications and the development of osseointegration seems well supported by this group of investigations. The contrary effect, i.e., drug-induced enhancement of osseointegration, has not been reported for any systemic medication.

There is a recurring theme in basic[17] and clinical[19] studies that osteoporosis at one particular site of the skeleton is not necessarily seen at another distant site. This site specificity of osteoporosis in the human skeleton has been well documented. Krolner and Nielsen[47] reported that although the correlation between the measures of bone mineral content of the lumbar spine and the forearm was significant for normal individuals, it is not significant in patients with osteoporosis. The lack of correlation of bone mass between trabecular bone and cortical bone in such patients was consistent with the results of several other studies.[48,49] This was confirmed by histomorphometric data showing that bone remodeling is focal, varying between skeletal sites at any given time, and varying from time to time within one site.[50,51] Thus, whether osteoporosis of any etiology (senile, menopausal, renal, disuse, arthritic, medication) affects bone quality, bone quantity, or osseointergation of orthopaedic implants in patients is suspect and a matter of continued controversy.

B. IMPLANT FACTORS AFFECTING BIOLOGIC FIXATION

A number of materials have been evaluated as potentially suitable for porous-coated implant devices.[3] Early studies concentrated on ceramics and polymers. Ceramics studied include porous forms of calcium aluminate, calcium titanate, calcium zirconate, titania (titanium oxide), Cerosium, and aluminum oxide. Polymers studied include polyvinyl sponge, porous polymethylmethacrylate, porous polysolfone, porous polyethylene, and Proplast. The limitations of the ceramic and polymeric materials under load led to investigations of porous-coated metals, principal of which were titanium and cobalt chrome. To facilitate biologic fixation, porous coatings on titanium and cobalt chrome substrates were developed from beads and wire mesh. The criteria for a porous coating to effectively promote osseous integration were developed by Klawitter and Hulbert.[52] These criteria include a pore size of 50 µm to promote osteoid ingrowth or 100 µm to promote ingrowth of mineralized bone. Additional requirements for osseointegration include close apposition of bone to the porous surface and a lack of movement at the developing interface of the tissue and the implant.

There is an abundance of information describing and defining these criteria for implants that will successfully undergo osseointegration in normal bone, but there is a paucity of information on the material properties of an implant that will facilitate biologic fixation in osteopenic bone. Many studies have explored the potential benefit of titanium over other substrates in promoting bone ingrowth, but of the two studies that address the performance of titanium in the face of osteopenia, neither study found any difference in bone ingrowth of a titanium implant between normal and osteoporotic bone.[53,54] No studies were identified that addressed the behavior of different surface textures, including beads and mesh, in the presence of osteoporosis.

A variety of adjuvant implants have been employed to augment the bony ingrowth process.[55] These implants include autogenous and allogeneic bone graft, synthetic calcium phosphates, demineralized bone matrix, growth factors [bone morphogenic protein (BMP), transforming growth factor beta (TGF-β)], and collagen. The functions of these adjuvant implants are to elicit an osteogenic response to accelerate the bony ingrowth process and/or serve as a grouting agent to further enhance the mechanical stability of the prosthesis.

Although bone autografts and allografts are routinely employed to augment the implantation of cementless total joint prostheses, few studies have been conducted to reveal the histologic response to these graft substances, and no studies were identified that addressed the behavior of bulk graft in osteopenic bone. Several studies were found that addressed the age of the recipient with respect to the induction of bone by demineralized bone powder.[56-60] These studies documented that bone induction decreases with increasing age of the recipient. Of interest, one of these studies addressed the age of the donor and documented that demineralized bone powder prepared from middle-aged adult rats was more inductive than that prepared from either prepubertal or young postpubertal animals, contradicting the widely held belief that demineralized bone matrix from younger donors is more inductive than that from older donors.[59] None of these studies addressed the behavior of demineralized bone powder in the presence of a porous-coated implant.

In contrast, there are numerous studies of the effect of ceramic surface coatings (hydroxyapatite, tricalcium phosphate) on porous-coated implants that promote biologic fixation in osteoporosis, all concluding that hydroxyapatite provides improved biologic fixation of porous-coated implants in osteopenic bone when compared to normal bone, while tricalcium phosphate alone displays little effect.[17,36,37,53,54,61-64] The only contemporary application for tricalcium phosphate as a surface coating of porous-coated implants appears to be that of a carrier for growth factors, a topic discussed in greater detail below. The role of bioglass as an implant coating has received considerably less attention, with only one study suggesting that the favorable environment bioglass provides for osteoblast proliferation in the presence of altered bone metabolism may make it a suitable adjunct to porous-coated implants in osteoporotic pathologies.[65] However, no studies were identified that actually tested a bioglass coating on a porous-coated surface in osteopenic bone.

Growth factors (BMP, TGF-β) represent another surface coating that has attracted attention as an adjunct to porous-coated implants.[66-72] In one investigation,[69] porous polyethylene specimens impregnated with a partially purified bovine BMP were implanted in rabbits, with no demonstrated benefit provided by the BMP. Two studies of porous-coated, ceramic-coated, titanium implants impregnated with TGF-β implanted in rabbits and dogs of indeterminate age and hormonal status (not likely to have osteoporotic bone) demonstrated increased fixation on mechanical testing and histologic analysis.[70,71] In a third study, in which the age and hormonal status of the animal, as well as the osteoporotic quality of the bone, were all documented, the addition of TGF-β to the porous-coated, ceramic-coated, cobalt chrome implant produced no improvement in mechanical test strength or histologic bone quality.[72] It is well documented that TGF-β and other growth factors that stimulate bone formation also increase bone resorption, an effect that is dose dependent.[66-68] It is also clear that the number of cells that are receptive to the effects of growth factor decreases with age.[73] It is not clear from the few studies available that growth factor will reliably stimulate new bone formation or augment the biologic fixation of porous-coated implants in the presence of osteoporosis.

One study of a porous polyethylene specimen filled with a purified bovine dermal collagen substance before implantation in rabbits demonstrated an increased amount of bony ingrowth 4 weeks after implantation.[74] It does not appear that this study has been repeated in osteopenic bone and there are no clinical correlates. It is possible, however, that collagen can serve as a stromal element to enhance osteoblast migration and/or attachment, providing a fertile area for future investigation.

When viewed together, the adjuvant implants and therapies described above appear to serve the purpose of either accelerating osseointegration (osteoinduction) or enhancing implant stability. Implant stability is enhanced when the material or adjuvant implant used functions like a grout. It has become increasingly evident that stability of the implant is a prerequisite for any osseointegration to occur, regardless of whether the bone is normal or osteoporotic. This requirement for stability may be more important in osteoporotic bone, where structural integrity is impaired and gaps develop between the implant and host during the process of implantation. Bone graft or bone graft substitutes in these gaps will form a biologic grout to stabilize the implant and provide a scaffold over which new host bone can form (osteoconduction). Synthetic calcium substitutes are under investigation for this purpose, but their role in promoting initial stability of porous-coated implants in osteoporosis remains to be demonstrated. As a general statement, very few animal or clinical studies of adjuvant implants and therapies have documented an improvement of osteoinduction or osteoconduction in osteopenic bone.

III. LOSS OF FIXATION/BONE MASS AFTER IMPLANT PLACEMENT

A. OSTEOPOROSIS/OSTEOLYSIS

The role of the development of osteoporosis following the successful osseointegration of a porous-coated implant, in the subsequent failure of the implant, has been investigated.[75] There appears to be no correlation between the loss of bone mass associated with osteoporosis and the loosening of the femoral component in total hip replacement. The principal cause of bone loss and the associated failure of well-fixed implants is osteolysis, a host response to particulate debris generated at the articular interface of the implant.[76] This biologic response to foreign material is not related to osteoporosis and is beyond the scope of this chapter.

B. ADAPTIVE REMODELING

Bone loss in the proximity of a successfully osseointegrated implant does occur over time and is age related, but it is not technically osteoporosis. This adaptive remodeling produces a natural cortical expansion measured in cemented femoral components, which is on average 0.33 mm per year.[77] There is also a decrease in cortical thickness and an associated increase in canal size.[78] These naturally occurring changes in the gross dimensions of the host bone have been suggested as a source of implant loosening.[78] In the context of a cemented arthroplasty, however, this process has not been deemed a threat to longevity of the implant because a neocortex forms to provide continued support to the cemented device.[79,80] Although not documented in the setting of a biologically fixed implant, this same process of neocortex formation has been invoked as an explanation for the long-term success of osseointegration.[76]

The adaptive remodeling of bone around biologically fixed implants is also related to certain design and material features of the implant. This aspect of adaptive remodeling, referred to as stress shielding, is largely determined by the stiffness of the implant relative to the host bone.[81] Dual-energy X-ray absorptiometry (DEXA) studies demonstrate a decrease in calcar bone mineral density (BMD) around cemented femoral stems[82] and a decrease in BMD in the proximal medial femur around cementless stems.[83] Maloney et al.[84] analyzed 48 autopsy femora from 24 patients with unilateral cemented and cementless femoral components and found the proximal medial cortex represented the specific region of maximal bone loss in both types of component fixation. Of note, these authors also found a strong correlation between the BMD of the control femur and the percentage decrease of BMD in the periprosthetic femur, i.e., stress shielding is correlated to coexisting host osteoporosis. However, no other studies were identified addressing adaptive remodeling in the context of coexisting osteoporosis. This issue of stress shielding and the associated loss of bone does not appear to affect the longevity of the implant, and few clinical problems have arisen from pronounced stress-related bone resorption.[78]

IV. CONCLUSION

There are very few studies, either animal or clinical, that address the long-term success or failure of orthopaedic implants in the setting of osteoporosis. By contrast, the long-term failure rate of orthopaedic implants used in the treatment of osteoporotic fractures is well documented.[85,86] It is high and increases dramatically with time. However, fracture results cannot be extrapolated to the field of osseointegration, because fracture implants are usually screwed in place, and their attachment mechanism to the bone and their mode of failure is completely different from that of an osseointegrated implant. Moreover, it has been well established that the overall success rate of osseointegrated fixtures in normal bone remains stable over time.[85,86] In contrast to fracture implants, however, the overall success rate of osseointegrated fixtures has not been well documented in osteopenic bone.

The works cited in this chapter suggest that osteoporosis associated with hormonal change may impact the early osseointegration of implants, and adjuvant therapies may counter this effect. It does not appear that age or senile osteoporosis alone will adversely affect the initial or long-term success of porous-coated implants, nor will adjuvant therapies necessarily improve the fixation of osseointegrated implants in the old, senile-osteoporotic recipient. There are insufficient studies upon which to make any additional conclusions. Further studies in all aspects of osteoinduction, osteoconduction, and maintenance of a stable bone–implant interface in osteoporosis need to be performed.

ACKNOWLEDGMENTS

The author thanks Mary Samson for proofreading and assistance with the literature search, and Edwin Baca for his assistance in gathering citations in preparation for this chapter.

REFERENCES

1. Grindlay, J.H. and Waugh, J.M., "Plastic sponge which acts as a framework for living tissue. Experimental studies and preliminary report of use to reinforce abdominal aneurysms," *Arch. Surg.*, 63, 288, 1951.
2. Struthers, A.M., "An experimental study of polyvinyl sponge as a substitute for bone," *Plast. Reconstr. Surg.*, 15, 274, 1955.
3. Haddad, R.J., Cook, S.D., and Thomas, K.A., "Biologic fixation of porous-coated implants," *J. Bone Joint Surg.*, 69A, 1459, 1987.

4. Cameron, H.U., Pilliar, R.M., and Macnab, I., "The rate of bone ingrowth into porous metal," *J. Biomed. Mater. Res.*, 10, 295, 1976.
5. Aberman, H.M., Bushelow, M., Dichiara, J.F., et al., "Retrieval analysis of Lord Madreporique stems implanted for up to 13 years," *J. Long Term Eff. Med. Implants*, 3, 119, 1993.
6. Soballe, K., Gotfredsen, K., Brockstedt-Rasmussen, H., et al., "Histologic analysis of a retrieved hydroxyapatite-coated femoral prosthesis," *Clin. Orthop.*, 272, 255, 1991.
7. Bobyn, J.D., Engh, C.A., and Glassman, A.H., "Histological analysis of a retrieved microporous coated femoral prosthesis. A seven-year case report," *Clin. Orthop.*, 224, 303, 1987.
8. Collier, J.P., Mayor, M.B., Chae, J.C., et al., "Macroscopic and microscopic evidence of prosthetic fixation with porous-coated materials, *Clin. Orthop.*, 235, 173, 1988.
9. Cook, S.D., Barrack, R.L., Thomas, K.A., and Haddad, R.J., Jr., "Quantitative analysis of tissue growth into human porous total hip components," *J. Arthroplasty*, 3, 249, 1988.
10. Cook, S.D., Thomas, K.A., and Haddad, R.J., Jr., "Histological analysis of retrieved human porous-coated total joint components," *Clin. Orthop.*, 234, 90, 1988.
11. Engh, C.A., Bobyn, J.D., and Petersen, T.L., "Radiographic and histologic study of porous-coated tibial component fixation in cementless total knee arthroplasty," *Orthopaedics*, 11, 725, 1988.
12. Magee, F.P., Longo, J.A., and Hedley, A.K., "The effect of age on the interface between porous coated implants and bones," *Orthop. Trans.*, 13, 455, 1989.
13. Aaron, J.E., Makins, N.B., and Sagreiya, K., "The microanatomy of trabecular bone loss in normal aging men and women," *Clin. Orthop.*, 215, 260, 1987.
14. Cummings, S.R., Kelsey, J.L., Nevitt, M.C., and O'Dowd, K.J., "Epidemiology of osteoporosis and osteoporotic fractures," *Epidemiol. Rev.*, 7, 178, 1985.
15. Faugere, M.C., Friedler, R.M., Fanti, P., and Malluche, H.H., "Bone changes occurring early after cessation of ovarian function in beagle dogs: a histomorphometric study employing sequential biopsies," *J. Bone Miner. Res.*, 5, 263, 1990.
16. Nakajima, I., Dai, K.R., Kelly, P.J., and Chao, E.Y., "The effect of age on bone ingrowth into titanium fibermetal segmental prosthesis: an experimental study in a canine model," *Orthop. Trans.*, 9, 296, 1985.
17. Eckhoff, D.G., Turner, A.S., and Aberman, H.M., "Effect of age on bone formation around orthopaedic implants," *Clin. Orthop.*, 312, 253, 1995.
18. Shaw, J.A., Bruno, A., and Paul, E.M., "The influence of age, sex and initial fit on bony ingrowth stabilization with the AML femoral component in primary THA," *Orthopaedics*, 15, 687, 1992.
19. Dao, T.T.T., Anderson, J.D., and Zarb, G.A., "Is osteoporosis a risk factor for osseointegration of dental implants?" *Int. J. Oral Maxillofac. Implants*, 8, 137, 1993.
20. Kondell, P.A., Nordenram, A., and Landt, H., "Titanium implants in the treatment of edentulousness: influence of patient's age on prognosis," *Gerodontics*, 4, 280, 1988.
21. Martin, R.B., Paul, H.A., Bargar, W.L., et al., "Effects of estrogen deficiency on the growth of tissue into porous titanium implants," *J. Bone Joint Surg.*, 70A, 540, 1988.
22. Turner, A.S., Eckhoff, D.G., Alvis, M.R., et al., "Failure of hydroxylapatite coating to promote biologic fixation in an estrogen-deficient model," *Orthop. Trans.*, 20, 598, 1996.
23. Mori, H., Manabe, M., Kurachi, Y., and Nagumo M., "Osseointegration of dental implants in rabbit bone with low mineral density," *J. Oral Maxillofac. Surg.*, 55, 351, 1997.
24. Fujimoto, T., Niimi, A., Nakai, H., and Ueda, M., "Osseointegrated implants in a patient with osteoporosis: a case report," *J. Oral Maxillofac. Implants*, 11, 539, 1996.
25. Gallagher-Albred, C.R. and Emley, S.J., "Specific dietary interventions. Diabetes, osteoporosis, renal disease," *Primary Care*, 21, 175, 1994.
26. Epstein, S., Shane, E., and Bilezikian, J.P., "Organ transplantation and osteoporosis," *Curr. Opin. Rheumatol.*, 7, 255, 1995.
27. Grotz, W.H., Mundinger, F.A., Gugel, B., et al., "Bone mineral density after kidney transplantation. A cross-sectional study in 190 graft recipients up to 20 years after transplantation," *Transplantation*, 59, 982, 1995.
28. Grotz, W.H., Mundinger, F.A., Gugel, B., et al., "Bone fracture and osteodensitometry with dual energy X-ray absorptiometry in kidney transplant recipients," *Transplantation*, 58, 912, 1994.
29. Sevastikoglou, J.A., Eriksson, U., and Larsson, S.E., "Skeletal changes of the amputation stump and the femur on the amputated side," *Acta Orthop. Scand.*, 40, 624, 1969.

30. Sevastikoglou, J.A. and Mattson, S., "Changes in composition and metabolic activity of the skeletal parts of the extremity of the adult rat following immobilization in a plaster cast," *Acta Chir. Scand. Suppl.*, 467, 21, 1976.

31. Sevastik, J.A. and Lindgren, J.U., "Osteoporosis: experimental and clinical studies," *Clin. Orthop.*, 191, 35, 1984.

32. Sevastikoglou, J.A. and Larsson, S.E., "Changes in composition and metabolic activity of the skeletal parts of the extremity of the adult rat following below-knee amputation," *Acta Chir. Scand. Suppl.*, 467, 9, 1976.

33. Hayashi, K., Uenoyama, K., Matsuguchi, N., et al., "The affinity of bone to hydroxyapatite and alumina in experimentally induced osteoporosis," *J. Arthroplasty*, 4, 257, 1989.

34. Soballe, K., Hansen, E.S., Rasmussen, H.B., and Dungen, C., "The effects of osteoporosis, bone deficiency, bone grafting, and micromotion on fixation of porous-coated vs. hydroxylapatite-coated implants," in *Hydroxylapatite Coating in Orthopaedic Surgery*, Geesink, R.G.T. and Manley, M.T., Eds., Raven Press, New York, 1993.

35. Soballe, K., Pedersen, C.M., Odgaard, A., et al., "Physical bone changes in Carragheenin-induced arthritis evaluated by quantitative computed tomography," *Skeletal Radiol.*, 20, 345, 1991.

36. Soballe, K., Hansen, E., Brockstedt-Tasmussen, H., et al., "Enhancement of osteopenic and normal bone ingrowth into porous coated implants by hydroxyapatite coating," *Orthop. Trans.*, 13, 446, 1989.

37. Soballe, K., Hansen, E.S., Brockstedt-Rasmussen, H., et al., "Fixation of titanium and hydroxyapatite coated implants in osteopenia," *J. Arthroplasty*, 6, 307, 1991.

38. Saville, P.D. and Kharmosh, O., "Osteoporosis of rheumatoid arthritis: influence of age and sex and corticosteroids," *Arthritis Rheum.*, 10, 423, 1967.

39. Ronningen, H., Urban, R.M., and Galante, J.O., "Bone ingrowth in a fiber metal implant in rabbits with steroid induced osteopenia," *Orthop. Trans.*, 7, 297, 1983.

40. Fujimoto, T., Niimi, A., Sawai, T., and Ueda, M., "Effects of steroid-induced osteoporosis on osseointegration of titanium implants," *Int. J. Oral Maxillofac. Implants*, 13, 183, 1998.

41. Keller, J.C., Trancik, T.M., Young, F.A., and St. Mary, E., "Effects of indomethacin on bone ingrowth," *J. Orthop. Res.*, 7, 28, 1989.

42. Longo, J.A., Magee, F.P., Hedley, A.K., et al., "The effect of indomethacin on fixation of porous implants to bone," *Orthop. Trans.*, 13, 367, 1989.

43. Trancik, T.M. and Mills, W., "The effect of several non-steroidal anti-inflammatory medications of bone ingrowth into a porous coated implant," *Orthop. Trans.*, 13, 61, 1989.

44. Lisecki, E.J., Callahan, B.C., Wolff, J.D., et al., "Attachment of hydroxyapatite-coated and uncoated porous implants is influenced by methotrexate and coumadin," *Orthop. Trans.*, 17, 1134, 1993.

45. Rivero, D.P., Skipor, A. K,. Singh, M., et al., "Effect of disodium etidronate (EHDP) on bone ingrowth in a porous material," *Clin. Orthop.*, 215, 279, 1987.

46. Starck, W.J. and Epker, B.N., "Failure of osseointegrated dental implants after diphosphonate therapy for osteoporosis: a case report," *Int. J. Oral Maxillofac. Implants*, 10, 74, 1995.

47. Krolner, B. and Nielsen, S.P., "Clinical application of dual photon absorptiometry of the lumbar vertebrae," in *Noninvasive Bone Measurements: Methodological Problems,* Dequeker, J. and Johnston, C.C., Eds., I.R.L. Press, Oxford, 1982, 201.

48. Wahner, H.W., Dunn, W.L., and Riggs, B.L., "Assessment of bone mineral, part 2," *J. Nucl. Med.*, 25, 1241, 1984.

49. Genant, H.K., Cann, E.E., Boyd, D.P., et al., "Quantitative computed tomography for vertebral mineral determination," in *Clinical Disorders of Bone and Mineral Metabolism*, Frame, B. and Potts, J.T., Jr., Eds., Excerpta Medica, Amsterdam, 1983, 40.

50. Charner, R.M., Bickerstaff, D.R., Wallace, W.A., et al., "The measurements of osteoporosis in clinical practice. Comparison of histologic and radiologic methods," *J. Bone Joint Surg.*, 71B, 661, 1989.

51. de Vernejoul, M.C., Belenguer-Prieto, R., Kuntz, D., et al., "Bone histologic heterogeneity in post-menopausal osteoporosis: a sequential histomorphometric study," *Bone*, 8, 339, 1988.

52. Klawitter, J.J. and Hulbert, S.F., "Application of porous ceramics for the attachment of load bearing internal orthopaedic applications," *J. Biomed. Mater. Res. (Symp.)*, 2, 161, 1971.

53. Hayashi, K., Uenoyama, K., Mashima, T., and Sugioka, Y., "Remodeling of bone around hydroxyapatite and titanium in experimental osteoporosis," *Biomaterials*, 15, 1, 1994.

54. Fini, M., Nicoli Aldini, N., Gandolfi, M.G., et al., "Biomaterials for orthopaedic surgery in osteoporotic bone: a comparative study in osteopenic rats," *Int. J. Artif. Organs*, 20, 291, 1997.

55. Spector, M., "Factors augmenting or inhibiting biological fixation," in *The Hip, Proceedings of the Fifteenth Open Scientific Meeting of the Hip Society*, Welch, R., Ed., C.V. Mosby, St. Louis, 1987, 213.

56. Jergesen, H.E., Chua, J., Kao, R.T., and Kaban, L.B., "Age effects on bone induction by demineralized bone powder," *Clin. Orthop.*, 268, 253, 1991.

57. Hosny, M. and Sharaway, M., "Osteoinduction in young and old rats using demineralized bone powder allografts," *J. Oral Maxillofac. Surg.*, 43, 925, 1985.

58. Irving, J.T., LeBolt, S.A., and Schneider, E.L., "Ectopic bone formation and aging," *Clin. Orthop.*, 154, 249, 1981.

59. Nishimoto, S.K., Chang, C.H., Gendler, E., et al., "The effect of aging on bone formation in rats: biochemical and histologic evidence for decreased bone formation capacity," *Calcif. Tissue Int.*, 37, 617, 1985.

60. Syftestad, G.T. and Urist, M.R., "Bone aging," *Clin. Orthop.*, 162, 288, 1982.

61. Hayashi, K., Uenoyama, K., Matsuguchi, N., et al., "The affinity of bone to hydroxyapatite and alumina in experimentally induced osteoporosis," *J. Arthroplasty*, 4, 257, 1989.

62. Soballe, K., "Hydroxyapatite ceramic coating for bone implant fixation," *Acta Orthop. Scand. Suppl.*, 255, 1, 1993.

63. Turner, A.S., Eckhoff, D.G., Dewell, R., et al., "Peri-apatite-coated implants improve fixation in osteopenic bone," *Orthop. Trans.*, 22, 665, 1998.

64. Rivero, D.P., Fox, J., Skipor, A.K., et al., "Effects of calcium phosphates and bone grafting materials on bone ingrowth in titanium fiber metal," *Orthop. Trans.*, 9, 295, 1985.

65. De Benedittis, A., Mattioli-Belmonte, M., Krajewski, A., et al., "*In vitro* and *in vivo* assessment of bone–implant interface: a comparative study," *Int. J. Artif. Organs*, 22, 516, 1999.

66. Goldring, M.B. and Goldring, S.R., "Skeletal tissue response to cytokines," *Clin. Orthop.*, 258, 245, 1990.

67. Centrella, M., McCarthy, T.L., and Canalis, E., "Current concepts review: transforming growth factor-beta and remodeling of bone," *J. Bone Joint Surg.*, 73A, 1418, 1991.

68. Trippel, S.B., Coutts, R.D., Einhorn, T.A., et al., "Growth factors as therapeutic agents," *J. Bone Joint Surg.*, 78A, 1272, 1996.

69. Kozinn, S.C., Hedley, A., Kim, W., and Urist, M., "Observations on bone ingrowth into bone morphogenetic protein (BMP) impregnated porous polyethylene implants," *Orthop. Trans.*, 6, 273, 1982.

70. Lind, M., Overgaard, S., Soballe, K., et al., "Transforming growth factor-β_1 enhances bone healing to unloaded tricalcium phosphate coated implants: an experimental study in dogs," *J. Orthop. Res.*, 14, 343, 1996.

71. Sumner, D.R., Turner, T.M., Purchio, A.F., et al., "Enhancement of bone ingrowth by transforming growth factor-β," *J. Bone Joint Surg.*, 77A, 1135, 1995.

72. Eckhoff, D.G., Turner, A.S., Clarke, R., et al., "Dose effect of rhTGF-β on bone growth around prosthetic implants in an age-controlled model," *Orthop. Trans.*, 20, 578, 1996.

73. Caplan, A.I., "The mesengenic process," *Clin. Plast. Surg.*, 21, 429, 1994.

74. Weinstein, A.M., Hedley, A.K., and Longo, J.A., "The effect of collagen on tissue growth into a porous polyethylene ingrowth model," in *Biological and Biomechanical Performance of Biomaterials*, Neumier, C.P. and Lee, A.J.C., Eds., Elsevier, Amsterdam, 1986.

75. Carlsson, A.S. and Nilsson, B.E., "The relationship of bone mass and loosening of the femoral component in total hip replacement," *Acta Orthop. Scand.*, 51, 285, 1980.

76. Rubash, H.E., Sinha, R.K., Shanbhag, A.S., and Kim, S.Y., "Pathogenesis of bone loss after total hip arthroplasty," *Orthop. Clin. North Am.*, 29, 173, 1998.

77. Poss, R., "Natural factors that affect the shape and strength of the aging human femur," *Clin. Orthop.*, 274, 194, 1992.

78. Comadoll, J.L., Sherman, R.E., Gustilo, R.B., and Bechtold, J.E., "Radiographic changes in bone dimensions in asymptomatic cemented total hip arthroplasties: results of nine- to thirteen-year follow-up," *J. Bone Joint Surg.*, 70A, 433, 1988

79. Jasty, M., Maloney, W.J., Bragdon, C.R., et al., "Histomorphologic studies of the long-term skeletal response to well fixed cemented femoral components," *J. Bone Joint Surg.*, 72A, 1220, 1990.

80. Wixson, R.L., Stulberg, S.D., and Mehihoff, M.A., "A comparison of the bone remodeling and radiographic changes between cemented and cementless total hip replacements," in Proceedings of the American Academy of Orthopaedic Surgeons 56th Annual Meeting, Las Vegas, NV, February 9–14, 1989.
81. Huiskes, R., "The various stress patterns of press fit, ingrown and cemented femoral stems," *Clin. Orthop.*, 261, 27, 1990.
82. Rushton, N. and Cohen B., "Bone remodeling in the proximal femur after Charnley total hip arthroplasty," *J. Bone Joint Surg.*, 77B, 815, 1995.
83. Kilgus, D.J., Shimaoka, E.E., Tipton, J.S., and Eberle, R.W., "Dual energy X-ray absorptiometry measurement of bone mineral density around porous coated cementless femoral implants," *J. Bone Joint Surg.*, 75B, 278, 1993.
84. Maloney, W.J., Sychterz, C., Bragdon, C., et al., "The Otto Aufranc Award. Skeletal response to well fixed femoral components inserted with and without cement," *Clin. Orthop.*, 333, 15, 1996.
85. Zarb, G.A. and Albrektsson, T., "Nature of implant attachments," in *Tissue-Integrated Prostheses: Osseointegration in Clinical Dentistry*, Branemark, P.I., Zarb, G.A., and Albrektsson, T., Eds., Quintessence, Chicago, 1985.
86. Noble, J., "Orthopaedic aspects of osteoporosis," in *Osteoporosis: A Multidisciplinary Problem*, Dixon, A.S.J., Russell, R.G.G., and Stamp, T.C.B., Eds., Royal Society of Medicine, London, 1983.

25 Periprosthetic Fractures and Osteoporosis

Kathleen A. Hogan and Harry A. Demos

CONTENTS

I. INTRODUCTION

A patch of black ice on a driveway. A throw rug on a wet bathroom floor. A child's toy left in the middle of a room. For millions of Americans with osteoporosis, even a small misstep can lead to a fracture with considerable consequences. For those who have had previous hip or knee arthroplasty, fractures occurring around the prosthesis are particularly devastating. Osteopenia, osteoporosis, female gender, rheumatoid arthritis, preoperative femoral deformities, revision surgeries, osteolysis, malpositioned prosthetic components, and prosthetic loosening are factors commonly associated with an increased risk of periprosthetic fractures.

Over 500,000 hip and knee arthroplasties are performed each year in the United States.[1] Many of these joint replacements are performed in women over the age of 65, the category of patients at highest risk for osteoporosis. Osteoporosis affects over 20 million people in the United States.[2] This condition weakens the structural integrity of bone and increases the potential for fracture. Intraoperative fractures can occur during total joint arthroplasty when a metal prosthesis is impacted into weakened bone. Postoperative fractures may result from stress shielding of the bone surrounding the stiff prosthesis, leading to further demineralization of the osteoporotic bone. The prosthesis also creates a stress riser at its end, which may contribute to fractures just below the prosthesis. These periprosthetic fractures represent technically difficult problems for total joint surgeons who

457

must attempt to provide stable fixation in already compromised bone. Periprosthetic fractures often require complex revision surgery, which may be poorly tolerated in an elderly patient with multiple medical problems. While the best treatment for periprosthetic fractures is prevention, some fractures may be inevitable because of the combination of bone weakened from osteoporosis and the stress risers created by stiff orthopaedic implants.

II. TOTAL HIP ARTHROPLASTY
AND PERIPROSTHETIC FRACTURES

Periprosthetic fractures related to total hip arthroplasty (THA) most commonly occur about the femoral stem. These fractures are relatively uncommon, complicating less than 1% of all primary THAs and 4.2% of revision cases.[3] Acetabular periprosthetic fractures are even more unusual. A retrospective analysis of the total joint registry of the Mayo Clinic in a 20-year period from 1971 to 1991 identified only 16 of 23,850 (0.07%) hip arthroplasties complicated by acetabular fractures.[4]

Osteoporosis, implant design, stress shielding by the prosthesis, osteolysis, aseptic loosening, and infection can all contribute to fractures of the proximal femur. Osteoporosis is a major risk factor for the early and late occurrence of fractures around the prosthesis. It is associated with femoral loosening, progressive varus alignment of hip prosthesis, femoral fractures, and trochanteric nonunions.[5] Cemented and uncemented femoral stems differ in the timing and location of their associated periprosthetic fractures. In an analysis of 93 periprosthetic femur fractures, Beals and Tower[6] found the majority (84%) to be associated with falls. Cemented stems had been in place an average 5.3 years and fractures usually occurred distal to the prosthesis when it was well fixed and always occurred at the stem tip when the prosthesis had loosened. Fractures around porous-coated stems occurred within 0.3 years and usually occurred along the stem or at the tip.[6] The risk of intraoperative fracture with uncemented femoral components has been shown in one series to be increased from 1.4 to 13% when the prosthesis was inserted into osteoporotic bone.[7]

Fracture risk can also be increased by prior surgical procedures. Cortical defects, created, for example, by hardware removal, tumors, or iatrogenic perforation, cause stress risers that are prone to fracture (Figure 25.1). The presence of an ipsilateral knee and hip prosthesis may leave only a small portion of normal diaphyseal bone interspersed between the stiff metal components. In such a case the integrity of the remaining bone is further weakened by the compromised blood supply and the modulus of elasticity of the bone, which is lower than that of the adjacent femoral canal filled with a metallic implant.[3] The combination of osteoporosis, progressive varus angulation, and subsidence of the femoral components may indicate that a prosthesis is at increased risk for an insufficiency fracture.[5]

Acetabular periprosthetic fractures may occur intraoperatively if a press-fit component is impacted into osteoporotic bone. Postoperative acetabular periprosthetic fractures usually are the result of severe osteolysis and loosening of the acetabular component and may result in a pelvic discontinuity. Because these fractures are rare and not commonly associated with osteoporosis, the following discussion mostly focuses on femoral periprosthetic fractures related to THA.

A. CLASSIFICATION

Classifications for fractures should have high inter- and intraobserver reliability and correlate to fracture treatment and outcome. Commonly used classification schemes are given in Table 25.1. The Johansson classification is one of the earlier classification schemes for periprosthetic femur fractures and describes the location of the fracture relative to the implant.[8] Type I fractures are proximal to the tip of the prosthesis, Type II are around the tip of the stem, and Type III are completely distal to the stem. However, the stability of the prosthesis and the bone quality are both factors that also must be considered when determining treatment. A newer classification scheme, developed by Duncan and Masri of Vancouver, incorporates fracture location with implant stability

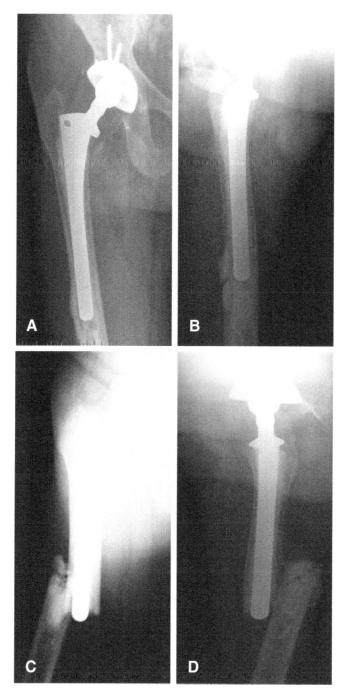

FIGURE 25.1 (A, B) This patient had an iatrogenic perforation of his femoral cortex during the insertion of the femoral stem. The extruded cement is visible on the postoperative radiographs. (C, D) He did well for 12 years until he stumbled and sustained a periprosthetic fracture through the cortical defect.

to create a useful guide for management of these fractures.[9] Type A fractures are located in the trochanteric region. They are subdivided into A_G and A_L indicating involvement of the greater or lesser trochanter, respectively. Type B fractures are located around or just distal to the implant stem. This group is divided by the stability of the prosthesis — stable (B1) or unstable (B2) — and

TABLE 25.1
Classification of Periprosthetic Femur Fractures

Johansson[8]	Cooke and Newman (cemented stems)[54]	Duncan and Masri[9]
I — Fracture that is entirely proximal to the distal tip of the prosthesis	I — Comminuted fracture around the stem; loose prosthesis and unstable fracture pattern	A — Proximal femur fracture (trochanteric region) A_G — Involving the greater trochanter A_L — Involving the lesser trochanter
II — Fracture extending beyond the tip of the prosthesis	II — Oblique or spiral fracture about stem; partially loose prosthesis but stable fracture	B — Involving diaphyseal bone around femoral component B1 — Well-fixed prosthesis B2 — Loose prosthesis B3 — Poor proximal bone
III — Fracture entirely distal to the tip of the prosthesis	III — Transverse fracture at distal tip of prosthesis; well-fixed prosthesis but unstable fracture IV — Distal fracture; well-fixed prosthesis but unstable fracture	C — Occurring entirely distal to femoral component

by the quality of the host bone. Fractures through osteoporotic or inadequate bone stock are classified as B3. Type C fractures are located distal to the tip of the prosthesis. The usefulness of this classification scheme in determining the management of these fractures will become evident later in this chapter when treatment options are discussed.

As previously mentioned, periprosthetic acetabular fractures are rare. They can be classified according to the stability of the implant. Type I fractures have stable implants, whereas Type II fractures are unstable.[4] The fracture pattern can also be described using the Letournel classification of acetabular fractures. Elementary pattern fractures are posterior wall, posterior column, anterior wall, anterior column, and transverse fractures. Associated patterns are T-shaped, posterior column and posterior wall, transverse and posterior wall, anterior column, posterior hemitransverse, and both column fractures.[10]

B. MANAGEMENT

1. Preoperative and Intraoperative Prevention

The management of periprosthetic fractures begins with an attempt at prevention. Preoperative planning and surgical technique in THA should anticipate potential problems — osteoporotic bone, cortical defects, and stress risers created between two implants, for example. Porous-coated stems are associated with a higher rate of intraoperative fracture (3.5%) than are cemented stems (0.4%).[11,12] Tapered, metaphyseal-fit porous stems have a higher incidence of fractures at the level of the calcar than do diaphyseal-fit porous femoral stems. Proximal femur fractures can occur during bone preparation or insertion of the prosthesis. Obtaining adequate exposure and minimizing force placed on osteoporotic bone with manipulation can minimize the intraoperative fracture risk. Some surgeons utilize prophylactic cerclage wiring of the proximal femur in patients considered to be at increased risk of fracture. Many surgeons prefer to use cemented implants in patients with osteoporosis, reserving ingrowth components for younger patients with stronger cortical bone.

2. Intraoperative Fractures

Intraoperative fractures of the greater trochanter may be a result of poor exposure of the entry site of the femoral component or excessive retraction for exposure. Intraoperative midprosthetic femur fractures are associated with excessive torque on bone during dislocation or relocation, osteoporotic bone, and the presence of contractures.[11] Careful preparation of the femur, osteotomy of the femoral neck prior to dislocation, and retention of preexisting hardware until after dislocation can help to minimize fracture risk. Intraoperative fractures of the portion of the femur around the tip of the prosthesis are typically a result of a mismatch between the shape of the prosthesis and bone. This may result from excessive reaming of the remaining cortex, or from a mismatch between a bowed femur and a straight femoral stem. Preoperative templating should minimize this type of fracture.[11] The rate of perioperative fractures with noncemented stems was reduced from 4 to 2% at the University of Maryland with preoperative templating, the use of fully fluted rigid reamers, and larger broaching instruments.[12]

For high-risk patients — the female with osteoporosis undergoing revision hip surgery, for example — added vigilance is needed to recognize fractures when they occur intraoperatively. The technical limitations of obtaining adequate radiographs intraoperatively can make recognizing these fractures challenging, however. If recognized intraoperatively, the stability of the prosthesis can be evaluated directly and fixation or revision can be preformed at that time if needed. Approximately 5% of intraoperative fractures involve only the greater trochanter. These fractures can either be managed nonoperatively or repaired with cerclage wires, cables, or other devices if displaced. Proximal cortical fractures involving the calcar can be treated with cerclage wiring.[11] Intraoperative fractures of the femur that extend beyond the tip of the prosthesis are usually treated with a longer stem, one that bridges the cortical defect by one to two times the diameter of the diaphysis to maximize torsional strength.[13] Allografts, plate, or cerclage wire fixation can be used to augment the fixation, if necessary. Cortical perforations or incomplete fractures distal to the stem that are noticed immediately after surgery may be stable and not require treatment. Larger defects or complete fractures may need revision with longer femoral component and possibly bone grafting. A comparison between patients who did and did not have an intraoperative fracture found no significant differences in pain scores, walking scores, or radiographic implant stability at a 2-year follow-up.[12]

3. Postoperative Fractures

When a periprosthetic fracture occurs postoperatively, management is based on fracture location, implant stability, and the patient's ability to tolerate treatment. A 1994 meta-analysis of 487 patients with postoperative periprosthetic femur fractures examined the relationship among fracture type, treatment, and outcome. The analysis found that proximal intertrochanteric periprosthetic fractures were rare and were usually treated with partial weight bearing without complications. Fractures along the proximal or distal aspect of the stem had the best outcomes when treated with either cerclage techniques (95 to 100% satisfactory results) or revision to long stem prosthesis (80 to 81% satisfactory results). These fractures did less well when treated with traction or screw and plate fixation (43 and 57% satisfactory results). Revision, cerclage techniques, and traction had similar outcomes in fractures distal to the tip of the stem in this study.[14] These data are of somewhat limited value, however. Published reports often do not describe factors such as the patient's medical condition, bone quality, the number of prior procedures, the type of prosthesis, the stability of the prosthesis, and pre- and postoperative hip scores, all of which influence treatment and outcomes. This analysis may also reflect older methods of treatment as it incorporates studies from 1964 to 1991. Nevertheless, it does give a basis of comparison to newer treatment innovations.

Fracture location, implant stability, and bone quality are important factors to consider in the treatment of periprosthetic fractures in the femur. The Duncan classification system,[9] as previously described, incorporates these factors and thus can be used as a guide for treatment decisions.

Proximal femur fractures involving the greater or lesser trochanter had an incidence of 4% in a series of 75 consecutive patients treated in Vancouver.[9] These Duncan Type A fractures may be treated conservatively if they are stable and nondisplaced. In a series of 30 patients with fractures of the greater trochanter (Duncan Type A_G) at the University of Washington, Seattle, 90% had stable

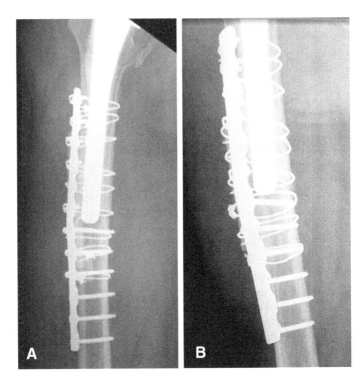

FIGURE 25.2 (A, B) The patient shown in Figure 25.1 was treated with an Ogden-type plate secured with cerclage cables. The fixation was reinforced with cortical strut allografts, also secured with cables. This construct provided adequate stabilization for early mobilization.

fractures and did well without treatment. Three patients required later surgical treatment for symptomatic displacement greater than 2 mm.[15]

Duncan Type B fractures occur along the femoral stem. These are the most commonly encountered periprosthetic femur fractures, comprising 86.7% of fractures treated in Vancouver over a 9-year period.[9] Treatment options depend on the stability of the prosthesis and the quality of the surrounding bone. This is the most difficult type of periprosthetic fracture to manage as it is often unstable and yet has a well-fixed femoral stem. If the implant is well fixed, removal is difficult and compromises bone stock, but the fracture itself usually requires repair.

Open reduction and internal fixation (ORIF) is typically used in Duncan B1 fractures where the prosthesis is stable (Figure 25.2). Fractures distal to the stem, Duncan Type C, do not involve the prosthesis and can also be treated with ORIF (Figure 25.3). A wide variety of techniques can be utilized for stabilization, but most involve combinations of various types of plates, screws, cerclage wires or cables, and cortical strut allografts.

The Mennen plate has been used in the past to provide semirigid fixation of femoral periprosthetic fractures. It is a paraskeletal clamp that supposedly can be placed with minimal surgical dissection or periosteal stripping. However, it is not a load-sharing or load-bearing device and it does not provide adequate stabilization to allow early mobilization. A report from Enfield, U.K., in 1999 reported a 100% implant failure at an average of 34 days in five of five patients.[16] Most surgeons have abandoned this plate in favor of more stable fixation.

The Ogden plate stabilizes the fracture with a side plate secured to the proximal fragment with bands and to the distal fragment with screws. Developed in 1976 by Ogden and Rendall, this technique rigidly fixes the fracture and allows early ambulation. The plate can be used in the presence of cemented stems. However, screw fixation leads to the development of stress risers and may increase the risk of subsequent fractures.[17] Zenni and colleagues[18] at the University of Cincinnati

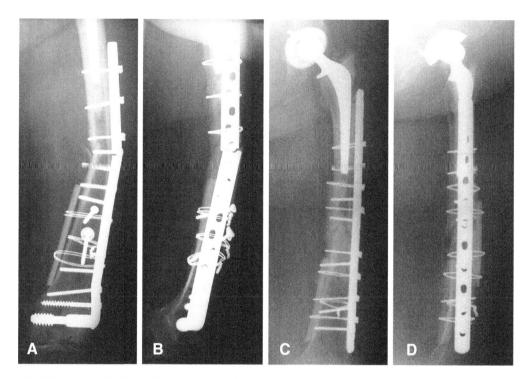

FIGURE 25.3 (A, B) This patient had previously undergone ORIF of a comminuted distal femoral fracture (Duncan C) with supplemental strut allograft. The distal-most fracture healed, but she had a nonunion of the more proximal fracture that eventually caused hardware failure. (C, D) This was treated with revision of the plate fixation and an additional strut allograft.

reviewed the outcomes of 19 periprosthetic fractures treated with the Ogden plate. Union occurred in 84% within 3.5 months. Excellent or satisfactory results were achieved in 16 of 19 patients.[18]

There are now numerous systems currently marketed that employ a plate fixed about bone using cerclage wires or cables. Originally described as a method for trochanteric reattachment, cables may also be used to provide fixation for femoral autograft and for the repair of proximal femur fractures. Two English groups have each recently published retrospective series of fractures treated by this technique. They found an average time to union of 3.5 and 4.4 months with successful treatment in 13 of 15 and 10 of 13 patients (86 and 77% union rate), respectively.[19,20] One potential advantage of cerclage over screw fixation is that stress risers are not created in bone already weakened by osteoporosis. Another advantage of the cerclage technique is that bicortical screws usually cannot be placed through the portion of the bone containing the canal-filling prosthesis. Screws, however, do provide superior axial stability and require less periosteal stripping. In most situations, the combination of proximal cerclage fixation and distal screw fixation, as described by Ogden, provides the most stable means of internal fixation for these fractures where the prosthesis is stable, but the fracture is unstable (Figures 25.2 and 25.3).

Fractures with unstable prosthesis (Duncan B2) often require a revision procedure using a long stem extending past the fracture site (Figure 25.4).[21] Bone grafting may be required. MacDonald et al.[22] recently reported midterm follow-up for a consecutive series of 14 patients with proximal femoral fractures and an unstable prosthesis. All fractures were treated with a long-stem, extensively porous-coated prosthesis (Solution Stem, Depuy, Warsaw, IN). Of the cases, 50% also required femoral strut grafts and cerclage wiring. Fractures occurred an average of 9.4 years following the index procedure. Fractures were classified as Johansson I (10/14) or Johansson II (4/14). All patients had radiographic union in an average of 4 months. Complications included posterior dislocation

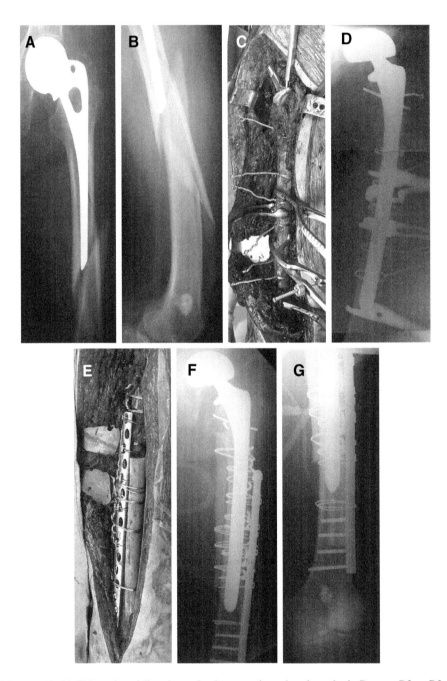

FIGURE 25.4 (A, B) This patient fell and sustained a comminuted periprosthetic Duncan B2 or B3 fracture around a hemiarthroplasty. (C, D) An intraoperative photograph and radiograph show the initial reduction after placement of a long stemmed femoral component. (E) This initial reduction was reinforced with cortical strut allograft and a plate. (F, G) The initial postoperative radiographs show anatomic alignment of the fracture and stable fixation to allow early mobilization.

(1 patient), a nonfatal myocardial infarction (1 patient), and anterior femoral perforation during reaming (1 patient). At an 8-year follow-up, 12 of 14 had stable bone ingrowth and 13 of 14 had distal diaphyseal fixation.[22] There is a risk of fracture propagation when a long femoral stem is inserted into weak and osteoporotic bone, however. [23]

If the surrounding bone is severely osteoporotic (Duncan B3) allograft supplementation is usually required (Figure 25.4). A cortical allograft secured to the femur with a plate and/or cerclage wiring has been used to treat fractures about well-fixed femoral stems. A 95% union rate has been reported.[24] The allograft bone provides structural support, may enhance healing, and does not create stress risers.[25] However, allografts are expensive, have a risk of disease transmission, and their strength weakens 4 to 6 months after surgery as they incorporate into host bone.[24] A retrospective review of 13 periprosthetic fractures fixed with allograft combined with the Dall-Miles cable and plate system (Howmedica, Allendale, NJ) found that union was achieved at an average of 4.4 months. Three fractures, each with greater than 6° of varus alignment of the femoral stem, required revision.[10] A recent study reported failure of Dall-Miles plating in 6 of 9 cases. Each of the failures was also associated with varus alignment.[26]

Finite-element modeling of a femur and femoral prosthesis has been used to compare the biomechanical results of these fixation techniques.[27] Revision to a longer stem was found to transfer stress distally as the stem length is increased but also progressively increased stress shielding at the fracture site and proximal to it. Allograft struts secured with cerclage wires experienced maximum stresses on the most distal wires, but these stresses did not exceed the theoretical failure threshold. As expected, stress shielding at the fracture was minimized. The Ogden plate resulted in high tensile stress at the fracture site and stress shielding occurred at the proximal lateral cortex. In this construct, the wires were loaded relatively evenly with a slight increase in stress at the most distal band.[27] Another biomechanical study compared the stability of fixation of an Ogden-type plate with proximal cables and distal bicortical screws vs. allograft struts and cerclage wiring.[17] Cooke Type III fractures (Duncan B1) were created distal to cemented Charnley hip prosthesis in embalmed femurs. Mechanical testing found a significant increase in torsional strength of the plate fixation. The Ogden plate typically failed through the proximal screw hole, whereas the allograft construct failed by either loss of fixation or fracturing of the allograft.[17]

The ultimate goal in the management of periprosthetic fractures is to provide the patient with a functional limb suitable for ambulation. Operative treatment of periprosthetic femoral fractures after THA is a major operation and complications are not uncommon. A review of 206 patients requiring revision THA for reasons other than infection found the following rates of complications: dislocation (9%), severe heterotopic bone formation (5.4%), postoperative fracture (4.2%), and deep infection (2%). In this series, the 35 patients who required revision for periprosthetic fractures had better clinical outcomes and Harris hip scores compared to those revised for loosening or recurrent dislocation.[28] Treatment of these fractures typically results in stable fixation. Crockarell et al.[29] reviewed the literature from 1974 to 1994 and found that the reported incidence of nonunion of femoral periprosthetic fractures following THA averaged 4% (range 0 to 18%). Although rare, nonunions occurring after treatment for a periprosthetic fracture are difficult to treat (see Figure 25.3). A retrospective review from the Mayo Clinic found that of the 27 patients treated for nonunion of periprosthetic fractures, 67% required additional operations for infection, persistent nonunion, or aseptic loosening.[29]

4. Acetabular Fractures

Fractures involving the acetabular component can be technically quite difficult to treat. Fortunately, they are rare. During a 6-year period at the Mayo Clinic, only 11 acetabular periprosthetic fractures were reported, 9 of which occurred around cemented components.[4] Most (72%) were related to either blunt trauma or a fall. Nonoperative treatment was initially attempted in eight fractures that were minimally displaced fractures. Patients were prevented from weight bearing for 6 to 12 weeks and progressively allowed to increase their weight-bearing status. Six of these patients ultimately required a revision procedure. Displacement of the acetabular component requires revision and usually reconstruction of the posterior column of the acetabulum. In this series from the Mayo Clinic only two patients had unstable fractures and both had immediate revisions. One patient did

TABLE 25.2
Distal Femur Fracture Classification

Neer Classification[34]	Lewis and Rorabeck Classification[35]
I — Fracture minimally displaced or impacted	I — Nondisplaced fracture; intact prosthesis
II — Displacement > 1 cm	II — Displaced fracture; intact prosthesis
A — Medial femoral shaft displacement	
B — Lateral femoral shaft displacement	
III — Displaced, comminuted fracture	III — Prosthesis loose or failing; fracture nondisplaced or displaced

well; the other required a subsequent revision for nonunion.[4] If a periprosthetic acetabular fracture results in pelvic discontinuity, a complex revision utilizing acetabular reconstruction cages will most likely be required.

III. TOTAL KNEE ARTHROPLASTY AND PERIPROSTHETIC FRACTURES

The risk of periprosthetic fracture is less in total knee arthroplasty (TKA) when compared with THA. Supracondylar distal femur fractures are the most common periprosthetic fracture associated with TKA. The reported incidence of these fractures following TKA ranges from 0.3 to 2.5%.[30] The risk of fracture is increased with female gender, osteoarthritis, rheumatoid arthritis, neurologic disorders, and notching of the anterior femoral cortex.[31,32] Periprosthetic fractures have also been associated with flexion contractures, revision TKA, stress risers at screw holes, the use of corticosteroids, and the presence of osteolysis. Long stemmed femoral components increase the load at the stem tip, which can contribute to diaphyseal fractures.[30,33] Fractures of the tibia are relatively rare and are often associated with stress fractures related to malalignment or component loosening.

A. CLASSIFICATION

Neer's classification of supracondylar femur fractures has frequently been adapted to describe periprosthetic fractures about the femoral implant in TKA. Fractures are described by the degree of displacement. Type I fractures are undisplaced, impacted, or minimally displaced but stable after closed reduction. Type II fractures are displaced greater than 1 cm with either medial (IIA) or lateral (IIB) displacement of the condyles. Type III fractures are displaced and comminuted high-energy injuries with conjoined supracondylar and shaft fractures.[34,35] The Neer classification, however, was not developed specifically for periprosthetic fractures and does not take into account implant stability. Digioia and Rubash[36] modified this classification to describe acceptable displacement in periprosthetic fractures as less than 5 mm translation, less than 5 to 10° of angulation, and less than 1 cm of shortening. Rorabeck and Taylor[35] later developed a new classification specifically to address periprosthetic supracondylar femur fractures occurring after TKA. In the Rorabeck classification, Type I and Type II are nondisplaced and displaced fractures, respectively, and do not involve the prosthesis. Fractures associated with loosening or failure of the implant are classified as Type III, regardless of the degree of fracture displacement.[35] This classification scheme can be used as a guide for treatment decisions as be discussed later in this chapter. The Neer and the Rorabeck classifications are outlined in Table 25.2.

Periprosthetic fractures of the tibia are most commonly described using the Felix-Stuart-Hanssen classification that was developed based on a review of treatment outcomes of 107 fractures treated at the Mayo Clinic. This classification is presented in Table 25.3. Fractures are described based on their location relative to the implant. Type I fractures involve the tibial plateau. Type II

TABLE 25.3
Periprosthetic Tibia Fracture Classification

Mayo Classification: Felix-Stuart-Hanssen[37]

I — Plateau fracture	A — Well-fixed prosthesis
II — Fracture adjacent to stem	B — Loose prosthesis
III — Fracture distal to stem	C — Intraoperative fracture
IV — Fracture of tibial tubercle	

TABLE 25.4
Periprosthetic Patellar Fracture Classification

Goldberg Classification[39]

I — Intact extensor mechanism and implant
II — Disruption of implant–bone interface or of extensor mechanism
III — Fracture of the inferior pole of the patella
   A — Rupture of patellar ligament
   B — Intact patellar ligament
IV — Fracture/dislocation of the patella

fractures are adjacent to the stem, while fractures distal to the implant are Type III. Each of these fracture types is modified as A — prosthesis well fixed, B — loose prosthesis, or C — occurring intraoperatively. Fractures of the tibial tubercle are classified as Type IV.[37] The Mayo classification can be used as a guide for treatment.

Hozack et al.[38] described patella periprosthetic fractures as being nondisplaced, displaced with or without an extensor lag, or having a displaced distal pole. Goldberg et al.[39] expanded on this classification, which is presented in Table 25.4. Type I fractures do not involve the implant, cement mantle, or quadriceps mechanism. Type II fractures do involve the implant. Fractures of the distal pole of the patella are Type III and are subdivided into A and B depending on the status of the patellar ligament. Fracture/dislocations of the patella are Type IV.[39]

B. MANAGEMENT

1. Supracondylar Fractures

Supracondylar fractures are the most common type of periprosthetic fracture complicating TKA. The goal of treating these fractures is to provide the patient with a functional painless knee with well-fixed components, allowing for a return to prefracture ambulatory status. The Rorabeck classification scheme, which incorporates implant stability, can be used as a guide to determining suitable treatment options. Supracondylar periprosthetic femur fractures with a stable prosthesis can be treated operatively or nonoperatively; controversy still exists regarding the optimal treatment. There are no large controlled studies comparing the two treatment options, and most of the literature consists of case reports of small series of patients.

Rorabeck Type I fractures are typically treated nonoperatively with a cast or cast brace and protected weight bearing. The fracture is nondisplaced and the implant is stable. A meta-analysis of 195 cases reported in the literature from 1981 to 1990 found no statistical significance in outcomes between operative and nonoperative management in Type I and Type II fractures. Between 67 and 69% of all patients had a successful outcome, but the overall complication rate was 30%. The overall rates of nonunion and malunion (10 and 12%, respectively) were not significantly different between the two treatment groups. Operative treatment was associated with a higher rate of major complications, however. Displaced fractures were more likely to be treated with surgical fixation than were nondisplaced fractures. Nonoperative treatment in Type I fractures resulted in higher patient satisfaction rates (87%) than did nonoperative management of Type II fractures (61 to 67% satisfaction).[32] In this analysis, prognosis was more dependent on the type of fracture than on the treatment. Union was achieved in 83% of Type I fractures compared to 64% of Type II fractures when treated nonoperatively. There was no significant difference in the outcomes of Type II fractures treated operatively vs. nonoperatively.[33] Successful nonoperative treatment of Neer Type I and II fractures has been associated with rotational deformity of less than 10°, shortening of less than 1 cm, and fracture angulation less than 15°.[33,40] Based upon experience with four patients, Hirsch et al.[31] initially advocated nonoperative management of supracondylar periprosthetic fractures in 1981. Although they reported that satisfactory union occurred in all fractures, radiographic findings and functional outcomes were not described. Sisto et al.[41] subsequently published a case report describing 15 fractures, 12 of which were minimally displaced and successfully treated with traction and casting. In a series by Merkel and Johnson[33] in 1986, 28 patients with Type I and Type II fractures were treated nonoperatively with traction followed by casting ($n = 19$) or by casting alone ($n = 6$). Nonunions occurred in 25% of these cases, requiring surgical correction.

Type II fractures are typically treated with internal fixation, as would be done if there were no TKA. Surgical fixation provides anatomic alignment and allows mobilization, which optimizes function of the knee and limits complications associated with immobilization.[42] A meta-analysis found complications of surgical treatment to include infection (7.4%), perioperative death (1.2%), nonunion (7.4%), and malunion (3%).[32] Commonly used fixation methods include stabilization with a plate or an intramedullary rod (Figure 25.5). Culp and colleagues[41] reported the retrospective experience of members of the Pennsylvania Orthopaedic Society with 61 fractures, classified as Types I and II. The union rate was 80% with operative treatment compared to 56% with conservative treatment. More recently, Healy and colleagues[42] reported union and a return to preexisting level of activity in 18 of 20 fractures treated with ORIF with blade plates or buttress plates and bone grafting, as needed. McLaren et al.[43] and Weber et al.[44] have both reported the successful treatment of displaced Type II fractures with a supracondylar retrograde nail in series of seven cases each.

Biomechanical studies have been conducted comparing the stiffness and strength of IM nails, blade plates, and buttress plates in the fixation of supracondylar fractures. A study on the use of retrograde IM nails for femoral supracondylar fractures showed no difference in bending stiffness among four different designs.[45] In osteoporotic embalmed cadaveric femurs with distal femoral osteotomy, a 95° supracondylar plate provided stiffer fixation in three-point bending than did retrograde or anterograde nails.[46] In a later study using a similar model, it was found that a condylar buttress plate with locked screws resulted in improved stability to axial compression and torsional loads compared to a 95° blade plate.[47] Biomechanical studies have also verified the clinical observation that notching of the anterior femoral cortex during a TKA increases subsequent fracture risk. Lesh et al.[48] found that notching significantly decreased the load to failure with torsional stress. During bending, fractures were initiated at the site of notching instead of occurring in the midshaft where non-notched femurs fractured.

Revision arthroplasty is required for most Rorabeck Type III fractures. The surgical options involve either bridging the fracture with a stemmed revision femoral component, or resecting and replacing the distal segment of the fracture. For revision TKA with a stemmed component, a tight fit in the femoral canal and a stem of at least 150 mm is recommended.[49] Kraay et al.[50] described the successful use of a large segment allograft with stemmed, nonlinked knee prosthesis to treat supracondylar fractures associated with significant bone loss. A review by McLaren et al.[43] of results following revision procedures found a successful outcome in 24 of 25 patients. A meta-analysis by Chen et al.[32] reports a 90% rate of successful union with revisions.

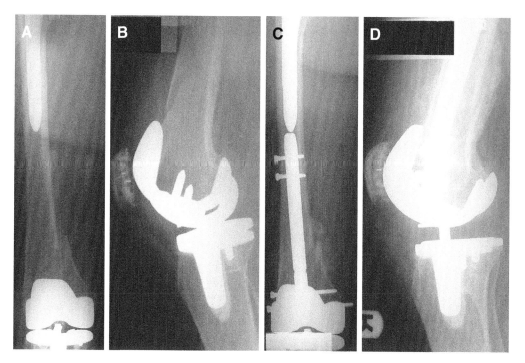

FIGURE 25.5 (A, B) This patient sustained a moderately displaced (Rorabeck II) supracondylar femoral fracture above a well-functioning TKA that remained well fixed. She also had a previous THA. (C, D) The fracture was fixed with a supracondylar nail and 8 weeks later, her fracture had healed. She is at risk, however, for fracturing her femoral shaft in the area between the intramedullary implants.

2. Tibial Fractures

Periprosthetic tibial fractures occur less frequently than femur fractures after a TKA. In a retrospective review at the Mayo Clinic, 102 tibial periprosthetic fractures were treated in a 25-year period. The overall incidence of late tibial fractures at the Mayo Clinic during that time period was 0.40% with the fractures occurring an average of 60 months postoperatively. Of the 102 fractures, 19 occurred intraoperatively. The overall incidence of intraoperative tibial fractures during this time period was 0.07% in primary cases and 0.36% in revisions.[37] As previously discussed, the Felix-Stuart-Hanssen classification evolved from the review of the management of the fractures identified in this study. Type I fractures, which involve the tibial plateau, occurred the most frequently, in 60% of the reported cases. Most of these fractures were associated with a varus alignment of the tibial component. When recognized postoperatively, the fracture was initially treated with avoidance of weight bearing, but in most cases ultimately required revision. Most of these fractures were Type IB with an unstable prosthesis. Type IC fractures recognized intraoperatively were fixed with screw fixation or by using a stem of sufficient length to provide fracture stability.[37]

The occurrence of Type II fractures, adjacent to the stem, was associated with a history of trauma. Nonoperative treatment was successful when the prosthesis was stable (Type IIA). Revision procedures for unstable components typically required extensive reconstruction with allograft. Type III fractures, distal to the stem, occurred in 16% of these patients. This fracture was typically stable and treated with a cast brace and weight-bearing restrictions.[38] In this study, only two patients sustained fractures of the tibial tubercle (Type IV) and both were successfully treated nonoperatively. In summary, the authors concluded that fractures with a stable prosthesis can be successfully treated nonoperatively, but those fractures with unstable implants (Type IB, IIB, IIIB) ultimately require revision procedures.[37] If the prosthesis is stable but the fracture itself is displaced or unstable, it can be treated with ORIF by conventional means (Figure 25.6).

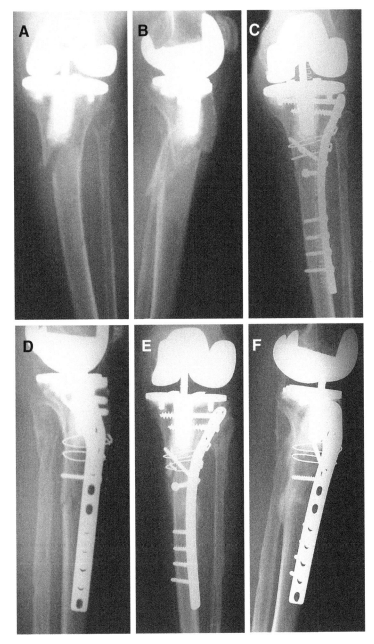

FIGURE 25.6 (A, B) This patient sustained a proximal tibial fracture below a well-fixed TKA. (C, D) This was treated with ORIF with a periarticular plate and cable. (E, F) The fracture healed uneventfully.

3.   Patellar Fractures

Fractures of the patella during or following a resurfacing procedure can occur because of trauma, excessive removal of native bone, avascularity, component malposition, inadequate soft tissue balancing, and osteoporosis. Treatment decisions are based on the degree of fracture displacement, the integrity of the extensor mechanism, and the quality of the remaining bone.[51] Goldberg and colleagues[39] examined the results of 36 patellar periprosthetic fractures. Those with the best outcomes did not involve the implant or the extensor mechanism (Type 1) or involved only the inferior pole of the patella (Type 3B). These were successfully treated nonoperatively. Operative repair was required in fractures involving the implant (Type 2), inferior pole fractures with rupture of the patella ligament (Type 3A), and fracture dislocations (Type 4). These fractures had lower knee scores, and less satisfactory results.[39]

IV. PERIPROSTHETIC FRACTURES BETWEEN HIP AND KNEE PROSTHESES

The presence of ipsilateral hip and knee prostheses can create a stress riser in the remnant of bone remaining between the two femoral stems. These fractures are quite rare, but the prevalence will undoubtedly increase as the incidence of ipsilateral hip and knee arthroplasty increases. Osteoporosis increases the risk of fracture. There is no established classification scheme for these fractures. Proposed treatments have included simultaneous ipsilateral revision THA and TKA with complete femoral allograft, customized metallic prosthesis spanning the length of the femur.[52,53] Creative preoperative planning is usually necessary (Figure 25.5).

V. CONCLUSIONS

Periprosthetic fractures around hip and knee prostheses pose difficult management problems for orthopaedic surgeons. As the baby-boomer generation in America ages, life expectancy increases, and those over age 65 lead more active lifestyles, the frequency at which these fractures occur will undoubtedly rise proportionally. Prevention is the most important step in treating these fractures — an understanding of the influence of metallic implants on the surrounding bone, the use of pharmacologic intervention to treat osteoporosis, and recognizing intraoperative fractures early can aid in limiting the prevalence of periprosthetic fractures. When confronted with a difficult fracture, the surgeon must take into account the technical challenges of the fracture but also consider the general health and ability of the patient to tolerate treatment.

REFERENCES

1. Beaty, J., Ed., *Orthopaedic Knowledge Update 6*, American Academy of Orthopaedic Surgeons, Rosemont, IL, 1999.
2. Lane, J., Riley, E., and Wirganowicz, P., "Osteoporosis: diagnosis and treatment," *Instr. Course Lect.* 46, 445, 1997.
3. Pellicci, P., Tria, A., and Garvin, K., Eds., *Orthopaedic Knowledge Update (Hip and Knee Reconstruction 2)*, American Academy of Orthopaedic Surgeons, Rosemont, IL, 2000.
4. Peterson, C. and Lewallen, D., "Periprosthetic fracture of the acetabulum after total hip arthroplasty," *J. Bone Joint Surg.*, 78A, 1206, 1996.
5. Gill, T.J., Sledge, J.B., Orler, R., and Ganz, R., "Lateral insufficiency fractures of the femur caused by osteopenia and varus angulation," *J. Arthroplasty*, 14, 982, 1999.
6. Beals, R.K. and Tower, S., "Periprosthetic fractures of the femur. An analysis of 93 fractures," *Clin. Orthop.*, 327, 238, 1996.
7. Toni, A., Ciaroni, D., and Sudanese, A., "Incidence of intraoperative femoral fracture. Straight stemmed vs. anatomic cementless total hip arthroplasty," *Acta Orthop. Belg.*, 60, 43, 1994.
8. Johansson, J., McBroom, R., Barrington, T., and Hunter, G., "Fracture of the ipsilateral femur in patients with total hip arthroplasty," *J. Bone Joint Surg.*, 63A, 1435, 1988.
9. Duncan, C.P. and Masri, B.A., "Fractures of the femur after hip replacement," in *Fractures of the Femur after Hip Replacement*, Vol. 44, Jackson, D., Ed., American Academy of Orthopaedic Surgeons, Rosemont, IL, 1995, 293.
10. Letournel, E., "Acetabulum fractures: classification and management," *Clin. Orthop.*, 151, 81, 1980.
11. Kelley, S.S., "Periprosthetic femoral fractures," *J. Am. Acad. Orthop. Surg.*, 2, 164, 1994.

12. Schwartz, J., Mayer, J., and Engh, C., "Femoral fracture during non-cemented total hip arthroplasty," *J. Bone Joint Surg.,* 71A, 1135, 1988.

13. Larson, J., Chao, E., and Fitzgerald, R., "Bypassing femoral cortical defects with cemented intramedullary stems," *J. Orthop. Res.,* 9, 414, 1991.

14. Mont, M. and Maar, D., "Fractures of the ipsilateral femur after hip arthroplasty. A statistical analysis of outcome based on 487 patients," *J. Arthroplasty,* 9, 511, 1994.

15. Pritchett, J., "Fracture of the greater trochanter after hip replacement," *Clin. Orthop.,* 390, 221, 2001.

16. Kamineni, S. and Ware, H.E., "The Mennen plate: unsuitable for elderly femoral periprosthetic fractures," *Injury,* 30, 257, 1999.

17. Dennis, M.G., Simon, J.A., Kummer, F.J., et al., "Fixation of periprosthetic femoral shaft fractures — a biomechanical comparison of two techniques," *J. Orthop. Trauma,* 15, 177, 2001.

18. Zenni, E.J., Pomeroy, D., and Caudle, R., "Ogden plate and other fixations for fractures complicating femoral endoprostheses," *Clin. Orthop.,* 231, 83, 1988.

19. Venu, K., Koka, R., Garikipati, R., et al., "Dall Miles cable and plate fixation for the treatment of peri-prosthetic femoal fractures — analysis of results in 13 cases," *Injury,* 32, 385, 2001.

20. Kamineni, S., Vindlacheruvu, R., and Ware, H.E., "Periprosthetic femoral shaft fractures treated with plate and cable fixation," *Injury,* 30, 261, 1999.

21. Jensen, J., Barfod, G., Hansen, D., et al., "Femoral shaft fracture after hip arthroplasty," *Acta Orthop. Scand.,* 59, 9, 1988.

22. Macdonald, S., Paprosky, W., Jablonsky, W., and Magnus, R., "Periprosthetic femoral fractures treated with a long stem cementless component," *J. Arthroplasty,* 16, 379, 2001.

23. Olerud, S. and Karlstrom, G., "Hip arthroplasty with an extended femoral stem for salvage procedures," *Clin. Orthop.,* 191, 64, 1984.

24. Chandler, H. and Tigges, R., "The role of allografts in the treatment of periprosthetic femoral fractures," *Instr. Course Lect.,* 47, 257, 1998.

25. Dall, D., "Cable techniques for trochanteric and femoral allograft fixation," *Tech. Orthop.,* 6, 7, 1991.

26. Tadross, T., Nanu, A., Buchanan, M., and Checketts, R., "Dall Miles plating for periprosthetic B1 fractures of the femur," *J. Arthroplasty,* 15, 47, 2000.

27. Mihalko, W., Beaudoin, A., Cardea, J., and Krause, W., "Finite element modeling of femoral shaft fracture fixation techniques post total hip arthroplasty," *J. Biomech.,* 25, 469, 1992.

28. Kavanagh, B., Ilstrup, D., and Fitzgerald, R., "Revision total hip arthroplasty," *J. Bone Joint Surg.,* 67A, 517, 1985.

29. Crockarell, J., Berry, D., and Lewallen, D., "Non union after periprosthetic femoral fracture associated with total hip arthroplasty," *J. Bone Joint Surg.,* 81A, 1073, 1999.

30. Sochart, D. and Hardinge, K., "Nonsurgical management of supracondylar fracture above total knee arthroplasty," *J. Arthroplasty,* 12, 830, 1997.

31. Hirsch, D., Bahalla, S., and Roffman, M., "Supracondylar fracture of the femur following total knee replacement," *J. Bone Joint Surg.,* 63A, 29, 1981.

32. Chen, F., Mont, M., and Bachner, R., "Management of ipsilateral supracondylar femur fractures following total knee arthroplasty," *J. Arthroplasty,* 10, 213, 1994.

33. Merkel, K. and Johnson, E., "Supracondylar fracture in the femur after total knee arthroplasty," *J. Bone Joint Surg.,* 68A, 29, 1986.

34. Neer, C., Grantham, S., and Shelton, M., "Supracondylar fracture of the adult femur. A study of one hundred and ten cases," *J. Bone Joint Surg.,* 49A, 591, 1967.

35. Rorabeck, C. and Taylor, J., "Classification of periprosthetic fractures complicating total knee arthroplasty," *Orthop. Clin. North Am.,* 30, 209, 1999.

36. Digioia, A. and Rubash, H., "Periprosthetic fractures of the femur after total knee arthroplasty," *Clin. Orthop.,* 271, 135, 1991.

37. Felix, N., Stuart, M., and Hanssen, A., "Periprosthetic fractures of the tibia associated with total knee arthroplasty," *Clin. Orthop.,* 345, 113, 1997.

38. Hozack, W., Goll, S., Lotke, P., et al., "Treatment of patellar fractures after TKA," *Clin. Orthop.,* 236, 123, 1988.

39. Goldberg, V., Figgie, H.E., Inglis, A., et al., "Patellar fracture type and prognosis in condylar total knee arthroplasty," *Clin. Orthop.,* 236, 115, 1988.

40. Culp, R., Schmidt, G., Hanks, G., et al., "Supracondylar fractures of the femur following prosthetic knee arthroplasty," *Clin. Orthop.,* 222, 212, 1987.

41. Sisto, D., Lachiewicz, P., and Insall, J., "Treatment of supracondylar fractures following prosthetic arthroplasty of the knee," *Clin. Orthop.,* 196, 265, 1985.

42. Healy, W., Siliski, J., and Incavo, S., "Operative treatment of distal femoral fractures proximal to knee replacements," *J. Bone Joint Surg.,* 75A, 27, 1993.

43. McLaren, A., Dupont, J., and Schroeber, D., "Open reduction and internal fixation of supracondylar fractures above total knee arthroplasties using the intramedullary supracondylar rod," *Clin. Orthop.,* 302, 194, 1994.

44. Weber, D., Pomeroy, D., Schaper, L., et al., "Supracondylar nailing of distal periprosthetic femoral fractures," *Int. Orthop.,* 24, 33, 2000.

45. Hora, N., Markel, D., Haynes, A., and Grimm, M., "Biomechanical analysis of supracondylar femoral fractures fixed with modern retrograde intramedullary nails," *J. Orthop. Trauma,* 13, 539, 1999.

46. Koval, K.J., Kummer, F., Bharam, S., et al., "Distal femoral fixation: a laboratory comparison of the 95 degree plate, antegrade and retorgrade inserted reamed intramedullary nails," *J. Orthop. Trauma,* 10, 378, 1996.

47. Koval, K.J., Hoehl, J., Kummer, F., and Simon, J.A., "Distal femoral fixation: a biomechanical comparision of the standard condylar buttress plate, a locked buttress plate, and the 95-degree blade plate," *J. Orthop. Trauma,* 11, 521, 1997.

48. Lesh, M., Schneider, D., Deol, G., et al., "The consequences of anterior femoral notching in total knee arthroplasty. A biomechanical study," *J. Bone Joint Surg.,* 82A, 1096, 2000.

49. Engh, G. and Ammeen, D., "Periprosthetic fractures adjacent to total knee implants: treatment and clinical results," *Instr. Course Lect.,* 47, 437, 1998.

50. Kraay, M., Goldberg, V., Figgie, M., and Figgie, H., "Distal femoral replacement with allograft/prosthetic reconstruction for treatment of supracondylar fractures in patients with total knee arthroplasty," *J. Arthroplasty,* 7, 7, 1992.

51. Bourne, R., "Fractures of the patella after total knee replacement," *Orthop. Clin. North Am.,* 30, 287, 1999.

52. Freedman, E. and Eckardt, J., "A modular endoprosthetic system for tumor and non-tumor reconstruction — preliminary experience," *Orthopaedics,* 20, 27, 1997.

53. Urch, S. and Moskal, J., "Simultaneous ipsilateral revision total hip arthroplasty and revision total knee arthroplasty with entire femoral allograft," *J. Arthroplasty,* 13, 833, 1998.

54. Cooke, P.H. and Newman, J., "Fractures of the femur in relation to cemented hip prosthesis," *J. Bone Joint Surg.,* 70B, 386, 1988.

26 The Prevention of Periprosthetic Osteoporosis

Michael S. Wildstein and Yuehuei H. An

CONTENTS

I. INTRODUCTION

One of the basic principles of osteodynamics is that trabeculae form in patterns best suited to counteract the forces imparted on them. Once a fracture callus has formed, an exquisite remodeling process ensues. Osteoblastic and osteoclastic cellular activity responds to the functional demands and muscle attachments of bone, strengthening where it is needed and resorbing where it is not. In 1868, the renowned German orthopaedist Dr. Julius Wolff first described his eponymous law which states that every change in the form or function of a bone is followed by adaptive changes in its internal architecture and its external shape. Following arthroplasty, the forces acting on and around the new joint change the stress that neighboring bone experiences. Bone, as Wolff observed, reacts by remodeling itself to meet these new demands.

Bone changes following joint arthroplasty are well documented in the literature.[1-4] Local osteopenia from stress shielding will be discussed below and is the most significant complication of total joint surgery leading to periprosthetic fracture. At the most basic level, the reason for periprosthetic osteopenia is low stress on the bone. Particularly in the hip, such changes are significant in the manner in which they affect implant fixation and result in mechanical loosening with subsequent failure of components. Component loosening, subsidence, and fracture (either of the bone or the prosthesis) all represent indications for revision arthroplasty. These entities can be attributed to one of three mechanisms to be discussed in this chapter.

II. STRESS SHIELDING

Two concepts that have risen to the forefront of remodeling theory are stress shielding and bone resorption. Although these terms are often used interchangeably, they are distinct entities. Stress shielding refers to a reduction in the stress level within bone and cannot be perceived per se. This entity sets up the conditions for local osteoporosis, which then can predispose bone to fracture. Bone resorption is the physical manifestation of stress shielding. Remodeling after intramedullary implant insertion most often occurs as stress shielding.[5,6] Preventing such a complication has been the source of much discussion in the orthopaedic community since the advent of arthroplasty.

Stress shielding in the hip occurs when, after arthroplasty, femoral load is transferred from the proximal-medial bone through the implant and down to the tip of the component which is firmly embedded in diaphyseal bone.[7,8] Dual-energy X-ray absorptiometry (DEXA) of this proximal-medial zone, also referred to as the femoral calcar, has demonstrated significant changes in bone mass after uncemented total hip arthroplasty (THA). Venesmaa et al.[1] measured periprosthetic bone mineral density (BMD) in seven Gruen zones around the femur over a 3-year span. During the first 3 months after arthroplasty, BMD decreased significantly in almost every Gruen zone. However, after the first postoperative year, periprosthetic bone loss was stable. Interestingly, the only factor shown to significantly affect periprosthetic bone loss has been preoperative BMD.[1] The challenge to the physician is preventing osteopenic changes from occurring once the arthroplastic surgery is complete.

III. COMPONENT PROPERTIES

Bobyn et al.[9] performed experimental studies on a canine model in which they successfully demonstrated that implantation of a stiff femoral component yielded greater cortical bone loss at 1, 2, and 3 years postoperatively when compared with implantation of an identical fully porous-coated, metallic femoral stem of increased flexibility. Investigators performed strain gauge studies demonstrating that increasing the stem flexibility of an implant caused strain to be more uniformly distributed over the cortical surface, resulting in a bone mineral content some 30% less than with the stiffer component.[9] Specifically, this study found the optimal bending stiffness of an implant to be about one half to one third that of a normal human femur. Additionally, stems greater than 13 mm in diameter and those with extensive porous coating showed a significant increase in bone resorption. Although significant osseointegration of a cementless femoral implant is the primary goal of total joint surgery, the resultant alteration in stress transfer to the femur causes adaptive femoral bone remodeling.

In an attempt to further promote the extent and reproducibility of osseointegration of implants, manufacturers use a hydroxyapatite (HA) coating. Numerous studies prove the effectiveness of HA in increasing both the rate and the extent of bone ingrowth while acting in a functional capacity at least as well as non-HA-coated implants. Some studies note that early radiographic analyses of HA-coated hip stems failed to demonstrate appreciable differences in bone quality.[10-12] However, this fact can be attributed to limitations in the roentgenographic technology of the time. Recent studies show that by the time a patient's plain radiographs demonstrate the appearance of osteopenia, fully one third of his BMD has already been lost.[13] However, with the advent of DEXA scanning, the ability to detect relatively small discrepancies in BMD has been greatly improved. In a series of 33 patients undergoing THA, Tanzer et al.[14] implanted 39 prostheses that utilized a proximally porous-coated cementless multilock stem (Figure 26.1). Individual hips were randomized to receive implants either with or without HA/tricalcium phosphate (TCP) coating. Following DEXA analysis of the prosthetic hips 2 years postoperatively, the HA/TCP-coated implants had significantly less bone loss than the non-HA/TCP counterparts.[14]

IV. DISUSE ATROPHY

In the weeks immediately following THA, a circumferential loss of bone has been described.[9,15] The main reason for this observation in cementless total hips is decreased physical activity of patients postoperatively. Presumably, disuse diminishes the amplitude of the factors that positively influence bone mass, thereby permitting resorptive factors (vitamin D or parathyroid hormone) to

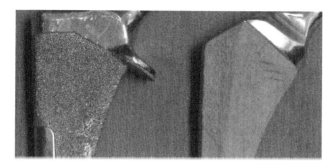

FIGURE 26.1 The proximally porous-coated femoral component (left, by Richards, Memphis, TN) and a similar design with HA-coating (right, by Howmedica/Osteonics, Rutherford, NJ).

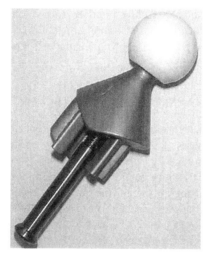

FIGURE 26.2 Femoral component of the hip prosthesis without medullary stem.

overwhelm the remodeling balance.[16] With the cementless THA, only partial weight bearing is normally allowed during the first 6 to 8 weeks following surgery. Over the ensuing months, full weight bearing is gradually approached until normal physical activity has resumed. Even in the case of cemented prostheses, patients, while permitted to engage in full weight-bearing activities virtually immediately postoperatively, rarely do so secondary to postoperative pain or simple reticence in testing their new joint. If no or reduced load bearing occurs in a limb for sufficient periods of time, bony character changes to meet the new, lightened demand for strength in the involved areas. Gross and Rubin[16] examined biochemical markers of bone resorption in weight-bearing joints of turkeys after disuse, and Inoue et al.[17] repeated this experiment later using humans. Both groups found elevations in the urine pyridinoline within 7 days of the loss of function. This chapter addresses several of the countermeasures that physicians have instituted in their attempts to combat periprosthetic osteopenia.

V. IMPLANT DESIGN

In an attempt to decrease the stress shielding mechanism described previously, Munting et al.[3] designed and implanted a stemless femoral component (Figure 26.2). The design, lacking a medullary stem and fitting into an angular resection of the femoral neck, also contains an HA layer on

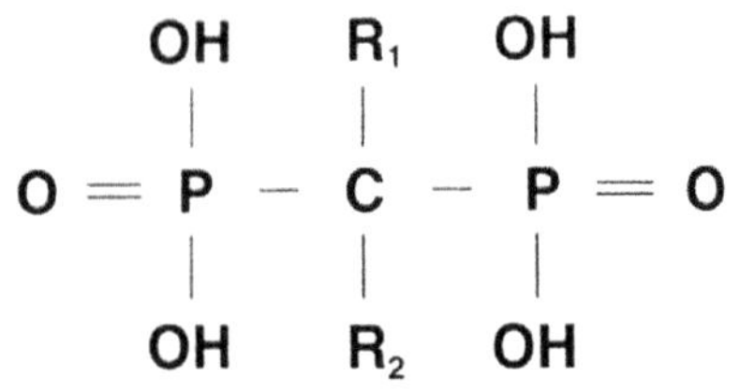

$$O = P - C - P = O$$

with OH and R_1 groups on top and OH and R_2 groups on the bottom of the phosphorus and carbon atoms.

FIGURE 26.3 Structure of the bisphosphonates.

the surface of the implant that comes in contact with the femoral neck. In a series of 48 hips, investigators showed that in patients who had low preoperative BMD, the proximal medial femoral calcar (PMFC) BMD actually increased on the operative side after surgery as compared with the level of the opposite, unaffected hip.[3]

This design not only prevented periprosthetic osteopenia, it also preserved bone stock in the femoral calcar, which is an invaluable asset for future revisions. Although this new implant has not been widely accepted into the mainstream of orthopaedics, it does appear to be a promising new addition to the hip implant arena, particularly in younger patients who will likely necessitate implant revision at some point in the future.

VI. PHARMACOLOGIC INTERVENTIONS

Another approach physicians have taken to combat post-arthroplasty osteopenia has been to focus on pharmacologic countermeasures. Although there currently exists no consensus regarding pharmacologic prophylaxis, initial studies by Wilkinson et al.[18] have shown promise with the use of the bisphosphonate pamidronate. Disodium pamidronate is an aminobisphosphonate compound that has the effect of inhibiting prenylation of the proteins necessary for osteoclast function (Figure 26.3).[19] Used to reduce bone loss in a number of osteopathologic conditions (such as Paget's disease, metastatic cancers, steroid-induced bone loss), a single dose of pamidronate delivered postoperatively exerts lasting effects on bone turnover. In a randomized, double-blind controlled trial, patients given 9 mg of pamidronate after THA had a significant reduction in acute-phase bone loss compared to placebo in both the proximal femur as well as the hip, both common areas of postimplant stress shielding. Unfortunately, extended follow-up of these patients has yet to be performed. Therefore, the long-term efficacy of bisphosphonates in preventing implant loosening remains unknown.

VII. SUMMARY

Sir John Charnley is credited with performing the first THA in 1960. Since that time, total joint surgery, while solving one dilemma for doctors and patients, has become a catalyst for the elucidation of several new pathologic entities in orthopaedic surgery. The phenomenon of stress shielding, undescribed before THA became so commonplace, is today an issue at the forefront of orthopaedic surgeons' agendas. With nearly 168,000 hip replacements performed each year,[20] the impetus for countermeasure development is tremendous. Through implant redesign, finite-element and biomechanic analysis and pharmacologic research, physicians and other scientists continue their search for more satisfactory answers to this "iatrogenic problem," periprosthetic osteopenia. Current research in these areas continues to offer promising results. Already, great advances have been made in understanding the genesis of these problems. It is only through the continued concerted efforts of physicians, biological researchers, and engineers that we will be able to develop superior implants resistant to bone loss for the next generation of patients.

REFERENCES

1. Venesmaa, P.K., Kroger, H.P., Miettinen, H.J., et al., "Monitoring of periprosthetic BMD after uncemented total hip arthroplasty with dual-energy X-ray absorptiometry — a 3-year follow-up study," *J. Bone Miner. Res.,* 16, 1056, 2001.

2. McCarthy, K., Steinberg, G., Agren, M., et al., "Quantifying bone loss from the proximal femur after total hip arthroplasty," *J. Bone Joint Surg.,* 73B, 774, 1991.

3. Munting, E., Smitz, P., and Van Sante, N., "Effect of a stemless femoral implant for total hip arthroplasty on the bone mineral density of the proximal femur. A prospective longitudinal study," *J. Arthroplasty,* 12, 373, 1997.

4. Kroger, H., Vanninen, E., Overmyer, M., et al., "Periprosthetic bone loss and regional bone turnover in uncemented total hip arthroplasty: a prospective study using high resolution single photon emission tomography and dual-energy X-ray absorptiometry," *J. Bone Miner. Res.,* 12, 487, 1997.

5. Huiskes, R., Weinans, H., and van Rietbergen, B., "The relationship between stress shielding and bone resorption around total hip stems and the effects of flexible materials," *Clin. Orthop.,* 274, 124, 1992.

6. Oh, I. and Harris, W.H., "Proximal strain distribution in the loaded femur: an *in vitro* comparison of the distributions in the intact femur and after insertion of different hip-replacement femoral components," *J. Bone Joint Surg.,* 60A, 75, 1978.

7. Nishii, T., Sugano, N., Masuhara, K., et al., "Longitudinal evaluation of time related bone remodeling after cementless total hip arthroplasty," *Clin. Orthop.,* 339, 121, 1997.

8. Kiratli, B.J., Checovich, M.M., McBeath, A.A., et al., "Measurement of bone mineral density by dual-energy X-ray absorptiometry in patients with the Wisconsin hip, an uncemented femoral stem," *J. Arthroplasty,* 11, 184, 1996.

9. Bobyn, J.D., Mortimer, E.S., Glassman, A.H., et al., "Producing and avoiding stress shielding. Laboratory and clinical observations of noncemented total hip arthroplasty," *Clin. Orthop.,* 274, 79, 1992.

10. Cook, K., Thomas, K.A., and Dalton, J.E., "Hydroxyapatite coating of porous implants improves bone ingrowth and interface attachment strength," *J. Biomed. Mater. Res.,* 26, 989, 1992.

11. Soballe, K., Hansen, E.S., Brockstedt-Rasmussen, H., and Bunger, C., "Hydroxyapatite coating converts fibrous tissue to bone around loaded implants," *J. Bone Joint Surg.,* 75B, 270, 1993.

12. Soballe, K., Hansen, E.S., Brockstedt-Rasmussen, H., et al., "Gap healing enhanced by hydroxyapatite coating in dogs," *Clin. Orthop.,* 272, 300, 1991.

13. Finsen, V. and Anda, S., "Accuracy of visually estimated bone mineralization in routine radiographs of the lower extremity," *Skeletal Radiol.,* 17, 270, 1988.

14. Tanzer, M., Kantor, S., Rosenthall, L., and Bobyn, D., "Femoral remodeling after porous-coated total hip arthroplasty with and without hydroxyapatite-tricalcium phosphate coating," *J. Arthroplasty,* 16, 552, 2001.

15. Kannus, P., Jarvinen, M., Sievanen, H., et al., "Osteoporosis in men with a history of tibial fracture," *J. Bone Miner. Res.,* 3, 423, 1994.

16. Gross, T.S. and Rubin, C.T., "Uniformity of resorptive bone loss induced by disuse," *J. Orthop. Res.,* 13, 708, 1995.

17. Inoue, M., Tanaka, H., Moriwake, T., et al., "Altered biochemical markers of bone turnover in humans during 120 days of bed rest," *Bone,* 26, 281, 2000.

18. Wilkinson, J.M., Stockley, I., Peel, N.F., et al., "Effect of pamidronate in preventing local bone loss after total hip arthroplasty: a randomized, double-blind, controlled trial," *J. Bone Miner. Res.,* 16, 556, 2001.

19. Russell, R.G. and Rogers, M.J., "Bisphosphonates: from the laboratory to the clinic and back again," *Bone,* 25, 97, 1999.

20. AAOS, Hip Implants, American Academy of Orthopaedic Surgeons Web Site, http://orthoinfo.aaos.org, 2001.

Part VI

Secondary or Other Forms
of Osteoporosis

27 Osteoporosis in Rheumatoid Arthritis

Qian K. Kang and Yuehuei H. An

CONTENTS

I. INTRODUCTION

Osteoporosis is a condition that can be defined as "diseases characterized by low bone mass, microarchitectural deterioration of bone tissue lead[ing] to enhanced bone fragility and a consequent increase in the fracture risk."[1] Osteoporosis is caused by many different events, including hormone depletion (menopause in women and hypogonadism in men), limb disuse or immobilization, steroid administration, and rheumatoid arthritis. Osteoporotic changes in rheumatoid arthritis (RA) were first described by Barwell in 1865.[2] It is known that both juxta-articular and generalized osteoporosis occur in RA. RA-related osteoporosis affects more women (both pre- and postmenopausal) than men and can lead to chronic immobility. RA osteoporosis is also a major determinant of the outcome of juvenile RA.[3,4] As shown by the overwhelming number of articles in the literature, the topic of osteoporosis in RA is a huge one, encompassing multiple specialties. Therefore, this chapter is intended only as a brief overview of osteoporotic changes in RA,[5-7] the mechanisms of these changes, animal models of inflammatory arthritis with osteoporotic changes,[8-10] and the impact of osteoporosis on medical and surgical management in patients with RA.[11]

II. PATHOGENESIS OF RA-RELATED OSTEOPOROSIS

Patients with early stage RA have osteoporotic changes to juxta-articular bone sites. Appendicular bone loss at sites distant from the affected joints does not occur in the early stage of RA. By contrast, diffuse, generalized osteoporosis of the axial and appendicular bones develops in the chronic stage of the disease. However, localized osteoporosis and generalized osteoporosis share most common pathogenic mechanisms; the latter has other confounding mechanisms such as menopause and the use of steroids and some other drugs. The common mechanisms include immobilization and the release of inflammatory factors due to rheumatoid synovial changes.

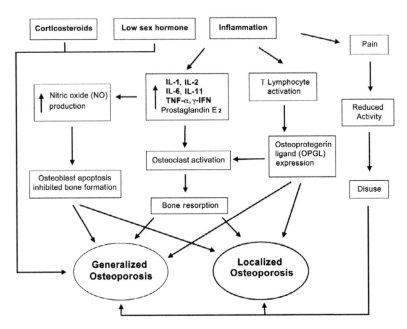

FIGURE 27.1 Schematic pathways of inflammation-mediated periarticular and generalized osteoporosis.

A. Juxta-Articular Osteoporosis

Juxta-articular osteoporosis can be defined as the osteoporotic changes in periarticular bones near the inflamed joint(s). The exact cause of juxta-articular osteopenic changes remains unclear, but several theories are offered by multiple investigations,[5,6,12-17] including the theories of (1) cytokine release (from activated lymphocytes and macrophages as major mediators of the localized osteoporosis), (2) disuse or immobilization, (3) osteoblast apoptosis and suppressed bone formation induced by increased level of nitric oxide (NO) synthase, and (4) a recent finding of osteoprotegerin ligand (OPGL)-mediated osteoclastogenesis (Figure 27.1).

The increased amount of inflammatory factors secreted by local inflammatory cells may contribute significantly to the development of periarticular osteopenia and osteoporosis. It is known that synovial tissues, which are enriched with cells of the monocyte/macrophage lineage, can be stimulated to differentiate into fully functional osteoclasts.[18,19] Local cytokines and other inflammatory factors, such as interleukin-1 (IL-1), interleukin-2 (IL-2), interleukin-6 (IL-6), IL-6 receptor, interleukin-11 (IL-11), tumor necrosis factor α (TNF-α), gamma interferon (γ-IFN), and prostaglandin E_2 (PGE$_2$), have been shown to stimulate bone resorption by activating osteoclast activity.[12,14,20-31] Many of these factors associated with increased osteoclastic bone resorption exert their effects on osteoclast differentiation indirectly, via effects on osteoblasts or bone lining cells, which in turn release products or express cell surface molecules that act on osteoclast precursors.[15,17] The factors acting through this mechanism include parathyroid hormone, parathyroid hormone-related peptide, 1,25-dihydroxyvitamin-D$_3$, prostaglandin E_2, IL-11, oncostatin M, estrogen, and glucocorticoids.[32,33] Interestingly, IL-1α or IL-β (which can act directly on osteoclasts) or TNF-α (which acts on osteoclast precursors) can also stimulate osteoblasts or bone lining cells to enhance osteoclastic function indirectly.[34]

However, the cytokine theory does not fully explain what causes the osteopenia at locations away from the arthritic joints such as the osteopenia of femoral head and distal tibia in a rabbit model of knee inflammation.[8] Bone mass is known to decrease in the absence of stimulation from gravity or weight-bearing ambulation.[35-37] As early as 1 to 2 weeks after the inflammatory arthritis developed (induced by carrageenan injection), the rabbits used their right legs less and less and some of them even carried their legs.[8] Osteopenia was found not only in the juxta-articular bones but also in locations away from the knee such as the femoral head and distal tibia of the same limb.

All these locations are subject to the effects of disuse, while the contralateral femur, tibia, and both humeri, which are not affected by disuse, had no osteopenic changes.

A recent study found that activation of the inducible NO synthase (iNOS) pathway contributes to inflammation-induced osteoporosis by suppressing bone formation and causing osteoblast apoptosis.[38] Cytokine-induced NO production has been shown to inhibit osteoblast growth and differentiation *in vitro*. In an *in vivo* inflammation-mediated osteoporosis model, compared to wild-type (WT) mice, the mice with inactivation of the iNOS gene (iNOS knockout mice) showed less inhibition of bone formation than WT mice and showed no significant increase in osteoblast apoptosis. Therefore, inducible NOS-mediated osteoblast apoptosis and depressed bone formation are seen to play important roles in the pathogenesis of osteoporosis related to inflammatory arthritis.[38]

Another major recent finding showed a role for T lymphocytes and their products in osteoclast-mediated bone loss.[39] Bone remodeling and bone loss are controlled by a balance between the tumor necrosis factor family molecule OPGL and its decoy receptor osteoprotegerin (OPG). The OPGL receptor RANK is expressed on chondrocytes, osteoclast precursors, and mature osteoclasts. OPGL expression in T cells is induced by antigen receptor engagement, which suggests that activated T cells may influence bone metabolism through OPGL and RANK. The study by Kong et al.[39] showed that activated T cells can directly trigger osteoclastogenesis through OPGL. Systemic activation of T cells *in vivo* leads to an OPGL-mediated increase in osteoclastogenesis and bone loss. In a T-cell-dependent model of rat adjuvant inflammatory arthritis with severe bone and cartilage destruction, blocking of OPGL through osteoprotegerin treatment at the onset of disease prevents bone and cartilage destruction but not inflammation.[39] These results show that both systemic and local T-cell activation can lead to OPGL production and subsequent bone loss, and they provide a novel paradigm for T cells as regulators of bone physiology.

B. GENERALIZED OSTEOPOROSIS

Generalized osteoporosis is often associated with long-standing, destructive, and disabling RA affecting both the cortical and trabecular bone, and the mechanisms for this clinical condition are still not fully understood.[5,6,12-15] The most typical patient at risk is the postmenopausal woman with severe, destructive RA who has impaired mobility, calcium malabsorption, and is vitamin D deficient. The relationship of bone formation, bone loss, and bone turnover to the decreased bone density is complex. There is certainly an increased overall rate of bone loss in RA, which means that the rate of bone resorption must exceed that of bone formation.[40] Several known mechanisms for the formation of generalized osteoporosis are similar to that of localized periarticular osteoporosis, but some are particular to RA (Figure 27.2). The latter include (1) long-term use of steroids and (2) estrogen depletion in postmenopausal women.

It is clear that generalized osteoporosis can result from long-term use of corticosteroid therapy for RA through changes in gonadal hormone secretion, calcium absorption, renal handling of calcium, and direct effect on bone.[41-45] Corticosteroid-induced osteoporosis remains a common and important problem in rheumatic disease, but controversy continues about the relative safety of "low-dose" corticosteroid therapy in regard to its effects on bone, which should be weighed against the beneficial effects of controlling synovitis and minimizing functional impairment.[43]

It is known that estrogen depletion may result in accentuated bone loss in RA. Postmenopausal women with RA have been shown to have increased serum phosphate and alkaline phosphatase (ALP), and increased urinary hydroxyproline and mucopolysaccharide excretion compared with normal postmenopausal women, suggesting higher metabolic activity.[46,47] In men with RA, it has been found that lower plasma testosterone concentrations are common and they were coexistent with spinal and femoral neck low bone mineral density (BMD).[48]

High disease activity, as shown by persistently increased erythrocyte sedimentation rate (>20 mm first hour), C reactive protein (>20 mg/l), and rheumatoid factor titer, is closely related

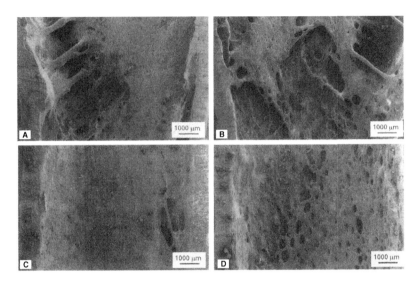

FIGURE 27.2 Morphologic changes of the endosteal surface of the femoral diaphysis by scanning electron microscopy (SEM) (mag: ×10, bar: 1000 μm). On the arthritic side in the proximal diaphyseal region (B) the trabecular portion of the cortex was diminished and looked more porous, with obvious thinner trabeculae compared to the control side (A). At the distal one third of the femur on the arthritic side (D) the endosteal surfaces were more porous than the control side (C) and many cavities were seen on the cortical sectional surface (D), which indicated subendosteal cavitations. (From Kang, Q. et al., *J. Mater. Sci. Mater. Med.*, 9, 463, 1998. With permission.)

to the degree of RA-related bone loss (as measured by total body calcium or local BMD, or recently studied biochemical markers of bone turnover in RA such as urinary pyridinoline and deoxypyridinoline).[43,49-53]

Physical activity is known to play a significant role in the development and maintenance of bone mass. Reduced physical activity and functional impairment have been shown to be related to osteopenia or osteoporosis in patients with RA.[8,43,53,54] High overall functional capacity in terms of physical activity (measured with a health assessment questionnaire, or HAQ) correlates with an increased BMD in the axial skeleton. The local functional capacity in terms of grip strength was found to be positively related to BMD in the appendicular skeleton.[54]

At the molecular level, in RA increased serum levels of hormonal factors or cytokines,[14] such as IL-6,[20,26] IL-2,[25] TNF-α,[27] γ-IFN,[21] and PGE$_2$,[28] in patients with active RA created the speculation that these factors may also contribute to generalized osteoporosis by directly and/or indirectly activating osteoclast activity.[12,22,24]

Again, the important recent finding based on the reports and reviews by Kong et al.[39,55] showed that activated T cells directly trigger osteoclastogenesis through OPGL, which aided the understanding of systemic osteoporotic change in RA. OPGL (TNFS11) and its receptor RANK (TNFRS11A) are essential for the development and activation of osteoclasts and critical regulators of physiologic bone remodeling and osteoporosis. Production of OPGL by activated T cells can directly regulate osteoclastogenesis and bone remodeling. This may explain why autoimmune diseases, cancers, leukemia, asthma, and chronic viral infections such as hepatitis and HIV result in systemic and local bone loss. OPGL is also the pathogenetic factor that causes bone and cartilage destruction and clinical crippling in arthritis. Inhibition of OPGL binding to RANK via the natural decoy receptor OPG prevents bone loss in postmenopausal osteoporosis and cancer metastases and completely blocks crippling in a rat model of arthritis.[39] Moreover, OPG expression is induced by estrogen,[56] which provides a molecular explanation of postmenopausal osteoporosis in women.

TABLE 27.1
**Selected Animal Models of Inflammatory Arthritis
with Demonstrated Juxta-Articular Osteoporosis**

Animal	Joint	Bone Evaluated	Inducing Factor	Route of Administration	Ref.
Rabbit	Knee	Femur, tibia	Carrageenan	Intra-articular	Bogoch et al.,[10,62] Kang et al.[8]
Canine	Knee	Femur	Carrageenan	Intra-articular	Bunger et al.,[63] Hansen et al.[64-67]
Rat	Polyarthritis	Tibia	Magnesium silicate	SC[b]	Minne et al.[68]
	Polyarthritis	Tibiotarsal	Adjuvant[a]	SC	Kong et al.[39]
	Knee	Femur, tibia	Carrageenan	Intra-articular	Hansra et al.[69]
	Polyarthritis	Tibia, vertebrae	Collagen type II	SC	Enokida et al.,[9] Hoshino et al.[70]
Mouse	Polyarthritis	Tibia	Magnesium silicate	SC	Armour et al.[38]

[a] Adjuvant: *Mycobacterium tuberculosis* emulsion in paraffin oil.
[b] SC = subcutaneous injection.

III. ANIMAL MODELS
OF INFLAMMATION-MEDIATED OSTEOPOROSIS

Many animal models are available for studying issues and questions related to inflammatory arthritis.[57-61] However, there are only a few animal models tested for investigating osteoporosis in chronic inflammatory arthritis (Table 27.1). Experimental animal models of secondary osteoporosis caused by induced inflammatory arthritis share similarities to human RA-related osteoporosis in certain aspects. These animal models are used in the investigation of the etiology, pathophysiology, and pharmaceutical treatment of RA-related osteoporosis.

Several animal models have pathologic findings similar to the human condition such as joint inflammation and juxta-articular osteoporosis.[61] So far, models using rabbits, dogs, rats, and mice have been well established. The parameters that have been studied include BMD, radiographic changes, histomorphometry, and mechanical properties of bone. It was believed that animal models of arthritis, regardless of the methods used for inducing disease, would provide some important information leading to the understanding of the etiologic and pathogenetic mechanisms of human secondary osteoporosis related to RA. However, none of the animal models exactly mirrors the entire spectrum of RA in humans, and it is difficult to mimic long-term human inflammatory arthritis in animals. Animal models of RA and related osteoporosis develop and progress much more rapidly than does human disease, so these models are characterized primarily on acute inflammatory changes. There have been no reports on the effects of long-term inflammatory arthritis on bone quality, although the effects had been noticed (not confirmed) in one earlier study conducted in our laboratory.[8]

Based on existing knowledge, generalized osteoporosis can be induced in animals after administration of steroids, which may shed some light on the understanding of osteoporosis in patients with RA who are taking significant dose of steroids.

IV. CHANGES OF BONE STRUCTURE

Juxta-articular osteoporosis is a common finding adjacent to joints affected by rheumatoid disease, extending for 1 to 2 cm from the articular surface of small joints and 4 to 5 cm from the surface of the knee joint.[71] It occurs early in the course of the disease before any breach of cortical bone is seen. Bone remodeling occurs continuously, more rapidly than normal and there is a delicate

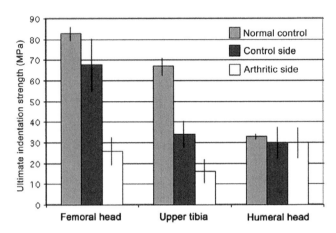

FIGURE 27.4 Comparison of indentation strength of cancellous bones from normal control and inflammatory arthritic osteoporosis in rabbits.

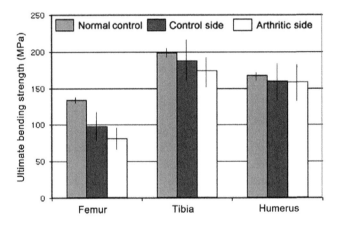

FIGURE 27.5 Comparison of bending strength of diaphyseal bones from normal control and inflammatory arthritic osteoporosis in rabbits.

be determined by the degree of immobilization (periarticular femur and tibial bones > contralateral femur and tibia > upper limb bones).

VI. CLINICAL CHALLENGES

A. DIAGNOSIS

Osteoporosis caused by RA occurs in the periarticular bones in the early stage of the inflammatory disease, and after 6 months generalized osteoporosis often develops.[45,52,88] The incidences of fractures were much higher than in the general population, ranging from 1.5 to 2.7 based on a limited literature search.[89-92] Apart from the underlying osteoporosis, patients with RA have an increased risk of falls.[93] The incidence of insufficiency fractures may not be low in RA, but they are thought to be underdiagnosed.[94-96] If long-term steroids were used, the risk of hip fracture was as high as 2.7. Numerous studies indicated increased risk of fracture associated with RA disease activity, increasing age, earlier age at diagnosis of RA, disability, impaired ambulation (immobility), steroid use, and thinness. If RA itself and all the above factors are considered as confounding factors, the prevention and treatment of the osteoporosis condition and osteoporotic fractures can be extremely complicated and challenging.

Awareness is the number one issue in the diagnosis, prevention, and management of osteoporosis related to RA. The fact is that the awareness of potential osteoporosis in general orthopaedic practice is still relatively limited, although it has become more prominent due to the enlarging elderly population and related problems.

Should we look for osteoporosis in patients with RA? Based on the above-mentioned facts, the answer is a resounding YES! However, a widely accepted set of criteria to decide which patients with RA should be evaluated for the presence of osteoporosis is currently not available.[97] One may consider using the Amsterdam Proposal, which depends on patient age, disease activity, and the degree of immobilization:[97]

1. High disease activity (C reactive protein > 20 mg/l, persistently increased erythrocyte sedimentation rate > 20 mm in first hour)
2. High age[98] (women > 50 years, men > 60 years)
3. Immobility (Steinbrocker score[89] > 3 or HAQ score < 1.25[99,100])

Based on this proposal, if a patient fulfills two of the three criteria, the bone density should be measured.

Although conventional radiology can show osteoporotic changes, it is not sufficient because losses of up to 30 to 40% can occur before changes appear on radiographs. X-ray photodensitometry is a useful method if the quality of the film can be controlled. SPA and DEXA have been used widely for screening and diagnosing osteoporotic conditions. SPA is applicable only to appendicular bone such as the distal one third radius or one tenth radius. DEXA is able to measure both appendicular and axial bone with an acceptable amount of radiation.[3] So far, DEXA has been used as the key method for measuring BMD both in basic research and clinical screening and diagnosis.

B. Surgical Interventions

Osteoporosis associated with RA impacts the practice of orthopaedic surgery on a daily basis. The orthopaedic surgeon must understand the effects of RA and its medical treatment on the outcome of surgical interventions and the effects of surgical intervention on the health and function of local bone.[11] Abnormalities of bone affect clinical decision making in the surgical treatment of patients with RA and must be considered for the optimal treatment of these patients. Several important and clinically prominent issues include fracture fixation and outcome, intraoperative fractures and prevention, bone ingrowth to cementless joint prostheses, and the general consideration of total joint replacement.

Bone healing (of fractures and bone grafts) is usually rapid,[11] but requires stable internal or external fixation. Fractures related to RA osteoporosis challenge surgical procedures and osteoporotic bone compromises bony fixation leading to serious complications. One study showed that the number of complications after internal fixation of femoral neck fractures was very high (12 of 20 patients), including nonunion, osteonecrosis, infection, and intertrochanteric fracture.[101] Theoretically, the insertion of fixation devices and prostheses creates stress shielding, which changes the normal loading pattern of the local bone resulting in further bone loss and local osteopenia. Methods of internal fixation of implants and other devices must be appropriate to the biomechanical properties of the bone. Techniques of surgery must be modified to prevent intraoperative fracture.[11]

Total joint replacement is perhaps the most successful surgical treatment for patients with RA in terms of pain relief, function restoration, and patient satisfaction. However, due to the poor bone quality and perhaps also the poor immune status, the long-term results of cemented prosthetic joint replacement in patients with RA has been reported to be relatively inferior to those patients who had prosthetic joint surgery with cement for the treatment of other diagnoses.[102,103] Relatively high rates of wound healing problems, aseptic loosening, and sepsis were found in patients with RA receiving joint prostheses, which may be due to the systemic immune nature of RA.[104-106] The existing studies indicate that improved techniques are still necessary to increase the long-term success of total hip replacement in the patient with RA, but no breakthrough improvement can be seen in the near future. RA is a bone-losing disease and has a high bone remodeling rate, which may jeopardize the bonding at the bone–cement or bone–implant interface. Other potentially harmful effects in patients with RA are the use of steroids, anti-inflammatory agents, and other drugs that are known to have the ability of causing osteoporosis or interfering with bone ingrowth to implant surfaces. These concerns still remain even after some recent successful short-term clinical reports on using cementless prostheses.[105,107-109]

Bone ingrowth into cementless joint prostheses in RA has been a major question in the field. Several studies have demonstrated limited bone ingrowth into cementless prosthesis, such as in the model of an antigen-induced arthritis in rabbits,[110] and the models of carrageenan-induced arthritis in dogs[67] and rabbits.[111] In the rabbit model induced by carrageenan, trabecular thickness (Tb.Th), trabecular number (Tb.N), and amount of bone apposition were all smaller or less on the arthritic side than the control side for all groups — titanium-beaded implant, beaded implant coated with hydroxyapatite (HA), and sandblasted titanium surface coated with HA. Mechanical testing showed a weaker interface shear strength on the arthritis side in all groups. The results suggest that carrageenan-induced inflammatory arthritis may influence the quality of local bone (osteoporotic changes), and hence the compromised bone apposition and mechanical stability of the implant–bone interface.[111] As long as the patient is in an active RA stage, bone remodeling is fast and osteopenic changes in periarticular bones are inevitable. Therefore, no solid bone–implant or bone–cement interfaces without potential loosening can be envisioned.

Future research may concentrate on medical prevention and treatment of RA and RA-related osteoporosis to improve the general health of the periarticular bone before a confident joint replacement procedure is performed. As a matter of fact, the awareness of the impact of RA-related osteoporosis has led to the initiation of several clinical trials designed to prevent bone loss and to increase bone mass in RA. Several animal and clinical investigations indicate that agents including estrogen, calcitonin, activated vitamin D products (alfacalcidol and calcitriol),[112-114] and bisphosphonates[86,115] may have clinical efficacy in preventing bone loss; hormones (such as parathyroid hormone) or growth factors with capacity of increasing bone formation may hold promise for the treatment of generalized bone loss in patients with RA.[15]

REFERENCES

1. "Proceedings of a symposium. Consensus Development Conference on Osteoporosis. October 19–20, 1990, Copenhagen, Denmark," *Am. J. Med.,* 91, 1S, 1991.
2. Barwell, H., *Disease of the Joints,* Hardwick, London, 1865.
3. Cassidy, J.T., Langman, C.B., Allen, S.H., and Hillman, L.S., "Bone mineral metabolism in children with juvenile rheumatoid arthritis," *Pediatr. Clin. North Am.,* 42, 1017, 1995.
4. McDonagh, J.E., "Osteoporosis in juvenile idiopathic arthritis," *Curr. Opin. Rheumatol.,* 13, 399, 2001.
5. Star, V.L. and Hochberg, M.C., "Osteoporosis in patients with rheumatic diseases," *Rheum. Dis. Clin. North Am.,* 20, 561, 1994.
6. Suzuki, Y. and Mizushima, Y., "Osteoporosis in rheumatoid arthritis," *Osteoporos. Int.,* 7, S217, 1997.
7. Dequeker, J., Westhovens, R., and Ravelingien, I., "Osteoporosis in rheumatoid arthritis," in *Management of Fractures in Severely Osteoporotic Bone: Orthopaedic and Pharmacologic Strategies,* Obrant, K., Ed., Springer, New York, 2000, 499.
8. Kang, Q., An, Y.H., Butehorn, H.F., and Friedman, R.J., "Morphological and mechanical study of the effects of experimentally induced inflammatory knee arthritis on rabbit long bones," *J. Mater. Sci. Mater. Med.,* 9, 463, 1998.

9. Enokida, M., Yamasaki, D., Okano, T., et al., "Bone mass changes of tibial and vertebral bones in young and adult rats with collagen-induced arthritis," *Bone*, 28, 87, 2001.

10. Bogoch, E., Gschwend, N., Bogoch, B., et al., "Juxtaarticular bone loss in experimental inflammatory arthritis," *J. Orthop. Res.*, 6, 648, 1988.

11. Bogoch, E.R. and Moran, E.L., "Bone abnormalities in the surgical treatment of patients with rheumatoid arthritis," *Clin. Orthop.*, 366, 8, 1999.

12. Joffe, I. and Epstein, S., "Osteoporosis associated with rheumatoid arthritis: pathogenesis and management," *Semin. Arthritis Rheum.*, 20, 256, 1991.

13. Jones, S.M. and Bhalla, A.K., "Osteoporosis in rheumatoid arthritis," *Clin. Exp. Rheumatol.*, 11, 557, 1993.

14. Roux, S. and Orcel, P., "Bone loss. Factors that regulate osteoclast differentiation: an update," *Arthritis Res.*, 2, 451, 2000.

15. Goldring, S.R. and Gravallese, E.M., "Mechanisms of bone loss in inflammatory arthritis: diagnosis and therapeutic implications," *Arthritis Res.*, 2, 33, 2000.

16. Goldring, S.R., "The final pathogenetic steps in focal bone erosions in rheumatoid arthritis," *Ann. Rheum. Dis.*, 59, S72, 2000.

17. Goldring, S.R. and Gravallese, E.M., "Pathogenesis of bone erosions in rheumatoid arthritis," *Curr. Opin. Rheumatol.*, 12, 195, 2000.

18. Fujikawa, Y., Sabokbar, A., Neale, S., and Athanasou, N.A., "Human osteoclast formation and bone resorption by monocytes and synovial macrophages in rheumatoid arthritis," *Ann. Rheum. Dis.*, 55, 816, 1996.

19. Chang, J.S., Quinn, J.M., Demaziere, A., et al., "Bone resorption by cells isolated from rheumatoid synovium," *Ann. Rheum. Dis.*, 51, 1223, 1992.

20. Kotake, S., Sato, K., Kim, K.J., et al., "Interleukin-6 and soluble interleukin-6 receptors in the synovial fluids from rheumatoid arthritis patients are responsible for osteoclast-like cell formation," *J. Bone Miner. Res.*, 11, 88, 1996.

21. DeGre, M., Mellbye, O.J., and Clarke-Jenssen, O., "Immune interferon in serum and synovial fluid in rheumatoid arthritis and related disorders," *Ann. Rheum. Dis.*, 42, 672, 1983.

22. Skerry, T. and Gowen, M., "Bone cells and bone remodeling in rheumatoid arthritis," in *Mechanisms and Models in Rheumatoid Arthritis*, Henderson, B., Edwards, J.C.W., and Pettipher, E.R., Eds., Academic Press, London, 1995, chap. 10.

23. Chambers, T.J., "The cellular basis of bone resorption," *Clin. Orthop.*, 151, 283, 1980.

24. Athanasou, N.A., "Cellular biology of bone-resorbing cells," *J. Bone Joint Surg. Am.*, 78, 1096, 1996.

25. McKenna, R.M., Ofosu-Appiah, W., Warrington, R.J., and Wilkins, J.A., "Interleukin 2 production and responsiveness in active and inactive rheumatoid arthritis," *J. Rheumatol.*, 13, 28, 1986.

26. Houssiau, F.A., Devogelaer, J.P., Van Damme, J., et al., "Interleukin-6 in synovial fluid and serum of patients with rheumatoid arthritis and other inflammatory arthritides," *Arthritis Rheum.*, 31, 784, 1988.

27. Saxne, T., Palladino, M.A., Jr., Heinegard, D., et al., "Detection of tumor necrosis factor alpha but not tumor necrosis factor beta in rheumatoid arthritis synovial fluid and serum," *Arthritis Rheum.*, 31, 1041, 1988.

28. Robinson, D.R., Tashjian, A.H., Jr., and Levine, L., "Prostaglandin-stimulated bone resorption by rheumatoid synovia. A possible mechanism for bone destruction in rheumatoid arthritis," *J. Clin. Invest.*, 56, 1181, 1975.

29. Lacey, D.L., Timms, E., Tan, H.L., et al., "Osteoprotegerin ligand is a cytokine that regulates osteoclast differentiation and activation," *Cell*, 93, 165, 1998.

30. Houssiau, F.A., "Cytokines in rheumatoid arthritis," *Clin. Rheumatol.*, 14, 10, 1995.

31. Mundy, G.R., "Cytokines and growth factors in the regulation of bone remodeling," *J. Bone Miner. Res.*, 8, S505, 1993.

32. Manolagas, S.C. and Jilka, R.L., "Bone marrow, cytokines, and bone remodeling. Emerging insights into the pathophysiology of osteoporosis," *N. Engl. J. Med.*, 332, 305, 1995.

33. Suda, T., Nakamura, I., Jimi, E., and Takahashi, N., "Regulation of osteoclast function," *J. Bone Miner. Res.*, 12, 869, 1997.

34. Kobayashi, K., Takahashi, N., Jimi, E., et al., "Tumor necrosis factor alpha stimulates osteoclast differentiation by a mechanism independent of the ODF/RANKL-RANK interaction," *J. Exp. Med.*, 191, 275, 2000.

35. Young, D.R., Niklowitz, W.J., Brown, R.J., and Jee, W.S., "Immobilization-associated osteoporosis in primates," *Bone*, 7, 109, 1986.
36. Wronski, T.J. and Morey, E.R., "Inhibition of cortical and trabecular bone formation in the long bones of immobilized monkeys," *Clin. Orthop.*, 181, 269, 1983.
37. Whedon, G.D., "Disuse osteoporosis: physiologic aspects," *Calcif. Tissue Int.*, 36, S146, 1984.
38. Armour, K.J., Armour, K.E., van't Hof, R.J., et al., "Activation of the inducible nitric oxide synthase pathway contributes to inflammation-induced osteoporosis by suppressing bone formation and causing osteoblast apoptosis," *Arthritis Rheum.*, 44, 2790, 2001.
39. Kong, Y.Y., Feige, U., Sarosi, I., et al., "Activated T cells regulate bone loss and joint destruction in adjuvant arthritis through osteoprotegerin ligand," *Nature (London)*, 402, 304, 1999.
40. Sambrook, P.N., Eisman, J.A., Champion, G.D., et al., "Determinants of axial bone loss in rheumatoid arthritis," *Arthritis Rheum.*, 30, 721, 1987.
41. Bjelle, A.O. and Nilsson, B.E., "Osteoporosis in rheumatoid arthritis," *Calcif. Tissue Res.*, 5, 327, 1970.
42. Lukert, B.P. and Raisz, L.G., "Glucocorticoid-induced osteoporosis: pathogenesis and management," *Ann. Intern. Med.*, 112, 352, 1990.
43. Henderson, N.K. and Sambrook, P.N., "Relationship between osteoporosis and arthritis and effect of corticosteroids and other drugs on bone," *Curr. Opin. Rheumatol.*, 8, 365, 1996.
44. Walsh, L.J., Wong, C.A., Pringle, M., and Tattersfield, A.E., "Use of oral corticosteroids in the community and the prevention of secondary osteoporosis: a cross sectional study," *Br. Med. J.*, 313, 344, 1996.
45. Verhoeven, A.C. and Boers, M., "Limited bone loss due to corticosteroids; a systematic review of prospective studies in rheumatoid arthritis and other diseases," *J. Rheumatol.*, 24, 1495, 1997.
46. Sambrook, P.N., Eisman, J.A., Champion, G.D., and Pocock, N.A., "Sex hormone status and osteoporosis in postmenopausal women with rheumatoid arthritis," *Arthritis Rheum.*, 31, 973, 1988.
47. Verstraeten, A. and Dequeker, J., "Vertebral and peripheral bone mineral content and fracture incidence in postmenopausal patients with rheumatoid arthritis: effect of low dose corticosteroids," *Ann. Rheum. Dis.*, 45, 852, 1986.
48. Stafford, L., Bleasel, J., Giles, A., and Handelsman, D., "Androgen deficiency and bone mineral density in men with rheumatoid arthritis," *J. Rheumatol.*, 27, 2786, 2000.
49. Eggelmeijer, F., Papapoulos, S.E., Westedt, M.L., et al., "Bone metabolism in rheumatoid arthritis; relation to disease activity," *Br. J. Rheumatol.*, 32, 387, 1993.
50. Sambrook, P.N., Ansell, B.M., Foster, S., et al., "Bone turnover in early rheumatoid arthritis. 2. Longitudinal bone density studies," *Ann. Rheum. Dis.*, 44, 580, 1985.
51. Gough, A., Sambrook, P., Devlin, J., et al., "Osteoclastic activation is the principal mechanism leading to secondary osteoporosis in rheumatoid arthritis," *J. Rheumatol.*, 25, 1282, 1998.
52. Gough, A.K., Lilley, J., Eyre, S., et al., "Generalised bone loss in patients with early rheumatoid arthritis," *Lancet*, 344, 23, 1994.
53. Laan, R.F., Buijs, W.C., Verbeek, A.L., et al., "Bone mineral density in patients with recent onset rheumatoid arthritis: influence of disease activity and functional capacity," *Ann. Rheum. Dis.*, 52, 21, 1993.
54. Hansen, M., Florescu, A., Stoltenberg, M., et al., "Bone loss in rheumatoid arthritis. Influence of disease activity, duration of the disease, functional capacity, and corticosteroid treatment," *Scand. J. Rheumatol.*, 25, 367, 1996.
55. Kong, Y.Y. and Penninger, J.M., "Molecular control of bone remodeling and osteoporosis," *Exp. Gerontol.*, 35, 947, 2000.
56. Hofbauer, L.C., Khosla, S., Dunstan, C.R., et al., "Estrogen stimulates gene expression and protein production of osteoprotegerin in human osteoblastic cells," *Endocrinology*, 140, 4367, 1999.
57. Brahn, E., "Animal models of rheumatoid arthritis. Clues to etiology and treatment," *Clin. Orthop.*, 265, 42, 1991.
58. Heymer, B., Spanel, R., and Haferkamp, O., "Experimental models of arthritis," *Curr. Top. Pathol.*, 71, 123, 1982.
59. Magilavy, D.B., "Animal models of chronic inflammatory arthritis," *Clin. Orthop.*, 259, 38, 1990.
60. Kaklamanis, P.M., "Experimental animal models resembling rheumatoid arthritis," *Clin. Rheumatol.*, 11, 41, 1992.

61. Bendele, A., McComb, J., Gould, T., et al., "Animal models of arthritis: relevance to human disease," *Toxicol. Pathol.,* 27, 134, 1999.

62. Bogoch, E.R., Moran, E., Crowe, S., and Fornasier, V., "Arthritis not immobilization causes bone loss in the carrageenan injection model of inflammatory arthritis," *J. Orthop. Res.,* 13, 777, 1995.

63. Bunger, C., Bunger, E.H., Harving, S., et al., "Growth disturbances in experimental juvenile arthritis of the dog knee," *Clin. Rheumatol.,* 3, 181, 1984.

64. Hansen, E.S., Soballe, K., Kjolseth, D., et al., "Microvascular hemodynamics in experimental arthritis: disparity between the distribution of microspheres and plasma flow in bone," *Microvasc. Res.,* 40, 206, 1990.

65. Hansen, E.S., Soballe, K., Henriksen, T.B., et al., "[99mTc]Diphosphonate uptake and hemodynamics in arthritis of the immature dog knee," *J. Orthop. Res.,* 9, 191, 1991.

66. Soballe, K., Pedersen, C.M., Odgaard, A., et al., "Physical bone changes in carragheenin-induced arthritis evaluated by quantitative computed tomography," *Skeletal Radiol.,* 20, 345, 1991.

67. Soballe, K., Hansen, E.S., Brockstedt-Rasmussen, H., et al., "Fixation of titanium and hydroxyapatite-coated implants in arthritic osteopenic bone," *J. Arthroplasty,* 6, 307, 1991.

68. Minne, H.W., Pfeilschifter, J., Scharla, S., et al., "Inflammation-mediated osteopenia in the rat: a new animal model for pathologic loss of bone mass," *Endocrinology,* 115, 50, 1984.

69. Hansra, P., Moran, E.L., Fornasier, V.L., and Bogoch, E.R., "Carrageenan-induced arthritis in the rat," *Inflammation,* 24, 141, 2000.

70. Hoshino, K., Hanyu, T., Arai, K., and Takahashi, H.E., "Mineral density and histomorphometric assessment of bone changes in the proximal tibia early after induction of type II collagen-induced arthritis in growing and mature rats," *J. Bone Miner. Metab.,* 19, 76, 2001.

71. Duncan, H. and Riddle, J.M., "Juxtaarticular osteoporosis," *Arthritis Rheum.,* 29, 149, 1986.

72. Shimizu, S., Shiozawa, S., Shiozawa, K., et al., "Quantitative histologic studies on the pathogenesis of periarticular osteoporosis in rheumatoid arthritis," *Arthritis Rheum.,* 28, 25, 1985.

73. Bogoch, E.R. and Moran, E., "Abnormal bone remodeling in inflammatory arthritis," *Can. J. Surg.,* 41, 264, 1998.

74. Deodhar, A.A. and Woolf, A.D., "Bone mass measurement and bone metabolism in rheumatoid arthritis: a review," *Br. J. Rheumatol.,* 35, 309, 1996.

75. Alenfeld, F.E., Diessel, E., Brezger, M., et al., "Detailed analyses of periarticular osteoporosis in rheumatoid arthritis," *Osteoporos. Int.,* 11, 400, 2000.

76. Takashima, T., Kawai, K., Hirohata, K., et al., "Inflammatory cell changes in Haversian canals. A possible cause of osteoporosis in rheumatoid arthritis," *J. Bone Joint Surg. Br.,* 71, 671, 1989.

77. Wordsworth, B.P., Vipond, S., Woods, C.G., and Mowat, A.G., "Metabolic bone disease among in-patients with rheumatoid arthritis," *Br. J. Rheumatol.,* 23, 251, 1984.

78. Njeh, C.F. and Genant, H.K., "Bone loss. Quantitative imaging techniques for assessing bone mass in rheumatoid arthritis," *Arthritis Res.,* 2, 446, 2000.

79. Keller, C., Hafstrom, I., and Svensson, B., "Bone mineral density in women and men with early rheumatoid arthritis," *Scand. J. Rheumatol.,* 30, 213, 2001.

80. Iwamoto, J., Takeda, T., and Ichimura, S., "Forearm bone mineral density in postmenopausal women with rheumatoid arthritis," *Calcif. Tissue Int.,* 70, 1, 2002.

81. Towheed, T.E., Brouillard, D., Yendt, E., and Anastassiades, T., "Osteoporosis in rheumatoid arthritis: findings in the metacarpal, spine, and hip and a study of the determinants of both localized and generalized osteopenia," *J. Rheumatol.,* 22, 440, 1995.

82. Kroot, E.J., Nieuwenhuizen, M.G., de Waal Malefijt, M.C., et al., "Change in bone mineral density in patients with rheumatoid arthritis during the first decade of the disease," *Arthritis Rheum.,* 44, 1254, 2001.

83. An, Y.H. and Draughn, R.A., "Mechanical properties and testing methods of bone," in *Animal Models in Orthopaedic Research,* An, Y.H. and Friedman, R.J., Eds., CRC Press, Boca Raton, FL, 1999, chap. 8.

84. An, Y.H., Barfield, W.R., and Draughn, R.A., "Mechanical properties of bone," in *Mechanical Testing of Bone and the Bone–Implant Interface,* An, Y.H. and Draughn, R.A., Eds., CRC Press, Boca Raton, FL, 2000, chap. 3.

85. Yang, J.P., Bogoch, E.R., Woodside, T.D., and Hearn, T.C., "Stiffness of trabecular bone of the tibial plateau in patients with rheumatoid arthritis of the knee," *J. Arthroplasty,* 12, 798, 1997.

86. Bellingham, C.M., Lee, J.M., Moran, E.L., and Bogoch, E.R., "Bisphosphonate (pamidronate/APD) prevents arthritis-induced loss of fracture toughness in the rabbit femoral diaphysis," *J. Orthop. Res.*, 13, 876, 1995.

87. An, Y.H., Kang, Q., and Friedman, R.J., "Mechanical symmetry of rabbit bones studied by bending and indentation testing," *Am. J. Vet. Res.*, 57, 1786, 1996.

88. Shenstone, B.D., Mahmoud, A., Woodward, R., et al., "Longitudinal bone mineral density changes in early rheumatoid arthritis," *Br. J. Rheumatol.*, 33, 541, 1994.

89. Hooyman, J.R., Melton, L.J., III, Nelson, A.M., et al., "Fractures after rheumatoid arthritis. A population-based study," *Arthritis Rheum.*, 27, 1353, 1984.

90. Urbanek, R., Tlustochowicz, W., Patola, J., and Glodzik, J., "[Incidence of osteoporosis in patients with rheumatoid arthritis]," *Przegl. Lek.*, 57, 103, 2000.

91. Wasnich, R., "Bone mass measurement: prediction of risk," *Am. J. Med.*, 95, 6S, 1993.

92. Cooper, C., Coupland, C., and Mitchell, M., "Rheumatoid arthritis, corticosteroid therapy and hip fracture," *Ann. Rheum. Dis.*, 54, 49, 1995.

93. Tinetti, M.E., Speechley, M., and Ginter, S.F., "Risk factors for falls among elderly persons living in the community," *N. Engl. J. Med.*, 319, 1701, 1988.

94. Alonso-Bartolome, P., Martinez-Taboada, V.M., Blanco, R., and Rodriguez-Valverde, V., "Insufficiency fractures of the tibia and fibula," *Semin. Arthritis Rheum.*, 28, 413, 1999.

95. Duston, M., "Osteolysis of the pelvis presenting as insufficiency fracture in a patient with rheumatoid arthritis," *J. Clin. Densitom.*, 3, 203, 2000.

96. Elkayam, O., Paran, D., Flusser, G., et al., "Insufficiency fractures in rheumatic patients: misdiagnosis and underlying characteristics," *Clin. Exp. Rheumatol.*, 18, 369, 2000.

97. Lems, W.F. and Dijkmans, B.A., "Should we look for osteoporosis in patients with rheumatoid arthritis?" *Ann. Rheum. Dis.*, 57, 325, 1998.

98. Ross, P.D., "Osteoporosis. Frequency, consequences, and risk factors," *Arch. Intern. Med.*, 156, 1399, 1996.

99. Kirwan, J.R. and Reeback, J.S., "Stanford Health Assessment Questionnaire modified to assess disability in British patients with rheumatoid arthritis," *Br. J. Rheumatol.*, 25, 206, 1986.

100. Eggelmeijer, F., Papapoulos, S.E., van Paassen, H.C., et al., "Increased bone mass with pamidronate treatment in rheumatoid arthritis. Results of a three-year randomized, double-blind trial," *Arthritis Rheum.*, 39, 396, 1996.

101. Bogoch, E., Ouellette, G., and Hastings, D., "Failure of internal fixation of displaced femoral neck fractures in rheumatoid patients," *J. Bone Joint Surg. Br.*, 73, 7, 1991.

102. Chmell, M.J., Scott, R.D., Thomas, W.H., and Sledge, C.B., "Total hip arthroplasty with cement for juvenile rheumatoid arthritis. Results at a minimum of ten years in patients less than thirty years old," *J. Bone Joint Surg. Am.*, 79, 44, 1997.

103. Creighton, M.G., Callaghan, J.J., Olejniczak, J.P., and Johnston, R.C., "Total hip arthroplasty with cement in patients who have rheumatoid arthritis. A minimum ten-year follow-up study," *J. Bone Joint Surg. Am.*, 80, 1439, 1998.

104. Severt, R., Wood, R., Cracchiolo, A., III, and Amstutz, H.C., "Long-term follow-up of cemented total hip arthroplasty in rheumatoid arthritis," *Clin. Orthop.*, 265, 137, 1991.

105. Tang, W.M. and Chiu, K.Y., "Primary total hip arthroplasty in patients with rheumatoid arthritis," *Int. Orthop.*, 25, 13, 2001.

106. Tang, W.M. and Chiu, K.Y., "Primary total hip arthroplasty in patients with ankylosing spondylitis," *J. Arthroplasty*, 15, 52, 2000.

107. Garcia Araujo, C., Fernandez Gonzalez, J., and Tonino, A., "Rheumatoid arthritis and hydroxyapatite-coated hip prostheses: five-year results. International ABG Study Group," *J. Arthroplasty*, 13, 660, 1998.

108. Lachiewicz, P.F., "Porous-coated total hip arthroplasty in rheumatoid arthritis," *J. Arthroplasty*, 9, 9, 1994.

109. Loehr, J.F., Munzinger, U., and Tibesku, C., "Uncemented total hip arthroplasty in patients with rheumatoid arthritis," *Clin. Orthop.*, 366, 31, 1999.

110. Sennerby, L. and Thomsen, P., "Tissue response to titanium implants in experimental antigen-induced arthritis," *Biomaterials*, 14, 413, 1993.

111. An, Y.H., Friedman, R.J., Jiang, M., et al., "Bone ingrowth to implant surfaces in an inflammatory arthritis model," *J. Orthop. Res.*, 16, 576, 1998.
112. Lakatos, P., Nagy, Z., Kiss, L., et al., "Prevention of corticosteroid-induced osteoporosis by alfacalcidol," *Z. Rheumatol.*, 59, 48, 2000.
113. Schacht, E., "[Osteoporosis in rheumatoid arthritis — significance of alfacalcidol in prevention and therapy]," *Z. Rheumatol.*, 59, 10, 2000.
114. Gukasian, D.A., Nasonov, E.L., Balabanova, R.M., et al., "[Effects of alfacalcidol on mineral density of bone tissue in patients with rheumatoid arthritis]," *Klin. Med.*, 79, 47, 2001.
115. Pysklywec, M.W., Moran, E.L., and Bogoch, E.R., "Zoledronate (CGP 42′446), a bisphosphonate, protects against metaphyseal intracortical defects in experimental inflammatory arthritis," *J. Orthop. Res.*, 13, 838, 1997.

28 Osteopenia and Related Fractures Caused by Immobilization

Kathleen A. Hogan and Yuehuei H. An

CONTENTS

I. INTRODUCTION

With a supersonic boom and a cloud of smoke, a space shuttle lifts off carrying supplies to astronauts living in the international space station. In the hospital below, an orthopaedic surgeon places a young child in a spica cast after a femur fracture. In the surgical intensive care unit, a patient lies paralyzed with respirators controlling his every breath. In each of these situations, prolonged periods of immobilization and lack of weight-bearing activities may adversely affect bone quality. Osteopenia, decreased calcification of bone, can occur in any age group. To maintain equilibrium between formation and resorption, bone must be stimulated. The universe is in a constant state of entropy, tending toward increased randomness in the absence of forces acting upon the system. The same concept applies to bone metabolism. Without mechanical loading forces, the forces of entropy will prevail and bone density in long bones will decrease. In primary osteoporosis, women and men lose bone density as a function of age and hormonal changes. Prevention of a critical drop in bone mass in part entails maximizing the bone mass obtained during the teenage and adult years. What effect does 2 months of immobilization in a spica cast at the age of 5 have upon the eventual peak bone density of that individual? Will the 3 months that a patient spends bedridden in the intensive care unit recovering from multiple extremity fractures after a motorcycle accident result in an increased risk of hip fractures when he reaches the age of 75? Will astronauts traveling to Mars ever be able to regain the bone mass they lose during the journey? These are important questions in orthopaedics today.

Osteopenia has been defined by the World Health Organization as a loss of bone mineral density (BMD) greater than 1 standard deviation below the adult mean. Osteoporosis represents a greater severity of bone loss, with a BMD greater than 2.5 standard deviations lower than the adult mean. It is classified as severe when associated with fractures. Osteoporosis is further subdivided into primary and secondary types, based on etiology. Primary osteoporosis is either postmenopausal (Type I) or age related (Type II). Secondary osteoporosis has an identifiable and usually preventable cause, such as alcohol or tobacco abuse, hypogonadism, hypercortisolism, hyperthyroidism, or immobilization. Pathologic fractures are associated with all types of osteoporosis. This chapter focuses on immobilization and disuse as causes of osteopenia and osteoporosis. The current literature on the effects of immobilization on bone is reviewed, with discussion of animal models and clinical studies.

II. FRACTURE RISK WITH IMMOBILIZATION

Biomechanically, osteopenic bone is more likely to fracture than is bone that is adequately mineralized. Cortical bone is thick, dense bone found in the diaphyses of long bones. The mechanical properties of cortical bone are dependent on the rate and direction of loading. It has been demonstrated that there is a 2% decline in the tensile strength and elastic modulus of cortical bone per decade.[1] Trabecular bone, in contrast, is found in the metaphyses and epiphyses. It is a porous structure with interconnected columns of bone. In trabecular bone, density does influence stress–strain properties. Loss of BMD has a greater effect on trabecular than on cortical bone. Compressive strength of trabecular bone is related to density by a power of 2 and to elastic modulus by a power of 2 to 3. A 25% reduction in trabecular density would therefore reduce strength by 44% and elastic modulus by 58%.[1] Fractures occur when applied forces exceed the yield point of the bone. The magnitude of the yield point is directly related to bone density, geometry, diameter, direction of applied force, and the rate of loading.

Once a fracture has occurred, recent studies suggest that osteoporotic bone may not heal as quickly as normal bone. Rats made osteoporotic by ovariectomy demonstrate poor early fracture healing with 40% less periosteal callus formation and decreased stiffness and strength of the fracture site.[2] In another study, when compared to young rats, older rats and ovariectomized rats demonstrated decreased mineralization by dual-energy X-ray absorptiometry (DEXA) scan of a femur fracture callus. Mechanical testing showed a corresponding decrease in bone strength.[3] Internal fixation may also be more complicated in this patient population. Experimental studies have shown significant decreases in screw pullout forces in osteoporotic spines.[4]

III. EFFECTS OF IMMOBILIZATION ON BONE

A. ANIMAL MODELS

Are there differences between primary osteoporosis resulting from hormonal changes and secondary osteoporosis resulting from immobilization or disuse? Although the clinical implications are the same, the basic science appears to differ. For example, Bagi and colleagues[5] compared histologic specimens of cortical bone obtained from rats after ovariectomy and immobilization. Both groups evidenced endosteal resorption of bone with expansion of the marrow cavity. In ovariectomized rats, periosteal bone formation increased, while in the immobilized rats there was significantly less periosteal reaction. Bone stiffness was decreased more in rats immobilized for 12 weeks than in ovariectomized rats and controls.[5] Immobilization appears to have a more rapid initial effect on loss of bone strength than does an acute loss of hormonal stimulation. Immobilization slows bone formation whereas primary osteoporosis speeds bone resorption. The end result in both types of osteoporosis is an uncoupling between forces of regeneration and destruction. Unlike primary osteoporosis, however, immobilization of one limb does not affect the other limbs. Loss of bone density is a local, not systemic, effect of immobilization and disuse.

There are many etiologies of immobilization and disuse-induced osteopenia. The forces generated on bone by muscles and soft tissues can differ depending on the environment. Conditions of weightlessness, spastic paralysis, or flaccid paralysis may affect bone metabolism differently than does cast immobilization in a limb with normal muscle tone. There have been several animal models developed by researchers in an attempt to mimic these specific physiologic conditions. There have been no investigations, however, that directly compare histologic or biochemical differences between these different models of immobilization. The results of studies done on each condition are discussed separately in this chapter.

Cast or tape immobilization is frequently used to study local effects of disuse on a single limb. Advantages to this procedure include reversibility, ease of obtaining fixation, and reproducibility of the technique. Tenotomy and external fixation can also be used for single limb immobilization.[6] Studies have demonstrated that bone loss with immobilization involves both periosteal and endosteal surfaces with a concurrent thinning of trabeculae.[7] In a classic 1978 study, Uhthoff and Jaworski[8] examined the histologic and radiographic effects of long-term cast immobilization in canines. A rapid initial loss of bone occurred in the first 6 weeks involving periosteal and endosteal bone. This loss was then reversed with a net gain in bone mass at weeks 8 through 12. The authors suggest that this increased bone density may represent an acute remodeling reaction. After week 12, there was a slow bone loss from the periosteum. Bone formation and resorption eventually reached an equilibrium state at week 24. After 40 weeks of immobilization, the canines had experienced a 30 to 50% loss of the bone mass in the immobilized hind limb.[8] Similar results have been seen in other animal populations. A 3-week immobilization resulted in significant decreases in BMD of rat femur.[9-11] Normal allometric relationships of bone mineral content to limb mass were also decreased, meaning that bone loss could not be explained merely by loss of muscle mass from limb atrophy.[10] Sheep immobilized in a cast for 12 weeks had a 29% decrease of trabecular bone volume in the immobilized calcaneus. There was no decline in the number of trabeculae, but a thinning of the trabeculae did occur.[12]

Another method to cause limb disuse is to paralyze one or more limbs. This model can mimic the physiologic conditions that exist after spinal cord injury or hemiplegic stroke. Animal models of paralysis are generated by spinal cord injury or by sectioning of the sciatic nerve. Resection of a 5-mm section of sciatic nerve results in lower limb paralysis, with loss of cancellous bone, which is evident within 10 days.[6] Bone resorption initially is markedly increased as demonstrated by an increase in osteoclasts during the first 72 hours after surgery.[13] The rate of periosteal bone formation decreases by day 7 and has been shown to be suppressed for as long as 2 months. Molecular markers of bone formation, including osteocalcin and alkaline phosphatase are likewise suppressed.[14] Mechanical testing reveals significant differences after 6 months of paralysis in the strength of the tibia and femur to compressive and torque loads.[15]

Unlike single limb immobilization, spaceflight affects all bones and also has systemic effects on the animal. The gold standard for studying the effects of spaceflight on bone is to send animals into orbit. Rats and mice have been flown aboard the Mir Space Station and on multiple space shuttle missions. There are many limitations to these studies, the first of which is the difficulty and cost of setting up the experiment. Researchers cannot always control the duration of the flight, data cannot be easily collected during spaceflight, and competition is fierce for experiments to be chosen for spaceflight. Furthermore, animal studies conducted in space have difficulties controlling for the potential systemic effects of the stress associated with a disruption in environment and the physiologic stress of takeoff and reentry. Despite the mentioned limitations, these experiments have provided valuable information to researchers. Cellular effects of spaceflight appear to occur even after a short period of weightlessness. Northern hybridization analysis of RNA from rats that traveled in space for only 4 days found significant reductions in aggrecan mRNA compared to Earth-bound animals. No change in long bone growth rate during this short flight was found as assessed by tetracycline labeling.[16] A week spent in space decreased mechanical strength of rat tibias in one study without evident histologic changes.[17] After 18 days in space the rate of periosteal bone formation decreased.[18] Histology at this time point demonstrated a growth arrest line in the periosteum and endosteum.[19]

Conditions of weightlessness encountered with space travel can be mimicked on Earth with a rat hind limb suspension model. The animal's tail and front limbs support its body weight; the hind limbs are suspended in midair.[6] This technique requires custom-designed cages and close monitoring of the animals. However, it is a simple, reversible, and reproducible means to study weightlessness without the difficulties involved in space missions. After 3 weeks of hind limb suspension, these animals show significant decrease of weight-adjusted BMD by DEXA scan.[10] Garber and colleagues[20] found that 2 weeks of weightlessness resulted in decreased cross-sectional area, percent mineralization, and surface calcification. Some researchers have performed identical experiments in space and on Earth to validate this model. In one such study, spaceflight and hind limb suspension resulted in similar changes in tibial mRNA expression: osteocalcin mRNA was decreased while alkaline phosphatase and insulin-like growth factor (IGF-1) increased.[21] Vico and colleagues,[22] however, discovered that bone resorption rate was increased in suspended rats but remained at a steady state during conditions of spaceflight. An important difference between immobilization and weightlessness is that while mechanical loading is removed during spaceflight, mobility is not impaired.

Based on these animal studies, several conclusions can be drawn. Although there have been no studies directly comparing bone mineralization in each model, there do not appear to be any striking differences in outcomes, regardless of the form of immobilization utilized in the study. Histology has demonstrated that immobilization by casting, paralysis, or weightlessness all result in decreased periosteal bone formation. Endosteal bone resorption also occurs. The rate of actual bone loss, however, may differ in each model. Immobilization with casting or surgical intervention results in an immediate increase in osteoclast activity not observed in a purely weightless environment of spaceflight. From a molecular perspective, immobilization has been found to cause downregulation of genes such as osteocalcin and bone sialoproteins that are involved in the regulation of bone formation.[14,21] Unlike primary osteoporosis where increased bone resorption is the primary cause of loss of bone mass, immobilization osteoporosis may be primarily the result of decreased formation secondary to loss of mechanical stimulation for bone growth.

B. Clinical Scenarios

Immobilization osteopenia is an area of active clinical research today. It has very important implications as NASA contemplates sending astronauts to Mars or to the international space station for prolonged tours of duty. Spinal cord injuries affect approximately 27 per 1 million persons per year, many of whom are age 14 to 24.[23] There are an estimated 3000 children diagnosed with cerebral palsy every year, many of whom will never be community ambulators. When chronic immobilization or disuse results in severe osteoporosis, a bone can fracture from the minor trauma of turning in bed or lifting a book. Even acute, short-term immobilization can result in osteopenia. Osteopenia resulting from limb immobilization during fracture healing, for example, may have important ramifications decades later on bone density and fracture risks when the patient develops primary osteoporosis. The clinical importance of bone density is seen in studies where the relative risk for hip fractures has been shown to be increased by a factor of 2.5 to 3.0 per standard deviation decrease in femoral neck BMD.[24]

1. Fracture Treatment

Orthopaedic surgeons immobilize patients every day in splints, casts, and external fixation devices. Standard treatment of fractures includes immobilization and limitation of weight-bearing activities until the bone begins to regain its original strength. Internal fixation often reduces the length of time that a patient is often protected from weight bearing. However, patients with multiple long bone fractures often must avoid weight bearing for several months. Tibia fractures treated with closed reduction and castings are often protected from full weight bearing for several months. This time period is reduced to days with the use of an IM nail for this fracture. Considerations of fracture stability are used to determine weight-bearing status. Intra-articular tibial plateau fractures, for example, even when internally fixed require 6 to 8 weeks of weight-bearing avoidance before protected partial weight bearing is allowed.

Avoidance of weight bearing or protected weight bearing prevents the patient from inadvertently overloading the weakened bone. Several studies demonstrate, however, that immobilization does have potentially significant consequences in relationship to long-term bone strength. One prospective study followed 37 patients with stable midshaft tibia fractures who were treated with either an external fixator or plaster cast. All patients were allowed to bear weight as tolerated. At 4 weeks, only 45% casted as compared to 70% of externally fixed fractures were weight bearing. At 8 weeks weight bearing had increased to 68 and 88% in the respective groups. At 16 weeks after the injuries, radiographic grading found a significantly increased severity of osteopenia in the group treated with casts.[25]

Osteoporosis associated with immobilization for fractures can be significant even years after the original injury has healed. A small prospective study of 11 patients with tibia fracture treated by either casting or intermedullary rod with a 12 to 14 week period avoiding weight bearing compared BMD of both hips at 1 and 5 years postinjury. At 1 year, BMD of the ipsilateral hip had decreased 12.5% compared to 1.4% on the contralateral hip. At 5 years postinjury, BMD was still 4.9% less than preinjury BMD compared to a 0.6% increase in the contralateral hip.[26] A larger study analyzed DEXA scans in patients identified retrospectively as having sustained a lower extremity fracture in the past (mean time from injury 9.3 years, mean age 81). A significant 4.7% difference in BMD of the trochanter on the injured compared with uninjured side was found.[26] Even 11 years after tibia fractures, small but significant decreases could be found between the BMD of the extremity with and without the prior injury with no change in the BMD of other parts of the skeleton.[27] Femoral shaft fractures occurring before puberty also result in a small but significant 2 to 5% loss of BMD in the affected extremity that persists into adulthood.[28] A history of anterior cruciate ligament injury has also been shown similarly to result in long-term decreases in bone density of the affected knee.[29]

Disuse osteopenia can affect even non-weight-bearing bones. After 6 weeks of immobilization following surgical repair of the rotator cuff or shoulder capsule, proximal humerus BMD decreased significantly at postoperative week 6. After 6 weeks of remobilization, BMD had not returned to preoperative levels in the proximal humerus, although trabecular bone area increased proportionally more than did cortical bone area.[30]

It is well accepted that bone remodeling occurs as a function of stress and strain upon bone and is thus directly affected by weight bearing. In a stabilized fracture, weight bearing causes compression at the fracture site, increased callus formation, and increased vascular profusion. Immobilization can have adverse effects on articular cartilage and tendons. All the data suggest benefits to early motion and protected weight bearing when fracture stability permits.

2. Prolonged Bed Rest

In the past, bed rest was prescribed as a treatment for the common cold, back injuries, angina, anxiety, and other common ailments. Although physicians today are less likely to encourage a patient to remain bedridden, there are exceptions. Patients hospitalized in the intensive care unit, for example, may remain supine for months as they recover. Mobility is intentionally limited after certain lower extremity skin-grafting procedures, severe burns, or while awaiting definitive fixation of spine or lower extremity fractures. The effects of prolonged immobilization on bone metabolism may be different depending on whether the underlying cause of immobilization is physiologic or neurologic. For example, a patient immobilized after a fracture still has muscle tone acting upon his or her bone whereas the normal resting muscle tone is absent in patients with spinal cord injury. Acutely ill patients have a hypermetabolic response to injury and stress. Therefore, when examining immobilization studies it is important to consider the patient population and not necessarily extrapolate the data to fit all immobilized patients.

There are several studies where volunteers adhered to strict bed rest for periods of time ranging from a few days to 30 weeks. The small number of participants limits most of these studies. As mentioned, this scenario differs greatly from clinical realities encountered in the intensive care unit. There is also a selection bias in the population willing to spend this much time confined to a bed! However, these studies do provide important information on the effects of immobilization on bone metabolism in human subjects and should be mentioned here. Markers of collagen breakdown are elevated within the first week of immobilization.[31-33] After 17 weeks of bed rest, BMD in six patients decreased significantly in the areas of total body, lumbar spine, femoral neck, trochanter, proximal tibia, and calcaneus. Rate of recovery of mineralization occurred more slowly than did its loss. At 6 months after the study only the calcaneus had regained preimmobilization mineralization.[34]

3. Paralysis

Many different types of patients are at risk for osteoporosis secondary to paralysis. Patients may have partial or complete inability to use a limb after a nerve, spine, or brain injury. The limb may be flaccid or spastic depending on the location of the injury and the enervation of muscles to that limb. Other patients, such as those with multiple sclerosis, muscular dystrophy, or AML, may experience progressive weakness that gradually impairs their ability to ambulate and to move their extremities. Other associated conditions, such as nutritional deficiencies, alterations in resting muscle tone (spastic or flaccid), age, hormone status, and duration of disuse will influence the development of osteoporosis in these patients. Unlike the other populations discussed in this chapter, these patients usually have chronic conditions. Although extremities may not be used for weight bearing, with severe osteopenia the yield point of bone is so decreased that forces generated from transferring from a bed to a chair can cause severe pathologic fractures. A study from Denmark on fracture incidence revealed a significant increase in the incidence of fractures in spinal cord–injured patients compared with the general population. These fractures were more likely to be low energy, involve the lower extremities, and occur in women. The femoral diaphysis and the supracondylar distal femur were two common sites of fractures in this population.[35]

There have been multiple studies documenting changes in bone mineralization acutely following spinal cord injury. Longitudinal studies of bone biochemical markers found early increases in bone resorption, peaking between 10 and 16 weeks after spinal cord injury, that did not return to baseline even 6 months after injury.[36] Fiore and colleagues[33] found a linear relationship with length of immobilization and markers of bone resorption. There was no corresponding increase in markers of bone formation. These data suggest that osteogenesis may not increase to compensate for the elevated bone degeneration associated with prolonged paralysis.[33]

Bone density loss after spinal cord injury occurs predominantly in the lower extremities, with the greatest loss in the distal femur. In a longitudinal study of eight patients with acute spinal cord injuries, at the level of C7 and below, decline in bone mineral content (BMC) of the tibia and femoral neck appeared to stop 2 years after the injury, at values 40 and 60% lower than normal, respectively. Femoral shaft BMC, however, appeared to be continuing to decline slowly.[37] Similar results were shown in a larger cross-sectional study. In the first year after injury, BMD decreased by 21 to 25% in the proximal and distal femur. After more than 5 years after the injury, bone loss in the proximal femur appeared to stabilize while density in the distal femur declined to 43% of ambulatory controls.[38] A recent study by Bauman et al.[39] reported findings on BMD in eight identical twins where one twin had suffered a spinal cord injury with resulting paralysis. Total BMD decreased by $18 \pm 7\%$ with loss greatest in the femur ($35 \pm 10\%$) and the pelvis ($30 \pm 9\%$) with slight increases in the BMD of the spine of the injured patients. Although limited by the small number of subjects, this study found a significant association between the duration of injury and the measured decrease in the total body BMD.[39] Lumbar spine BMD, in contrast, was not found to be significantly affected by osteoporosis after spinal injury.[37,39,40]

Strokes are a nontraumatic etiology of lower extremity paralysis, which typically occur in elderly patients who are already at high risk for primary osteoporosis by age and/or loss of hormone stimulation. Loss of bone mass in a patient with hemiplegia can be correlated to length of immobilization and time since menopause. Postmenopausal women experience greater bone loss in the paralyzed limb than do men.[41] Loss of mobility and balance after a stroke places these patients at an increased risk of falls. It is not surprising to find, therefore, that the risk of hip fracture in this population is four times greater than age-matched controls.[42] The overall hip fracture incidence in a study in Sweden was 0.5 to 0.7% of persons over age 65; this more than doubled to 1.27 to 1.96% in patients with previous strokes. In patients over the age of 85, the incidence was even higher. Fractures occurred an average of 5.4 years following the stroke and occurred on the affected side in 62.5%.[43] Biochemical markers of bone formation were decreased and markers of bone resorption were increased in patients studied at 1 and 2 years after a stroke.[44]

4.   Space Travel

The effect of weightlessness on bone density has been an area of interest for scientists since the pioneering days of space exploration. Although bone still experiences forces generated by muscle contraction, the mechanical load of weight is eliminated. The effects of spaceflight on bone are believed to be secondary to the freefall experienced by astronauts and the resulting lack of weight-bearing activity. Bone loss does not occur because of a lack of gravity. Gravity is merely a force exerted by a larger mass on a smaller one. During Earth orbit, there remains a gravitational force of the Earth on the spacecraft and its occupants; this force keeps the spacecraft in orbit. Studies that attempt to mimic conditions of weightlessness have used centrifugation of *in vitro* cultures, hind limb suspension in animal models, or enforced bed rest in human volunteers. Clinical studies performed in space are difficult to design well because of researchers' inability to control for variations such as the length of time of the mission, activity levels of astronauts while in space, and the inability to perform long-term studies without an operational space station. Several of the clinical studies performed on astronauts have investigated calcium metabolism and bone density. For example, in an early experiment, astronauts in *Skylab* were monitored for calcium balance. Calcium loss ranged from 50 to 200 mg per day. Negative calcium balance persisted up to 18 days after return to Earth. Secretion of hydroxyproline in urine was increased by 30% during an astronaut's first 30 days in space and then equilibrated.[45] Other studies have also reported that astronauts have negative calcium balances after even 1 week of space travel and calcium balance does not return to baseline for several weeks after spaceflight.[46,47]

In an attempt to minimize the effects of prolonged spaceflight on bone and muscle composition, cosmonauts inhabiting the *Mir* space station were required to participate in daily exercises including resistance training and bicycle and treadmill aerobic exercise. Despite these measures, DEXA scans revealed bone loss in the spine, femur, and pelvis, which was related to duration of time in space. Bone loss in the spine and femur occurred at a steady rate of 1.0 to 1.6% per month over 6 months. Two cosmonauts who were in space over 10 months had continuous bone loss at the femur but a considerably lower rate of bone loss in the spine.[47] The clinical relevance of increased calcium metabolism and loss of BMD is not clear, at least on spaceflights of short duration. To date, there have been no reports of fractures occurring either in space or during the immediate postflight period. As astronauts spend increasingly longer periods of time in space, however, efforts will be needed to limit bone loss and prevent the sequelae of pathologic fractures on return to Earth's atmosphere.

IV. EFFECTS OF CHRONIC IMMOBILIZATION

There is still considerable debate regarding the effect of long-term weightlessness or immobilization on BMD. The process of bone resorption occurs almost immediately. After 7 days of strict bed rest, significant increases occur in the ratio of hydroxyproline and calcium to creatine in the urine, serum calcium levels, and the products of collagen breakdown, pyridinoline and deoxypyridino-line.[32,48] Does this bone loss continue indefinitely? Evidence from canine studies demonstrated that rate of bone loss with disuse eventually slowed to reach a new equilibrium balance with bone formation.[8] This research is supported by clinical data on osteoporosis in spinal cord injuries, which found that chronic bone loss in the femoral neck and midshaft was less than 2% per year compared to an initial decline of 17 to 21% in the first year after injury.[38] The same study also found a greater loss of bone in the distal compared to proximal femur. BMD in this region decreased 25% in the first year and continued a steady rate of decline to an average of 45% 5 years after the injury. The authors hypothesized that the increased rate of bone loss in the distal femur may reflect an increased bone loss in areas of the femur that were previously subjected to higher mechanical loading during ambulation. The difference between the rate of bone loss in the proximal and distal femur may also be secondary to a mechanical load on the proximal femur with wheelchair sitting.[27]

In an attempt to determine the effects of chronic disuse on bone metabolism, some researchers have measured the effects of prolonged immobilization on markers of bone resorption and formation. In one such study, urinary calcium, hydroxyproline, and pyrophosphate excretion, all markers of bone resorption, rose initially to a maximum value during week 7 of bed rest, and remained elevated during a 30-week period of bed rest in three patients. Levels subsequently began to decline but did not return to baseline even after 2 weeks of remobilization.[31] However, conflicting data are reported in a similar study in which urinary calcium returned to baseline levels by week 15, after an initial rise.[32] In that study, other markers of collagen breakdown, pyridinoline and deoxypyrid-inoline, remained elevated throughout the 120-day period. The carboxy terminal propeptide of type I collagen, a marker of bone formation, decreased beginning on day 50 and did not return to baseline levels until day 10 of remobilization.[32] These studies indicate that the bone loss that occurs during disuse may initially be due to an increase in bone resorption but at later time points is also a result of a decrease in bone formation.

V. TREATMENT AND PREVENTION

What happens when astronauts return from space or cast immobilization is discontinued? Investigators have sought to determine if the body can accelerate bone formation with resumption of mechanical stimulation to the bone. Studies of the effects of immobilization in animal models suggest that complete reversal of disuse osteopenia may not be easily attained. With resumption of normal activity, for example, rats immobilized for 2 months failed to show increased bone even after over more than 2 months of remobilization.[9] Kannus and colleagues[49] investigated the effects of the intensity of activity on bone regeneration in young rats that had been immobilized for 3 weeks. Rats were randomized to normal cage activity, low-intensity running (20 cm/s velocity, 10° incline), or high intensity running (30 cm/s velocity, 30° incline). Rats were exercised twice per day, for a 20-min time period, which was increased gradually to 45 min per day. Immobilization produced a 9.6% change in BMD. Rats allowed normal cage activity had significant differences in BMD between the hind limbs that persisted for 8 weeks after immobilization had been discontinued. Rats that were exercised daily also had a 5% BMD deficit on the previously immobilized leg. However, in the exercised rats the BMD of both limbs was higher than in the limbs of the rats that did not run.[49] In a follow-up study, rats exercised daily for 8 weeks after immobilization were returned to cage level ambulation. After 18 weeks, these rats still had a lower BMD than age-matched controls that had never been immobilized.[11]

Studies in other animal models have verified that a time period greater than the duration of immobilization is needed to regain bone mass. In a canine study, immobilization decreased BMD by 22% in cancellous bone and 17% in cortical bone.[11] At 32 weeks after remobilization, BMD of trabecular bone was still 9% less on the previously immobilized limb compared to the control limb. Trabecular thickness was decreased 13 to 17% with immobilization but recovered with exercise.[11] Tests of mechanical strength in canines found that immobilization decreased the mechanical properties of cancellous bone significantly more than cortical bone. After immobilization, failure stress of cortical bone was reduced by 12%, whereas in trabecular bone it decreased by 56% compared to controls. After remobilization, however, mechanical strength parameters were restored.[50] Age also is a factor in the recovery following disuse. A study in canines found that after 32 weeks of immobilization followed by 60 weeks of normal mobilization, only 40% of older canines recovered significant bone mass compared to 70% of younger dogs.[51]

Even if a bone density equal to preimmobilization density can be obtained, evidence clearly indicates that considerable activity at an intensity above the normal daily activity level is required. Treatment of disuse osteopenia should therefore begin with prevention. Animal studies have shown that the detrimental effects of immobilization can be mediated by performing loading activities during periods of immobilization. Mechanical loading three times per week in a rat hind limb suspension model has been found to prevent some of the loss of BMD. Although endosteal bone was still lost, histology showed increased periosteal bone at the sites of loading and an increase in mechanical strength.[10] Zerath and colleagues[52] in France applied electrical stimulation to the limb muscles of immobilized rats. After 3 weeks of treatment, bone loss was significantly less than seen in the untreated but immobilized animals. Researchers were unable to determine if these effects were related to mechanical loading or to increased muscle activity.[52]

Weight-bearing exercise increases bone mass in loaded extremities. What happens when patients of limited mobility increase their weight-bearing activities? One risk is that muscles may become stronger than the osteoporotic bone to which they attach and fractures may result. The potential benefit is that bone-loading activities will stimulate osteogenesis. In one clinical study, non-ambulating children with spastic cerebral palsy were started on a monitored load-bearing physical activity program. After 8 weeks, BMD increased significantly in the activity group in the proximal femur and femoral neck. Femoral neck BMD increased 5.6% compared to baseline in the activity group and decreased 6.7% without intervention.[53] Weight-bearing physical therapy activities in spinal cord injuries prevented the loss of bone density, which occurred in patients without this intervention. Electrical stimulation (FES cycle ergometry) has been shown in some studies to increase tibial bone density if performed at a high intensity level for 30 min, three times per week.[54] Other studies have not found changes in femoral bone density except for a nonsignificant trend toward increase in bone density in those patients capable of generating "high loading intensity."[55]

Increasing weight-bearing activity is difficult in paralyzed patients and cumbersome for astronauts during spaceflight. Pharmacologic options for prevention of bone loss have thus been investigated. Considerable research has been done on agents to prevent or slow primary osteoporosis. The role of these agents in preventing or reducing disuse-related osteoporosis is currently under investigation. Individuals at risk for bone loss should, at minimum, meet daily nutritional requirements especially for vitamin D and calcium. Nutritional supplements should be used if needed.

Vitamin D affects bone by increasing absorption of calcium from the gastrointestinal tract. This hormone, formed by the action of ultraviolet light on 7-dehydrocholestrol in the skin, stimulates intestinal cells to produce calcium-binding proteins. It also may suppress secretion of parathyroid hormone.[56] When given to immobilized rats, vitamin D increased femoral calcium content and cortical thickness.[57] Clinically, vitamin D supplementation has been shown to increase BMD in children with spastic cerebral palsy being treated with antiseizure drugs, medications that are known to decrease calcium absorption.[58] Calcium (750 mg/day) and vitamin D supplementation in elderly patients have been shown to prevent bone density loss.[59] Use of this supplement may benefit those at risk for vitamin D deficiency, particularly hospitalized patients who are at risk for nutritional depletion and whose exposure to sunlight is minimal. Daily calcium (500 to 1000 mg/day) is recommended for all adults to help obtain optimal peak bone density. Another vitamin, vitamin K, acts as a cofactor in the carboxylation of osteocalcin and other bone matrix proteins, which occurs prior to binding with hydroxyapatite. In one study, vitamin K supplementation (menatetrenone) was given to patients with osteoporosis who had hemiplegia secondary to a stroke in a randomized, prospective study. Patients treated with 45 mg/day of menatetrenone had a significant increase in femoral BMD on both the hemiplegic and intact sides compared to the untreated controls.[60]

Calcitonin is a hormone secreted by the parafolicular cells in the thyroid gland. This hormone, activated naturally under conditions of increased serum calcium levels, binds to osteoclasts and prevents bone resorption. It is now used clinically in the treatment of osteoporosis, particularly if a patient cannot take estrogen. This medication has also been shown to decrease pain after vertebral fractures.[56] Calcitonin has been mostly ineffective in preventing postfracture osteopenia, however. In a sheep immobilization model, it was unable to prevent bone loss.[61] In a randomly controlled trial, patients with internally fixed ankle fractures were treated with calcitonin nasal spray daily for 3 months. A smaller decline of BMD of the injured ankle was noted; however, the difference was not statistically significant.[62] Furthermore, administration of calcitonin did not change markers of bone metabolism when administered to patients with CVA-induced hemiplegia.[63] There may be some benefits to using this medication to prevent increases in bone resorption rates with acute immobilization. For example, calcitonin, when given to patients immobilized for only 10 days, reduced the decreases in vitamin D and the increases in markers of bone resorption that were found in the untreated group.[64] Similar results were found when calcitonin was given acutely to patients immobilized after a hip fracture.[65]

Bisphosphonates are medications approved by the Food and Drug Administration (FDA) for the treatment of osteoporosis. Studies in women with postmenopausal osteoporosis show significant reductions in the incidence of hip, wrist, and vertebral fractures after 1 year of treatment with alendronate.[66] Bisphosphonates are absorbed by bone. They are then released locally and inhibit resorption of bone. These drugs inhibit osteoclast activity by interfering with activation of precursors, inducing osteoclast apoptosis, and decreasing the concentration of enzymes released by these cells.[56] Bisphosphonates have been shown to reduce immobilization-related bone loss in animal studies.[67,68] Paraplegic rats treated with a bisphosphonate had a significant increase in bone calcium content and trabeculae in the metaphysis compared to animals treated with calcitonin and untreated controls.[69] Clinically, bisphosphonates have been used to halt the resorption of bone in spinal cord–injured patients. In a double-blind randomized study, patients with a traumatic spinal cord injury received tiludronate for 3 months, initiated in the first 2 weeks after injury. Iliac bone biopsies were obtained pre- and post-treatment to assess histologic changes. Osteoclast number was decreased in patients treated with tiludronate but the small increase in trabecular bone volume in this group was not significant.[70] Alendronate has also been shown to prevent immobilization-related loss of bone density in the radius when immobilized for fracture treatment.[71] As multiple studies seem to suggest that bone resorption in spinal cord injury occurs during the first postinjury year, this type of pharmacologic intervention may provide the best results if initiated acutely.

VI. CONCLUSION

With disuse, muscles atrophy, tendons tighten, cartilage becomes less hydrated, and bone mineralization decreases. Immobilization causes an initial increase in bone resorption by osteoclasts. The formation of new periosteal bone in the long bones of the extremities is slowed in the absence of mechanical stimulation. Animal studies clearly demonstrate endosteal resorption, thinning of trabeculae, and loss of periosteal bone formation. On a cellular level, these effects begin almost immediately. Radiographic changes in bone density may appear in the following weeks or months if disuse continues. Clinical evidence of decreased bone strength, manifested by fracture, may not occur until years later. Even short periods of disuse can affect bone strength years later, making bone more susceptible to fracture with subsequent immobilization or with the bone loss associated with primary osteoporosis. The best method for preventing disuse osteopenia is prevention. Immobilization should be prevented unless absolutely necessary. Patients with conditions resulting in chronic disuse of their extremities should have aggressive steps undertaken early in their disease to prevent pathologic fractures from occurring years later. Prevention can be with mechanical loading or pharmacologic agents. At minimum, these patients should all receive daily calcium and vitamin D supplementation. When dealing with patients with prolonged immobilization, clinicians need to realize the increased fracture risk and screen these patients appropriately for evidence of osteoporosis. More research is needed to find optimal methods of preventing bone loss during prolonged periods of disuse.

REFERENCES

1. Hayes, W. and Bouxsein, M., "Biomechanics of cortical and trabecular bone — implications for assessment of fracture risk," in *Basic Orthopaedic Biomechanics,* Mow, V. and Hayes, W., Eds., Lippincott-Raven, Philadelphia, 1997, 69.
2. Namkung-Matthai, H., Appleyard, R., Jansen, J., et al., "Osteoporosis influences the early period of fracture healing in a rat osteoporotic model," *Bone,* 28, 80, 2001.
3. Meyer, R., Tsahakis, P., Marvin, D., et al., "Aging and ovariectomy impair both the normalization of mechanical properties and accumulation of mineral by the fracture callus in rats," *J. Orthop. Res.,* 19, 428, 2001.
4. Halvorson, T., Kelley, L., and Thomas, K., "Effects of bone mineral density on pedicle screw fixation," *Spine,* 19, 2415, 1994.
5. Bagi, C., Mecham, M., Weiss, J., et al., "Comparative morphometric changes in rat cortical bone following ovariectomy and/or immobilization," *Bone,* 14, 877, 1993.
6. Kimmel, D., Moran, E., and Bogoch, E., "Animal models of osteopenia or osteoporosis," in *Animal Models in Orthopaedic Research*, An, Y. and Friedman, R., Eds., CRC Press, Boca Raton, FL, 1999, 279.
7. Gross, T. and Rubin, C., "Uniformity of resorbtive bone loss induced by disuse," *J. Orthop. Res.,* 13, 708, 1995.
8. Uhthoff, H.K. and Jaworski, Z.F., "Bone loss in response to long term immobilization," *J. Bone Joint Surg.,* 60B, 420, 1978.
9. Lindgren, U. and Matheson, S., "The reversibility of disuse osteoporosis. Studies of bone density, bone formation, and cell proliferation in bone tissue," *Calcif. Tissue Int.,* 23, 179, 1977.
10. Sievanen, H., Kannus, P., and Jarvinen, T., "Immobilization distorts allometry of rat femur: implications for disuse osteoporosis," *Calcif. Tissue Int.,* 60, 387, 1997.
11. Kannus, P., Teppo, L., Sievanen, H., et al., "Effects of immobilization, three forms of remobilization, and subsequent deconditioning on bone mineral content and density in rat femora," *J. Bone Miner. Res.,* 11, 1339, 1996.
12. Thomas, T., Vico, L., Skerry, T., et al., "Architectural modifications and cellular response during disuse related bone loss in calcaneus of the sheep," *Am. J. Physiol.,* 8, 198, 1996.
13. Weinreb, M., Rodan, G., and Thompson, D., "Osteopenia in the immobilized rat hind limb is associated with increased bone resorption and decreased bone formation," *Bone,* 10, 187, 1989.
14. Wakley, G., Portwood, J., and Turner, R.T., "Disuse osteopenia is accompanied by down regulation of gene expression for bone proteins in growing rats," *Am. J. Physiol.,* 263, E1029, 1992.
15. Sugawara, H., Linsenmeyer, T., Beam, H., et al., "Mechanical properties of bone in a paraplegic rat model," *J. Spinal Cord. Med.,* 21, 302, 1998.
16. Sibonga, J.D., Zhang, M., Evans, G.L., et al., "Effects of spaceflight and simulated weightlessness on longitudinal bone growth," *Bone,* 27, 535, 2000.
17. Shaw, S., Vailas, A., Grindeland, R.E., et al., "Effects of a one week spaceflight on morphologic and mechanical properties of growing bone," *Am. J. Physiol.,* 254, R78, 1988.

18. Wronski, T. and Morey, E., "Effect of spaceflight on periosteal bone formation in rats," *Am. J. Physiol.,* 244, R305, 1983.

19. Morey, E. and Baylink, D., "Inhibition of bone formation during spaceflight," *Science,* 22, 1138, 1978.

20. Garber, M., McDowell, D., and Hutton, W., "Bone loss during simulated weightlessness: a biomechanical and mineralization study in the rat model," *Aviat. Space Environ. Med.,* 71, 586, 2000.

21. Bikle, D. and Halloran, B., "The response of bone to unloading," *J. Bone Miner. Metab.,* 17, 233, 1999.

22. Vico, L., Novikov, V., Very, J., et al., "Bone histomorphometric comparison of rat tibial metaphysis after 7 day tail suspension vs. 7 day spaceflight," *Aviat. Space Environ. Med.,* 62, 26, 1991.

23. Burke, D., Linden, R., Zhang, Y., et al., "Incidence rates and populations at risk for spinal cord injury — a regional study," *Spinal Cord,* 39, 274, 2001.

24. De Laet, C., Van Hout, B., Burger, H., et al., "Hip fracture prediction in elderly men and women — validation in the Rotterdam Study," *J. Bone Miner. Res.,* 13, 1587, 1998.

25. Tandon, S., Gregson, P., Thomas, P., et al., "Reduction of post traumatic osteoporosis after external fixation of tibial fractures," *Injury,* 26, 459, 1995.

26. van der Poest, C., van der Wiel, H., Patka, P., et al., "Long-term consequences of fracture of the lower leg: cross-sectional study and long-term longitudinal follow-up of bone mineral density in the hip after fracture of lower leg," *Bone,* 24, 131, 1999.

27. Leppala, J., Kannus, P., Sievanen, H., et al., "A tibial shaft fracture sustained in childhood or adolescence does not seem to interfere with attainment of peak bone density," *J. Bone Miner. Res.,* 14B, 988, 1999.

28. Leppala, J., Kannus, P., Niemi, S., et al., "An early life femoral shaft fracture and bone mineral density at adulthood," *Osteoporos. Int.,* 10, 337, 1999.

29. Kannus, P., Sievanen, H., Jarvinen, M., et al., "A cruciate ligament injury produces considerable, permanent osteoporosis in the affected knee," *J. Bone Miner. Res.,* 7, 1429, 1992.

30. Marchetti, M., Houde, J., Steinberg, G.G., et al., "Humeral bone density loss after shoulder surgery and immobilization," *J. Shoulder Elbow Surg.,* 5, 471, 1996.

31. Donaldson, C., Hulley, S., Vogel, J., et al., "Effect of prolonged bedrest on bone mineral," *Metabolism,* 19, 1071, 1970.

32. Inoue, M., Tanaka, H., Moriwake, T., et al., "Altered biochemical markers of bone turnover in humans during 120 days of bedrest," *Bone,* 26, 281, 2000.

33. Fiore, C., Pennisi, P., Ciffo, F., et al., "Immobilization dependent bone collagen breakdown appears to increase with time: evidence for lack of a new bone equilibrium in response to reduced load during prolonged bedrest," *Horm. Metab. Res.,* 31, 31, 1999.

34. LeBlanc, A., Schneider, V., Evans, H.J., et al., "Bone mineral loss and recovery after 17 weeks of bed rest," *J. Bone Miner. Res.,* 5, 843, 1990.

35. Vestergaard, P., Krogh, K., Rejnmark, L., et al., "Fracture rates and risk factors for fractures in patients with spinal cord injuries," *Spinal Cord,* 36, 790, 1998.

36. Roberts, D., Lee, W., Cuneo, R., et al., "Longitudinal study of bone turnover after acute spinal cord injury," *Clin. Endocrinol. Metab.,* 83, 415, 1998.

37. Biering-Sorensen, F., Bohr, H.H., and Schaadt, O.P., "Longitudinal study of bone mineral content in the lumbar spine, the forearm, and the lower extremities after spinal cord injury," *Eur. J. Clin. Invest.,* 20, 330, 1990.

38. Kiratli, B.J., Smith, A.E., Nauenberg, T., et al., "Bone mineral and geometric changes through the femur with immobilization due to spinal cord injury," *J. Rehabil. Res. Dev.,* 37, 225, 2000.

39. Bauman, W.A., Spungen, A.M., Wang, J., et al., "Continuous loss of bone during chronic immobilization: a monozygotic twin study," *Osteoporos. Int.,* 10, 123, 1999.

40. Sabo, D., Blaich, S., Wenz, W., et al., "Osteoporosis in patients with paralysis after spinal cord injury. A cross sectional study in 46 male patients with dual-energy X-ray absorptiometry," *Arch. Orthop. Trauma Surg.,* 121, 75, 2001.

41. del Puente, A., Pappone, N., Mandes, M., et al., "Determinants of bone mineral density in immobilization — a study on hemiplegic patients," *Osteoporos. Int.,* 6, 50, 1996.

42. Ramnemark, A., Nyberg, L., Borssen, B., et al., "Fractures after stroke," *Osteoporos. Int.,* 8, 92, 1998.

43. Ramnemark, A., Nilsson, M., Borssen, B., et al., "Stroke, a major and increasing risk factor for femoral neck fracture," *Stroke,* 31, 1572, 2000.

44. Sato, Y., Kuno, H., Kaji, M., et al., "Increased bone resorption during the first year after stroke," *Stroke,* 29, 1373, 1998.
45. Rambaut, P. and Goode, A., "Skeletal changes during spaceflight," *Lancet,* 9, 1050, 1985.
46. Miyamoto, A., Shigematsu, T., Fukunaga, T., et al., "Medical baseline data collection on bone and muscle change with spaceflight," *Bone,* 22, 79, 1998.
47. LeBlanc, A., Shackelford, L., and Schneider, V., "Future human bone research in space," *Bone,* 22, 113, 1998.
48. van der Wiel, H., Lips, P., Nauta, J., et al., "Biochemical parameters of bone turnover during ten days of bed rest and subsequent mobilization," *Bone Miner.,* 13, 123, 1991.
49. Kannus, P., Sievanen, H., Jarvinen, T., et al., "Effects of free mobilization and low to high intensity treadmill running on the immobilization induced bone loss in rats," *J. Bone Miner. Res.,* 9, 1613, 1994.
50. Kaneps, A., Stover, S., and Lane, N., "Changes in canine cortical and cancellous bone mechanical properties following immobilization and remobilization with exercise," *Bone,* 21, 419, 1997.
51. Jaworski, Z., "Reversibility of nontraumatic disuse osteoporosis during its active phase," *Bone,* 7, 431, 1986.
52. Zerath, E., Canon, F., Guezennec, C., et al., "Electrical stimulation of leg muscles increases tibial trabecular bone formation in unloaded rats," *J. Appl. Physiol.,* 79, 1889, 1995.
53. Chad, K., Bailey, D., McKay, H., et al., "The effect of a weight bearing physical activity program on bone mineral content and estimated volumetric density in children with spastic cerebral palsy," *J. Pediatr.,* 135, 115, 1999.
54. Mohr, T., Podenphant, J., Biering-Sorensen, F., et al., "Increased bone mineral density after prolonged electrically induced cycle training of paralyzed limbs in spinal cord injured men," *Calcif. Tissue Int.,* 61, 22, 1997.
55. Bloomfield, S., Mysiw, W., and Jackson, R., "Bone mass and endocrine adaptations to training in spinal cord injured individuals," *Bone,* 19, 61, 1996.
56. Watts, N., "Pharmacology of agents to treat osteoporosis," in *Primer on the Metabolic Bone Diseases and Disorders of Mineral Metabolism,* 4th ed., Favus, M., Ed., Lippincott/Williams & Williams, New York, 1999, 223.
57. Izawa, Y., Makita, T., Hino, S., et al., "Immobilization osteoporosis and active vitamin D-effect of active vitamin D analogs on the development of immobilization osteoporosis in rats," *Calcif. Tissue Int.,* 33, 623, 1981.
58. Jekovec-Vrhovsek, M., Kocijancic, A., and Prezelj, J., "Effect of vitamin D and calcium on bone mineral density in children with CP and epilepsy in full-time care," *Dev. Med. Child Neurol.,* 42, 403, 2000.
59. Peacock, M., Liu, G., Carey, M., et al., "Effect of calcium or 25-OH vitamin D dietary supplementation on bone loss at the hip in men and women over the age of 60," *J. Clin. Endocrinol. Metab.,* 85, 3011, 2000.
60. Sato, Y., Honda, Y., Kuno, H., et al., "Menatetrenone ameliorates osteopenia in disuse-affected limbs of vitamin D- and K-deficient stroke patients," *Bone,* 23, 291, 1998.
61. Thomas, T., Skerry, T., Vico, L., et al., "Ineffectiveness of calcitonin on a local disuse osteoporosis in the sheep — a histomorphometric study," *Calcif. Tissue Int.,* 57, 224, 1995.
62. Peterson, M., Lauritzen, J., Schwarz, P., et al., "Effect of nasal salmon calcitonin on post traumatic osteopenia following ankle fractures," *Acta Orthop. Scand.,* 69, 347, 1998.
63. Uebelhart, D., Hartmann, D., Barbezat, S., et al., "Effect of calcitonin on bone and connective tissue metabolism in hemiplegic patients: a two year prospective study," *Clin. Rehabil.,* 13, 384, 1999.
64. van der Wiel, H., Lips, P., Nauta, J., et al., "Intranasal calcitonin suppresses increased bone resorption during short term immobilization," *J. Bone Miner. Res.,* 8, 1459, 1993.
65. Tsakalakos, N., Magiasis, B., Tsekoura, M., et al., "The effect of short term calcitonin administration on biochemical bone markers in patients with acute immobilization following hip fracture," *Osteoporos. Int.,* 3, 337, 1993.
66. Black, D., Thompson, D., Bauer, D., et al., "Fracture risk reduction with alendronate in women with osteoporosis — the fracture intervention trial," *J. Clin. Endocrinol. Metab.,* 85, 4118, 2000.
67. Thompson, D., Seedor, J., Weinreb, M., et al., "Aminohydroxybutane bisphosphonate inhibits bone loss due to immobilization in rats," *J. Bone Miner. Res.,* 5, 279, 1990.

68. Li, J., Mashiba, T., Kaji, Y., et al., "Preadministration of icadronate disodium can prevent bone loss in rat proximal tibial metaphysis when induced by hindlimb immobilization by bandage," *Bone,* 23, 459, 1998.

69. Schoutens, A., Verhas, M., Dourov, N., et al., "Bone loss and bone blood flow in paraplegic rats treated with calcitonin, diphosphonate, and indomethacin," *Calcif. Tissue Int.,* 42, 136, 1988.

70. Chappard, D., Minaire, P., Privat, C., et al., "Effects of tiludronate on bone loss in paraplegic patients," *J. Bone Miner. Res.,* 10, 112, 1995.

71. van der Poest, C., Patka, P., Vandormael, K., et al., "The effect of alendronate on bone mass after distal forearm fracture," *J. Bone Miner. Res.,* 15, 586, 2000.

29 Osteoarthritis and Osteoporosis — The Interface

Raymond Lau and Philip N. Sambrook

CONTENTS

I. INTRODUCTION

Osteoarthritis (OA) and osteoporosis (OP) are diseases of increasing incidence and prevalence with age and both are associated with considerable morbidity. In general terms, OP is usually considered to be primarily a disease of the bone whereas OA a disease of the cartilage, although increasingly it is believed that the subchondral bone plays an important role in the pathogenesis of OA as well. Interestingly, both cartilage and bone cells are in a constant state of turnover and it has been suggested that abnormal turnover is a common theme that underlies the pathophysiology of OP and OA.

The relationship between the two diseases was first suggested to be an inverse one almost 30 years ago[1,2] and a large number of studies have generally shown a lower incidence or prevalence of osteoporosis in subjects with OA, and vice versa. In three recent literature reviews of the relationship of OA and OP and bone mineral density (BMD), there is agreement that the majority of studies showed an increase in BMD in OA cases compared with age- and sex-matched controls. Correction for anthropometric characteristics did not change these results.[3-5] However, not all studies, especially earlier ones, have shown this relationship and this probably reflects increasing sophistication of the methodology used to assess BMD over time as well as differences in the populations studied. The nature of this relationship between OA and OP is addressed in this chapter.

II. IS THERE AN INVERSE RELATIONSHIP BETWEEN OA AND OP?

The evidence for an inverse relationship comes mainly from cross-sectional studies, although a few longitudinal studies have recently been published looking at the association between OA and OP.

TABLE 29.1
Period and Number of Publications with Positive or Negative Findings Concerning the Inverse Relationship of Osteoarthritis/Osteoporosis

Period	Positive	Negative	None
1970–1979	5	3	—
1980–1989	2	2	1
1990–	25	4	1
Total = 43	32	9	2

Source: Dequeker, J., *J. Rheumatol.*, 24, 795, 1997. With permission.

In interpreting those studies that have examined the relationship, it is important to note that measures of OA are complicated by the heterogeneous nature of the disease. It is likely that the association may be different for OA at different joints and different between localized OA and primary generalized OA. Most studies have relied on radiologic grading of OA rather than self-reported or clinical diagnosis and there is generally only a modest correlation between osteoarthritic symptoms and radiologic signs. Early studies have relied on plain radiographs to obtain measures of OP whereas more recent studies have used bone densitometry and even ultrasound measurement. In some studies, BMD was measured at the same joint that was assessed for OA and in other studies BMD was measured at sites distant from the site of OA. All these points must be taken into consideration when looking at the evidence for and against an inverse relationship between OA and OP.

Table 29.1 shows the period of publication and the number with positive or negative findings between the relationship of OA/OP with BMD. Table 29.2 summarizes the results concerning bone mass in OA compared to matched controls.

III. WHAT SPECIFIC EVIDENCE SUPPORTS AN ASSOCIATION?

A number of large epidemiologic studies, designed primarily to examine OP, but in which data about OA at various sites have been collected, have been examined to determine if there exists an inverse relationship between OA and OP.

Sowers et al.[7] conducted a prospective study looking at the relationship between bone mass and hand OA. As part of the Tecumseh Community Health Study, women were examined twice for radiographic evidence of OA of the hands, in 1962–1965 and 20 years later in 1985. Bone mass was estimated from the hand radiographs using metacarpal cortical area width, medullary cavity, and periosteal width. It was found that women who were classified as having OA in 1985, based on the highest score assigned to any 32 wrist/hand joints and the sum of scores for all wrist/hand joints, had a greater mean metacarpal bone mass two decades earlier. The authors pointed out that radiographs were the only method available to estimate bone mass for longitudinal studies in the general population at the start of the study. Although age and body size were adjusted for, other relevant factors occurring between the two time points (such as menopause and medication use) were not examined.

More recently, Sowers et al.[8] looked at a random population of pre- and perimenopausal women from the Michigan Bone Health Study. This 3-year longitudinal study looked for the presence of hand and knee OA, and all women had BMD measured at the hip and spine. The period prevalence of OA (Kellgren/Lawrence grade ≥ 2 in the knees or the dominant hand) was 15.3% (92 of 601), with 8.7% for the knees and 6.7% for the hand. The 3-year incidence of knee OA was 1.9% (9 of 482) and hand OA was 3.3% (16 of 482). Women with incident knee OA had greater mean BMD (z-scores 0.3 to 0.8 higher for the three BMD sites) than women without knee OA ($p < 0.04$ at the femoral neck). Women with incident knee OA had less change in their mean BMD z-scores over

TABLE 29.2
Summary of the Positive and Negative Results Concerning
Bone Mass in Osteoarthritis Compared to Matched Controls
According to Technique to Evaluate BMD

Technique	Increased Bone Mass	No Difference in Bone Mass
Metacarpal radiogrammetry	5	5
Single-photon absorptiometry		
Radius trabecular	5	
Radius cortical	5	5
Femur shaft		1
Calcaneus	1	
Peripheral QCT		
Radius trabecular	1	
Radius cortical		1
Singh index	2	
Neutron activation analysis		1
Iliac crest histomorphometry		3
QCT L1	2	
Dual-photon or dual-energy X-ray absorptiometry		
Spine	14	
Femur	12	
Total body	3	
Total	53	13

QCT: quantitative computed tomography.

Source: Dequeker, J., *J. Rheumatol.,* 24, 795, 1997. With permission.

the 3-year study period. Mean BMD z-scores for women with prevalent knee OA were greater (0.4 to 0.7 higher) than for women without knee OA ($p < 0.002$ at all sites). There was no difference in mean BMD z-scores or their change in women with and without hand OA. The authors concluded that women with radiographically defined knee OA have greater BMD than do women without knee OA and are less likely to lose that higher level of BMD.

The Chingford Study is a population survey of women examining, among other end points, the relationship between OA at a number of sites and BMD measured at the lumbar spine and femoral neck.[9] A total of 979 women had radiographs taken of the hands and knees, and 579 had radiographs taken of the lumbar spine. Mean BMD was compared between those with radiologic OA and those without disease. Those with OA were divided into five groups: distal interphalangeal OA (DIP), carpometacarpal OA (CMC), knee OA, lumbar spine OA, and generalized OA. Generalized OA was defined as the combination of radiologic DIP, CMC, and knee OA. For lumbar spine BMD, all positive individuals in each joint group with OA showed a significant increase in BMD compared with controls. Affected individuals in CMC, knee, and lumbar spine OA groups also had significantly higher femoral neck BMD compared with nonaffected controls. The increase in femoral neck BMD was not statistically significant in the group with generalized OA. The results were adjusted for age, body mass index (BMI), and, in the case of lumbar spine BMD, for lumbar spine OA. Additional adjustment for smoking status, hormone replacement therapy use, age of menopause, alcohol, social class, and physical activity made no important differences to the results.

As part of the Rotterdam Study, 700 men and 1000 women from the general population underwent weight-bearing knee and hip radiography.[10] The radiographs were graded (0 to 4) using the Kellgren method. The subjects also had baseline femoral BMD and serial measurements, on average 2.2 years later. With the exception of knee OA in men, radiographic OA (knee OA in women and hip OA) was associated with significantly increased femoral neck BMD (3 to 8%) at baseline. BMD increased significantly according to the number of affected sites and higher Kellgren score. Both men and women showed a significant trend toward increasing BMD with increased number of affected OA sites. Of interest, the serial BMD results in men found hip OA (but not knee OA) was associated with significantly increased bone loss with age and, in women, significantly increased bone loss was associated with OA in both joints. The authors suggest that if osteoarthritic subjects had higher bone density but also lost bone at a greater rate, then it should follow that the differences in BMD between subjects with and without osteoarthritis would be present from early in life. This result contrasts that of Sowers et al.[8] where bone loss appears to be less in the OA group. The difference may be due to the older population of the Rotterdam study (mean age 68) compared with the pre- and perimenopausal population of the Sowers study. Moreover, the presence of OA may have contributed to a more sedentary lifestyle and therefore more rapid loss of bone in a more elderly population.

The Study of Osteoporotic Fractures (SOF)[11] reported the association between radiographic features of hip OA and BMD of the hip, spine, and appendicular skeleton in a cross-sectional analysis of 4855 Caucasian American women aged 65 and older. Pelvic radiographs were assessed for individual radiographic features of hip OA. Women with Grade 3 to 4 hip OA had a higher age-adjusted BMD at the femoral neck and Ward's triangle (9 to 10%; $p < 0.0001$), trochanter (4%; $p < 0.01$), lumbar spine (8%; $p < 0.0001$), distal radius and calcaneus (5%; $p < 0.0001$) compared with those with Grade 0 to 1 OA in the worse hip. Elevations in BMD were greatest in the femoral neck of hips with OA, in women with bilateral hip OA, and in women with hip osteophytes. Hip BMD was not elevated in the normal hips of women with Grade 3 to 4 OA on the contralateral side. The presence of osteophytes influenced the association, as joint space narrowing alone was not associated with increased BMD. Important confounders such as age, weight, and other determinants of bone mass were adjusted for.

The SOF group reported again in 1999[12] with longitudinal data on these subjects, looking particularly at bone loss and fractures. Those who had OA in 1995 appeared to lose bone more slowly than those without OA ($p = 0.018$), with mean femoral neck BMD loss per year for Grade 0 to 1 being approximately 0.5%, Grade 2 approximately 0.3%, and Grade 3 to 4, 0.15%.

Antoniades et al.[13] performed a matched case-control study using twin pairs discordant for OA to assess the relationship between hip OA and BMD at the affected hip and at more distal sites. They also evaluated the bone density differences within pairs discordant for hip OA. The main advantage of using twins is the close matching for genetic and environmental factors within pairs, which markedly reduces the effect of confounding variables, including potential confounding due to genetic factors. Pelvic radiographs of 1252 women (170 monozygotic and 456 dizygotic pairs) were assessed for features of hip OA. The Croft grading scale was used to assess the individual radiographic features of minimal joint space, presence of osteophytes, maximum thickness of subchondral sclerosis, and cyst formation. BMD was measured at the nondominant hip (femoral neck, total hip), lumbar spine (L1–L4), and the total body. Twins with radiographic features of hip OA had 3 to 4% higher BMD at the femoral neck area than their cotwins. However, the relationship was confined to the femoral neck and localized to the ipsilateral hip. There was no clear association of radiographic hip OA features with BMD in the contralateral hip, lumbar spine, or total body. Of the individual features of OA, severe osteophytosis was associated with 5 to 6% higher BMD at the ipsilateral hip. There was no association with joint space narrowing. Adjustment for potential confounding variables such as BMI, lifetime physical activity, menopausal status, estrogen use, and smoking had no important effect on the results. The comparatively lower percentage elevation in femoral neck BMD (3 to 4%) and the lack of association with lumbar spine and whole-body BMD seen in this study vs. that by Nevitt et al.[11] may be explained by the use of the twin model with matching for genetic factors.

Stewart et al.[14] looked at elderly women with either hip OA ($n = 30$) or OP ($n = 30$), or controls ($n = 30$). In this cross-sectional study the BMD was higher in both the hip (neck of femur +5.7%, $p < 0.001$) and total body (+9.2%, $p = 0.012$) in the OA group compared with controls.

The study by Cooper et al.[15] is typical of earlier studies that used plain radiography rather than densitometry to assess OP. Hip radiographs of 314 men and women aged 50 and over who consecutively visted the hospital for radiography for nonskeletal indications were reviewed. Bone mass was assessed using the Singh index grading system of the femoral neck trabecular pattern, and the degree of OA of the hip was graded as normal, mild, or marked. There was a statistically significant negative association between the two disorders, but the analysis did not adjust for the important confounder of weight.

One interesting study by Li and Aspden[16] looked at subchondral bone from the femoral head of subjects with OP and OA and compared these with controls. The subchondral bone plate appears to be less stiff in OP than in OA. Generalized changes in bone composition in subjects with OA are thought to support the hypothesis that OA is a disease of bone rather than simply of articular cartilage.

Knee OA has also been shown to be associated with higher BMD. As mentioned above, knee OA has been shown to be associated with higher lumbar spine and femoral neck BMD.[9,10] In a recently published cross-sectional analysis of 573 women aged 24 to 45,[8] looking at the association of BMD and OA of the hands and knees, OA was classified using two methods: (1) the highest joint grade in any of the joints of the hand and knee and (2) the presence of a joint grade of >2. Total-body BMD was found to be significantly associated with knee OA for both methods of classifications. A number of important confounders were taken into account such as age, BMI, previous injury, smoking, alcohol consumption, hormonal levels, and use of hormone replacement therapy (HRT). It is worth noting that the association between BMD and OA was shown in this study in a relatively young group of women with a consequent lower prevalence of OA, compared with most other studies.

The association between BMD and knee OA was also evaluated in the Framingham Study cohort.[17] Knee OA was assessed radiographically and graded on a scale from 0 (no OA) to 4 (severe OA) in 572 women and 360 men, age range 63 to 91. Osteophytes and joint space narrowing were also assessed separately. BMD was measured at the proximal femur and radius by densitometry 4 years later. Mean femoral neck BMD (adjusted for potential confounders such as age, BMI, and physical activity) was higher in women with both Grade 1 and Grade 2 compared with no knee OA ($p < 0.0001$). Higher femoral neck BMD was also observed in Grade 3 OA, although this was not statistically significant compared with those with no OA, and mean OA was not increased at all. It may have been that in higher grades of OA other factors, which were not adjusted for, influenced BMD. Only men with Grade 1 knee OA had significantly higher BMD of the femoral neck. There was no statistically significant difference in the femoral neck BMD of men with higher-grade knee OA compared with no OA. The inverse relationship between OP and OA was stronger in women than in men in this study. The authors hypothesized that these differences may be due to dissimilar risk factor profiles for knee OA, that women may be more affected by a metabolic factor while men may be more influenced by joint injury. Radius BMD was not associated with knee OA in either gender. It was suggested that the lack of positive findings in the radius may be because radial bone is primarily cortical and is not very active metabolically.

The relationship between lumbar spine OA and OP at the spine and other sites has also been examined in a number of studies, but it is important to note that lumbar osteophytosis and apophyseal OA can spuriously elevate lumbar BMD readings. In a study of 375 women aged 50 to 85, radiographs were taken of the thoracic and lumbar spine.[18] BMD measurements were obtained for the lumbar spine, total body, and femoral neck. Both absolute values of BMD and z-scores were found to be significantly higher in the women with spinal OA for all three sites. The mean increase in BMD was 7.9% at the lumbar spine, 6.4% at the femoral neck, and 8.4% for the total body. The authors noted that these findings could reflect a generalized increase in BMD or may reflect OA at sites other than the spine in association with spinal OA. Radiographs were not taken of other skeletal sites. In another study of 93 postmenopausal women who presented to an OP clinic with at least one vertebral fracture, a significant increase (8.2%) in femoral neck bone density was seen in women with spinal osteophytosis.[19] The more severe the osteophytosis, the greater the femoral bone density in comparison with the women with no spinal osteophytosis.

In a further population-based sample of 113 male and 187 female subjects over 60 years of age, participating in the Dubbo Osteoporosis Epidemiology Study, where BMD was measured on two occasions (mean interval 2.5 years) and spinal radiographs were performed on one occasion, baseline lumbar BMD and the rate of change in lumbar BMD were related to the degree of osteophytosis in both sexes.[20] However, in the femoral neck, although the presence of spinal OA was associated with a modest increase in baseline BMD, there was no effect on its rate of change.

Another recent study by Liu et al.[21] studied the BMD and radiograph of the hip and spine of 120 men and 314 women aged 60 to 99 years. Using stepwise multiple regression analysis of age, weight, height, osteophytes, sclerosis, and joint space narrowing, the authors concluded that lumbar osteophytosis accounted for 16.6% of variation in lumbar spine BMD in women and 22.4% in men. Hip osteophytes had minimal effect on hip BMD. Therefore, diagnosis of osteoporosis and assessment of osteoporotic fracture risk should be based on hip BMD and not on anteroposterior lumbar spine, unless spinal osteoarthritis has been excluded.

Hand OA is considered to be part of the spectrum of primary generalized OA. However, the evidence for an association with this form of OA and OP is not as strong, and the results of studies reporting an apparent association have yielded discrepancies. For example, in a study by Marcelli et al.,[22] hand osteoarthritic (HOA) score was assessed in 300 healthy women aged over 75 and BMD was measured at a number of sites. Total-body BMD, upper limb BMD, lower limb BMD, and spinal BMD were positively associated with the combined HOA score, but there was no significant association with femoral neck or Ward's triangle BMD. When the data were analyzed by dividing into low-grade and high-grade OA, the findings were similar. Interestingly, the HOA score was significantly lower in the 23% of women who reported a history of osteoporotic fracture compared with women with no history of fracture. The study by Sowers et al.[23] also looked at the association between hand OA and BMD. The highest grade of OA in the hand was associated with an increased risk of high total-body bone density, but when OA was defined by the Kellgren grading system (Grade > 2), no association with BMD was found. Hordon et al.[24] compared the bone density of 20 postmenopausal women with primary generalized OA with 89 normal controls. Women with osteoarthritis had significantly increased BMD at the spine and distal forearm and increased total-body bone mass, but there was no difference in the femoral BMD. The controls, however, were not from the same population base as the cases. Sowers et al.[8] also confirmed the lack of association of hand OA and OP in the study discussed above. Relevant from a pathophysiologic point of view is a series of studies demonstrating that the density, stiffness, compressive strength, and osteocalcin content of bone from the iliac crest is significantly increased in patients with hand OA compared with controls.[25,26] Hand OA was used as an indicator of generalized OA and the changes in iliac bone, a site distant from the site of OA, were considered to reflect the association of generalized skeletal changes with OA, but only 30 patients were studied and cases and controls were not matched for other variables.

IV. WHAT EVIDENCE DOES NOT SUPPORT AN ASSOCIATION?

Although a number of studies above have shown an association between large joint OA and OP, there are a number of studies, particularly of hand OA, that have failed to show an association with OP. The association of appendicular bone mass with hand OA was studied in 238 Caucasian females aged 40 and over in the Baltimore Longitudinal Study.[27] Bilateral hand radiographs were graded for OA using the Kellgren–Lawrence scales. The two measures of appendicular bone mass were the percentage of cortical area of the second metacarpal and the BMD of the distal radius measured with single-photon absorptiometry. After adjustment for age and BMI, neither of these measures of appendicular bone mass was significantly associated with grade of hand OA. In an earlier publication on men from the same study, 886 males had hand radiographs taken and bone mass was measured as a percentage of cortical area of the second metacarpal. No association was found between the age-adjusted percent cortical area and either the presence or severity of hand OA.[28] When the bone mass was expressed as absolute bone mass, male OA cases had more bone than those without OA. The authors pointed out that the participants in this study were volunteers and not a random sample of the general population. In addition, few were employed in manual labor where sustained microtrauma of the hand may influence the incidence of hand OA and, in turn, influence the association between bone density and OA. Some of the earlier studies of hand OA using a smaller sample size also found no significant association between hand OA and OP.[29-31]

Similarly, not all studies on hip and knee OA have shown a significant association with OP. Hochberg et al.[32] analyzed longitudinal data to examine the association of several measures of upper extremity bone mass, size, and BMD with radiologic changes of knee OA in 430 men and 266 women. Plain radiographs of the hand were used to estimate cortical thickness, total metacarpal width, and percentage of cortical area of the second metacarpal. Single-photon absorptiometry was used to calculate the BMD of the distal third of the radius. In women, none of the measures of bone mass, size, or density differed significantly according to the presence of definite knee OA. In men, adjusted mean bone mineral content and radial width were both significantly greater in the presence of definite knee OA; however, adjusted mean radial BMD and all bone measures of the second metacarpal were not significantly higher in the presence of definite knee OA. The same pattern of results was found when the analyses were repeated on men and women aged 60 or over. These results were consistent with the report of Hannan et al.[17] using data from the Framingham Study, where no association between knee OA and radial BMD could be shown.

It is possible that reduced activity associated with more advanced OA, aging, or other factors could lead to bone loss over time, which may mask the relationship between OA and OP.[33] This theory is supported by the evidence that radiographic hip and knee OA is associated not only with higher BMD but also with increased rate of bone loss.[10]

In summary, the evidence for an inverse relationship between OA and OP is stronger at the axial skeleton (lumbar and femoral) than for the appendicular skeleton (hand and radius). Data from the Framingham Study[17] and Baltimore Study[27] showed that knee OA was not associated with radial or hand BMD but an increase in adjusted lumbar spine BMD was found in women with definite knee OA. Appendicular sites are composed primarily of cortical bone and the influence of circulating factors may be different in the axial skeleton where there is more trabecular bone. The influence of increased BMD on the weight-bearing axial skeleton compared with the non-weight-bearing appendicular skeleton may play a role as well.

V. POSSIBLE MECHANISMS FOR THE RELATIONSHIP BETWEEN OA AND OP

At present there is no unifying theory to account for the inverse relationship between OA and OP observed in the studies discussed above. This is not surprising considering the differing results of the studies and the fact that OA is a heterogeneous disease. As shown above, the relationship between OA and OP is not the same at each joint; the association can even vary between unilateral and bilateral OA of the same joint. For example, in a cross-sectional study of the factors associated with hip OA, it was found that obesity was associated with bilateral hip OA but not unilateral hip OA.[34] It may be that in bilateral hip OA, obesity is a risk factor by maintaining BMD and preventing OP, whereas in unilateral OA local factors such as a history of trauma or hip dysplasia predominate.[35] Therefore, it is possible that different mechanisms are involved in the pathogenesis of OA at different joints.

It is likely that genetic influences play a significant role in mechanisms for the inverse relationship between OA and OP. It is well established that there are strong familial and genetic influences on adult BMD. For example, studies in twins suggest that genetic factors contribute around 80% of the total variance in peak adult BMD.[36] Other recent twin studies have also suggested important genetic influences on OA of the knee and hand[37] and OA of the hip and spine.[38,39] Genetic factors contribute significantly to OA at the hip in women and account for 60% of the variation in population liability to the disease.

As yet there are no clear data on the relative influence of genetic and environmental factors in hip OA. It may be that the OA and OP share common genetic determinants. People may inherit a tendency to "softer" bone leading to OP and "stiffer" bone resulting in OA. In response to repeated loading, these differences could result in fractures in OP and cartilage damage in OA.

Another explanation for the inverse relationship is that both OA and OP share common risk factors. It may be that risk factors for one disease are protective for the other disease. Dequeker et al.[40] showed that women with osteoporosis were shorter, slenderer, and had less fat, muscle girth, and strength whereas women with osteoarthritis of comparable age and skeletal size were more obese and had more fat, muscle mass, and strength. Higher body weight in the osteoarthritic group may increase the force on bone leading to increased bone mass. The associated increased subcutaneous fat in the osteoarthritic group may also affect BMD by preserving a better postmenopausal estrogen status due to the peripheral conversion of androstenedione to estrone in subcutaneous fat.[41] Most recent studies on the relationship between OA and OP have therefore adjusted for variables such as age, weight, height, muscle strength, and menopausal status, and in many cases have still shown a significant association.

Although cartilage pathology is generally thought to be the primary mechanism behind OA, a role for subchondral bone changes has also been hypothesized. Radin and Rose[42] suggested that subchondral bone changes may have a role in the initiation and progression of cartilage damage and suggested that OA may initially be a bone disease rather than cartilage disease. Subchondral bone stiffness may be part of a generalized inherited increase in BMD. Once cartilage damage is initiated, the stiffness of the subchondral bone may contribute further to progression and chondrocyte dysfunction.[41] Higher bone density may increase and osteoporotic bone may decrease the peak mechanical stress on cartilage during impact loading. Once OA is established, it could in turn influence bone remodeling. Nevitt et al.[11] suggest a number of mechanisms for the changes in bone remodeling secondary to hip OA, such as altered distribution of mechanical stresses, reduced area and shock absorbing capacity of cartilage, stiffening and increased vascularization of periarticular bone, and changes in musculature and weight bearing through the joint. However, Li and Aspden[16] found subchondral bone of surgically removed femoral heads from age- and sex-matched patients with OA and OP to be less stiff than normal controls. They postulated that subchondral bone by itself could not explain the preserving of the overlying cartilage in OP while aiding in the destruction in OA. Changes in the cancellous bone need to be considered as well.

Bone scintigraphy has been shown to predict the outcome of OA of the knee joint.[43] In this study, 100 patients with established symptomatic OA of the knee joint had baseline plain radiographs of each knee and bone scan images of each knee. Outcome data were obtained on 75 of these subjects 5 years later. In particular, the need for a major operation on the knee in the intervening 5 years and changes in the radiographic appearances of each knee were evaluated. Only those patients with positive bone scans at baseline showed progression to surgery or radiographic changes of OA. The positive bone scans were felt to reflect increased subchondral bone remodeling.

A number of studies have shown the radiologic features of osteophytosis rather than joint space narrowing (reflecting cartilage loss) to be specifically associated with increased BMD. In a study discussed above, examining the association of hip OA with BMD, isolated moderate or large osteophytes were associated with a significant increase in BMD[11,13,21] and the increase in BMD was at all sites, not just the hip.[11] However, there was no significant increase in BMD for the radiologic feature of moderate to severe joint space narrowing of the hip.[13] In a study of knee OA by Hannan et al.,[17] women with radiologic knee osteophytes had higher femoral BMD than those with no osteophytes. Again, joint space narrowing had less of an influence on BMD. The authors in this study concluded that perhaps subjects with higher BMD were "bone formers" and thus present with an increased tendency towards osteophytosis in contrast to subjects with lower BMD who were "bone-resorbers" who may have more OA changes of attrition and atrophy. A higher prevalence of vertebral fractures in patients with atrophic hip OA compared with those with osteophytes in the hip joint has been shown.[44] Hand osteophytosis seems to have less of a specific association with BMD, and it may be that genetic factors predominate in this form of arthritis compared with local mechanical factors in knee and hip OA.

Insulin-like growth factor (IGF) receptors exist on bone and cartilage and *in vitro* work has suggested an anabolic effect of IGF-1 on chondrocytes and osteoblasts.[45] Serum IGF-1 has also been shown to be associated with body composition, muscle strength, and adiposity. These known associations have led to the hypothesis that IGF-1 may be a factor in both OP and OA. It has been proposed that increased levels of growth factors may stimulate bone formation accounting for the inverse association between OA and OP. A higher level of a growth factor may account for both a higher bone density and osteophyte formation.

It may also explain the findings of increased bone mass and BMD at sites distant from the site of OA. It has been reported that generalized OA is associated with increased IGF-2 and transforming growth factor beta (TGF-β) in extracts of cortical bone from the iliac crest.[46,47] The results from population studies, however, are conflicting. In a 12-year longitudinal study of 141 subjects with radiologic OA of the knee, circulating IGF-1 at follow-up was found to be related to osteophyte growth and overall progression of knee OA. The relationship was still present after adjustment for age, gender, and baseline.[48] The authors concluded that the results of the study might explain the inverse relationship found between OP and OA. No clear relationship was found with cartilage loss. On the other hand, Hochberg et al.,[49] using data from the Baltimore Study, found that when serum IGF-1 levels were adjusted for age there was no significant difference in these levels between those with radiographic changes of definite knee OA and those with normal radiographs.

Lloyd et al.[45] assessed the association between serum IGF-1 concentrations, OA, BMD, and fractures in a large group of middle-aged women in the general population using data from the Chingford study. The study suggested that serum IGF-1 was associated with severe knee OA and hand OA. There was no association of IGF-1 with bone density. The authors concluded, however, that serum IGF-1 levels do not reflect a systemic tendency to OA, OP, or fractures. Meulenbelt et al.[50] studied a population-based cohort of 1040 unrelated people from the Rotterdam study and also concur that IGF-1 locus was significantly associated with the presence of radiologic OA of hip, knee, hand, and spine — overall adjusted odds ratio (OR) for heterozygous subject = 1.9, 95% confidence interval (CI) = 1.2 to 3.1, and for homozygous subjects 3.6, 95% CI = 0.8 to 16.2. Cases containing the A3 allele were more frequently represented in the OA group (homozygous genotype 3.5 times frequency, heterozygous genotype almost 2 times frequency), which appears to be the most likely allele associated with OA. When each site affected by OA is considered separately, the association still holds; the strongest association is with hip OA. However, an association between the IGF-1 gene and BMD was not found.

One other candidate gene is the vitamin D receptor gene, although the results are controversial. Although polymorphisms in the vitamin D receptor gene have been previously associated with BMD, a recent paper has described an association of the same Taq polymorphism with knee OA and higher BMD.[51] In this study of 351 postmenopausal women, a Taq 1 polymorphism was associated with an increased risk of knee OA (RR 2.82; 95% CI = 1.16 to 6.85). The Rotterdam Study group also found similar results. However, in the Dubbo study, an association was also found, but in the opposite direction, with a decreased risk of spinal OA with presence of the relevant allele.[52] When the results were adjusted for bone density, the findings were not changed, indicating the association between the polymorphism and OA is not mediated through BMD. Videman et al.[53] also investigated the role of intragenic polymorphisms of the Vitamin D receptor gene in lumbar spine degeneration and BMD. The strongest associations were with signal intensity and annular tears on magnetic resonance (MR) imaging, which were worse for the subjects with tt genotypes than for those with TT genotypes in the L4–S1 spine discs. Conversely, the prevalence of disc bulges and osteophytes was lowest for the tt genotype. Bone density, disc height, and herniations did not differ significantly by genotype. The strongest association of Vitamin D receptor TaqI polymorphisms with degeneration in nonmineralized connective tissues suggests that the underlying mechanism of TaqI polymorphisms is not specific to bone.

Markers of bone formation and resorption have been compared between subjects with OA and normal controls. The urinary excretion of pyridinium cross-links has been shown to be increased in patients with large joint OA and hand OA, suggesting an increased rate of bone resorption.[14,54,55] However, none of these studies allowed for the fact that there may have been an increased skeletal mass to account for the increase in cross-link excretion. On the other hand, Peel et al.[18] found a decrease in both resorption and formation markers in women with spinal OA. The urinary excretion of deoxypyridnoline was found to be lower in women with spinal OA compared with women without the disease. Unlike other studies, bone mass was taken into account. Sowers et al.[23] examined osteocalcin as a measure of bone formation and found osteocalcin levels to be lower (–16.1%) in those with knee OA, suggesting that bone formation is lower in the OA group, but this was not significant ($p = 0.14$). In patients with hand OA, osteocalcin levels were on mean 25 to 30% lower ($p < 0.007$), suggesting significantly reduced bone formation in the hand OA group. A lower rate of bone turnover in OA may reflect protection against bone loss. The presence of hand OA in young women has been thought by many authors to be part of a different disease spectrum and this may explain these differing results.

VI. WHAT IS THE INCIDENCE AND PREVALENCE OF OA IN OP?

If there is an inverse relationship between OP and OA, it may be asked what is the incidence and prevalence of one disease in the presence of the other? One of the earliest reports examining how frequently OA occurs in the presence of OP was by Foss and Byers.[1] These authors examined 100 femoral heads resected for the treatment of hip fractures and noted that the cartilage changes usually seen in hips that had been resected for treatment for hip joint OA, were not evident. In a more population-based, case-controlled study of subjects aged 65 to 79, the prevalence of self-reported arthritis of the hip was much lower in patients with hip fracture than controls randomly selected from the community,[56] with an age- and gender-adjusted OR of 0.33 (95% CI, 0.15 to 0.74). The relationship between OA and OP was also studied in the MEDOS study, a large prospective epidemiologic study of patients with femoral neck fractures and age-matched controls in the Mediterranean area. In the study questionnaire, patients were asked if they had ever been told they suffered from OA. OA was self-reported in 49% of women and 26% of men with hip fracture.[46] However, in a prospective study of risk factors for hip fracture, where women aged 65 and over were followed for a mean of 4 years, self-reported OA was not significantly associated with hip fracture.[57]

The limitations in answering the question of the prevalence of OA in OP is the fact that in many studies the prevalence of OA is based upon self-reported symptoms rather than radiologic OA. Data on the incidence of OA are limited by the fact that no large longitudinal studies exist where subjects with OP have been followed with serial radiology to determine the incidence of OA.

VII. WHAT IS THE INCIDENCE AND PREVALENCE OF OP IN OA?

There have been a number of studies comparing BMD between subjects with OA and controls without OA. Few of these studies, however, have presented data on the actual prevalence of OP in these cases of OA. Certainly, no recent study has attempted to analyze cases of arthritis based on the current WHO criteria for OP. Longitudinal studies on large groups of subjects with OA of various joints are needed to determine the incidence of OP in OA.

In the MEDOS study, the age-adjusted risk for hip fracture associated with definite OA was 0.68 ($p < 0.001$) for women and 0.48 ($p < 0.001$) for men.[46] When cases of probable OA were included, the negative relative risk remained highly significant. The authors concluded that OA was protective for hip fracture. They also found that if subjects with osteoarthritis develop osteoporotic fracture, they do so at a later age.

However, OA, despite being associated with higher BMD, may not necessarily lead to a lower incidence of osteoporotic fractures. Jones et al.,[59] in a longitudinal population based study of fracture risk, observed that individuals with self-reported OA, despite higher bone density, were not protected against nonvertebral osteoporotic fractures, due to worsened postural stability and thus an increased tendency to fall.

The SOF study reported in 1999 that patients with self-reported OA were not associated with a higher fracture risk (RR = 1; 95% CI = 0.9 to 1.1). However, there was an increased risk of falling in those with self-reported OA (RR 1.4; 95% CI = 1.2 to 1.5). Interestingly, this was the inverse of those with radiographic OA, where a decreased risk of falling was seen (Grade 2 RR = 0.7, 95% CI = 0.5 to 0.95; Grade 3 to 4 RR = 0.6, 95% CI = 0.4 to 1.0). In addition, in patients who had definite OA on radiographs, there was no difference in risk of osteoporotic fracture. When examining all nonvertebral fractures, the relative risk of fracture was 0.8 (95% CI = 0.7 to 1.0, p = not significant) for Grade 2 OA and 0.8 (95% CI = 0.6 to 1.1, p = not significant) for Grade 3 and 4 OA. Examining the relative risk by different types of fractures still resulted in no significant decreased fracture risk despite that these women with OA have increased BMD. This may be due to increased risk of falling. The failure of the observed increase in BMD to translate into a reduced fracture risk may be due, in part, to the number and type of falls sustained by subjects with OA. Patients with OA should not be considered to be at a lower risk of fracture than the general population.

VIII. DOES TREATING OP INCREASE THE RISK OF OA?

In theory, increasing bone density, and in particular subchondral bone density, could lead to increased mechanical load through the cartilage of weight-bearing joints, thereby increasing the risk of OA. None of the large randomized control trials on agents used in the prevention or treatment of OP has looked closely at either arthritic symptoms or radiologic features of OA in their outcome measures.

Calcium supplementation recommended in the prevention of OP has not been shown to increase the risk of OA. Physical activity is often recommended as a preventative measure for OP and may have benefits on peak bone mass.[59] It is possible that the increased load through weight-bearing joints could lead to an increased risk of OA, but there is little evidence for this. In one study, involving a comparison of long-distance runners with community controls, running was found to be associated with higher BMD.[60] There was no difference between the groups in the prevalence of radiologic OA of groups were compared 2 years later.[61] A recent editorial by the same author[62] concluded that only individuals who participate in sports with abnormal or injured joints or at a highly competitive level appear to be at risk of developing OA.

Estrogen is prescribed for both prevention and treatment of OP. A recent study examined the cross-sectional association of postmenopausal estrogen replacement with the prevalence of radiographic findings of OA of the hip in a large cohort of 4366 elderly Caucasian women.[63] A number of possible confounders, including BMI and physical activity, were adjusted for. Women who were currently using oral estrogen had a significantly reduced risk of OA of the hip. Current users who had taken estrogen for 10 years or longer had a greater reduction in the risk of any OA of the hip compared with those who had used estrogen for less than 10 years. Analysis of the female participants in the Framingham study concluded that estrogen use in women is not associated with an increased risk of radiographic knee OA.[64] In contrast, another cross-sectional study on younger women aged 25 to 45 found current use of HRT, including use among women with oophorectomy and hysterectomy, was significantly associated with higher radiographic knee OA scores.[23] Longitudinal studies are needed to adequately assess the effect of HRT on OA.

There are no reports of increased risk of OA with the use of the bisphosphonates, calcitonin, or vitamin D metabolites. In the study referred to above in which higher serum IGF-1 levels were observed in subjects with radiologic OA, the authors concluded that use of IGF-1 to treat OP had the potential of worsening OA.[48]

IX. DOES TREATING OA INCREASE THE RISK OF OP?

The medical treatment of OA usually involves the principles of adequate pain relief, where appropriate, with simple analgesics or short-term nonsteroidal anti-inflammatory drugs (NSAIDs) and ensuring mobility by exercise programs and physiotherapy. With regard to drug therapy, there is evidence that prostaglandins, including prostaglandin E2, are produced by osteoblasts and osteoblast-like cells and may regulate bone formation and resorption. NSAIDs could therefore theoretically affect bone formation and/or resorption by decreasing the production of prostaglandins. Interestingly, in one small study of eight postmenopausal women with high rates of bone resorption, diclofenac sodium was observed to reduce markers of bone resorption to the same degree as conjugated estrogens.[65] Also, in a randomized trial, piroxicam was compared with placebo in 42 postmenopausal women treated with a below-elbow plaster for 4 weeks after reduction of a displaced Colles' fracture. When BMD was measured 8 weeks after the initial fracture, there was no significant difference between the two groups.[66] These two studies suggest it is unlikely that NSAIDs would increase the risk of OP; however, there is a need for longitudinal studies to assess BMD on patients on long-term NSAIDs.

X. SUMMARY

The evidence for an inverse relationship between OA and OP comes mainly from cross-sectional studies and a few recent longitudinal studies. The evidence for an association with OP is stronger for hip and knee OA than for hand OA and primary generalized OA. The different mechanisms involved in the pathogenesis of OA at different joints are reflected in the variable and sometimes conflicting results seen in these studies. Twin and family studies have shown that both OA and OP have a strong genetic influence, but a common genetic determinant is yet to be shown. Gene polymorphisms have been associated with OA, but their influence appears not to be mediated through BMD. Rather, their effect may be linked to osteophyte formation or progression. OA and OP are influenced by a number of similar risk factors such as age and anthropometric measures. These need to be taken into account in examining any relationship between the two diseases. OA is not only a disease of cartilage but of the underlying subchondral bone as well. Higher bone density is associated with stiffer subchondral bone. This can result in increased mechanical load through the cartilage. The results of studies on the role of growth factors in the pathogenesis of OA and increased bone density have been conflicting.

Cross-sectional studies show a lower prevalence of OA in subjects with hip fractures. There have been no longitudinal studies looking at the incidence of OA in OP. Current methods of measuring bone density have not been performed on large groups of subjects with the aim of studying the incidence and prevalence of OP in OA. There is no evidence that current treatments of one disease can increase the risk of the other.

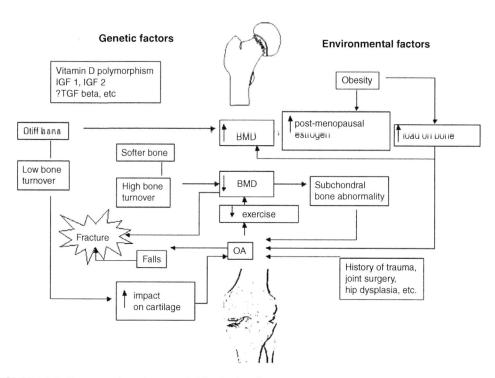

FIGURE 29.1 Osteoporosis and osteoarthritis: the interface.

We conclude this chapter with Figure 29.1, a summary diagram integrating the effects of different genetic and environmental factors on osteoporosis and osteoarthritis. Several practice points and future research directions are also listed below.

Practice points

- Different mechanisms are involved in the pathogenesis of OA at different joints.
- Lumbar osteophytosis and apophyseal OA can spuriously elevate lumbar BMD readings.
- Increased bone density associated with OA may not result in decreased fracture risk because of the increased risk of falling.
- An inverse relationship is observed in populations of patients, but does not necessarily have practical implications in individuals; for example, in a patient with multiple risk factors for OP, the presence of OA does not mean further assessment and treatment are unnecessary.

Research agenda

- Further longitudinal studies need to be undertaken to study the association between OA and OP.
- Do OA and OP share common genetic determinants?
- Long-term therapeutic measures to treat one disease should monitor for possible increased risk of the other.

REFERENCES

1. Foss, M.V. and Byers, P., "Bone density, osteoarthritis of the hip and fracture of the upper end of the femur," *Ann. Rheum. Dis.*, 31, 259, 1972.
2. Roh, Y.S., Dequeker, J., and Mulier, J.C., et al., "Bone mass in osteoarthrosis, measured *in vivo* by photon absorption," *J. Bone Joint Surg.*, 56A, 587, 1974.
3. Sambrook, P. and Naganathan, V., "What is the relationship between osteoarthritis and osteoporosis?" *Bailliere's Clin. Rheumatol.*, 11, 695, 1997.
4. Dequeker, J., Boonen, S., Aerssens, J., and Westhovens, R., "Inverse relationship osteoarthritis-osteoporosis: what is the evidence?" *Br. J. Rheumatol.*, 35, 813, 1996.
5. Steward, A. and Black, A.J., "Bone mineral density in osteoarthritis," *Current Opinion Rheumatol.*, 12, 464, 2000.
6. Dequeker, J., "Inverse relationship of interface between osteoporosis and osteoarthritis," *J. Rheumatol.*, 24, 795, 1997.
7. Sowers, M.F., Zobel, D., Weissfeld, L., et al., "Progression of osteoarthritis of the hand and metacarpal bone loss. A twenty-year follow up of incident cases," *Arthritis Rheum.*, 34, 36, 1991.
8. Sowers, M.F., Lachance, L., Jamadar, D., et al., "The association of bone mineral density and bone turnover markers with osteoarthritis of the hand and knee in pre and perimenopausal women," *Arthritis Rheum.*, 42, 483, 1999.
9. Hart, D.J., Mootoosamy, L, Doyle, D.V., and Spector, T.D., "The relationship between osteoarthritis and OP in the general population: the Chingford study," *Ann. Rheum. Dis.*, 53, 158, 1994.
10. Burger, H., van-Daele, P.L., Odding, E., et al., "Association of radiographically evident osteoarthritis with higher bone mineral density and increased bone loss with age. The Rotterdam study," *Arthritis Rheum.*, 39, 81, 1996.
11. Nevitt, M.C., Lane, N.E., Scott, J.C., et al., "Radiographic osteoarthritis of the hip and bone mineral density. The Study of Osteoporotic Fractures Research Group." *Arthritis Rheum.*, 38, 907, 1995.
12. Arden, N.K., Nevitt, M.C., Michael, C., et al., "Osteoarthritis and risk of falls, rate of bone loss, and osteoporotic fractures," *Arthritis Rheum.*, 42, 1378, 1999.
13. Antoniades, L., MacGregor, A.J., Matson, M., and Spector, T.D., "A co-twin control study of the relationship between hip osteoarthritis and bone mineral density," *Arthritis Rheum.*, 43, 1450, 2000.
14. Stewart, A., Black, A., Robins, S.P., and Reid, D., "Bone density and bone turnover in patients with osteoarthritis and osteoporosis," *J. Rheumatol.*, 26, 622, 1999.
15. Cooper, C., Cook, P.L., Osmond, C., et al., "Osteoarthritis of the hip and osteoporosis of the proximal femur," *Ann. Rheum. Dis.*, 50, 540, 1991.
16. Li, B. and Aspden, R.M., "Material properties of bone from the femoral neck and calcar femorale of patients with osteoporosis or osteoarthritis," *Osteoporos. Int.*, 7, 450, 1997.
17. Hannan, M.T., Anderson, J.J., Zhang, Y., et al., "Bone mineral density and knee osteoarthritis in elderly men and women. The Framingham study," *Arthritis Rheum.*, 36, 1671, 1993.
18. Peel, N.F., Barrington, N.A., Blumsohn, A., et al., "Bone mineral density and bone turnover in spinal osteoarthrosis," *Ann. Rheum. Dis.*, 54, 867, 1995.
19. Masud, T., Langley, S., Wiltshire, P., et al., "Effect of spinal osteophytosis on bone mineral density measurements in vertebral OP," *Br. Med. J.*, 307, 172, 1993.
20. Jones, G., Nguyen, T., Sambrook, P.N., et al., "A longitudinal study of the effect of spinal degenerative disease on bone density in the elderly." *J. Rheumatol.*, 22, 932, 1995.
21. Liu, G., Peacock, M., Eilam, O., et al., "Effect of osteoarthritis in the lumbar spine and hip on bone mineral density and diagnosis of osteoporosis in elderly men and women," *Osteoporos. Int.*, 7, 564, 1997.
22. Marcelli, C., Favier, F., Kotzki, P.O., et al., "The relationship between osteoarthritis of the hands, bone mineral density, and osteoporotic fractures in elderly women," *Osteoporos. Int.*, 5, 382, 1995.
23. Sowers, M.F., Hochberg, M., Crabbe, J.P., et al., "Association of bone mineral density and sex hormone levels with osteoarthritis of the hand and knee in premenopausal women," *Am. J. Epidemiol.*, 143, 38, 1996.
24. Hordon, L.D., Stewart, S.P., Troughton, P.R., et al., "Primary generalized osteoarthritis and bone mass," *Br. J. Rheumatol.*, 32, 1059, 1993.

25. Gevers, Q., Dequeker, J., Geusens, P., et al., "Physical and histomorphologic characteristics of iliac crest bone differ according to the grade of osteoarthritis at the hand," *Bone*, 10, 173, 1998.
26. Gevers, G., Dequeker, J., Martens, M., et al., "Biomechanical characteristics of iliac crest bone in elderly women according to osteoarthritis grade at the hand joints," *J. Rheumatol.*, 16, 660, 1989.
27. Hochberg, M.C., Lethbridge-Ceiku, M., Scott, W.W., et al., "Appendicular bone mass and osteoarthritis of the hands in women: data from the Baltimore Longitudinal Study of Aging," *J. Rheumatol.*, 21, 1532, 1994.
28. Hochherg, M.C., Lethbridge-Ceiku, M., Plato, C.C., et al., "Factors associated with osteoarthritis of the hand in males: data from the Baltimore Longitudinal Study of Aging," *Am. J. Epidemiol.*, 134, 1121, 1991.
29. Reid, D.M., Kennedy, N.S., and Smith, M.A., "Bone mass in nodal primary generalised osteoarthrosis," *Ann. Rheum. Dis.*, 43, 240, 1984.
30. Price, T., Hesp, R., and Mitchell, R., "Bone density in generalized osteoarthritis," *J. Rheumatol.*, 14, 560, 1987.
31. Cooper, C., Poll, V., McLaren, M., et al., "Alteration in appendicular mass in patients with rheumatoid, psoriatic and osteoarthropathy," *Ann. Rheum. Dis.*, 47, 481, 1998.
32. Hochberg, M.C., Lethbridge-Cejku, M., Scott, W.W., Jr., et al., "Upper extremity bone mass and osteoarthritis of the knees: data from the Baltimore Longitudinal Study of Aging," *J. Bone Miner. Res.*, 10, 432, 1995.
33. Lane, N.E. and Nevitt, M.C., "Osteoarthritis and bone mass," *J. Rheumatol.*, 21, 1393, 1994.
34. Tepper, S. and Hochberg, M.C., "Factors associated with hip osteoarthritis: data from the First National Health and Nutrition Examination Survey (NHANES-1)," *Am. J. Epidemiol.*, 137, 1081, 1993.
35. Lane, N.E., Lin, P., Nevitt, M.C. et al., "Association of mild acetabular dysplasia with an increase risk of incident hip osteoarthritis in elderly white women. The study of osteoporosis of fractures," *Arthritis Rheum.*, 43, 400, 1999.
36. Pocock, N.A., Eisman, I.A., Hopper, L.L., et al., "Genetic determinants of bone mass in adults: a twin study," *J. Clin. Invest.*, 80, 706, 1987.
37. Spector, T.D., Cicuttini, F., Baker, J., et al., "Genetic influences on osteoarthritis: a twin study," *Br. Med. J.*, 312, 940, 1996.
38. MacGregor, A.J., Antoniades, L., Matson, M., et al., "The genetic contribution to radiographic hip osteoarthritis in women: result of a classic twin study," *Arthritis Rheum.*, 43, 2410, 1999.
39. Sambrook, P., MacGregor, A.J., and Spector, T.D., "Genetic influences on cervical and lumbar disc degeneration: a magnetic resonance imaging study in twins," *Arthritis Rheum.*, 42, 366, 1999.
40. Dequeker, J., Goris, P., and Uytterhoeven, R., "Osteoporosis and osteoarthritis (osteoarthrosis). Anthropometric distinctions," *J. Am. Med. Assoc.*, 249, 1448, 1983.
41. Dequeker, J., Mokassa, L., and Aerssens, J., "Bone density and osteoarthritis," *J. Rheumatol. Suppl.*, 43, 98, 1995.
42. Radin, E.L. and Rose, R.M., "Role of subchondral bone in the initiation and progression of cartilage damage," *Clin. Orthop.*, 213, 34, 1986.
43. Dieppe, P., Cushnaghan, I., Young, P., and Kirwan, J., "Prediction of the progression of joint space narrowing in osteoarthritis of the knee by bone scintigraphy," *Ann. Rheum. Dis.*, 52, 557, 1993.
44. Schnitzler, C.M., Mesquita, J.M., and Wane, L., "Bone histomorphometry of the iliac crest, and spinal fracture prevalence in atrophic and hypertrophic osteoarthritis of the hip," *Osteoporos. Int.*, 2, 186, 1992.
45. Lloyd, M.E., Hart, D.J., Nandra, D., et al., "Relation between insulin-like growth factor-1 concentration, osteoarthritis, bone density, and fractures in the general population: the Chingford study," *Ann. Rheum. Dis.*, 55, 870, 1996.
46. Dequeker, J. and Johnell, O., "Osteoarthritis protects against femoral neck fracture: the MEDOS study experience," *Bone*, 14, S51, 1993.
47. Dequeker, J., Mohan, S., Finkelman, R.D., et al., "Generalized osteoarthritis associated with increased insulin-like growth factor types 1 and II and transforming growth factor beta in cortical bone from the iliac crest. Possible mechanism of increased bone density and protection against OP," *Arthritis Rheum.*, 36, 1702, 1993.
48. Schouten, J.S., Van-den-Ouweland, F.A., Valkenburg, H.A., et al., "Insulin-like growth factor 1: a prognostic factor of knee osteoarthritis," *Br. J. Rheumatol.*, 32, 274, 1993.

49. Hochberg, M.C., Lethbridge-Ceiku, M., Scott, W.W., Jr., et al., "Serum levels of insulin-like growth factor in subjects with osteoarthritis of the knee: data from the Baltimore Longitudinal Study of Aging," *Arthritis Rheum.*, 37, 1177, 1994.

50. Meulenbelt, I., Bijkerk, C., Miedema, H.S., et al., "A genetic association study of the IGF-1 gene and radiologic osteoarthritis in a population-based cohort study (the Rotterdam study)," *Ann. Rheum. Dis.*, 57, 371, 1998.

51. Keen, R.W., Hart, D.J., Lanchbury, J.S., and Spector, T.D., "Early osteoarthritis of the knee is associated with a Taq1 polymorphism of the vitamin D receptor gene," *Arthritis Rheum.*, 40, 1444, 1997.

52. Jones G., White, C., Sambrook, P., and Eisman, J., "Allelic variation in the vitamin D receptor, lifestyle factors and lumbar spinal degenerative disease," *Ann. Rheum. Dis.*, 57, 94, 1998.

53. Videman, T., Gibbons, L.E., Battie, M.C., et al., "The relative roles of intragenic polymorphisms of the vitamin D receptor gene in lumbar spine degeneration and bone density," *Spine*, 26, A1, 2001.

54. Thompson, P.W., Spector, T.D., James, I.T., et al., "Urinary collagen cross-links reflect the radiographic severity of knee osteoarthritis," *Br. J. Rheumatol.*, 31, 759, 1992.

55. MacDonald, A.G., McHenry, P., Robins, S.P., and Reid, D.M., "Relationship of urinary pyridinium cross-links to disease extent and activity in osteoarthritis," *Br. J. Rheumatol.*, 33, 16, 1994.

56. Cumming, R.G. and Klineberg, R.J., "Epidemiological study of the relation between arthritis of the hip and hip fractures," *Ann. Rheum. Dis.*, 52, 707, 1993.

57. Cummings, S.R., Nevitt, M.C., Browner, W.S., et al., "Risk factors for hip fracture in white women. Study of Osteoporotic Fractures Research Group," *N. Engl. J. Med.*, 332, 767, 1995.

58. Jones, G., Nguyen, T., Sambrook, P.N., et al., "Osteoarthritis, bone density, postural stability, and osteoporotic fractures: a population based study," *J. Rheumatol.*, 22, 921, 1995.

59. Welten, D.C., Kemper, F.I.C., Post, G.B., et al., "Weight-bearing activity during youth is a more important factor for peak bone mass than calcium intake," *J. Bone Miner. Res.*, 9, 1089, 1994.

60. Lane, N.E., Bloch, D.A., Jones, H.H., et al., "Long-distance running, bone density and osteoarthritis," *J. Am. Med. Assoc.*, 255, 1147, 1986.

61. Lane, N.E., Bloch, D.A., Hubert, H.H., et al., "Running, osteoarthritis and bone density: initial 2-year longitudinal study," *Am. J. Med.*, 88, 452, 1990.

62. Lane, N.E., "Exercise: a cause of osteoarthritis," *J. Rheumatol. Suppl.*, 43, 3, 1995.

63. Nevitt, M.C., Cummings, S.R., Lane, N.E., et al., "Association of estrogen replacement therapy with the risk of osteoarthritis of the hip in elderly white women. Study of Osteoporotic Fractures Research Group," *Arch. Intern. Med.*, 156, 2073, 1996.

64. Hannan, M.T., Felson, D.T., Anderson, J.J., et al., "Estrogen use and radiographic osteoarthritis of the knee in women: The Framingham Osteoarthritis Study," *Arthritis Rheum.*, 33, 525, 1990.

65. Bell, N.H., Hollis, B.W., Shary, J.R., et al., "Diclofenac sodium inhibits bone resorption in postmenopausal women," *Am. J. Med.*, 96, 349, 1994.

66. Adolphson, P., Abbaszadegan, H., Jonsson, U., et al., "No effects of piroxicam on osteopenia and recovery after Colles' fracture. A randomised, double-blind, placebo-controlled, prospective trial," *Arch. Orthop. Trauma Surg.*, 112, 127, 1993.

Part VII

Prevention and Management of Osteoporotic Conditions

crippling disease. Imagine a 17-year-old female, attending the teen clinic for pregnancy prevention, taking the birth control Depo-Provera, not knowing that over time it is a "bone killer." Years later she takes a ski trip and falls on the slopes with outstretched hands sustaining a fractured wrist. A radiograph shows her to be osteopenic, defined as "any state in which bone mass is reduced below normal."[1] She has no understanding of why, and only later realizes she has been on a steroid containing progesterone for pregnancy prevention. Then there are the individuals who increase their risk factors multifold because they smoke at least a pack per day, drink two to three soft drinks per day, drink alcohol with their friends on weekends, and of course they are dieting to stay slim. Not to mention they were never really fond of milk or dairy products as well as green leafy vegetables. Are they taking their multivitamins daily? Of course not! Does this sound like the general American adolescent population? How about the female soccer athlete who has been amenorrheic throughout the season or her friend competing for homecoming queen who is bulimic? Let's not forget the 19-year-old asthmatic male football player who has had severe asthma since childhood and is taking inhaled corticosteroids, but has never been compliant on his preventive asthma medications and takes a puff of his inhaler as needed and seems to puff away taking the easier route to give him immediate relief to breathe. Long-term use of inhaled corticosteroids for asthma control results in decreased bone mineral density (BMD). Is he now osteoporotic? Finally, consider the frail elderly woman admitted to the emergency room because she fell, sustaining a hip fracture, who mentions to the physician she has been getting shorter yearly, but really has not taken her height recently. She is now a candidate for an open reduction internal fixation or even total hip replacement, which increases her risk for morbidity or mortality threefold. How many physicians' offices take their patients' heights and keep an ongoing record to monitor whether their patients are shrinking?

Osteoporosis is a serious, degenerative, potentially crippling disorder that causes many people to suffer as they get older. Bone substance is lost over the years and eventually causes painful fractures and limits the person's activities. There is no cure for this disease; however, with early intervention, preferably when a person is between 10 and 20 years of age, we can prevent it. Interventions can be implemented easily through use of orthopaedic nurses in the role of educator. An example of such an intervention specific to this author is utilization of a nurse practitioner who is a member of the National Association of Orthopaedic Nurses (NAON) as a site coordinator for an osteoporosis prevention project for teenagers called the OPTIONS (Osteoporosis Prevention: Teaching in Our Nation's Schools) program.[2] The purpose of this program is to teach teenagers the importance of food selections, weight-bearing exercises, and healthy lifestyle to develop healthy bones and prevent osteoporosis.

A. OSTEOPOROSIS OVERVIEW

Osteoporosis is characterized by low bone mass and structural deterioration of bone tissue, leading to bone fragility and an increased susceptibility to fractures of the hip, spine, and wrist.[3] Orthopaedic physicians also define osteoporosis as an unexplained fracture of one major long bone.[4] Men, women, and children suffer from osteoporosis, a disease that can be prevented and treated. Osteo-malacia is defined as a disturbance in the metabolism of calcium and phosphorus that results in impaired and decreased mineralization of bone. A variety of underlying disorders may result in osteomalacia, including a nutritional deficiency of vitamin D and other vitamin D disturbances, renal disorders, and congenital errors in metabolism. Patients generally present with diffuse bone pain, generalized weakness, and malaise. Radiographically, diffuse osteopenia is seen as any state in which bone mass is reduced below normal.[1]

B. BASIC BONE PHYSIOLOGY

Boning up on osteoporosis involves taking a look at bone definition and bone loss. According to the National Institutes of Health, bone is living, growing tissue. It is made mostly of collagen, a protein that provides a soft framework, and calcium phosphate, a mineral that adds strength and hardens the framework. This combination of collagen and calcium makes bone strong yet flexible to withstand stress. More than 99% of the body's calcium is contained in the bones and teeth. The remaining 1% is found in the blood.[5]

Throughout life bone constantly remodels itself through bone resorption (which is a process of losing calcium and bone matrix from the skeleton) and bone formation (building up of calcium in bone or new bone added to the skeleton). Cells called osteoclasts break the bone down, while cells called osteoblasts remodel it. Between birth and age 2 the bone mass changes substantially, doubling through increased work of osteoblasts far exceeding the osteoclasts. During childhood and the teenage years bone mass doubles again as new bone is added faster than old bone is removed so that by the time the teenager reaches the age of 18 he or she has acquired 90% of maximum bone mass. As a result of this growth, bones become larger, heavier, and denser. Bone formation continues at a pace faster than resorption until peak bone mass; maximum bone density and strength is reached around age 30. After age 30, bone resorption slowly begins to exceed bone formation. Osteoporosis occurs because the rate of bone resorption is greater than the rate of bone formation. There is a greater loss of trabecular bone (the honeycombed mesh found inside bones) than of cortical bone. The loss of trabecular bone can lead to injuries such as vertebral compression fractures, fracture of the neck of the femur, and, most commonly, fractures of the distal end of the radius.

In females, bone loss is most rapid in the first few years after menopause but persists into the postmenopausal years. Osteoporosis develops when bone resorption occurs too quickly or replacement occurs too slowly. Osteoporosis is more likely to develop in an individual who did not reach optimal bone mass during the bone-building years. In a healthy adult, a complete remodeling cycle takes about 4 months but in a person with osteoporosis, that same remodeling cycle may take 2 years.

The effect of this change in resorption and rebuilding is that women in their mid-30s begin to lose bone at a rate of 0.5 to 1% every year. After menopause the rate increases to 1.5% of bone mass per year in the 5 years following menopause. By her late 80s a woman may have only half the bone mass she did when her bones were at their peak.

Men should not just consider this as only a woman's problem; 1 to 2 million men in the United States have osteoporosis and up to 13 million have osteopenia. Men begin losing bone mass in their late 30s to early 40s. The bone loss rate in men is more gradual than that in women until the age of 65. After age 65 a man's bone loss rate may be greater than a woman's. The rate for osteoporosis-related fracture in men is 13 to 25%.

This chapter shares some facts about the disease and presents an overview of osteoporosis and how it develops, signs and symptoms to watch for, prevention by prudent lifestyle changes, and the importance of a clinical history, physical, and diagnostic exam to determine the severity and treatment of the disease.

C. Facts about Osteoporosis

- Osteoporosis has been present in the human population since prehistoric times.[4]
- "Oral contraceptive use and estrogen replacement therapy were the only variables studied that were statistically significant for prediction of osteoporosis."[6]
- Spine and hip fractures are the most common. The wrist fracture is the third most common fracture.[4]
- Estimated national direct expenditure (hospitals and nursing homes) for osteoporosis and related fractures is $4 billion each year.[3] Increased morbidity and mortality is associated with hip fractures resulting in chronic complications. Approximately 50% of fracture patients require help with activities of daily living, 15 to 25% are institutionalized, and 12 to 20% die within 2 years after a hip fracture.[4]

- Ninety percent of cases of primary osteoporosis can be expected in women over 50 years of age. The primary factor is loss of ovarian function.[4]
- Osteoporosis is a major public health threat affecting 28 million Americans in 1996, 80% of whom are women.
- One of every two women and one in eight men over 50 will have an osteoporosis-related fracture at some time in their life.[5]
- More than 2 million American men suffer from osteoporosis, and millions more are at risk. Each year 80,000 men suffer a hip fracture and one third of these men die within a year.[7]
- Osteoporosis can strike at any age; however, as the population ages osteoporosis becomes increasingly prevalent.
- Osteoporosis is responsible for more than 1.5 million fractures annually, including 300,000 hip fractures, and approximately 700,000 vertebral fractures, 250,000 wrist fractures, and more than 300,000 fractures at other sites including pelvis, humerus, tibia, and distal femur.[8]
- The National Osteoporosis Foundation estimates the number of people diagnosed with osteoporosis will increase to 41 million by 2015.[9]
- In 2015, estimates predict 2.25 million fractures with a possible cost of more than $60 billion.[10]

II. CLINICAL ASPECTS

A. CLINICAL HISTORY AND PHYSICAL EXAMINATION

Osteoporosis is often called a "silent disease" because bone loss occurs without symptoms. People may not know that they have osteoporosis until their bones become so weak that a sudden strain, bump, or fall causes a hip fracture or a vertebra to collapse. Collapsed vertebrae may initially be felt or seen in the form of severe back pain, loss of height, spinal deformities such as kyphosis, or severely stooped posture.

For a patient with osteoporosis, the following subtle signs can be seen at the clinic:

- No early warnings, with a fracture often the first sign
- Gradual height loss more than 1.5 in. in height
- Dorsal kyphosis with "dowager's hump"
- Protuberant lower abdomen
- Acute or chronic upper or middle back pain
- Pulmonary dysfunction
- Low skeletal mass and/or atraumatic fractures

B. DIAGNOSIS AND DETECTION

Following a comprehensive medical assessment, a bone mass index or a BMD test may be ordered. BMD tests measure bone density in the spine, wrist, and/or hip (the most common sites of fractures due to osteoporosis), while other diagnostic tests such as ultrasound measure bone in the heel or hand. These tests are painless, noninvasive, and safe. A BMD test measures the amount of mineral in a specific area of bone and is the only way to diagnose osteopenia or osteoporosis. The World Health Organization defines osteoporosis as a BMD of more than 2.5 standard deviations below the mean bone mineral content for young adults (Table 30.1). A measurement of more than 1 standard deviation but less than 2.5 indicates osteopenia.

TABLE 30.1

World Health Organization Definition of Osteoporosis Based on Bone Density Levels

Normal Bone Mass	Within 1 Standard Deviation of the Young Adult Mean
Low bone mass	1 to 2.5 standard deviations less than the young adult mean
Osteoporosis	>2.5 standard deviations less than the young adult mean
Severe osteoporosis	>2.5 standard deviations less than the young adult mean and there have been one or more fractures

Sequential BMD testing can be helpful in the following:

- Detecting low bone density before a fracture occurs
- Confirming a diagnosis of osteoporosis after a fracture
- Predicting the chances of experiencing a fracture in the future
- Determining the rate of bone loss and/or monitoring the effects of treatment if the test is conducted at intervals of a year or more

C. OSTEOPOROSIS IN CHILDREN

BMD increases most during the first 3 years of life and in late puberty. Bone mass and bone density increase the most during childhood and adolescence. By age 20, 90% of peak bone mass is achieved.

Bone density can continue to increase into the 30s, although much more slowly.[11] Late menarche at age 14 or older can lead to decreased peak bone mass because there is no increase in estrogen levels. The higher the peak bone mass, the lower the risk for osteoporosis. Factors that affect peak bone mass can be categorized as genetic or lifestyle.

Present lifestyles of adolescents leave them predisposed to osteoporosis later in life. Educating teens about osteoporosis including the causes and risk factors and the ways that teens can reduce their risks may prevent this condition in later life. Adolescence is the most critical period for calcium absorption because the calcium content of bones triples during the adolescent growth spurt. Special attention is given to diets rich in calcium and exercise that will strengthen bone during adolescence. Dietary supplements will affect their bone health.

The number of adolescents who smoke is increasing. Approximately 50% of males and 49% of females have used tobacco during their high school years.[12] Each year of smoking is equivalent to about a 1 to 1.5% deficit in bone density. The more a person smokes, the more bone mass is affected.[13]

In 1998, the National Fluid Milk Processor Promotion Board found that 85% of teenage girls and 60% of boys do not get the U.S. RDA (recommended dietary allowance) of calcium.[14] The U.S. RDA for teenagers is more than 1 quart of milk per day, approximately 1000 mg of calcium. The average milk consumption in America is about 1 quart per week. Soft drinks are consumed at a rate of about 4 quarts per week. The high intake of phosphates and sodium increases urinary excretion of calcium. Some sources say that high caffeine intake also increases urinary excretion of calcium.

Eating disorders also contribute to osteoporosis, and 95% of females with eating disorders are in the adolescent age range. Eating disorders include anorexia nervosa and bulimia. The mean age of onset of anorexia nervosa is 13.75 years. These eating disorders deplete the body of needed nutrients and can also cause delayed menarche or amenorrhea because of decreased levels of estrogen.

The National Osteoporosis Foundation recommends that teens be taught risk factors, the need for sunshine and vitamin D, the effects of smoking and alcohol use on bone, dietary calcium needs and dietary assessment, the need for appropriate exercise, and good body alignment and mechanics.

The National Association of Orthopaedic Nurses (NAON) is dedicated to education for the prevention of osteoporosis. Toward that goal it has developed a short educational program (called OPTIONS) to teach teenagers the importance of food selection, weight-bearing exercise and healthy lifestyle in developing healthy bones and preventing osteoporosis. The target of the pilot study is to give 900 high school students a presentation and questionnaire taking 15 to 20 minutes. Posters and information flyers about calcium and osteoporosis will be delivered to the classrooms.[2]

Adolescents and children are very much at risk for osteoporosis, and not knowing the facts about this disease means that they are even more at risk. Nursing educators can expose these young adults by teaching them risk factors and how to live a more prudent lifestyle. This information will give them the tools to take charge of their bone health. The hope is that this will prevent epidemic numbers of fractures happening early in their lives. This research project will give us the knowledge needed to incorporate this information in the schools for the students with very little monetary cost. Lastly, the students will appreciate learning the necessary information needed to change their lifestyles.

D. Osteoporosis in Men

Although osteoporosis has been considered for decades to be a disease of women, it is known that the age-related increase in fractures seen in women is also present in men. The subject of osteoporosis in men is gaining international attention because it has become a significant public health issue. Hip fractures in men account for one third of all hip fractures and have a higher mortality than in women. In fact, men are three times more likely to die after a hip fracture than women.[15] One study found that 1 year after a hip fracture, 80% of men are in long-term care facilities.[16]

Osteoporosis in men is much more common than previously believed. Most men view osteoporosis as a women's disease. More than seven in ten men think that a woman is at least "likely" to develop the disease. The differences between women and men are that the increase in fractures in men begins about 10 years later than in women. Men are not as prone to long bone fractures as women. In fact, 1 to 2 million American men have osteoporosis and 8 to 13 million men have osteopenia.[11] The age-specific incidence of hip fractures is increasing, which means the public health burden will increase. Peak bone mass is higher in men than in women because men have bigger bones. Peak bone density is the same. The absolute trabecular bone loss at the spine and iliac crest during aging is similar in men and women. Cortical bone loss is less in men because endocortical resorption is less and periosteal formation is greater. Bone fragility is less in men because the cross-sectional surface of the vertebral body is larger, and the trabecular bone loss is less as a percentage of the higher peak bone mass. Trabecular bone loss occurs by thinning rather than perforation and periosteal appositional growth compensated for endocortical resorption by maintaining the bending strength of bone.[17]

Hypogonadism and testosterone replacement are currently the subject of much interesting research. Testosterone levels decline with age, but do not undergo the dramatic drop that menopause causes for estrogen in women. A study was conducted in Yugoslavia of men castrated after conviction for sexual crimes.[18] The results showed that once the gonads no longer function, men have early rapid bone loss and then a gradual decline afterward. Treating hypogonadism with testosterone is one option.

It is important to assess osteoporosis in men with a complete history, physical evaluation, and risk assessment. Any secondary causes related to diseases with an increased risk of generalized osteoporosis should be ruled out. Past medical and behavioral history of heavy smoking or high alcohol intake as well as back pain should alert the clinician to potential risk factors. Bone density testing is the gold standard for diagnosing osteoporosis. Laboratory testing helps identify biochemical indication of altered bone turnover. Blood and urine analysis for parathyroid hormone level, vitamin D level, and urine calcium content can also indicate altered bone metabolism and risk or presence of osteoporosis.

Osteoporosis in men is a growing issue in the public eye. It is a source of great health-care expense and a common cause of increased morbidity and mortality. The highest incidence of osteoporosis in men is secondary to disease or drug therapy; however, some men are diagnosed with idiopathic osteoporosis. The future of prevention and treatment of male osteoporosis will depend greatly on awareness and research findings.

III. PREVENTION OF OSTEOPOROSIS AND RELATED FRACTURES

A. AWARENESS AND IMPORTANCE

Office patients should be screened regularly to determine whether they are at risk of osteoporosis. "Women over the age of 65 years old who weigh less than 140 pounds at menopause or have never used estrogen for more than 6 months [should] be screened for osteoporosis."[6] "All physicians need to make their patients aware of osteoporosis and the importance of it, and then, by looking at the risk factors, determine who is cost effective to screen."[6] Height and weight should be recorded and a questionnaire be filled out by patients to determine their risk factors. A screening tool has been developed to remind the clinician of the key elements to ask the patient to see whether or not that patient should be concerned about osteoporosis. The age of the patient, bone stock, and whether or not the patient is or has been on estrogens, are among the key elements in targeting this population. A mnemonic, ABONE, has been developed to remind the clinician to ask those specific questions: A = age; B = bulk; and ONE = or never estrogens. This is one way to identify those women who are at risk.[4]

Osteoporosis can be primary or secondary. Primary osteoporosis involves trabecular bone loss, most commonly related to an estrogen deficiency. It mostly affects women in the first decade after menopause. Men who develop osteoporosis without a known cause can also fall into this group. Secondary osteoporosis involves cortical and trabecular bone loss, and occurs in association with certain diseases and treatments as mentioned in the case scenarios in the introduction. These diseases include cancer, hormonal or gastrointestinal disorders, alcoholism, and use of anticonvulsants, glucocorticoids, and chemotherapy. In the case of an individual with asthma, even low doses of corticosteroids are associated with accelerated bone loss and increased fracture risk. The most rapid bone loss occurs during the first 6 to 12 months of systemic therapy, and the loss continues at a slower rate with prolonged therapy. Senile osteoporosis, also known as primary osteoporosis, develops after the age of 70. This is mostly affected by the decreased calcium and vitamin D intake and lack of activity.

B. RISK FACTORS

Many people with osteoporosis have several risk factors contributing to the disease. Some of these risk factors are modifiable and others are not. However, people with no identifiable risk factors can also develop osteoporosis. Extensive research to identify risk factors for osteoporosis is under way with the hope that identification of all potential risk factors will facilitate earlier intervention to limit the devastating consequences of this disease.

1. Genetic and Biologic Risk Factors

- *Gender* — Females are at greater risk than males. Women have 25% less bone mass and lose bone more rapidly than men because of the changes involved in menopause. Women will lose 25% of their bone mass after age of 50. Men lose only about 12% because they do not go through the hormonal changes of menopause.
- *Age* — The older one is, the greater the risk of osteoporosis. Bones become less dense and weaker as an individual ages.
- *Body Size* — Higher risks are associated with small slender body build. Asian women are thought to be at a higher risk because of their smaller frames.[5]

- *Ethnicity* — Caucasian and Asian women are at highest risk. African-American and Latino women have a lower but significant risk. Northern European blonde women with a history of scoliosis, fair skin, a small and flexible frame with easy bruisability are at higher risk. Black women have 10 to 15% more bone mass than Caucasians.[13]
- *Family History* — Heredity may play a part in being susceptible to fractures. People whose parents have a history of fractures also seem to have reduced bone mass and may be at risk for fractures.
- *Late Menarche* — A late first menstrual period, occurring later than 12 to 14 years of age, can increase the risk of developing osteoporosis.
- *Irregular Menses* — Irregular menstrual periods, oophorectomy, and early or current menopause are all associated with low estrogen level, which is a risk factor for osteoporosis.

2. Behavioral and Environmental Risk Factors

- *Sex Hormones* — A major factor in women is the low level of estrogen associated with menopause. Women athletes who diet and train to decrease fat and increase muscle mass have an abnormal absence of menstrual periods (amenorrhea) and are at increased risk. Also to be considered are those agents that suppress estrogen for birth control, contributing to lack of menses. Low testosterone levels in men are a risk factor.
- *Dietary Causes* — Low calcium intake and/or malnutrition, high fiber, high phosphate, and high protein diets are all risk factors. People with gastrointestinal absorption problems such as anorexia nervosa, bulimia, and dietary fads, a lifetime diet low in calcium and vitamin D, and low body weight are at risk. Those who suffer from eating disorders in their teens and early 20s may never reach optimal bone mass. Many studies show that low calcium intake appears to be associated with low bone mass, rapid bone loss, and high fracture rate.[3] National nutrition studies have shown that many people consume less than half the amount of calcium recommended for building and maintaining healthy bones.[6]
- *Sedentary Lifestyle* — Lack of exercise, extended bed rest, immobilization, or paralysis all speed bone loss from lack of stress on the bones. Immobilization after sustaining a fracture is also a risk factor.
- *Cigarette Smoking* — Compounds in cigarette smoke have a toxic effect on the ovaries causing loss of function and accelerated aging. Smoking alters metabolism of sex hormones, decreasing conversion of hormones to an inactive form.
- *Excessive Use of Alcohol* — Alcohol inhibits osteoblasts, the bone-building cells. Men do get osteoporosis, usually secondary to alcoholism. In men, alcohol abuse is the main cause of calcium diuresis and depression of osteoblast function.
- *Medication Use* — Many medications such as glucocorticoids used to treat patients with asthma affect bone mass throughout their lifetime; this places them at a higher risk for developing osteoporosis. Other secondary causes are those patients needing long-term glucocorticoid steroids, anticonvulsant drugs, long-term use of heparin or warfarin, thyroid supplements, antacids that contain aluminum, and certain cancer treatment medications.[4] Caffeine has also been stated in the literature to contribute to bone loss.

C. PRUDENT LIFESTYLE CHANGES AND DIETARY CONSIDERATIONS

To reach optimal peak bone mass and continue building new bone tissue as one ages, there are several factors to be considered. Calcium supplementation is key in the management of osteoporosis and is well tolerated and inexpensive. It appears to limit bone loss but has not been shown to increase bone mineral mass.[19]

1. Nutrition

Diet is an important factor in osteoporosis prevention. The foods we eat contain a variety of vitamins, minerals, and other important nutrients that help keep our bodies healthy. All these nutrients are needed in a balanced proportion. Adequate amounts of calcium and vitamin D are the building blocks for strong bones as well as for heart, muscles, and nerves to function properly.

2. Calcium Intake

Good sources of calcium include low-fat dairy products, such as milk, yogurt, cheese, and ice cream; dark green leafy vegetables, such as broccoli, collards, bok choy, and spinach; sardines and salmon with bones; tofu; almonds; and foods fortified with calcium, such as orange juice, cereals, and breads.[3]

Calcium supplementation is also a source of calcium replacement. Most multivitamins only contain 162 mg or 16% of U.S. RDA, calcium tablets generally contain 330 mg, and chewable candies, which come in a multitude of flavors, provide 500 mg of calcium. The recommended daily allowance of calcium is 1300 mg/day for the child and adolescent (ages 9 to 18), when the skeleton is rapidly growing. Individuals from 19 to 50 years old are recommended to take 1000 mg/day of calcium. Pregnant women and those who are breastfeeding require 1200 to 1500 mg/day. Post-menopausal women and older men are at greater risk of inadequate calcium intake because of multiple factors. They consume an inadequate amount of vitamin D, a necessary vitamin needed for intestinal absorption of calcium. Aging causes the body to become less efficient at absorbing calcium and other nutrients. Older adults with chronic diseases may take multiple medications that may impair calcium absorption or deplete the calcium store. Thus, individuals 51 years and older are recommended to take 1200 to 1500 mg of calcium per day.

3. Vitamin D

Vitamin D plays an important role in calcium absorption and in bone health. It is synthesized in the skin through exposure to sunlight. While many people are able to obtain enough vitamin D naturally, studies show that vitamin D production decreases in elderly people, in people who are housebound, and during the winter. These individuals may require vitamin D supplementation to ensure a daily intake of 400 to 800 IU. Massive doses are not recommended.

4. Weight-Bearing Exercise

Bone is a living tissue that responds to exercise by becoming stronger. Bones must act against resistance to grow stronger. The best exercise for bones is weight-bearing exercise that forces the individual to work against gravity. These exercises include walking, hiking, jogging, stair climbing, weight training, tennis, and dancing. Exercise is an important component of an osteoporosis prevention and treatment program as it not only improves bone health, but it also increases muscle strength, coordination, and balance and leads to better overall health. Although exercise is good for someone with osteoporosis, one should not put any sudden or excessive strain on bones.

5. Smoking Cessation

Smoking is harmful to the health of bones as well as that of heart and lungs. Women who smoke have lower levels of estrogen compared with nonsmokers and frequently go through menopause earlier. Postmenopausal women who smoke may require higher doses of hormone replacement therapy and consequently may have more side effects. Smokers also may absorb less calcium from their diets.

6. Alcohol

Regular consumption of 2 to 3 ounces a day of alcohol may be damaging to the skeleton, even in young women and men. Those who drink heavily are more prone to bone loss and fractures, both because of poor nutrition as well as increased risk of falling.

7. Medications That Cause Bone Loss

The long-term use of glucocorticoids (prescribed for a wide range of diseases, including arthritis, asthma, Crohn's disease, lupus, and other diseases of the lungs, kidneys, and liver) can lead to a loss of bone density and fractures. Other forms of drug therapy that can cause bone loss include long-term treatment with certain antiseizure drugs, such as phenytoin and barbiturates; gonadotropin releasing hormone (GnRH) analogues used to treat endometriosis; excessive use of aluminum-containing antacids; certain cancer treatments (chemotherapy); and excessive thyroid hormone or insulin. It is important for patients to discuss the use of these drugs with their physician and not to stop or alter the medication dose on their own.

D. Fall Prevention

This is a special concern for men and women with osteoporosis. Falls can increase the likelihood of fracturing a bone in the hip, wrist, spine, or other part of the skeleton. In addition to the environmental factors listed below, falls can also be caused by impaired vision and/or balance, chronic diseases that impair mental or physical functioning, and certain medications such as sedatives and antidepressants. It is important that individuals with osteoporosis be aware of any physical changes they may be experiencing that affect their balance or gait, and that they discuss these changes with their health-care provider.

1. Outdoors

Recommendations for avoiding falls outdoors include the following. Use a cane or walker for added stability; wear rubber-soled shoes for traction; walk on grass when sidewalks are slippery; in winter carry salt or kitty litter to sprinkle on slippery sidewalks.

2. Indoors

Recommendations for avoiding falls indoors include the following. Keep rooms free of clutter, especially floors; keep floor surfaces smooth but not slippery; be careful on highly polished floors that become slick and dangerous when wet and use plastic or carpet runners when possible; be sure carpets and area rugs have skid-proof backing or are tacked to the floor; wear supportive, low-heeled shoes even at home; avoid walking in socks, stockings, or slippers; be sure stairwells are well lit and that stairs have handrails on both sides; install grab bars on bathroom walls near tub, shower, and toilet; use a rubber mat in the shower or tub; keep a flashlight with fresh batteries beside the bed; if using a step stool for hard-to-reach areas, use a sturdy one with a handrail and wide steps; add ceiling fixtures into rooms lit by lamps; consider a cordless telephone to eliminate the rush to answer the phone when it rings or to use to call for help in case of a fall.

E. Medication for Prevention and Treatment

Various medications are available for the prevention and treatment of osteoporosis (see Chapter 32 for recommended medications). A comprehensive osteoporosis treatment program includes a focus on proper nutrition, exercise, and safety issues to prevent falls that may result in fractures. In addition, medication may be prescribed to slow or stop bone loss, increase bone density, and reduce fracture risk.

IV. SUMMARY

Osteoporosis occurs in all cultural populations and age groups. Medical experts agree that osteoporosis is highly preventable. The clinician must work to optimize bone health during the adolescent years, because bone mass attained early in life is perhaps the most important determinant of lifelong skeletal health.[20] Screening should be individualized, rather than using a universal approach. Careful attention to adequate calcium and vitamin D intake is essential. Multiple treatment options, appropriate diagnosis, and risk assessment are essentials in prevention of this disease.

REFERENCES

1. Pope, M.H., Phillips, R.B., Haugh, L.D., et al., "A prospective randomized three-week trial of spinal manipulation, transcutaneous muscle stimulation, massage and corset in the treatment of subacute low back pain," *Spine*, 19, 2571, 1994.
2. National Association of Orthopaedic Nurses, "OPTIONS Research Program (Osteoporosis Prevention: Teaching in Our Nation's Schools)," Released on January 14, 2002; available at http://naon.inurse.com.
3. Osteoporosis and Related Bone Diseases National Resource Center, "Osteoporosis Overview," National Institutes of Health, Bethesda, MD, 2000; available at www.osteo.org.
4. Eady, J.L., *Metabolic Disease Slides*, University of South Carolina School of Medicine, Columbia, 1997.
5. Osteoporosis and Related Bone Diseases National Resource Center, "Fast Facts on Osteoporosis," National Institutes of Health, Bethesda, MD, 2000; available at www.osteo.org.
6. Weinstein, L. and Ullery, B., "Identification of at-risk women for osteoporosis screening," *Am. J. Obstet. Gynecol.*, 183, 547, 2000.
7. Lucas, T.S. and Einhorn, T.A., "Osteoporosis: the role of the orthopaedist," *J. Am. Acad. Orthop. Surg.*, 1, 48, 1993.
8. Einhorn, T.A., "Bone metabolism and metabolic bone disease," in *Orthopaedic Knowledge Update IV*, Frymoyer, J.W., Ed., American Academy of Orthopaedic Surgeons, Rosemont, IL, 1993, 69.
9. National Osteoporosis Foundation, Osteoporosis Report, Vol. 14(4), Washington, D.C., winter, 1998.
10. "1996 and 2015 Osteoporosis Prevalence Figures: State-by-State Report," National Osteoporosis Foundation, Washington, D.C., 1997.
11. Poor, G., Atkinson, E.J., Lewallen, D.G., et al., "Age-related hip fractures in men: clinical spectrum and short-term outcomes," *Osteoporos. Int.*, 5, 419, 1995.
12. "Tobacco use continues to rise among high school students in the U.S.," Centers for Disease Control, Office on Smoking and Health, Press Release, Atlanta, GA, 1998.
13. Luke, B., *Good Bones*, Bull Publishing Co., Palo Alto, CA, 1998.
14. www.whymilk.com, "Milk U Nutrition 101," 2002.
15. Orwoll, E., "Men with osteoporosis," presented at the World Congress on Osteoporosis 2000, Chicago, IL, June 15–18, 2000.
16. Seeman, E., "The dilemma of osteoporosis in men," *Am. J. Med.*, 98, 76S, 1995.
17. Bilczikian, J.P., "Osteoporosis in men," *J. Clin. Endocrinol. Metab.*, 84, 3431, 1999.
18. Stepan, J.J., Lachman, M., Zverina, J., et al., "Castrated men exhibit bone loss: effect of calcitonin treatment on biochemical indices of bone remodeling," *J. Clin. Endocrinol. Metab.*, 69, 523, 1989.
19. Rosenthal, R.E., "Osteoporosis," *Arch. Am. Acad. Orthop. Surg.*, 2, 52, 1998.
20. NIH Consensus Statement, "Osteoporosis Prevention, Diagnosis, and Therapy," National Institutes of Health, Bethesda, MD, 17(1), 1–36, 2000.

31 Exercise for Prevention of Osteoporotic Fractures

Ilkka Vuori and Pekka Kannus

CONTENTS

I. INTRODUCTION

Human survival and physical performance depend to a large extent on locomotion. The bony skeleton provides a sturdy framework for other locomotive organs and functions. To provide this framework, bones should be strong enough to resist both ordinary and exceptional forces imposed on them, but at the same time weigh as little as possible. The requirements on bone mass and architecture and on functional demands are matched by a lifelong functional adaptation, which maintains sufficient bone mass, adequate material properties, and favorable architecture to resist all loading possibilities without fracture. The principle of functional adaptation to physical loading was stated by Wolff in 1892: "Every change in the form and function of bone or of their function alone is followed by certain definite changes in their internal architecture and equally definite alteration in their external conformation, in accordance with mathematical laws."[1]

After reaching a peak in early adulthood, bone mass and strength decrease due to normal aging, disuse, and eventually, various pathologic processes. Because an increasing number of people now live to old age, the number of people with weak bones is increasing. Consequently, both the potential and the actual number of osteoporotic fractures are increasing (Figure 31.1). However, most osteoporotic fractures are caused by a combination of two factors: weak bones and a sudden external force, most often a fall. Therefore, prevention of osteoporotic fractures includes two main strategies: maintenance of adequate bone strength and maintenance of the capability of safe locomotion, especially gait.

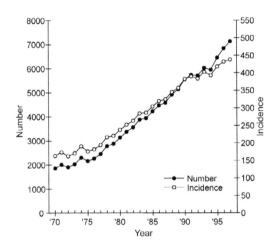

FIGURE 31.1 Number and incidence (per 100,000 persons) of hip fractures in people aged 50 years or older between 1970 and 1997. (From Kannus, P. et al., *Lancet*, 353, 802, 1999. With permission.)

II. EXERCISE FOR PREVENTION OF OSTEOPOROSIS

A. ADAPTATION OF BONE TO MECHANICAL LOADING — BASIC BIOLOGY

A primary condition for functional skeletal adaptation is a relevant feedback mechanism between the load on the bone and the processes influencing the bone mass, material properties, and architecture. The feedback variable is the mechanical strain or deformation in the matrix. Strain is defined as relative deformation or percentage change in length caused by the applied force. A 1% change in bone length is equivalent to 0.01 strains, and 1000 microstrains correspond to 0.1% in length. Bone strength can be expressed in terms of strains, i.e., the fracture strength of a normal lamellar bone is about 25,000 ± 5,000 microstrains, corresponding to a 2.5% change in bone length under compression or tension. For many limb bones the peak dynamic strain range is 2000 to 4000 microstrains.

The strain may be the only feedback variable that confers the necessary information to allow relation of the existing bone structure to the imposed loads. It is likely that the strains mediate information to the effector cells, the osteoblasts and osteoclasts, at the bone surface. The effector cells then bring about the appropriate changes in bone mass, material, and architecture to return matrix strain to some predetermined optimum level at each location within the skeleton.[2] Increasing evidence suggests that osteocytes are the strain-sensitive cells, because they, together with the surface osteoblasts, respond to changes in the strain environment by releasing prostacyclin and prostaglandin E2.[3] The subsequent cascade is likely to result in an increased rate of osteogenesis and a decreased rate of resorption by osteoclasts.[4] In postmenopausal osteoporosis there is a failure of homeostatic adaptation to functional load bearing expressed as weak or no response of the bone to mechanical loading. Mechanical strain exerts its effect at least in part through estrogen receptors, and downregulation of the estrogen receptors following estrogen withdrawal may seriously decrease the adaptive potential of bone to mechanical loading.[5]

Physical loading influences bone mass, geometry, and internal architecture through the three bone turnover processes of growth, modeling, and remodeling. Growth is strongly controlled by genetic factors; it is also influenced by physical loading. In modeling, bone is removed and formed simultaneously at different sites by resorption and formation. Modeling determines the cross-sectional size and shape as well as the longitudinal shape of bones and trabeculae. Modeling seems to be the primary method of increasing the strength of a bone. When mechanical strains exceed a modeling threshold range at a bone site, modeling increases bone strength to reduce subsequent strains toward that range. The threshold range lies below the ultimate strength of the bone. Therefore, modeling by mechanical strains makes healthy bones stronger than needed for their peak voluntary loads.[1]

Bone remodeling is a process that turns bone over in small packets in which osteoclasts resorb some bone and osteoblasts then fill the resulting void with new bone. The resorption and formation take place at the same bone site. Remodeling can take place in at least two modes. In the "conservation mode," approximately equal amounts of bone are removed and formed resulting in no significant change or only a small loss of bone. This type of remodeling maintains the functional competence of bone by replacing aged bone with new bone and repairing microcracks on bone surfaces. In the "disuse mode," less bone is formed than is absorbed, resulting in bone loss. This process can occur in both children and adults, and it removes only endocortical and trabecular bone. This mode of remodeling is thought to be the cause of the 40% decrease in bone mass that occurs in healthy subjects between ages 25 and 75 years.[1] "Disuse-pattern osteopenia" is characterized by less spongiosa, an enlarged marrow cavity, and a thinned cortex, but not a decreased outside bone diameter. The remodeling threshold lies well below the modeling threshold. Therefore, even rather low mechanical loads, such as those produced by walking, can still be sufficient to induce the conservation mode remodeling to maintain the existing bone strength.

The mechanical control of modeling and remodeling seems to be driven mainly by large strains that exceed the threshold range, and the lesser, more usual strains have little effect. The thresholds would be internal standards, possibly genetically determined, in some skeletal cells. When mechanical load is imposed on bone, the strain-induced signals would be compared to the internal standards. If a mismatch is detected, a signal arises to start modeling or remodeling to change the bone characteristics to bring the strain to the customary level. Thus, within the customary strain level, or "lazy zone," bone turnover is in balance, but with overloading, e.g., in exercise, formation exceeds resorption and with underloading or disuse, e.g., in bed rest, resorption exceeds formation.[6] Bones are thought to function as mechanostats that keep bones healthy enough and strong enough to resist spontaneous fracturing due to chronically subnormal, normal, or supranormal voluntary loads.

Bones are loaded and strained by gravitational forces in different activities that involve weight bearing. Lack of these forces (e.g., during spaceflight) leads to osteopenia. Loads even greater than gravitational forces are produced by muscular contractions. This explains why strong muscles usually make strong bones and weak muscles usually make weak bones. This is one factor that explains the usually weaker bones of women as compared to men. Weakening of muscles is likely to be one reason for the decrease in bone strength with aging. On the other hand, the weak muscles of elderly people cause serious limitations to increasing bone mass by exercise. When examining the relationship between muscle strength and bone strength, it is important to note that changes in muscle strength, especially an increase, occur much faster than changes in bone mass and strength.

B. EFFECTIVE LOADING STIMULUS

Animal experiments have revealed several characteristics of an effective osteogenic stimulus:

- *Strain magnitude:* Strains of approximately 1000 microstrains stop bone loss and maintain bone mass. Increasing strain magnitude above that level produces a proportional increase in bone mass. The osteogenic range begins at about 1500 microstrains. In ordinary daily activities the strain range is from 200 to 2500 microstrains. Very recent findings challenge the old views by showing that very low magnitude, high-frequency mechanical stimuli are also osteogenic.[7,8]
- *Strain type:* Only dynamic strains are osteogenic. Static strains are no different from disuse. Within the physiologic strain rate range, the osteogenic response increases by about 70% by increasing the strain rate from low to high. Rate of strain change is a major determinant of the adaptive osteogenic/antiresorptive response to mechanical loading.[9]

- *Number of strains:* A relatively small number (10 to 40) or short period of strains of sufficient magnitude (~2000 microstrains) at a time is sufficient to elicit the full osteogenic response.[10-12] However, when the strain magnitude is low, increasing the number of loading cycles increases the osteogenic effect.[13]
- *Strain distribution:* Strains from unusual directions that cause "error signals" in the bone are much more effective than customary strains.
- *Strain site:* The osteogenic response need not be greatest at the site of the greatest strain and the signals appreciated by one site may not be relevant to another site.

These findings suggest that bones may not be concerned with the entire strain history. The effective subset of strains is dominated by high-magnitude strains applied in unusual distributions. Such strains are infrequent, and therefore it is not surprising that relatively few cycles are sufficient for full osteogenic response.

C. EFFECTS OF EXERCISE ON BONE

Mechanical loading can substantially increase bone mass, apparent density, and strength, up to 30 to 50%. In addition, exercise can improve bone structure (geometry, architecture) and material properties (strength, stiffness, and energy-absorbing capacity). Bone tissue shows different sensitivity to the loading stimulus at different ages, and three distinct periods are evident: childhood and adolescence, premenopausal, and postmenopausal years.

1. Exercise in Childhood and Adolescence

Bone mass accumulates during childhood and adolescence, and reaches its peak at about age 20. High peak bone mass is important for subsequent development of bone strength, because of its contribution in determining bone mass at age 70. Thus, attainment of high peak bone mass is an important goal in the prevention of osteoporosis.

Numerous studies have demonstrated substantially greater (up to 30 to 50% greater) BMD (bone mineral density) and BMC (bone mineral content) at the most-loaded bone sites of athletes as compared with the findings in nonathletes.[14] At nonloaded bone sites the differences between these groups have consistently been small. The effect of mechanical loading on bones has been shown even more convincingly by comparing the side-to-side differences of BMD and BMC in bones of the same individuals, such as athletes practicing unilaterally loading sports such as tennis and squash (Figure 31.2). The side-to-side differences in BMD and BMC depend greatly on the age of starting intensive sports training. It has become evident that the maximal effect of mechanical loading on bone can be attained by starting intensive training before or at puberty. In female tennis players, the benefits in bone mass and dimension are two to four times greater if the training is started before or at puberty (12 to 45%) rather than after it (3 to 12%) (Figure 31.3). The optimal age period to obtain these benefits seems to be relatively short, i.e., during the period of rapid longitudinal growth at puberty or Tanner stages II to IV (corresponding approximately to ages 11 to 14 years in girls).[15,16] At this time the increasing estrogen content probably induces a positive bone balance by inhibiting resorption and enhancing formation of bone, thus adding to the effect of mechanical loading.[17] The increased levels of insulin-like growth factor-1 (IGF-1), growth hormone, and androgen also enhance growth of bone mass at this time. It seems that before or after the growth spurt the bone loading activity needs to be more intense, more frequent, and needs to last for a longer period to induce substantial adaptations in bone.

The growing bones respond to physical loading not only by increasing their mass but also by increasing their size.[18,19] Studies on young tennis players using quantitative computerized tomography have shown that the extra bone mineral gained in the playing-arm bones was, in large part, due to increased bone dimensions, total cross-sectional area, and cortical wall thickness, and not

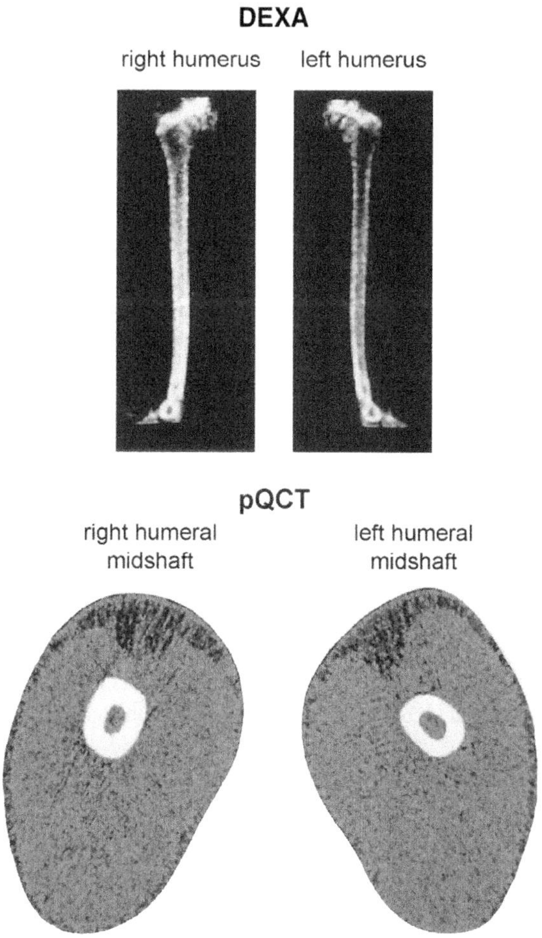

DEXA

right humerus   left humerus

pQCT

right humeral   left humeral
midshaft   midshaft

FIGURE 31.2 Demonstration of the effect of mechanical loading on bone by comparing DEXA and peripheral computed tomographic (pQCT) images of the playing (right) and nonplaying (left) arm humeri of an adult male tennis player. The mineral content and cross-ssectional area of the humerus are 32 and 40% higher on the playing than on the nonplaying side. (From Kannus, P. and Sievänen, H., in *Management of Fractures in Severely Osteoporotic Bone*, Obrant, K., Ed., Springer, London, 2000, 383. With permission.)

to an increase of volumetric cortical or trabecular bone density. Also, the changes in bone geometry seem to be highly site specific. At the proximal humerus, for example, the bone marrow cavity area (side-to-side difference: +18.5%) contributed to most of the increase in total cross-sectional area, whereas at the shaft of the humerus the increase in total cross-sectional area was attributable to the increase of cortical area. In the radial shaft, both the cortical (side-to-side difference: +14.8%) and marrow cavity areas (side-to-side difference: +28.6%) were increased.

The observed loading-induced bone adaptations correspond well with the principle stated in Wolff's law. At the different bone sites the loadings increase the strength of the bones in a logical manner to resist the primary forces imposed on them. The shaft of a bone has to resist bending and torsional forces in particular, and this means a hollow, cylindrical bone with the mineral mass distributed away from the center of gravity is a desirable structure. For bones that have to resist axial, compressive forces, a large cross-sectional area is appropriate.

Loading-induced changes are not readily apparent in mature bones. The difference in response to loading between growing and mature bone can be explained by the apposition of bone to both

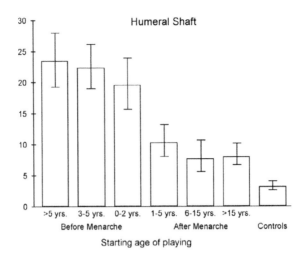

FIGURE 31.3 The effect of starting age of playing tennis on the BMC of the dominant arm (humeral shaft). The BMC of the playing arm was about two times greater if the girls started playing at or before, rather than after, menarche. The bars represent the 95% confidence intervals. (From Kannus, P. et al., *Ann. Intern. Med.*, 123, 27, 1995. With permission.)

inner and outer sides of the bone cortex by endosteal and periosteal processes only during the growth spurt. After the growth spurt, the endosteal apposition ceases.[20]

In addition to cross-sectional studies, controlled intervention trials also show significant loading-induced changes in the bones of children and adolescents, although the magnitude of the change has remained somewhat lower than that seen in the cross-sectional studies. The difference is mainly due to differences in the type, intensity, and duration of training. Studies that have used high-impact loadings corresponding to the characteristics of effective loading stimulus based on findings from animal experiments, and that have continued the training for a sufficiently long period to allow the remodeling cycle to complete, have shown bone mass increases of several percent over that in the control subjects in the lumbar spine and in the femoral neck region.[14] The importance of the age period, i.e., before menarche rather than after it, is corroborated in these studies.[21] The much smaller bone gain in the training studies as compared to the findings of cross-sectional studies is likely to be due to lower intensity and volume and shorter duration of training in the trials.

High peak bone mass attained by physical activity can contribute to osteoporosis prevention if it is maintained until old age. Follow-up studies of male weight and power lifters have shown that part of the large bone mass was retained for decades, but at the end of middle age the bone mass of the athletes was no longer greater than in nonathletes.[22,23] Prospective follow-up of female tennis and squash players has shown that the side-to-side differences of BMC between the playing and nonplaying arm in the athletes are well maintained in both young starters (mean starting age 10.5 years) and old starters (starting age 26.4 years) despite a very substantial decrease in training volume and intensity.[24] Cross-sectional comparison of nonathletic women who had been continuously either physically active or sedentary during their leisure time from childhood on showed that between the ages 25 and 65 years the femoral neck BMD was about 5% higher in the active as compared with the sedentary women. The femur shaft width of the active women was also larger and this bone was mechanically more competent (cross-sectional moment of inertia, section modulus) and these differences increased with age.[25] These findings suggest that the benefits to bone strength that are obtained in youth can be maintained thereafter by moderate physical activity. Further studies are needed, however, to see if and to what extent the higher peak bone mass attained by exercising in childhood and youth can be maintained.

2. Exercise during Premenopausal Years

Strong evidence indicates that bone also responds to loading in adulthood. In the premenopausal years exercise is effective in preserving the existing bone at clinically important sites, but bone gain is modest at best.[14] Many studies have failed to show any effect of exercise on bone mass because they have been of too short duration or the training mode has been inadequate to stimulate bone growth.[14] Only high-intensity exercise programs have been effective in premenopausal women. It seems, however, that the positive effects of exercise training on bone mass can be maintained with less-demanding exercise than that used in the original study. Although the average age-related decrease of bone mass during the premenopausal years is small, the average 1% per year difference in bone mass change in favor of physically active subjects[26,27] is potentially important regarding future fracture risk, as small differences in bone mass translate to substantial difference in fracture risk.[28,29]

Competitive athletes are exposed to large amounts of high-intensity training for prolonged periods. This stress, often combined with low body and fat mass and eating disorders, can lead to disruption of normal ovarian function and consequently decreased estrogen levels. These athletes develop oligomenorrhea or amenorrhea and bone mass gradually decreases or remains low in young athletes. The low bone mass increases the risk of stress fractures, but it is not yet known if the risk of osteoporosis later in life is also increased.[30,31]

3. Exercise during Postmenopausal Years

During the early postmenopausal years, bone loss is accelerated because of decreased estrogen levels, leading to increased osteoclast activation frequency and bone resorption. In addition, at this time muscle mass and especially the number of Type II (fast twitch) muscle fibers and consequently muscle strength decrease. These changes are partly due to biological aging and partly to less and less intensive physical activity. Whether exercise is effective in curtailing the rapid postmenopausal bone loss remains unclear because of lack of data, but one study suggests that exercise may be effective at this time.[32] However, the bones seem to be less sensitive to mechanical loading at and after menopause than before it as shown by studies using the same exercise program at various times.[33-35] In later postmenopausal years, exercise has been shown to be effective in maintaining or even increasing BMD at the clinically relevant sites, while in control subjects BMD decreased. Several meta-analyses and systematic reviews of the published studies indicate that both impact and nonimpact exercise programs produce on average about 1% net gain of bone mass in post-menopausal women,[14,26,27,36-39] although there is great variation in the results from different studies. Positive responses have been seen also in frail and osteoporotic subjects.[40-42] The response seems to be of the same magnitude in both women and men.[43] Exercise may enhance the bone-conserving effect of estrogen replacement therapy,[40,41,44,45] although this effect has not been seen in all studies.[46,47] Sufficient calcium intake, at least 1000 mg per day, seems to be a necessary condition for exercise to influence bone mass,[48] but the benefit of large amounts of supplemental calcium in addition to exercise seems questionable.[49]

III. EXERCISE FOR PREVENTION OF FALLS

The public health burden of osteoporosis is mainly due to fractures. A great majority of osteoporotic fractures (including 90% of hip fractures) result from falls.[50,51] Although only about 5% of falls in older persons lead to fracture,[52] the high incidence of falls among elderly people make falls a great hazard. In the community-dwelling population 65 years and older, 35 to 40% of generally healthy subjects fall at least once annually and about half of these do so recurrently.[53,54] Incidence rates of falls among residents of hospitals and nursing homes are about three times the rates for community-

TABLE 31.1

Most Common Risk Factors for Falls Identified in 16 Studies, and the Corresponding Relative Risks (RR) or Odds Ratios (OR)

Risk Factor	Mean RR or OR	Range
Muscle weakness	4.4	1.5–10.3
History of falls	3.0	1.7–7.0
Gait deficit	2.9	1.3–5.6
Balance deficit	2.9	1.6–5.4
Use of assistive device	2.6	1.2–4.6
Visual deficit	2.5	1.6–3.5
Arthritis	2.4	1.9–2.9
Impaired ADL	2.3	1.5–3.1
Depression	2.2	1.7–2.5
Cognitive impairment	1.8	1.0–2.3
Age over 80 years	1.7	1.1–2.5

ADL = activities of daily living.

Source: "Guideline for the presentation of falls in older persons," *J. Am Geriatr. Soc.,* 49, 664, 2001. With permission.

dwelling subjects 65 years and older.[55] Alarmingly, the incidence of fall-induced injuries (including hip and other osteoporotic fractures)[52,56] and deaths among older subjects is increasing at a rate that cannot be explained simply by demographic changes.[52] Falls are responsible for two thirds of deaths resulting from unintentional injuries, and these injuries are the fifth leading cause of death in older adults in the United States.[57] These data indicate that prevention of falls has to be an important public health goal.

A. Risk Factors for Falls

Falls are caused by the simultaneous interaction of several factors. More than 130 factors that relate to the risk of fall have been listed.[58] They are commonly grouped into two main categories: (1) intrinsic or host factors that increase a person's liability to fall, and (2) extrinsic or environmental factors that increase the opportunity for falling. Table 31.1 shows the ranking of the most common risk factors according to the size of their relative risk or odds ratio. Table 31.2 summarizes the findings of some studies that have reported specific impairments (loss or abnormality of structure or function) and disabilities (restriction or lack of ability, resulting from impairment, to perform an activity to the manner or within the range considered normal) that predispose to falls, and the corresponding relative risks.[59]

B. Effects of Exercise on Risk Factors

Several of the listed intrinsic risk factors are amenable to change by exercise, e.g., muscle strength (6 to 174% improvement in different studies), range of motion (0.5 to 18% improvement), balance (7 to 53% change), gait (12 to 48% improvement), and reaction time (0 to 4% improvement).[58] Even more importantly, most of the recent randomized controlled trials showed significant decrease and the rest of these trials showed a trend of decrease of falls among elderly subjects as a result of an exercise training program.[57,59] However, the available information does not allow us to determine the optimal type, duration, intensity, and frequency of exercise for fall prevention. At any rate, on the basis of the positive evidence, the Guideline for the Prevention of Falls in Older

TABLE 31.2
Impairments and Disabilities
as Risk Factors for Falls

Risk Factor	Relative Risk for Falls (range between studies)
Impairment	
Lower limb strength	0.5–10.3
Upper limb strength	1.5–4.3
Lower limb range of motion	1.9
Sensation	0.6–5.0
Vestibular function	4.0
Vision	1.3–1.6
Cognition	1.2–5.0
Disability	
Static balance	1.5–4.1
Dynamic balance/gait	1.6–3.3

Source: Based on Carter, N.D. et al., *Sports Med.,* 31, 427, 2001.

Persons,[57] issued by several professional and scientific societies, gives the following recommendations:

- In multifactorial interventions among community-dwelling older persons, the interventions should include, among other components, gait and balance training and, for persons in long-term care and assisted living settings, should include gait training.
- In single interventions, older people who have had recurrent falls should be offered long-term exercise training. The evidence is strongest for balance and weaker for resistance and aerobic training. The programs should be prolonged, and for sustained benefits the exercise needs to be sustained. Individual programs seem to be more effective than generic ones.

IV. PRACTICAL CONSIDERATIONS

Scientific evidence on the role of exercise in prevention of osteoporosis and related fractures is incomplete. The evidence is sufficient, however, for several recommendations to use the potential of exercise for bone health. The practical implications based on the current knowledge can be summarized as follows:

- Mechanical loading is an essential biological stimulus for bone formation in all phases of life. Bone adapts continuously to loading applied on it. Natural skeletal loading is caused by gravity and muscular activity. Both of these loading modes should be used continuously throughout life to maintain adequate bone strength.
- The optimal amount and characteristics of bone loading are not definitively known, but effective loading must be dynamic as opposed to static, and strong enough to cause microscopic, transient deformation (strain) in the bone structure, either compression or lengthening. This means that effective loading stimuli for normal adult bones have to be forceful, especially when muscles effectively dampen the loading on bones in most physical activities. On the other hand, if the dampening effect of active muscle function is prevented, the risk of acute and chronic injury is increased. Impacts caused by landing from a jump and hitting a ball with a racquet are examples of effective — but also

risky — loading stimuli. Forces that load the bone from many and unusual directions are more effective than customary, repetitive loadings from one or few directions. Therefore, fast ball games offer effective loading stimuli for hips. Relatively few strong stimuli saturate the local bone formation capacity for a time. In case of weak stimuli, their effectiveness seems to be increased by increasing their number. The optimal frequency to repeat the loading stimuli is not known, but it is likely to be two to three times a week. Taken together, aerobic dancing, fast ball games, gymnastics, and weight lifting are effective exercises for loading bones, whereas track running, cycling, and especially swimming lack important bone-loading characteristics.

- Weak bones are strained by less force than strong bones. Therefore, less force is needed to elicit osteogenic response in otherwise healthy but weakened bone, e.g., in elderly subjects, and for them fast walking can be an effective bone exercise.

- The effects of mechanical loading are limited to the site of the resulting strain. Therefore, bone-strengthening exercises have to be designed to affect relevant sites, most often the hip and lumbar spine. Ideal exercises that meet the requirements of effectiveness, safety, and site specificity are not easy to design and apply, especially for middle-aged and older people. It is also worth emphasizing that the effects of exercise on bones should be assessed not only by measuring bone mass and "density" by dual-energy X-ray absorptiometry (DEXA) but also by studying changes in bone geometry and architecture. These changes may have substantial influence on bone strength without noticeable changes in DEXA results.

- The optimal time in life to increase bone mass is at or just before puberty. This period should be used effectively, i.e., in school physical education. At later times of life the main goal of exercise in terms of bone is to maintain its mass and strength or to deter age-related decline.

- Favorable hormonal milieu and sufficient availability of calcium are essential conditions for exercise to be effective.

- With advancing age, especially after 60 to 65 years, increasing emphasis should be directed to exercises that decrease the risk of falls. Strong evidence supports the benefits of gait and balance training. Maintenance and even a substantial increase of muscle strength is possible and important both for maintenance of bone strength and for decreasing the risk of falling.

- Effective exercise programs for increasing bone strength and for decreasing the risk of falls include the risk of acute and chronic injury as an inherent problem. This risk can be decreased to a very acceptable level by emphasizing the right goals and corresponding components of the exercise programs at different ages, by assessing the individual abilities by appropriate tests, by choosing exercises that have been shown to be safe for the participating subjects, and by habituating the subjects gradually to the program.

Rational application of the principles above will decrease the likelihood of osteoporosis and related fractures significantly and safely, and at the same time bring other valuable health benefits.

REFERENCES

1. Frost, H.M., "From Wolff's law to the Utah paradigm: insights about bone physiology and its clinical applications," *Anat. Rec.,* 262, 398, 2001.
2. Rubin, C.T., "Skeletal strain and the functional significance of bone architecture," *Calcif. Tissue Int.,* 36, S11, 1984.
3. Rawlinson, S.C., el-Haj, A.J., Minter, S.L., et al., "Loading-related increases in prostaglandin production in cores of adult canine cancellous bone *in vitro*: a role for prostacyclin in adaptive bone remodeling?" *J. Bone Miner. Res.,* 6, 1345, 1991.

4. Mosley, J.R., "Osteoporosis and bone functional adaptation: mechanobiological regulation of bone architecture in growing and adult bone, a review," *J. Rehabil. Res. Dev.*, 37, 189, 2000.

5. Damien, E., Price, J.S., and Lanyon, L.E., "The estrogen receptor's involvement in osteoblasts' adaptive response to mechanical strain," *J. Bone Miner. Res.*, 13, 1275, 1998.

6. Carter, D.R., "Mechanical loading history and skeletal biology," *J. Biomech.*, 20, 1095, 1987.

7. Rubin, C., Turner, A.S., Bain, S., et al., "Anabolism. Low mechanical signals strengthen long bones," *Nature (London)*, 412, 603, 2001.

8. Rubin, C., Xu, G., and Judex, S., "The anabolic activity of bone tissue, suppressed by disuse, is normalized by brief exposure to extremely low-magnitude mechanical stimuli," *FASEB J.*, 15, 2225, 2001.

9. Mosley, J.R. and Lanyon, L.E., "Strain rate as a controlling influence on adaptive modeling in response to dynamic loading of the ulna in growing male rats," *Bone*, 23, 313, 1998.

10. Rubin, C.T. and Lanyon, L.E., "Regulation of bone mass by mechanical strain magnitude," *Calcif. Tissue Int.*, 37, 411, 1985.

11. Umemura, Y., Ishiko, T., Yamauchi, T., et al., "Five jumps per day increase bone mass and breaking force in rats," *J. Bone Miner. Res.*, 12, 1480, 1997.

12. Mosley, J.R., March, B.M., Lynch, J., and Lanyon, L.E., "Strain magnitude related changes in whole bone architecture in growing rats," *Bone*, 20, 191, 1997.

13. Cullen, D.M., Smith, R.T., and Akhter, M.P., "Bone-loading response varies with strain magnitude and cycle number," *J. Appl. Physiol.*, 91, 1971, 2001.

14. Vuori, I.M., "Dose–response of physical activity and low back pain, osteoarthritis, and osteoporosis," *Med. Sci. Sports Exerc.*, 33, S551, 2001.

15. Kannus, P., Haapasalo, H., Sankelo, M., et al., "Effect of starting age of physical activity on bone mass in the dominant arm of tennis and squash players," *Ann. Intern. Med.*, 123, 27, 1995.

16. Haapasalo, H., Kannus, P., Sievanen, H., et al., "Effect of long-term unilateral activity on bone mineral density of female junior tennis players," *J. Bone Miner. Res.*, 13, 310, 1998.

17. Lanyon, L.E., "Using functional loading to influence bone mass and architecture: objectives, mechanisms, and relationship with estrogen of the mechanically adaptive process in bone," *Bone*, 18, 37S, 1996.

18. Haapasalo, H., Sievanen, H., Kannus, P., et al., "Dimensions and estimated mechanical characteristics of the humerus after long-term tennis loading," *J. Bone Miner. Res.*, 11, 864, 1996.

19. Morris, F.L., Naughton, G.A., Gibbs, J.L., et al., "Prospective ten-month exercise intervention in premenarcheal girls: positive effects on bone and lean mass," *J. Bone Miner. Res.*, 12, 1453, 1997.

20. Parfitt, A.M., "The two faces of growth: benefits and risks to bone integrity," *Osteoporos. Int.*, 4, 382, 1994.

21. Heinonen, A., Sievanen, H., Kannus, P., et al., "High-impact exercise and bones of growing girls: a 9-month controlled trial," *Osteoporos. Int.*, 11, 1010, 2000.

22. Karlsson, M.K., Johnell, O., and Obrant, K.J., "Is bone mineral density advantage maintained long-term in previous weight lifters?" *Calcif. Tissue Int.*, 57, 325, 1995.

23. Karlsson, M.K., Hasserius, R., and Obrant, K.J., "Bone mineral density in athletes during and after career: a comparison between loaded and unloaded skeletal regions," *Calcif. Tissue Int.*, 59, 245, 1996.

24. Kontulainen, S., Kannus, P., Haapasalo, H., et al., "Good maintenance of exercise-induced bone gain with decreased training of female tennis and squash players: a prospective 5-year follow-up study of young and old starters and controls," *J. Bone Miner. Res.*, 16, 195, 2001.

25. Uusi-Rasi, K., Sievanen, H., Vuori, I., et al., "Associations of physical activity and calcium intake with bone mass and size in healthy women at different ages," *J. Bone Miner. Res.*, 13, 133, 1998.

26. Wolff, I., van Croonenborg, J.J., Kemper, H.C., et al., "The effect of exercise training programs on bone mass: a meta-analysis of published controlled trials in pre- and postmenopausal women," *Osteoporos. Int.*, 9, 1, 1999.

27. Wallace, B.A. and Cumming, R.G., "Systematic review of randomized trials of the effect of exercise on bone mass in pre- and postmenopausal women," *Calcif. Tissue Int.*, 67, 10, 2000.

28. Cummings, S.R., Black, D.M., Nevitt, M.C., et al., "Bone density at various sites for prediction of hip fractures. The Study of Osteoporotic Fractures Research Group," *Lancet*, 341, 72, 1993.

29. Hui, S.L., Slemenda, C.W., and Johnston, C.C., Jr., "Age and bone mass as predictors of fracture in a prospective study," *J. Clin. Invest.*, 81, 1804, 1988.

30. Bennell, K.L., Malcolm, S.A., Wark, J.D., and Brukner, P.D., "Skeletal effects of menstrual disturbances in athletes," *Scand. J. Med. Sci. Sports,* 7, 261, 1997.

31. Gibson, J.H., Harries, M., Mitchell, A., et al., "Determinants of bone density and prevalence of osteopenia among female runners in their second to seventh decades of age," *Bone,* 26, 591, 2000.

32. Pruitt, L.A., Jackson, R.D., Bartels, R.L., and Lehnhard, H.J., "Weight-training effects on bone mineral density in early postmenopausal women," *J. Bone Miner. Res.,* 7, 179, 1992.

33. Bassey, E.J. and Ramsdale, S.J., "Weight-bearing exercise and ground reaction forces: a 12-month randomized controlled trial of effects on bone mineral density in healthy postmenopausal women," *Bone,* 16, 469, 1995.

34. Bassey, E.J. and Ramsdale, S.J., "Increase in femoral bone density in young women following high-impact exercise," *Osteoporos. Int.,* 4, 72, 1994.

35. Bassey, E.J., Rothwell, M.C., Littlewood, J.J., and Pye, D.W., "Pre- and postmenopausal women have different bone mineral density responses to the same high-impact exercise," *J. Bone Miner. Res.,* 13, 1805, 1998.

36. Kelley, G.A., "Aerobic exercise and bone density at the hip in postmenopausal women: a meta-analysis," *Prev. Med.,* 27, 798, 1998.

37. Kelley, G. A, "Aerobic exercise and lumbar spine bone mineral density in postmenopausal women: a meta-analysis," *J. Am. Geriatr. Soc.,* 46, 143, 1998.

38. Kelley, G.A., "Exercise and regional bone mineral density in postmenopausal women: a meta-analytic review of randomized trials," *Am. J. Phys. Med. Rehabil.,* 77, 76, 1998.

39. Layne, J.E. and Nelson, M.E., "The effects of progressive resistance training on bone density: a review," *Med. Sci. Sports Exerc.,* 31, 25, 1999.

40. Kohrt, W.M., Ehsani, A.A., and Birge, S.J., Jr., "HRT preserves increases in bone mineral density and reductions in body fat after a supervised exercise program," *J. Appl. Physiol.,* 84, 1506, 1998.

41. Kohrt, W.M., Yarasheski, K.E., and Holloszy, J.O., "Effects of exercise training on bone mass in elderly women and men with physical frailty," *Bone,* 23, S499, 1998.

42. Iwamoto, J., Takeda, T., Otani, T., and Yabe, Y., "Effect of increased physical activity on bone mineral density in postmenopausal osteoporotic women," *Keio J. Med.,* 47, 157, 1998.

43. Welsh, L. and Rutherford, O.M., "Hip bone mineral density is improved by high-impact aerobic exercise in postmenopausal women and men over 50 years," *Eur. J. Appl. Physiol. Occup. Physiol.,* 74, 511, 1996.

44. Notelovitz, M., Martin, D., Tesar, R., et al., "Estrogen therapy and variable-resistance weight training increase bone mineral in surgically menopausal women," *J. Bone Miner. Res.,* 6, 583, 1991.

45. Prince, R.L., Smith, M., Dick, I.M., et al., "Prevention of postmenopausal osteoporosis. A comparative study of exercise, calcium supplementation, and hormone-replacement therapy," *N. Engl. J. Med.,* 325, 1189, 1991.

46. Heikkinen, J., Kurttila-Matero, E., Kyllonen, E., et al., "Moderate exercise does not enhance the positive effect of estrogen on bone mineral density in postmenopausal women," *Calcif. Tissue Int.,* 49, S83, 1991.

47. Heikkinen, J., Kyllonen, E., Kurttila-Matero, E., et al., "HRT and exercise: effects on bone density, muscle strength and lipid metabolism. A placebo controlled 2-year prospective trial on two estrogen-progestin regimens in healthy postmenopausal women," *Maturitas,* 26, 139, 1997.

48. Specker, B.L., "Evidence for an interaction between calcium intake and physical activity on changes in bone mineral density," *J. Bone Miner. Res.,* 11, 1539, 1996.

49. Friedlander, A.L., Genant, H.K., Sadowsky, S., et al., "A two-year program of aerobics and weight training enhances bone mineral density of young women," *J. Bone Miner. Res.,* 10, 574, 1995.

50. Grisso, J.A., Kelsey, J.L., Strom, B.L., et al., "Risk factors for falls as a cause of hip fracture in women. The Northeast Hip Fracture Study Group," *N. Engl. J. Med.,* 324, 1326, 1991.

51. Parkkari, J., Kannus, P., Palvanen, M., et al., "Majority of hip fractures occur as a result of a fall and impact on the greater trochanter of the femur: a prospective controlled hip fracture study with 206 consecutive patients," *Calcif. Tissue Int.,* 65, 183, 1999.

52. Kannus, P., Parkkari, J., Koskinen, S., et al., "Fall-induced injuries and deaths among older adults," *J. Am. Med. Assoc.,* 281, 1895, 1999.

53. Campbell, A.J., Borrie, M.J., and Spears, G.F., "Risk factors for falls in a community-based prospective study of people 70 years and older," *J. Gerontol.,* 44, M112, 1989.

54. Campbell, A.J., Spears, G.F., and Borrie, M.J., "Examination by logistic regression modeling of the variables which increase the relative risk of elderly women falling compared to elderly men," *J. Clin. Epidemiol.,* 43, 1415, 1990.
55. Rubenstein, L.Z. and Powers, C., "Falls and mobility problems: potential quality indicators and literature review," in *ACOVE Project,* RAND Corporation, Santa Monica, CA, 1999, 1.
56. Kannus, P., Niemi, S., Palvanen, M., et al., "Continuously rising problem of osteoporotic knee fractures in elderly women: nationwide statistics in Finland in 1970–1999 and predictions until the year 2030," *Bone,* 29, 419, 2001.
57. "Guideline for the prevention of falls in older persons. American Geriatrics Society, British Geriatrics Society, and American Academy of Orthopaedic Surgeons Panel on Falls Prevention," *J. Am. Geriatr. Soc.,* 49, 004, 2001.
58. Myers, A.H., Young, Y., and Langlois, J.A., "Prevention of falls in the elderly," *Bone,* 18, 87S, 1996.
59. Carter, N.D., Kannus, P., and Khan, K.M., "Exercise in the prevention of falls in older people: a systematic literature review examining the rationale and the evidence," *Sports Med.,* 31, 427, 2001.

32 Pharmacologic Management of Osteoporotic Conditions

Thomas F. Oppelt

CONTENTS

I. INTRODUCTION

Osteoporosis (a combination of the Greek terms *osteo*, meaning bone, and *poros*, meaning passage or pore) is a systemic disease in which there are structural changes in the latticework of bone. The poverty of bone, defined as osteopenia, affects 16 to 20 million Americans and is responsible for almost 1.3 million fractures in the United States each year.[1,2] The subsequent cost of this common phenomenon exceeds $10 billion annually.[1] An issue confounding the targeting of osteoporosis has become clinically evident: the progression of this condition is often occult until the patient suffers a fracture (or multiple fractures) in the presence of little to no stress or trauma. However, the recognition of various risk factors and preemptive bone mineral density (BMD) measures *may* improve future morbidities related to bone loss.[3,4] Therefore, it is the role of the orthopaedic health provider to recognize the prevalence of this disease and target those patients who may benefit from preventative and/or treatment measures. The purpose of this chapter is to provide a basic overview of osteoporosis and to focus on the pharmacologic options available to such health-care providers.

II. PATHOPHYSIOLOGY

The skeleton consists of a 4:1 ratio of cortical to trabecular bone.[5] Under normal conditions, the trabecular, or cancellous, bone is remodeled at a general rate of 25% annually.[5] The cortical bone

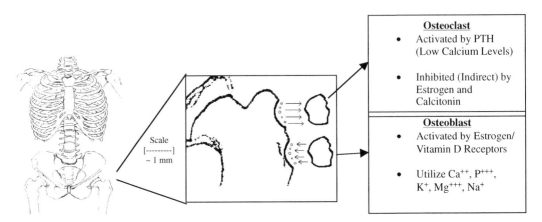

FIGURE 32.1 Bone turnover. (Adapted from Manolagas, S.C. and Jilka, R.L., *N. Engl. J. Med.,* 332, 305, 1995; Kanis, J.A., *Am. J. Med.,* 91, 295, 1991; Raisz, L.G., *N. Engl. J. Med.,* 318, 818, 1988; and Teitelbaum, S.L., *Science,* 289, 1504, 2000.)

has a more conservative constructive process of 3 to 4% per year.[5] This continuous bone evolution is directed by a balance between osteoblastic (bone-forming cells) and osteoclastic (multinucleated cells that resorb bone) activity (Figure 32.1). There is a coupling of these antagonizing forces that functions, in part, based on serum calcium levels, various hormones, certain immunomodulating pathways, and the physiologic condition of bone.[6-8] The goal of understanding the pharmacotherapy utilized in preventing and treating osteoporosis stems from how medications target this equilibration of bone turnover.

Osteoclasts, derived from monocytes, follow a stepwise progression in the resorption phase of bone (Figure 32.1).[6-8]

Step 1: Osteoclasts are regulated via estrogen and calcitonin receptors.
Step 2: If activated, these cells attach to the bone surface.
Step 3: Proteolytic enzymes, in concert with H-ATPase and carbonic anhydrase II-derived acids, dissolve bone. This results in an aperture upon the surface of the bone and a release of the mineral components.

Osteoblasts also follow a logical sequence of events (Figure 32.1).[6-8]

Step 1: Osteoblasts are synchronized via receptors for estrogen, androgen, and vitamin D, as well as parathyroid and growth hormones to rebuild osteoclastic-derived pores.
Step 2: The introduction of collagen and alkaline phosphatase by osteoblasts begins to mend the foraminal space.
Step 3: The addition of ions including calcium, phosphorus, sodium, magnesium and potassium assists in the solidification of the newly formed bone.

Note: This is an oversimplified version of this process, and a more comprehensive description of these mechanisms may be found in other chapters.

III. EPIDEMIOLOGY

A. OSTEOPOROSIS CLASSIFICATION

Osteoporosis has been categorized by its various differences and manifestations (Table 32.1). Type I (postmenopausal osteoporosis) is described by loss of trabecular bone that occurs upon the onset

TABLE 32.1
Osteoporosis Classification

Type	Definition	Cause
I	Postmenopausal osteoporosis	Estrogen deficiency
II	Senile osteoporosis	*Age-Related Changes in:*
		Calcium metabolism
		Vitamin D metabolism
		PTH levels
		Others
III	Secondary osteoporosis	*Diseases:*
		Hyperthyroidism
		Hyperparathyroidism
		Rheumatoid arthritis
		Hypogonadism
		Chronic renal/liver failure
		Alcoholism/smoking
		Multiple myeloma
		Others
		Medications:
		Corticosteroids
		Excessive thyroid hormone
		Heparin (>4–6 mo)
		Anticonvulsants
		Aluminum-containing antacids
		Furosemide
		Cyclosporine A
		Others

Source: Adapted from Riggs, B.L. and Melton, L.J., *N. Engl. J. Med.*, 314, 1676, 1986 and Prince, R.L. et al., *J. Bone Miner. Res.*, 10, 835, 1995.

of menopause. The pathophysiology (discussed further in the following section) is believed to be associated with an increase in osteoclastic activity.[5] Postmenopausal osteoporosis is thought to progress for one to two decades from the start of decreased endogenous estrogen levels and presents as vertebral compression, distal radius fractures, or hip/pelvic fractures.

Type II (senile osteoporosis) consists of a more global alteration in bone matrix, equally affecting cortical and trabecular bone. These patients may have markedly decreased osteoblastic activity leading to untoward changes.[5] Of note, this classification can be observed in men and women over the age of 70, with women having a higher prevalence.[9]

Type III (secondary osteoporosis) has been shown to be the product of various chronic disease states or medication use. The underlying process typically results in changes in calcium/vitamin D utilization or parathyroid hormone (PTH) levels. Furthermore, this form of bone loss is independent of age or sex.

B. GLUCOCORTICOID-INDUCED BONE LOSS

Although there is an expansive list of medications that can lead to osteoporosis, corticosteroids deserve an especially close examination. The incidence of fracture in patients on this class of medication (including those with rheumatic or pulmonary diseases) may reach 50%, and the common practice of preventative measures is often underutilized.[11,12] The proposed mechanism of bone loss in the presence of corticosteroids is multivariate (Figure 32.2), and can be clinically

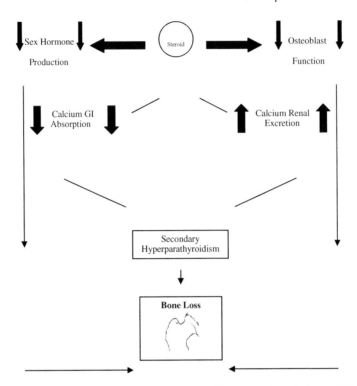

FIGURE 32.2 Corticosteroid-induced osteoporosis. (Adapted from American College of Rheumatology Task Force on Osteoporosis Guidelines, *Arthritis Rheum.,* 39, 1791, 1996.)

relevant at doses ≥7.5 mg (prednisone) a day. The greatest degree of bone loss is typically during the first 6 to 12 months of therapy.[11] In 1996, the American College of Rheumatology developed specific guidelines for the prevention of this particular medication-induced disorder.[13] These recommendations include the following:

1. Baseline measurement of bone density *before* long-term corticosteroids
2. Periodic reassessment of bone density *after* medication administration
3. Calcium intake at 1500 mg per day
4. Vitamin D supplementation at 400 to 800 IU per day
5. Consideration of hormone replacement therapy (HRT), bisphosphonates (see Table 32.4 below), or calcitonin where appropriate

C. OSTEOPOROSIS IN MEN

There is a list of reasons women are predisposed to develop osteoporosis (see Table 32.1). Osteoporosis, however, is not completely gender biased. Males inherently have a higher peak bone mass (by approximately 10%) and physiologically larger bones than females.[14] They also have a subtler decline in hormone production, as well as a decreased risk of fall.[14] Nevertheless, men have a 15 to 25% risk of developing this disease.[2] Although this percentage is related more to advanced age and secondary causes, it must be addressed in treating male patients (see Table 32.4 below).

Glucocorticoid treatment, hypogonadism, and excessive alcohol consumption are considered three of the most common causes of secondary osteoporosis in men.[15] Age-related decreases in insulin-like growth factor-1 (IGF-1), changes in calcium or vitamin D metabolism, or idiopathic causes may also play a role.[14,15] The prevalence of osteoporosis in men is growing and is further discussed in other chapters. Therapeutic options in treating men with osteoporosis are described in the following section.

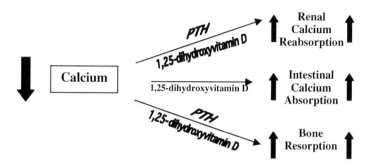

FIGURE 32.3 Serum calcium effects. (Adapted from Manolagas, S.C. and Jilka, R.L., *N. Engl. J. Med.,* 332, 305, 1995 and Riggs, B.L. and Melton, L.J., *N. Engl. J. Med.,* 314, 1676, 1986.)

IV. PREVENTION AND TREATMENT

There is a distinct difference between the prevention and treatment of osteoporosis. For orthopaedic health-care providers, treatment may typify the most common course of action. This is largely because they most often see patients after a trauma fracture. It is important to note, however, that prevention tends to have much higher success rates than treatment. Therefore, both modalities are discussed.

A. CALCIUM AND VITAMIN D

Serum calcium levels are one of the common influences on osteoclastic bone resorption (typically when concentrations fall below 9 to 11 mg/dl) (Figures 32.1 and 32.3).[5,7] Therefore, adequate calcium intake can help minimize (although not eliminate) bone resorption via sustained serum concentrations.[16] Defining *adequate* has been the focus of several nutritional and clinical studies. The current consensus on daily calcium requirements in premenopausal women attempts to obtain maximum peak bone density prior to endogenous hormonal changes.[17] This directive *may* alter the rate of bone deficit and fracture in the later years.

An opposing viewpoint proposes that women who maintain a sufficient amount of dietary calcium will not show conclusive benefit of additional supplementation. Common dietary sources of calcium include dairy products, fortified juices, certain fish, and a number of green vegetables (including collards and broccoli). Although these foods are readily available, American diets still tend to require supplementation to reach the current recommendations.[18-20] Therefore, the common clinical standard states that the benefit of unintentionally exceeding recommended calcium requirements via supplementation outweighs the consequences. Additional calcium is typically inexpensive and well tolerated by most patients. In fact, absorption of calcium is regulated by serum concentrations (Figure 32.3), making adverse reactions including hypercalciuria and renal calculi atypical. One common complaint is constipation, although this rarely precludes patient compliance.

The National Institutes of Health (NIH) have developed a specific recommended intake of calcium based on generalized patient populations (Table 32.2).[18,19] These guidelines have been compared to various other expert sources (including the recommended dietary allowance, or RDA) and are commonly seen as the most aggressive, based on the aforementioned risk vs. benefit. This is especially evident in young adults, postmenopausal women not taking estrogen, and all patients over 65 years of age.

There are some specific considerations when selecting a calcium supplement. An understanding of the percent of elemental calcium and gut absorption characteristics of each product will help maximize serum concentrations.

TABLE 32.2
Daily Calcium Requirements

Patient Demographics	NIH Consensus Elemental Calcium (mg/day)
Infant	
Birth–6 mo	400
6–12 mo	600
Children	
1–5 yr	800
6–10 yr	800–1200
Adolescents	
11–18 yr	1200–1500
Women	
19–24 yr	1200–1500
25–50 yr (premenopause)	1000
>50 yr with estrogen	1000
>50 yr without estrogen	1500
>65 yr	1500
Pregnant or nursing	1200–1500
Men	
19–24 yr	1200–1500
25–65 yr	1000
>65 yr	1500

Source: From *J. Am. Med. Assoc.,* 272, 1942, 1994; NIH Consensus Statement, 12, 1, 1994.

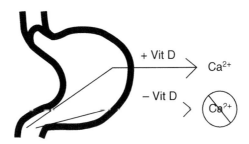

FIGURE 32.4 Effect of vitamin D on calcium absorption. (Adapted from NIH Consensus, *J. Am. Med. Assoc.,* 272, 1942, 1994; NIH Consensus Statement, 12, 1, 1994; and Ensrud, K.E. et al., *Ann. Intern. Med.,* 132, 345, 2000.)

Calcium carbonates (available as generic, OsCal® or Tums®) and tribasic calcium phosphate (Posture®) commonly provide the highest amount of elemental calcium at approximately 40%. These formulations tend to have absorptive rates proportional to gut acidity. Therefore, taking these compounds with meals will increase availability to the serum.

Calcium citrate (generic or Citracal®) and calcium lactate (generic) contain approximately 18 to 20% elemental calcium, and have acid-independent absorptive characteristics. Therefore, elderly patients or those on H_2 blockers or proton-pump inhibitors may benefit more from these formulations.

Serum calcium concentrations may fluctuate over time. It is with this in mind that most calcium regimens should be divided (by 3 to 4) throughout the day.[16] This will help elevate total serum availability and maximize tolerability. One must also realize that the full benefits of calcium often require corresponding weight-bearing exercise, adequate vitamin D levels (Figure 32.4), and, potentially, other osteoporosis medications.[16]

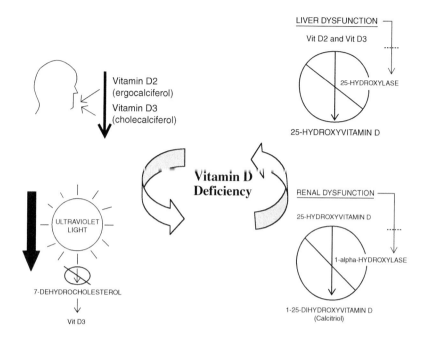

FIGURE 32.5 Causes of vitamin D deficiency. (Adapted from NIH Consensus, *J. Am. Med. Assoc.*, 272, 1942, 1994; NIH Consensus Statement, 12, 1, 1994; and Ensrud, K.E. et al., *Ann. Intern. Med.*, 132, 345, 2000.)

Vitamin D deficiency is associated with elderly patients, poor dietary intake, prolonged sun avoidance, or renal or liver dysfunction (Figure 32.5). Unfortunately, specific supplement guidelines for these patients and sustained benefit studies remain elusive.[16]

The 1997 Summary Statement on Calcium and Related Nutrients, from the Institute of Medicine,[22] suggests daily Vitamin D 200 IU for most patients. There is a higher recommended allowance for postmenopausal women and all patients over 70 years old of 400 and 600 IU, respectively.

The prescribing of Vitamin D supplementation requires a detailed review of the patient's medical history. Patients with renal or liver insufficiency may require the activated vitamin D product calcitriol (1,25-dihydroxyvitamin D) since normal vitamin D metabolism may be altered (Figure 32.5). Also, the risk of hypercalcemia and kidney stones can be exaggerated with vitamin D supplementation, necessitating a decrease in daily calcium intake and appropriate monitoring.

B. HORMONE REPLACEMENT THERAPY (HRT)

The "gold standard" for the prevention and treatment of osteoporosis in women is estrogen. Estrogen (as HRT or birth control) has consistently displayed the ability to minimize bone loss, increase BMD, and decrease fracture rates by as high as 25 to 50%.[23-26] These beneficial effects have been seen in common osteoporotic sites including the radius, vertebrae, and hip, in a variety of different female demographics (Table 32.3).[24-26]

In premenopausal women, serum 17-β-estradiol (the most potent endogenous estrogen) levels range from approximately 150 pmol/L (early follicular phase) to 2600 pmol/L (midcycle).[28] The liver provides the site of metabolism for estradiol to estrone and estriol. In women, 10 to 15% of total bone mass is dependent on the collective serum concentrations of these estrogen constituents.[29] This explains why the postmenopausal phase of life can be so detrimental to bone integrity, and the FDA approval of estrogen for prevention *and* treatment. Currently, the conjugated equine estrogens (at doses ≥0.625 mg/day) are indicated for treatment and the esterified estrogens (≥0.3 mg/day) for prevention. 17-β-Estradiol is also available orally (at recommended doses of 0.5 to 1 mg/day) and transdermally (0.05 mg/day), with suggested bone maintenance benefit.

TABLE 32.3
Estrogen Considerations: Benefits of Estrogen (as compared to placebo)

A decrease in risk of wrist fractures (RR, 0.39; 95% CI, 0.24 to 0.64)

A decrease in risk for all nonvertebral fractures (RR, 0.66; 95% CI, 0.54 to 0.80)

Beneficial results are similar using estrogen or an estrogen/progestin combination

Estrogen is most effective in preventing hip fractures in patients 75 years and older, although a trend of risk reduction is
seen in all ages

The response of bone formation to estrogen begins to fade on discontinuation of the hormone replacement therapy

Source: Adapted from Cauley, J.A. et al., *Ann. Intern. Med.*, 122, 9, 1995 and Ettinger, B. and Grady, D., *N. Engl. J. Med.*,
329, 1192, 1993.

Estrogen may have several simultaneous mechanisms in the development and preservation on
bone (see Figure 32.1). Osteoblasts have estrogen-specific binding sites that stimulate the production of bone matrix.[30] The hormone also influences the availability of osteoclast-dependent
cytokines — interleukin-1 (IL-1), IL-6, and tumor necrosis factors (TNF) — resulting in a decrease
in bone resorption.[31] Increased calcium absorption, decreased renal calcium excretion, and inhibition
of PTH also occur more consistently in the presence of sustained estrogen levels.[32]

Although the advantageous attributes of estrogen for bone turnover are clear, there are a number
of considerations in prescribing these compounds to women. The decisions of "when" to begin
HRT and "how long" are undecided.[33-35] Some postmenopausal women will take several years to
actually have clinically significant changes in bone matrix. Therefore, it may seem rational to
withhold HRT for a period of time after menopausal cessation.[26] However, estrogen is effective as
a preventative *and* treatment modality.[23-26] Also, patients may develop estrogen-related bone density
changes at different rates. Ultimately, the decision should focus on the current degree of low bone
density, as defined by the World Health Organization,[36] and risk factors for osteoporosis. The
Women's Health Initiative (WHI), an ongoing osteoporosis trial of 10,000 subjects, will help clarify
some of theses issues when it is completed (scheduled for 2007).

The presence or absence of an intact uterus will also influence HRT selection. Progestin therapy,
either continuous or cyclic, will decrease the risk of estrogen-induced endometrial hyperplasia or
cancer.[26] Therefore, women who have not had a hysterectomy should receive progestin, as medroxy-
progesterone acetate 2.5 mg (continuous) or 5 mg (cyclic) per dose, with their estrogen replacement.
Also, the presence of progestin may improve patient adherence by altering side effects often related
to estrogen use.

There are a number of risks, other than the endometrial effects previously mentioned, associated
with estrogen supplementation. Documented contraindications to HRT include estrogen-agonized
cancer (i.e., forms of breast and cervical cancer), unexplained vaginal bleeding, significant liver
disease, and recent thromboembolic disease. There are warnings to avoid use in patients who smoke,
suffer chronic or migraine headaches, have a family history of breast cancer, or a history of
thrombosis associated with HRT or oral contraceptives. Common side effects of HRT can include
breast tenderness, edema, weight gain, and vaginal bleeding. It is the recognition of these contraindications, warnings, and patient risk factors, coupled with adequate monitoring, that should direct
HRT initiation. Postmenopausal women may also continue to develop osteoporosis in the presence
of hormone replacement, justifying the utilization of other treatment options.[34]

C. SELECTIVE ESTROGEN RECEPTOR MODULATORS

The benefits of estrogen on bone density and fracture risk have led to an increased understanding
of osteoporosis prevention and treatment. HRT, however, has historically had a number of adverse
effects that decrease patient compliance and physician prescribing practices. The long-term use of

these compounds has also been scrutinized.[27] This collection of clinical issues has led to the development of selective estrogen receptor modulators (SERMs) that may offer the benefits of hormone replacement without some of the risks. Because the relationship of estrogen and certain cancers has been continually questioned, the research into SERMs has been justified.[26,37]

Tamoxifen is one of the earliest medications of this class. It is primarily used as an estrogen-antagonist in the treatment of certain breast cancers.[38] It has an interesting mix of activity, however, with some proestrogenic activity in other tissue sites. It was this duality of mechanisms that resulted in a noted beneficial activity of estrogen in bone, with the opposite potential in areas where adverse effects may ensue (namely, the breast). Unfortunately, tamoxifen still presents the possible risk of endometrial hyperplasia.[38]

Raloxifene (Evista®) is an SERM that has been approved by the FDA for prevention of osteoporosis. It has a combination of estrogen agonistic and antagonistic traits that may maximize its bone maintenance potential. Raloxifene, with effects that differ from estradiol, is believed to induce conformational changes in estrogen receptors.[39,40] The changes seem to be tissue specific, leading to gene expression of receptors that allow activation at one site and blockade in another.[41] The tissue specificity seems to antagonize estrogen response of the breast and endometrium, which differs from tamoxifen.[38,42] This is an oversimplification of the SERM mechanism, but allows a basic understanding of why these compounds may be safer than their hormone predecessors.

Raloxifene should be dosed at 60 mg per day, with calcium supplementation added, as needed, for maximum benefit. This combination has been shown to significantly increase BMD at sites including the lumbar spine, hip and total body at 2 years.[42,43] The MORE trial, published in 1999, attempted to evaluate further the benefits of raloxifene by focusing on fracture risk.[44] At 36 months, risk of vertebral fracture was significantly reduced with raloxifene — RR (relative risk), 0.7; 95% CI (confidence interval), 0.5 to 0.8 — compared to placebo. Also, raloxifene increased bone density in the femoral neck by 2.1% and the spine by 2.6% in relation to the control group ($p < 0.001$). This trial confirmed the potential utility of SERMs as an alternative to HRT. It should be mentioned, however, that vitamin D supplementation was often included in the above trial. This addition may have independently altered the overall benefit of bone maintenance.

There are some clinical deliberations for this class of medications. The adverse effect profile, as seen in literature with raloxifene, is mild but noteworthy.[38-44] Common complaints were hot flashes approximately 10% of the time and leg cramps 7%.[44] The risk of thromboembolic events including deep vein thrombosis (DVT), pulmonary embolism (PE), and retinal vein thrombosis may be elevated in patients taking raloxifene.[42] With this, raloxifene should be avoided in patients with a history of any of these complications.

Finally, there is a vast amount of literature on estrogens, which suggests that they may increase BMD more than their SERM counterpart.[26] This will force a practitioner to weigh the total benefits of HRT with the risk of certain cancers, as mentioned above. It is this observed difference in efficacy, coupled with a need to consider the male patient population, that has led to other treatment options in the prevention and treatment of osteoporosis.

D. BISPHOSPHONATES

Bisphosphonates are a class of medications with an interesting history. They have been recognized in various European countries since the mid-1800s. Their role during that time was to prevent the scaling of pipes by adding small amounts of the compound (via soap products) to the water supply. The purpose was to minimize the precipitation, and subsequent binding, of calcium carbonate. This would prolong the viability of water lines. Today, bisphosphonates including risedronate (Actonel®) and alendronate (Fosamax®) are prescribed for the prevention and treatment of osteoporosis (Table 32.4). [45-47]

The clinical mechanism of bisphosphonates relates to their antagonism of osteoclasts (Figure 32.6).[48] As shown below, there are different targeted sites that decrease bone resorption and

TABLE 32.4
The Uses of Bisphosphonates: Indication and Dosing

Indication	Risedronate[45]	Alendronate[46]
Prevention of postmenopausal osteoporosis	5 mg p.o./day	5 mg p.o./day or 35 mg p.o./once weekly
Treatment of postmenopausal osteoporosis	5 mg p.o./day	10 mg p.o./day or 70 mg/once weekly
Treatment of glucocorticoid-induced osteoporosis	5 mg p.o./day	5 mg p.o./day
Treatment of osteoporosis in men[47]	Not at present indicated	10 mg/day

p.o. = oral.

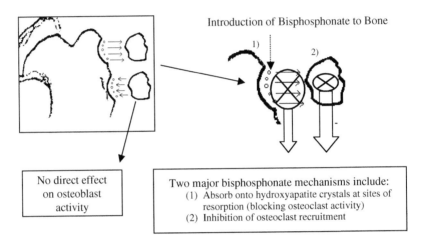

FIGURE 32.6 Bisphosphonate mechanisms of action. (Adapted from Fisher, J.E. et al., *Proc. Natl. Acad. Sci. U.S.A.,* 96, 133, 1999 and Hughes, D.E. et al., *J. Clin. Invest.,* 83, 1930, 1989.)

ultimately increase BMD. Also, a number of other potential effects on calcium, osteoclasts, and bone turnover are being investigated, although these are beyond the scope of this chapter.

The therapeutic role of the bisphosphonates includes the treatment of tumor-related osteolysis, malignancy-induced hypercalcemia, Paget's disease, and, of course, osteoporosis.[45-49] In terms of the last, there are a number of clinical trials to provide insight into the potential role of these medications.

The VERT trial, published in 1999, assessed the ability of risedronate to prevent fractures in postmenopausal women.[51] Risedronate, at 5 mg per day (with calcium and vitamin D supplementation added as needed), reduced the incidence of new vertebral fractures by 41%, and nonvertebral fractures by 39%, over a 3-year period ($p = 0.003$ and $p = 0.02$, respectively, compared to placebo). BMD at the lumbar spine, femoral neck, femoral trochanter, and midshaft of the radius increased significantly and was defined as histologically normal.

A variety of studies have examined the effects of risedronate in preventing and treating corticosteroid-induced osteoporosis.[52,53] These trials suggest that the medication can preserve BMD and minimize this form of drug-related osteoporosis in males and females. There have also been results concluding that markers of bone turnover and risk of fracture have been significantly reduced with the use of risedronate.

Data from the FIT trial, published in 1998, offer an evaluation on the effectiveness of alendronate in postmenopausal osteoporosis.[54] Alendronate (with the addition of calcium and vitamin D) significantly decreased the risk of fractures and vertebral degradation in women with low BMD who have not had a previous fracture. This 4-year trial concluded that alendronate was a safe and effective alternative in preventing osteoporosis in women at risk.

The efficacy of alendronate in glucocorticoid-induced osteoporosis has also been measured.[55] The medication offered a dose-related increase in BMD at the lumbar spine, trochanter, femoral neck, and total body. This bone maintenance was independent of steroid intake or duration. As the result of an overall lack of incidence, alendronate failed to show significant decreases in actual fracture rates compared to placebo. Nevertheless, the authors concluded that the therapy was a rational option for prevention and treatment of steroid-induced osteoporosis.

In one additional study, alendronate was administered to 241 men with significantly decreased BMD compared with healthy young men.[47] A mean increase in lumbar spine, femoral neck, and total body densities was noted ($p < 0.001$, compared to baseline). Furthermore, the incidence of vertebral fractures was lower with treatment than placebo ($p < 0.02$). The trial proved to be one of the few evaluations solely dedicated to males with osteoporosis.

The bisphosphonates, as a class, have the potential to cause esophageal irritation and ulceration.[56,57] The severity of this phenomenon may be related to its chemical structure, with alendronate having the most documented cases. To minimize this localized reaction, bisphosphonates should be taken at least 30 to 60 min before breakfast, with a full glass of water.[46] The patient should be instructed to remain in an upright position for at least 30 min after taking the medication. Following this regimen of administration may also decrease common side effects including nausea and diarrhea. Finally, oral bisphosphonates should not be taken at the exact same time as any other medication, including calcium and vitamin D.[46]

The bisphosphonates become an actual part of the bone matrix (Figure 32.6), with an estimated efficacy half-life of several years. Therefore, alendronate has received approval as a once-per-week medication.[58] This dosing schedule may improve patient compliance, in terms of proper administration, and tolerability.[58]

E. Calcitonin

Calcitonin (Calcimar® or Miacalcin®) is an endogenous hormone produced by the parafollicular cells of the thyroid, in response to serum calcium concentrations.[59] Calcitonin inhibits osteolysis secondary to PTH and interacts directly with osteoclast receptors.[60,61] The end result is decreased osteoclast adhesion, motility, and overall resorptive ability. Clinically, this medication has increased BMD, decreased fracture rates, and improved symptoms of bone pain often associated with osteoporosis and fractures.[62,63] These properties have led the FDA to approve calcitonin for the treatment of postmenopausal osteoporosis. The medication is generally recommended for those who have a contraindication to HRT or a bisphosphonate (as these two latter options tend to have more impressive results). Furthermore, calcitonin may play a role in the glucocorticoid-induced osteoporosis and in treating males with the disease.

Current routes of administration for calcitonin include intranasal (200 IU, one spray per day; subcutaneous or intramuscular, 100 IU SC/IM per day).[64,65] The medication is not available orally because of its absorption and chemical characteristics. The intranasal route is relatively well tolerated, but may cause rhinitis or mild nasal irritation.[64] The SC/IM routes have been associated with nausea/vomiting, diarrhea, anorexia, rash, edema, and pain at the site of injection.[65] The gastrointestinal side effects may be minimized by administering the medication at bedtime, or may diminish over time. Concomitant calcium and vitamin D, if needed, should be included with any of the aforementioned treatment regimens.

Ellerington et al.[66] described the effect of intranasal salmon calcitonin on BMD and markers of bone turnover. In the study, 117 postmenopausal women with reduced BMD at baseline maintained their existing bone matrix significantly more than their placebo counterparts ($p < 0.02$). The medication was also well tolerated.

The PROOF study, presented in 1998, evaluated salmon calcitonin nasal spray and fracture in 1255 postmenopausal women with osteoporosis.[67] This 5-year trial offered a 36% reduction in the relative risk of new vertebral fractures compared to placebo (RR = 0.643; 95% CI, 0.443 to 0.934; $p = 0.02$). A significant decrease in multiple vertebral fractures and deterioration of spinal deformity was also noted in the treatment group.

There have also been a number of studies measuring the analgesic properties of calcitonin.[63,68] They have shown significantly improved pain intensity, duration of immobility secondary to pain, and need for other analgesic medications in patients with vertebral fractures. The actual mechanism of altered pain may include effects on prostaglandins, endorphins, serum calcium fluctuations, and/or neuromodulation.[69,70]

F. FLUORIDE

Fluoride has the ability to activate osteoblastic formation of bone, stimulate calcium deposition, and chemically alter hydroxyapatite crystals (incorporating fluoride into bone). These changes lead to an increased bone density that may have an inherent resistance to future resorption.[71] The most common utilization of this phenomenon is in fluoridating water and toothpaste to decrease the risk of dental caries. The quality of bone formulated by this process (mostly trabecular vs. cortical), however, remains questionable. The texture, mineralization, and strength of this new bone are not believed to be consistent with bone developed from normal production. These concerns, coupled with an uncertainty about appropriate dosing and side effects, places fluoride on an investigational status in osteoporosis.[72]

Sodium fluoride treatment doses in osteoporosis typically range from 50 to 60 mg (approximately 20 to 30 mg elemental fluoride) divided per day.[73,74] The resulting therapeutic levels of fluoride should be maintained at 95 to 190 ng/ml, and may be reached most consistently with sustained-release formulations.[75] The addition of calcium and vitamin D (given at separate times from fluoride) is also encouraged in patients that may have low levels and poor intake.

In 1994, Riggs et al.[76] showed an increase in spinal bone density and decreased fractures in postmenopausal women on fluoride doses less than 75 mg/day (as opposed to higher doses given in the trial). These conclusions were secondary outcomes that were later identified from the original publication. Nevertheless, this study showed that higher doses of fluoride are not necessarily associated with improved bone mechanics.

In 1995, Pak et al.[77] treated 110 postmenopausal women with osteoporosis with slow-release fluoride, 25 mg twice a day. This study supplemented with calcium citrate (400 mg twice a day) and included 14-month cycles with 2-month drug-free periods between each cycle. The treatment group had lower vertebral fracture rate and higher bone densitometry compared to the placebo group.

A more recent trial, in 1999, compared HRT (estradiol/norethisterone), fluoride, HRT plus fluoride, and placebo in 100 healthy postmenopausal women.[78] The results showed that the HRT plus fluoride group had significant increases in spinal BMD compared to HRT alone ($p < 0.05$), fluoride, or placebo. There was also a clear decrease in the markers of bone resorption in the HRT and HRT-plus-fluoride arms. The authors commented that adverse effects of any treatment group were mild and rare.

The common side effects of fluoride supplementation include epigastric pain, nausea, and vomiting. Antacids or H_2-blockers may alleviate these symptoms. Musculoskeletal pain of the knees, ankles, or feet has also been associated with fluoride. All these adverse reactions are typically dose related and may be less frequent with the low-dose sustained-release products.

There is also the possibility that fluoride therapy may *increase* the incidence of stress and hip fractures.[79,80] This may be due to decreases in cortical bone mineralization and overall poor bone quality. This reaction, suspected to be dose related, is not conclusive and is being further evaluated as it relates to fluoride supplementation.

The future of fluoride use in osteoporosis is still speculative, inconsistent among different patients, and requires further research before it will gain acceptance as a regularly prescribed treatment modality.

G. INVESTIGATIONAL THERAPIES

Although fluoride probably falls into this heading, there are a number of other treatments that are undergoing clinical review.

Phytoestrogens, which are similar to endogenous estrogens (although much less potent), are found in soybeans, soyflour, tofu, and certain vegetables.[81] The most common form, known as isoflavones, may have mixed activity and antagonism that potentiates estrogen in various tissues (not unlike the SERMs mentioned previously).[82] This may result in an inhibitory effect on osteoclast production and promote osteoblast maturation.[83] Studies have shown the protective effect of this compound on bone, but the appropriate dose and comparative studies are lacking.[81] Ongoing trials may help determine the future role that these compounds will have in the prevention or treatment of osteoporosis.

Evidence of the clinical utility of testosterone and anabolic steroids in osteoporosis has been conflicting.[84-86] It has been shown that osteoblasts have androgen receptors (Section II), which are stimulatory in nature.[86,87] The improvement in bone density periodically seen in studies may derive from this osteoblastic activity, or be secondary to increased muscle strength and mass associated with these hormones. The most hopeful, however, may be in treating hypogonadal men. This is especially relevant when considering the minimum number of options currently available for males with osteoporosis (i.e., calcium/vitamin D, bisphosphonates, and calcitonin, as mentioned previously). The most significant adverse effects of this class include liver dysfunction (cholestatic jaundice, hepatitis, hepatocellular cancer), untoward changes in high-density lipoprotein, acne, hirsutism, and myalgias. The variety of doses (usually 200 mg intramuscularly every 2 weeks), study group, duration, site of proposed action (spine, hip, radius, etc.), and inconsistent results have left these compounds at an investigational status.[84-86]

PTH is a major participant in serum calcium homeostasis and bone turnover (Figure 32.3). Increasing levels of this hormone, in response to low calcium levels, activate bone resorption. Other endogenous modulators, including growth hormone (GH, i.e., somatotropin) and IGF, have an opposing purpose of stimulating bone formation and bone resorption.[83] Changes in any of these serum levels may play an important role in the pathogenesis of osteoporosis.[88] Daily injections of PTH have been shown to improve trabecular bone formation, but inhibit cortical matrix.[83,89] Postmenopausal women with osteoporosis have had improved BMD and decreased vertebral fractures when PTH is added to a typical HRT regimen.[90]

The use of GH has also been periodically studied in 27 postmenopausal females treated with GH for 6 to 12 months.[91] There were noted changes in markers of bone formation, although BMD did not significantly change. These hormonal supplements have shown some promise, but their respective trials are limited and inconclusive. Further understanding of the endogenous roles of these chemicals is expanding, and may lead to their future clinical impact in certain patients.

Last, there have been a number of case control studies that suggest that HMG-CoA reductase inhibitors (commonly referred to as "statins") may have a secondary benefit in reducing fracture risk.[92-94] The role of statins, including simvastatin, pravastatin, and atorvastatin, is typically their ability to treat hyperlipidemias and/or alter cardiovascular morbidities and mortalities.[95] Meier et al.[93] conducted an analysis of patients on these lipid lowering medications to determine if there was any impact on fracture risk. After measuring confounding characteristics, including steroid use, estrogen use, and smoking, a significant risk reduction was noted in the statin group (RR = 0.55; 95% CI = 0.44 to 0.69). The authors concluded that patients over the age of 50 may show secondary benefits in bone stability with the use of HMG-CoA reductase inhibitors.

A similar study by Wang et al.[94] examined Medicare/Medicaid patients on this class of medication. The objectives focused on change in hip fracture risk in elderly patients on a statin. The results displayed a 71% reduction in risk for the treatment group. The authors admit, however, that a large number of variations among the study patients justify further examination before this possible benefit can be fully elucidated.

With this, HMG-CoA reductase inhibitors remain in an investigational category for fracture risk. The limitations of currently published studies, and some conflicting studies, have justified future trials to determine any role these medications may have for the orthopaedic health-care provider.

V. SUMMARY

There are a number of factors that may lead to osteoporosis, and an equally significant number of options in the prevention and treatment of the disease. However, there is a common question that may help clarify why these modalities remain underutilized. Who is more responsible for the prevention and treatment of osteoporosis, the primary care physician or the orthopaedic health-care provider? The answer is *both*. Typically, an orthopaedic surgeon is consulted after some event has already resulted in bone fracture. This becomes a pivotal point in future treatment, as the orthopaedic health-care provider must decide if bone formation and matrix may have played a role in the insult. If there is clinical suspicion, consider beginning therapy or contacting the primary care physician. Either way, studies have shown that there are several choices, based mostly on patient demographics, that can decrease further morbidity/mortality as it relates to osteoporosis.

ACKNOWLEDGMENT

The author thanks Dr. Xin Huang for his artistic contributions to this chapter.

REFERENCES

1. Consensus Development Conference, "Prophylaxis and treatment of osteoporosis," *Am. J. Med.,* 90, 107, 1991.
2. Looker, A.C., Orwoll, E.S., Johnston, C.C., Jr., et al., "Prevalence of low femoral bone density in older U.S. adults from the NHANES III," *J. Bone. Miner. Res.,* 12, 1761, 1997.
3. Ross, P.D., "Prediction of fracture risk II: other risk factors," *Am. J. Med. Sci.,* 312, 260, 1996.
4. Ross, P.D., Davis, J.W., Epstein, R.S., et al., "Preexisting fractures and bone mass predict vertebral fracture incidence in women," *Ann. Intern. Med.,* 114, 919, 1991.
5. Manolagas, S.C. and Jilka, R.L., "Bone marrow, cytokines, and bone remodeling. Emerging insights into the pathophysiology of osteoporosis," *N. Engl. J. Med.,* 332, 305, 1995.
6. Kanis, J.A., "The restoration of skeletal mass: a theoretic overview," *Am. J. Med.,* 91, 29S, 1991.
7. Raisz, L.G., "Local and systemic factors in the pathogenesis of osteoporosis," *N. Engl. J. Med.,* 318, 818, 1988.
8. Teitelbaum, S.L., "Bone resorption by osteoclasts," *Science,* 289, 1504, 2000.
9. Riggs, L. and Melton, J., "Involutional osteoporosis," *N. Engl. J. Med.,* 314, 1676, 1986.
10. Prince, R.L., Dick, I., Devine, A., et al., "The effects of menopause and age on calcitropic hormones: a cross-sectional study of 655 healthy women aged 35–90," *J. Bone Miner. Res.,* 10, 835, 1995,
11. Adachi, J.D., "Corticosteroid-induced osteoporosis," *Am. J. Med. Sci.,* 313, 41, 1997.
12. Buckley, L.M., Marquez, M., Feezor, R., et al., "Prevention of corticosteroid-induced osteoporosis," *Arthritis Rheum.,* 42, 1736, 1999.
13. American College of Rheumatology Task Force on Osteoporosis Guidelines, "Recommendations for the prevention and treatment of glucocorticoid-induced osteoporosis," *Arthritis Rheum.,* 39, 1791, 1996.
14. Bilezikian, J.P., "Osteoporosis in men," *J. Clin. Endocrinol. Metab.,* 84, 3431, 1999.
15. Siddiqui, N.A., Shetty, K.R., and Duthie, E.H., "Osteoporosis in older men: discovering when and how to treat it," *Geriatrics,* 54, 20, 1999.
16. Reid, I.R., "Therapy of osteoporosis: calcium, vitamin D, and exercise," *Am. J. Med. Sci.,* 312, 278, 1996.

17. Dawson-Hughes, B., Dallal, G.E., Krall, E.A., et al., "A controlled trial of the effect of calcium supplementation on bone density in postmenopausal women," *N. Engl. J. Med.,* 323, 878, 1990.

18. NIH Consensus Development Panel on Optimal Calcium Intake, "Optimal calcium intake," *J. Am. Med. Assoc.,* 272, 1942, 1994.

19. "Optimal calcium intake," NIH Consensus Statement, 12, 1, 1994.

20. Calvo, M.S. and Park, Y.K., "Changing phosphorus content of the U.S. diet: potential for adverse effects on bone," *J. Nutr.,* 126, 1168S, 1996.

21. Ensrud, K.E., Duong, T., Cauley, J.A., et al., "Low fractional calcium absorption increases the risk for hip fracture in women with low calcium intake. Study of Osteoporotic Fractures Research Group," *Ann. Intern. Med.,* 132, 345, 2000.

22. Institute of Medicine, National Research Council, "Summary Statement on Calcium and Related Nutrients," 1997, S1; available at www.nas.edu/new.

23. Eastell, R., "Treatment of postmenopausal osteoporosis," *N. Engl. J. Med.,* 338, 736, 1998.

24. Grady, D., Rubin, S.M., Petitti, D.B., et al., "Hormone therapy to prevent disease and prolong life in postmenopausal women," *Ann. Intern. Med.,* 117, 1016, 1992.

25. Grodstein, F., Stampfer, M.J., Colditz, G.A., et al., "Postmenopausal hormone therapy and mortality," *N. Engl. J. Med.,* 336, 1769, 1997.

26. Writing group for the PEPI Trial, "Effects of hormone therapy on bone mineral density: results from the postmenopausal estrogen/progestin interventions (PEPI) trial," *J. Am. Med. Assoc.,* 276, 1389, 1996.

27. Cauley, J.A., Seeley, D.G., Ensrud, K., et al., "Estrogen replacement therapy and fractures in older women," *Ann. Intern. Med.,* 122, 9, 1995.

28. Carr, B.R., "The ovary," in *Textbook of Reproductive Medicine,* Blackwall, R.E. and Carr, B.R., Eds., Appleton & Lange, Norfolk, VA, 1993, 199.

29. Ettinger, B. and Grady, D., "The waning effect of postmenopausal estrogen therapy on osteoporosis," *N. Engl. J. Med.,* 329, 1192, 1993.

30. Eriksen, E.F., Colvard, D.S., Berg, N.J., et al., "Evidence of estrogen receptors in normal human osteoblast-like cells," *Science,* 241, 84, 1988,

31. Horowitz, M., "Cytokines and estrogen in bone: anti-osteoporotic effects," *Science,* 260, 625, 1993.

32. Duursma, S.A., Raymakers, J.A., Boereboom, F.T. J., et al., "Estrogen and bone metabolism," *Obstet. Gynecol. Surg.,* 47, 38, 1991.

33. Stevenson, J.C., "Is there a case for targeting hormone replacement therapy for osteoporosis at the menopause?" *Osteoporos. Int.,* 8, 47, 1998.

34. Notelovitz, M., "Estrogen therapy and osteoporosis: principles and practice," *Am. J. Med. Sci.,* 313, 2, 1997.

35. Ettinger, B., Genant, H.K., and Cann, C.E., "Long-term estrogen replacement therapy prevents bone loss and fractures," *Ann. Intern. Med.,* 102, 319, 1985.

36. WHO, "Assessment of fracture risk and its application to the screening of postmenopausal osteoporosis," *WHO Technical Report Series,* World Health Organization, Geneva, 1994.

37. Colditz, G.A., Hankinson, S.E., Hunter, D.J., et al., "The use of estrogens and progestins and the risk of breast cancer in postmenopausal women," *N. Engl. J. Med.,* 332, 1589, 1995.

38. Tamoxifen Citrate, Package insert, AstraZeneca, Wilmington, DE, 1999.

39. Gradishar, W.J. and Jordan, V.C., "Clinical potential of new antiestrogens," *J. Clin. Oncol.,* 15, 840, 1997.

40. Mitlak, B.H. and Cohen, F.J., "In search of optimal long-term female hormone replacement: the potential of selective estrogen receptor modulators," *Horm. Res.,* 48, 155, 1997.

41. Brzozowski, A.M., Pike, A.C.W., Hubbard, D.Z., et al., "Molecular basis of agonism and antagonism in the estrogen receptor," *Nature (London),* 389, 753, 1997.

42. Raloxifene, Package insert, Eli Lilly and Company, Indianapolis, 1997.

43. Delmas, P.D., Bjarnason, N.H., Mitlak, B.H., et al., "Effects of raloxifene on bone mineral density, serum cholesterol concentrations, and uterine endometrium in postmenopausal women," *N. Engl. J. Med.,* 337, 1641, 1997.

44. Ettinger, B., Black, D.M., Mitlak, B.H., et al., "Reduction of vertebral fracture risk in postmenopausal women with osteoporosis treated with realxifene: for the multiple outcomes of raloxifene evaluation (MORE) investigators," *J. Am. Med. Assoc.,* 282, 637, 1999.

45. Actonel, Package Insert, Proctor & Gamble Pharmaceuticals, Cincinnati, OH, 2000.

46. Fosamax, Package Insert, Merck & Co., Inc., Whitehouse Station, NJ, 2000.

47. Orwoll, E., Ettinger, M., Weiss, S., et al., "Alendronate for the treatment of osteoporosis in men," *N. Engl. J. Med.*, 343, 604, 2000.

48. Fisher, J.E., Rogers, M.J., Halasy, J.M., et al., "Alendronate mechanism of action: geranylgeraniol, an intermediate in the mevalonate pathway, prevents inhibition of osteoclast formation, bone resorption, and kinase activation *in vitro*," *Proc. Natl. Acad. Sci. U.S.A.*, 96, 133, 1999.

49. Fleish, H., "Biphosphonates: pharmacology and use in the treatment of tumor-induced hypercalcemia and metastatic bone diseases," *Drugs*, 42, 919, 1991.

50. Hughes, D.E., MacDonald, B.R., Russell, R.G.G., et al., "Inhibition of osteoclast-like cell formation by biphosphonates in long-term cultures of human bone marrow," *J. Clin. Invest.*, 83, 1930, 1989.

51. Harris, S.T., Watts, N.B., Genant, H.K., et al., for the Vertebral Efficacy with Risedronate Therapy (VERT) study group, "Effects of risedronate treatment on vertebral and nonvertebral fractures in women with postmenopausal osteoporosis," *J. Am. Med. Assoc.*, 282, 1344, 1999.

52. Cohen, S., Levy, R.M., Keller, M., et al., "Risedronate therapy prevents corticosteroid-induced bone loss," *Arthritis Rheum.*, 42, 2309, 1999.

53. Wallach, S., Cohen, S., Reid, D.M., et al., "Effects of risedronate treatment on bone density and vertebral fracture in patients on corticosteroid therapy," *Calcif. Tissue Int.*, 67, 277, 1999.

54. Cummings, S.R., Black, D.M., Thompson, D.E., et al., "Effect of alendronate on risk of fracture in women with low bone density but without vertebral fractures. Results from the fracture intervention trial (FIT)," *J. Am. Med. Assoc.*, 280, 2077, 1998.

55. Saag, K.G., Emkey, R., Schnitzer, T.J., et al., "Alendronate for the prevention and treatment of glucocorticoid-induced osteoporosis," *N. Engl. J. Med.*, 339, 292, 1998.

56. De Groen, P.C., Lubbe, D.F., Hirsch, L., et al., "Esophagitis associated with the use of alendronate," *N. Engl. J. Med.*, 335, 1016, 1996.

57. Kelly, R. and Taggart, H., "Incidence of gastrointestinal side effects due to alendronate is high in clinical practice [letter]," *Br. Med. J.*, 315, 1235, 1997.

58. Bone, H.G., Adami, S., Rizzoli, R., et al., "Weekly administration of alendronate: rationale and plan for clinical assessment," *Clin. Ther.*, 22, 15, 2000.

59. Wolffe, H.J., "Calcitonin: perspective in current concepts," *J. Endocrinol. Invest.*, 5, 523, 1982.

60. Holtrop, M.E., Raisz, L.G., and Simmons, H.A., "The effects of parathyroid hormone, colchicine and calcitonin on the ultrastructure and the activity of osteoclasts in organ culture," *J. Cell. Biol.*, 60, 346, 1974.

61. Reynolds, J.J. and Dingle, J.T., "A sensitive *in vitro* method for studying the induction and inhibition of bone resorption," *Calcif. Tissue Res.*, 4, 339, 1970.

62. Overgaard, K., Hansen, M.A., Jensen, S.B., et al., "Effect of salcatonin given intranasally on bone mass and fracture rates in established osteoporosis: a dose–response study," *Br. Med. J.*, 305, 556, 1992.

63. Pun, K.K. and Chan, L.W.L., "Analgesic effect of intranasal salmon calcitonin in the treatment of osetoporotic vertebral fractures," *Clin. Ther.*, 11, 205, 1989.

64. Mialcalcin Nasal Spray, Package Insert, Sandoz, East Hanover, NJ, 1997.

65. Mialcalcin Injection, Package Insert, Novartis Pharmaceuticals Corp., East Hanover, NJ, 1999.

66. Ellerington, M.C., Hillard, T.C., Whitcroft, S.I., et al., "Intranasal salmon calcitonin for the prevention and treatment of postmenopausal osteoporosis," *Calcif. Tissue Int.*, 59, 6, 1996.

67. Silverman, S.L., Chestnut, C., Andriano, K., et al., "Salmon calcitonin nasal spray reduces risk of vertebral fracture in established osteoporosis and has continuous efficacy with prolonged treatment. Accrued 5 year worldwide data of the PROOF study," *Bone*, 23, 174, 1998.

68. Lyritis, G.P., Paspati, I., Karachalios, T., et al., "Pain relief from nasal salmon calcitonin in osteoporotic vertebral crush fractures," *Acta Orthop. Scand.*, 68, 112, 1997.

69. Silverman, S.L., "Calcitonin," *Am. J. Med. Sci.*, 313, 13, 1997.

70. Gennari, C., "Calcitonins in osteogenic pain," *Osteoporosis*, 30, 5, 1987.

71. Kleerekoper, M., "The role of fluoride in the prevention of osteoporosis," *Endocrinol. Metab. Clin. North Am.*, 27, 441, 1998.

72. Sögaard, C.H., Mosekilde, L., Richards, A., et al., "Marked decrease in trabecular bone quality after five years of sodium fluoride therapy — assessed by biomechanical testing of iliac crest bone biopsies in osteoporotic patients," *Bone*, 15, 393, 1994.

73. Joysey, J., "Effect of combined therapy with sodium fluoride, vitamin D and calcium in osteoporosis," *Am. J. Med.*, 53, 43, 1972.

74. Parkins, F.M., "Fluoride therapy for osteoporotic lesions," *Ann. Otol. Rhinol. Laryngol.*, 83, 626, 1974.

75. Pak, C.Y.C., Shakaheee, K., Rubin, C.D., et al., "Sustained-release sodium fluoride in the management of established postmenopausal osteoporosis," *Am. J. Med. Sci.*, 313, 23, 1997.

76. Riggs, B.L., O'Fallon, W.M., Lane, A., et al., "Clinical trial of fluoride therapy in postmenopausal osteoporotic women: extended observations and additional analysis," *J. Bone Miner. Res.*, 9, 265, 1994.

77. Pak, C.Y., Sakhaee, K., Adams-Huet, B., et al., "Treatment of postmenopausal osteoporosis with slow-release sodium fluoride," *Ann. Intern. Med.*, 123, 401, 1995.

78. Alexandersen, P., Riis, B.J., and Christiansen, C., "Monofluorophosphate combined with hormone replacement therapy induces a synergistic effect on bone mass by dissociating bone formation and resorption in postmenopausal women: a randomized study," *J. Clin. Endocrinol. Metab.*, 84, 3013, 1999.

79. Hedlund, L.R. and Gallagher, J.C., "Increased incidence of hip fracture in osteoporotic women treated with sodium fluoride," *J. Bone Miner. Res.*, 4, 223, 1989.

80. Riggs, B.L., Baylink, D.J., Kleerekoper, M., et al., "Incidence of hip fractures in osteoporotic women treated with sodium fluoride," *J. Bone Miner. Res.*, 2, 123, 1987.

81. Knight, D.C. and Eden, J.A., "A review of the clinical effects of phytoestrogens," *Obstet. Gynecol.*, 87, 897, 1996.

82. Fitzpatrick, L.A., "Selective estrogen receptor modulators and phytoestrogens: new therapies for the postmenopausal woman," *Mayo Clin. Proc.*, 74, 601, 1999.

83. Reginster, J.Y., Taquet, A.N., and Gosset, C., "Therapy for osteoporosis: miscellaneous and experimental agents," *Endocrinol. Metab. Clin. North Am.*, 27, 453, 1998.

84. Finkelstein, J., Klibanski, A., Neer, R., et al., "Osteoporosis in men with idiopathic hypogonadotropic hypogonadism," *Ann. Intern. Med.*, 106, 354, 1987.

85. Wang, C., Eyre, D.R., Clark, R., et al., "Sublingual testosterone replacement improves muscle mass and strength, decreases bone resorption, and increases bone formation markers in hypogonadal men: a clinical research center study," *J. Clin. Endocrinol. Metab.*, 81, 3654, 1996.

86. Watts, N.B., Motelovitz, M., Timmons, M.C., et al., "Comparison of oral estrogens and estrogens plus androgen on bone mineral density, menopausal symptoms, and lipid-lipoprotein profiles in surgical menopause," *Obstet. Gynecol.*, 85, 529, 1995.

87. Colvard, D., Eriksen, E., Keeting, P., et al., "Identification of androgen receptors in normal human osteoblast-like cells," *Proc. Natl. Acad. Sci. U.S.A.*, 86, 854, 1989.

88. Wüster, C.H.R., Blum, W.F., Sclemilch, S., et al., "Decreased serum levels of insulin like growth factors 1 and 2 and IGF binding protein-3 in patients with osteoporosis," *J. Intern. Med.*, 234, 249, 1993.

89. Cosman, F. and Lindsay, R., "Is parathyroid hormone a therapeutic option for osteoporosis? A review of the clinical evidence," *Calcif. Tissue Int.*, 62, 476, 1998.

90. Lindsay, R., Nieves, J., Formica, C., et al., "Randomised controlled study of effect of parathyroid hormone on vertebral-bone mass and fracture incidence among postmenopausal women on estrogen with osteoporosis," *Lancet,* 280, 1067, 1998.

91. Holloway, L., Butterfield, G., Hintz, R., et al., "Effects of recombinant human growth hormone on metabolic indices, body composition, and bone turnover in healthy elderly women," *J. Endocrinol. Metab.*, 79, 470, 1994.

92. Meier, C.R., Schlienger, R.G., Kraenzlin, M.E., et al., "HMG-CoA reductase inhibitors and the risk of fractures," *J. Am. Med. Assoc.*, 283, 3205, 2000.

93. van Staa, T.P., Wegman, S., de Vries, F., et al., "Use of statins and risk of fractures," *J. Am. Med. Assoc.*, 285, 1850, 2001.

94. Wang, P.S., Solomon, D.H., Mogun, H., et al., "HMG-CoA reductase inhibitors and the risk of hip fractures in elderly patients," *J. Am. Med. Assoc.*, 283, 3211, 2000.

95. Corsini, A., Bellosta, S., Baetta, R., et al., "New insights into the pharmacodynamic and pharmacokinetic properties of statins," *Pharmacol. Ther.*, 84, 413, 1999.

Index

Printed and bound by CPI Group (UK) Ltd, Croydon, CR0 4YY

23/10/2024

01778247-0006